ESSENTIALS OF CLINICAL PATHOLOGY

Dr. Disha Arora

ALLIED HEALTH PRESS

Essentials of Clinical Pathology

Author: **Dr. Disha Arora**

Allied Health Press
4164 Lakeshore Road
Burlington ON L7L 1A4
Canada
www.alliedhealthpress.com
Email: orders@arclereducation.com

ISBN: 978-1-77956-782-6

ABOUT THE AUTHOR

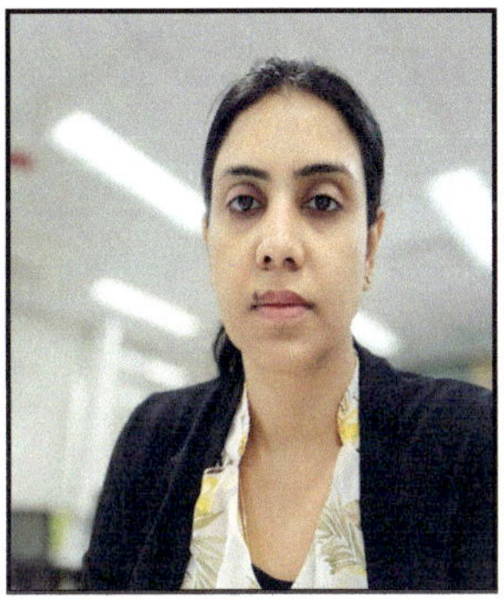

Dr. Disha Arora, MD, MPH, is a pathologist with extensive experience in hematology, transfusion medicine, histopathology, and cytopathology. Trained at the National Institute of Pathology (ICMR), New Delhi, she has worked as Senior Resident at Safdarjung Hospital and as Consultant Pathologist in private practice. She also holds a Master of Public Health from the University of Toronto, bringing a population health perspective to her diagnostic expertise.

Brief Table of Contents

Getting Started with This Book

Chapter Openers

A list of Chapter Outline is presented providing a brief Introduction to what will be covered in the chapter.

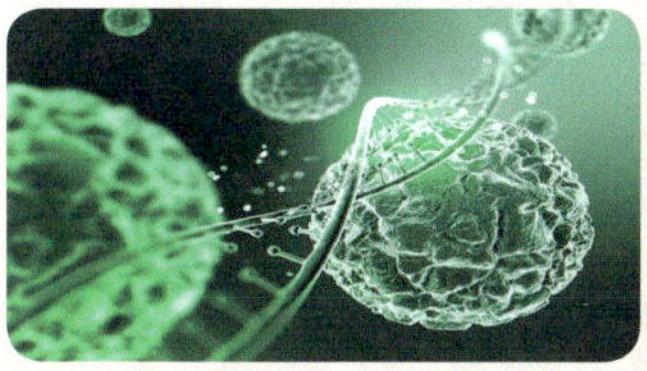

LEARNING OBJECTIVES

After studying this chapter, you will be able to:

1. Discuss the scientific method in biology;
2. Explain the cell theory;
3. Discuss the genetics and heredity;
4. Evolution and natural selection;
5. Focus on ecology and ecosystems;
6. Learn about human biology;
7. Evaluate the plant biology;
8. Explain the microbiology;
9. Focus on current trends in biology.

Introduction

Often referred to as the science of life, biology is a broad field of study aimed at comprehending the several kinds of life on Earth, from tiny creatures to sophisticated multicellular entities. Comprising several subfields, including molecular biology, ecology, and evolutionary biology, each of which advances our knowledge of living systems, this field clarifies the mechanisms controlling life events, including development, reproduction, and interaction with the surroundings, which is the central goal of biology. Moreover, biology fills in the void between the natural sciences and medicine by offering a necessary understanding of health, illness, and the interactions between organisms and their environments. Dealing with urgent global issues such as climate change, biodiversity loss, and new diseases depends on an awareness of these complex biological interactions, therefore highlighting the critical part biology plays in modern civilization. Fundamentally, biology explores and tests ideas about the living world using the scientific method. Through methodical observation and experimentation,

1.1. The Scientific Method in Biology

Learning Outcome

1. Describe the steps of the scientific method;
2. Focus on hypothesis formation;
3. Learn about experimental design.

Learning Outcomes

The beginning of each section of every chapter contains a set of Learning Outcomes that inform students of concepts they should understand. These outcomes help students understand what they should be able to do if they have mastered the material in that section.

Test Your Knowledge

Throughout each chapter, Test Your Knowledge cues you to note which topics have been covered and to self-test your understanding of the material presented.

Test Your Knowledge

1. Explain why correlation does not imply causation in scientific experiments.
2. How does the scientific method help reduce the influence of personal opinions in research?

Chapter Summary

The Summary Section appear at the end of each chapter and summarize main concepts covered throughout the chapter. These points provide key concepts in an engaging and meaningful way.

Summary

The investigation of biological principles highlights the importance of a comprehensive view of life by reflecting the intricate interactions that occur within living systems. The complexity of biology goes beyond individual species or systems, as this essay highlights; it also includes the interactions that mold ecosystems and affect biodiversity. Researchers can conduct in-depth analyses of metabolomic data using sophisticated technologies like MetaboAnalyst, which offer insights into the molecular mechanisms underlying these interactions. As demonstrated by the developments in MetaboAnalyst, for example, the integration of diverse omics data promotes a thorough understanding of metabolic pathways and helps identify important biological markers necessary for research on development and disease (Chong et al., 2018). Additionally, the phenomenon of ecological invasions is a key component of biological research and a vital field of study. The introduction of non-native species into unfamiliar habitats has significant ramifications and calls for multidisciplinary management strategies. Examining the origins and effects of these biological incursions, invasion science has become a crucial field that highlights the need to comprehend ecological dynamics and community interactions. As interest in biological invasions increases, new findings are emerging that put conventional ecological theories and practices to the test. The importance of incorporating various scientific viewpoints is shown by this developing discipline, which also highlights how invasive species shape ecosystems and advances our knowledge of ecological resilience (David et al., 2013). When taken as a whole, these discoveries from invasion science and metabolomics highlight the value of multidisciplinary biology research. Fostering cross-disciplinary collaboration and utilizing technological breakthroughs to improve our comprehension of intricate biological interactions are crucial as we look to the future of biological research. In addition to deepening our understanding of the complexities of life, this method lays the groundwork for tackling urgent environmental issues. Future studies can ensure the continued relevance of biology in a world that is constantly changing by acknowledging the interconnection of biological systems and opening the door to creative solutions that support sustainability and biodiversity conservation. We might imagine a thorough comprehension of life that serves both academia and society at large through ongoing investigation and integration of scientific knowledge.

Knowledge Assessment

The chapter includes material designed to review and reinforce each content. It includes Critical Thinking Questions to help test of your understanding of information presented in the chapter and Short answer Questions to review your understanding of the key concepts presented in the chapter.

Critical Thinking Questions

1. **Who is known as the "Father of Modern Biology"?**
   a. Aristotle
   b. Charles Darwin
   c. Gregor Mendel
   d. Louis Pasteur
2. **What is the basic unit of life?**
   a. Atom
   b. Molecule
   c. Cell
   d. Organism
3. **Which branch of biology studies the interaction of organisms with their environment?**
   a. Genetics
   b. Ecology
   c. Physiology
   d. Botany
4. **Which macromolecule is the main source of energy for living organisms?**
   a. Proteins
   b. Lipids
   c. Carbohydrates
   d. Nucleic acids
5. **DNA is primarily responsible for which function in living organisms?**
   a. Energy production
   b. Protein synthesis
   c. Storing genetic information
   d. Regulating body temperature

Short Answer Questions

1. What is biology, and why is it important to study biology?
2. What are the three main domains of life, and how are they different from one another?
3. Define homeostasis and give an example of how it works in living organisms.
4. What is the cell theory, and why is it fundamental to biology?
5. How do autotrophs and heterotrophs differ in the way they obtain energy?
6. What is the scientific method, and how is it applied in biological research?
7. Discuss how biology helps address global challenges such as climate change, disease, and food security.
8. Explain the levels of biological organization from the smallest unit to the largest. Provide examples at each level.
9. Describe the relationship between structure and function in biology, giving specific examples from cells or organs.
10. How has the discovery of genetics shaped our understanding of inheritance and variation among organisms?

Supplementary Materials

Key Terms: A list of key terms is given for quick reference

KEY TERMS FROM THIS CHAPTER

Annotation enrichment analysis	Biological structure	Cell
Cell theory	Cellular structure	Ecology
Ecosystems	Genetics	Human biology
Microbiology	Natural selection	Organism
Plant biology		

Further Resources: Recommendations for additional readings, websites, and multimedia resources.

References

1. Argelaguet, R., Velten, B., Arnol, D., Dietrich, S., Zenz, T., Marioni, J. C., Buettner, F., et al. (2018). Multi-omics factor analysis—A framework for unsupervised integration of multi-omics data sets. *Molecular Systems Biology, 14*. https://doi.org/10.15252/msb.20178124.
2. Bacher, S., Blackburn, T. M., Essl, F., & Genovesi, P. (2017). *Socio-Economic Impact Classification of Alien Taxa (SEICAT)*. https://core.ac.uk/download/286567949.pdf (accessed on 8th March 2025).
3. Barnett, R., Brace, S., Cucchi, T., & Dobney, K. (2013). *Divergent Evolutionary Processes Associated with Colonization of Offshore Islands*. https://core.ac.uk/download/20664364.pdf (accessed on 8th March 2025).

Detailed Table of Contents

CHAPTER 5

Anemia: Classification and Diagnosis 137

CHAPTER 6

White Blood Cell Disorders 171

CHAPTER 12

Urinalysis 385

CHAPTER 13

Examination of Cerebrospinal Fluid (CSF) 415

LIST OF FIGURES

PREFACE

Clinical pathology continues to be at the forefront of modern medical diagnosis, transducing biochemical, hematologic, immunologic, microbiologic, and molecular data into clinical decision-making. It is the sequential study of body fluids and tissues for the detection of abnormalities, which point to disease processes ranging from simple infections to complex genetic diseases. The discipline demands adherence to laboratory safety practices, quality control policies, and data validation methods so that results can be relied upon by clinicians. By integrating advances in instrumentation—i.e., spectrophotometry, chromatography, automated analyzers, and intricate microscopy—with a thorough understanding of physiologic norms, clinical pathology ensures accurate diagnosis and monitoring of therapeutic interventions.

The expanding universe of laboratory medicine has placed on the front lines of patient care powerful technologies for early disease detection and tailored therapy. High-throughput systems and digital image analysis expedite test turnaround times without compromising standards of accuracy. In addition to the traditional assays, the field now comprises genetic and immunologic testing that influences prognosis and guides targeted therapies. Professionals here must combine technical proficiency with ethical concern, such as ensuring test appropriateness, maintaining confidentiality, and following regulations. The lab is thus a critical interface between scientific discovery and patient care, distilling raw data into useful information that adds value to clinical outcomes.

With this goal in mind, *Essentials of Clinical Pathology* presents a thorough survey of the fundamental concepts and clinical applications of laboratory medicine. The book provides core subjects in a focused, logical sequence, with attention to both theoretical concepts and practical techniques. Each chapter begins with learning objectives and concludes with review questions, which are designed to reinforce learning and self-testing. Case-based examples give real-life applications of laboratory findings, and algorithmic flowcharts guide test ordering and interpretation. Demonstrations and photos depict instrumentation, slide preparation, and key morphologic observations. Alignment with current guidelines of professional organizations ensures conformity with regulatory needs, and cross-references highlight the relationship between numerous tests and common clinical conditions.

Chapter 1 explains the history, purpose, and structure of clinical laboratories and covers safety protocols, regulatory standards, and principles of quality assurance.

Chapter 2 describes light, fluorescence, and electron microscopy; spectrophotometric assays; chromatographic separation technology; immunoassay platforms; and automated analyzers, with teaching guidelines on calibration, reagent preparation, and troubleshooting.

Chapter 3 discusses red blood cell and white blood cell biology, platelet physiology, functions of plasma proteins, hemoglobin structure and gas transport, osmotic equilibrium, and complement pathways.

Chapter 4 includes protocols for automated cell counts, differential leukocyte count, slide staining techniques, reference ranges determination, and interpretation of instrument flags and abnormal morphologies.

Chapter 5 discusses the etiologies and laboratory evaluation of microcytic, macrocytic, hemolytic, and aplastic anemias, including reviewing iron tests, vitamin B_{12} and folate testing, reticulocyte count, and bone marrow exam.

Chapter 6 addresses leukemias, lymphomas, neutropenia, and leukemoid reactions, including classification by cell lineage and morphology, immunophenotyping, molecular diagnosis, and prognostic scoring systems. Chapter 7 addresses platelet plug formation, intrinsic and extrinsic coagulation pathways, prothrombin time assays, activated partial thromboplastin time assay, fibrinogen level assays, and D-dimer assays, and bleeding and thrombotic disorder evaluation.

Chapter 8 covers serum creatinine and blood urea nitrogen measurement, calculation of glomerular filtration rate, urine osmolality testing, electrolyte excretion ratios, and tubular reabsorption tests to evaluate glomerular and tubular function.

Chapter 9 evaluates serum transaminases, alkaline phosphatase, gamma-glutamyl transferase, bilirubin, albumin synthesis, and coagulation factors to distinguish hepatocellular injury from cholestasis profiles and monitor chronic liver disease.

Chapter 10 covers glucose oxidase and hexokinase assays, oral glucose tolerance tests, measurement of glycated hemoglobin, and continuous glucose monitoring systems, along with diagnostic criteria for type 1 and type 2 diabetes. Chapter 11 describes enzymatic and direct measurement of total cholesterol, LDL and HDL fractions, triglycerides, lipoprotein(a), and calculated atherogenic indices, against current guidelines on risk stratification and lipid-lowering therapy.

Chapter 12 covers macroscopic inspection, dipstick chemical testing for pH and proteins, glucose, ketones, and bilirubin, and microscopic inspection of cells, casts, crystals, bacteria, and yeasts with remarks on culture and sensitivity testing in urinary tract infections.

Chapter 13 covers the procedure for lumbar puncture, measurement of opening pressure, cell count and differential, glucose, and protein, cytochemical stains, and immunologic assays for detecting infections, hemorrhage, and inflammatory disorders of the central nervous system. Chapter 14 covers sample collection and handling, macroscopic and microscopic examination, chemical assays for proteins and enzymes, and examination for inflammatory and neoplastic markers to diagnose reproductive, joint, and serous membrane disease. Chapter 15 discusses concepts of antibody-antigen interactions, direct and indirect agglutination methods, enzyme-linked immunosorbent assay, immunofluorescence, flow cytometry, serum protein electrophoresis, measurement of complement, autoantibody detection tests for infectious and autoimmune diseases.

Essentials of Clinical Pathology is written for medical students, pathology residents, and clinical laboratory scientists who desire a solid foundation in the practice of diagnostic medicine. It will be a working resource for practicing clinicians, laboratory managers, and quality officers responsible for test selection, protocol development, and regulatory compliance. Educators will appreciate the case studies and review questions as teaching aids, and researchers will benefit from using the complete protocols to prepare experimental methods to correlate with standard diagnostic methods.

INTRODUCTION TO CLINICAL PATHOLOGY

1

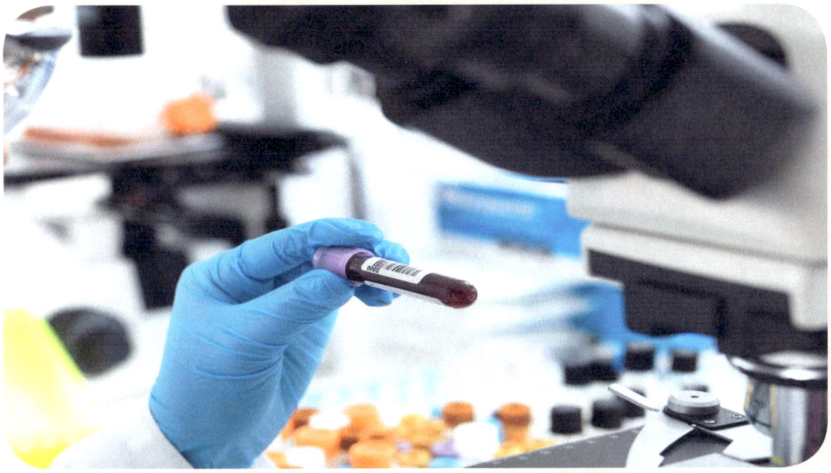

LEARNING OBJECTIVES

After studying this chapter, you will be able to:

1. Give historical development of clinical pathology;
2. Define the role of clinical pathologists;
3. Explore the diagnostic techniques in clinical pathology;
4. Describe common diseases diagnosed through clinical pathology;
5. Explain quality assurance in clinical pathology;
6. Discuss the future trends in clinical pathology.

Introduction

The human body has a tendency to catch us off guard, and we have to make a connection between what we observe in the clinic and what our laboratory results show us. That is essentially where clinical pathology is. It is test-running and analyzing body fluids to see if something is amiss or to see how healthy or unhealthy a person is overall. By looking closely at blood, tissues, and other body fluids, pathologists receive clues that guide treatment. They do not just aid in diagnosis, but track shifting disease and watch a therapy's progress. With modern medicine, having these objective, discrete measurements is nearly the cornerstone of quality care. A clinical pathologist consumes years of education in order to sift through lab reports that flash up in-patient care. Their task diversifies into fields such as hematology, microbiology, and even chemistry, each with its own revelations. It is not a purely reactive career; rather, these specialists guide patient management with in-depth lab reports. They bore into things like blood work, metabolic panels, and cultures, and they are almost always conversing with other healthcare individuals. This kind of cooperation provides a better picture of a patient's health and shows that the lab's function goes so much beyond merely swapping numbers—it is about doctors, pathologists, and specialists collaborating for better outcomes (Srivastava et al., 2020). The clinical pathology history demonstrates how essential it has become in addressing new medical challenges, especially with diseases more complex than ever. With advances in molecular diagnostics and digital technologies, the practice has skipped into new territory, making medicine more precise and targeted. Developments such as next-generation sequencing and liquid biopsies best describe how the discipline develops to address current needs. And as such issues like infectious diseases and chronic illnesses keep on piling up, good clinical pathology just gets louder in terms of demand. In its very nature, standards like quality control, ethical conduct, and continuous learning keep the discipline effective and responsive making it a force to reckon with in patient care (Rebecca et al., 2020) (Figure 1.1).

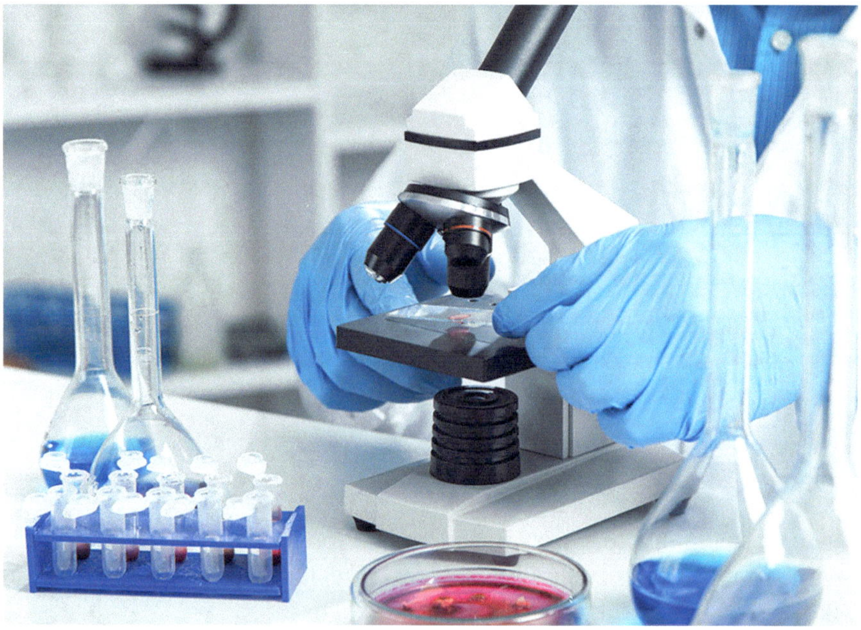

Figure 1.1. Clinical pathology.

Source: https://external-content.duckduckgo.com/iu/?u=https%3A%2F%2Fwww.fvhospital.com%2Fwp-content%2Fuploads%2F2020%2F02%2FThe-anatomopathological-testing.jpg&f=1&nofb=1&ipt=a9b68338df6a5834e81b83be1c5f27518a955582d4b29194fdde54bc4224f767.

Overview of clinical pathology as a medical specialty

Clinical pathology has also become a key support of modern medicine today, indeed revolutionizing patient care. It is all about detecting disease by analyzing specimens like blood, tissue, and other body fluids. Using modern methods—picture molecular diagnostics and genome scans—it not only detects illness, but also helps determine treatment strategies tailored to individual individuals (most of the time). The skill that pathologists have to interpret laboratory tests is the foundation of clinical decisions in most cases, all to make treatments both effective and suitable.

New diagnostic technology continues to emerge, which compels these specialists to constantly learn new techniques and technology; all of this contributes a lot toward allowing doctors to provide care that is patient-focused and based on the latest science advancements. The application of clinical pathology is more than simply calling a disease by name. Let us consider the example of fighting antimicrobial resistance (AMR): it is an enormous problem that threatens public health. A wider perspective on AMR shows some staggering statistics—such as an estimated 4.95 million deaths attributed to bacterial resistance in 2019 (Christopher et al., 2022). With numbers like these, doctors count heavily on clinical pathologists to sift through intricate microbiological data and make the right choice of antibiotics. Such collaboration not only cures infections but also helps implement protocols for infection avoidance. As these experts continue to improve their diagnosing methods, their recommendations ultimately inform healthcare policy and standard medical practice, always underpinned by good science to help battle recalcitrant pathogens. Beyond the proverbial making a diagnosis stick, clinical pathology really values putting together findings from various lab tests to give a better picture of the health of a patient. When you aggregate and crossmatch data from various tests, you have a comprehensive picture that can inform smarter clinical decisions. Advances in artificial intelligence and machine learning have also taken this process to the next level, with more accurate predictions for the fate of patients. For instance, some studies show that such advanced models can assist in clinical decision and medical training, even sometimes scoring at or below the passing grade for exams like the USMLE (Tiffany et al., 2023). So, with time, the combination of cutting-edge technology and established laboratory experience is set to disrupt entrenched habits and make patient treatment even more accurate and efficient in all types of medical environments.

Importance of Clinical Pathology in Patient Diagnosis

Technology's rapid advancements have actually flipped clinical pathology and its contribution to patient diagnosis on its head. Molecular techniques, now integrated into routine pathology, have inverted our worldview of disease—cancer, for instance, is treated in a whole different way these days. Next-generation sequencing has been like a big game-changer; it enables us to dive into the tumor genome and point to more accurate diagnostic and therapeutic avenues. Consider the 100,000 Genome Project in England, for example – they are attempting to bring whole-genome sequencing into normal clinical practice. To stay relevant to cellular pathology, pathologists are usually forced to bridge the skills gap, towards what is colloquially known as 'morphomolecular pathology.' When these ideas come together, the whole specialty not only lifts its game when it comes to the handling of cancer, but also generates the buzz for precision medicine, at last enhancing patient outcomes (Jones et al., 2018). Recent case reports also show the way that clinical pathology becomes a determining factor. One of the patients, for instance, came in with long-standing back pain and eventually received an unexpected diagnosis – a gastric antral mass that was found to be early gastric cancer. This kind of situation especially emphasizes the need to drill down with pathological tests despite symptoms seeming too nonspecific. By embracing a broad-dish diagnostic model that utilizes wide-scale pathology exams, medical practitioners are able to identify underlying conditions which would otherwise be missed. In essence, clinical pathology proves to be more than a mere tool but a significant cog in managing overall patient health—albeit, at times, the signs are obscured (Cardriche et al., 2020). Today, diagnosis of patients is all about understanding the combination of clinical pathology and everyday care. As therapy gets more individualized, more is expected from pathologists to be adept at molecular diagnosis. For the most part, it is not merely about increasing precision, but also helps pathology as a core member of multidisciplinary teams towards patient care. Pathologists who delve into genomic and molecular data find that their role in disease management becomes increasingly critical in response to the growing demand for treatments tailored to each individual patient. Also, in summary, the pivotal role played by clinical pathology in diagnosing the patient simply cannot be overlooked if we are to truly lead the way in modern medicine (Figure 1.2).

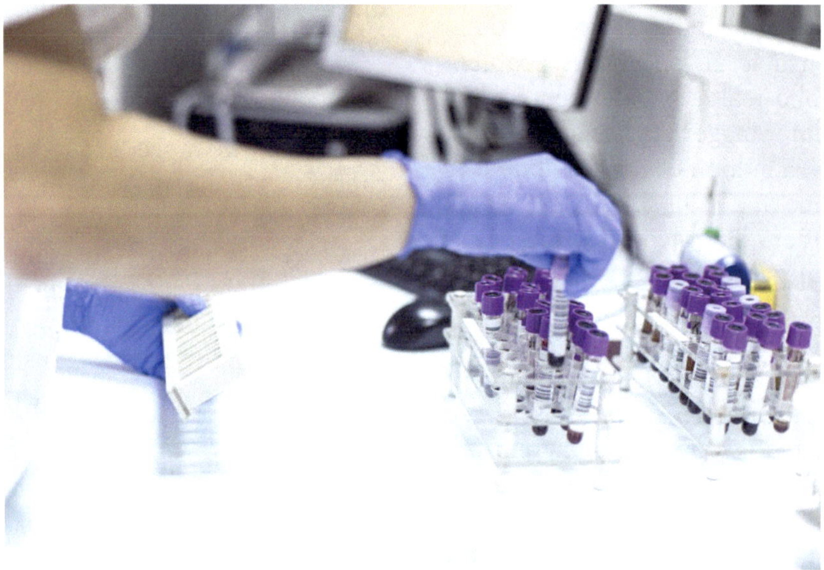

Figure 1.2. The most important pathology tests that help in correct diagnosis.

Source: https://external-content.duckduckgo.com/iu/?u=https%3A%2F%2Fregencyhealthcare.in%2Fwp-content%2Fuploads%2F2019%2F04%2FBlog-image_26_apr-1200x800.jpg&f=1&nofb=1&ipt=47c9ce5a6eaa64f75d2a37dca7c02082e625e698b4b3ab440930b38c6c5d5d88.

Distinction Between Clinical Pathology and Other Pathology Branches

Clinical pathology is a ground-level convergence point where lab experimentation converges with everyday patient care. It diverges from anatomic pathology, which has its focus primarily on structural changes within tissues and organs. Clinical pathology delves into a wider range of diagnostic tests—such as lab work examining blood and other fluids in the body—and then tries to interpret those to guide treatment. In contemporary evidence-based medicine, this approach is often the clincher, particularly where such quick action turns the outcome for the patient in diabetes or infection. Its focus on functional analysis, in a sense, complements the structural information acquired through anatomic investigation, making it a critical element of total care. All types of pathology do not do that, though. For example, forensic pathology is really about piecing together causes of death and sometimes finds itself working for legal teams in cases that are ethically ambiguous. Molecular pathology, conversely, digs deep into the finest minutiae through advanced genetic and protein testing, which has a tendency to illuminate the mechanisms of disease at the molecular level—findings that sometimes lead to targeted therapies. In most cases, though, such specialties are not directly focused on patient care like clinical pathology is. Instead, they bring their own expertise-based views with them, bringing to prominence the way different sections of pathology, with their different visions, come together in healthcare practice in a teamwork context. In the broader health scene, incidentally, the role of clinical pathology has contributed to major diagnostic gains. With new methods like liquid biopsies and next-generation sequencing, tests in the lab are now quicker and more precise. Take, for instance, evaluating amyloid β-protein aggregates in Alzheimer's: this is no longer a question of identifying markers but actually determining treatment protocols to slow down the development as compared to just addressing the symptoms. Similarly, the management of issues like pathologic nipple discharge today rely on a blend of techniques, including ductoscopy and imaging—apparatus that guide more sophisticated surgical procedures. In general, as technology becomes increasingly embedded in laboratory activity, clinical pathology always sets its standards higher to better care for patients and redefine quietly yesterday's standards of diagnosis.

1.1. Historical Development of Clinical Pathology

Learning Outcome

- Early practices and the evolution of laboratory medicine;
- Key figures in the history of clinical pathology;
- Milestones in the advancement of diagnostic techniques.

Clinical pathology has evolved with colossal changes in medicine that transformed how we detect and deal with disease. It did not start with high technology equipment but with the early, descriptive efforts of the ancient Greeks—then, relatively suddenly in the 1800s, there were laboratory tests. Think of individuals such as Rudolf Virchow; his plunge into cells essentially shifted things from pure theory to a more practical, empirical mindset. In many ways, those early, quite uncoordinated approaches eventually settled into a crude toolkit that still has an impact on clinical decisions today. Technological innovations and better knowledge about how diseases really work over the course of the years, especially throughout the 20th century, essentially refined the field. A whole array of tests were available in labs, which, understandably enough, made diagnosis far more accurate. A good case in point here would be the De Ritis ratio-biomarker that was a quite significant marker for liver issues, as many studies have proven (Suhail et al., 2024). Pathologists, once in the back rooms behind microscopes, began getting confused with multidisciplinary groups of a sort quite naturally; they began using lab test results and patient histories in treatment decisions, another sign of how complexity of disease required more specialized expertise. In the past few years, however, increased developments in molecular biology and other technology have just taken it to the next level. New imaging techniques and high-throughput sequencing have transformed traditional diagnostics to an extent where clinicians are now able to personalize treatments on a genetic and biochemical level. Studies such as PREOPANC-4, for instance, highlight this new, interdisciplinary model of patient care (Stoop et al., 2025). Overall, clinical pathology's history is a roundabout journey of ongoing adaptation—both reflecting sweeping technology advances and mounting constant pressure to move faster toward individualized medicine—and still maps a model for future innovation in the specialty (Figure 1.3).

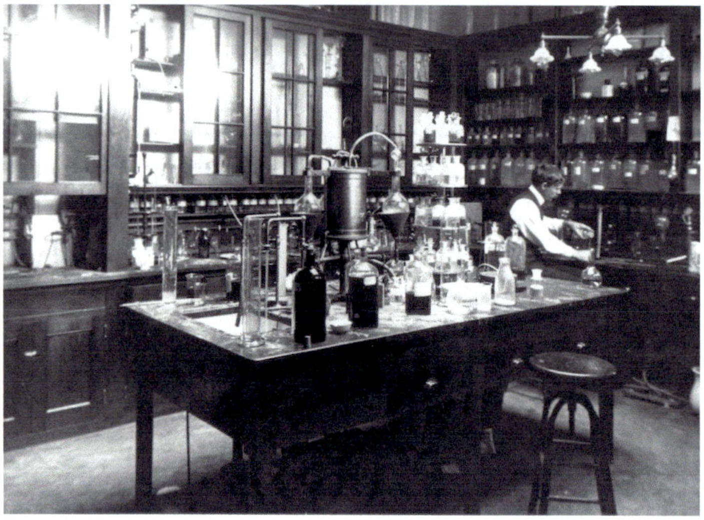

Figure 1.3. History of pathology.

Source: https://www.massgeneral.org/assets/mgh/images/pathology/history-lab.jpg.

1.1.1. Early practices and the evolution of laboratory medicine

Way back when, lab medicine started nearly by happenstance – a combination of experiment, blunder, and plain observation. Even way back in history, individuals would analyze body fluids to obtain hints concerning health, and our early physicians, such as the Egyptians, would categorize diseases merely by inspecting urine and even stool. They did not have sophisticated tests, but these early experiments gradually laid the foundation for what we today refer to as clinical pathology. In most instances, there was a gradual movement from exclusive dependence on personal opinion to adopting techniques that were less based on guesswork and more on hard facts, resulting in today's standards in laboratory procedures. By the 19th and early part of the 20th century, things began to change on a grand scale. Microscopes and chemical tests entered the scene, allowing us to observe things about the human body that had been concealed previously. It was not rare, say, to discover that pioneers such as Louis Pasteur and Robert Koch were attributing illness to small microorganisms – something that made laboratory tests a prerequisite to diagnose and treat disease. That era also witnessed the establishment of the first clinical labs, where not only was testing born but even standardized. Through this, a more intimate relationship between clinicians and lab technicians became established, which quite literally started to position lab results at the forefront of medical decision-making. The evolution of laboratory medicine just kept on going, as well. Quality assurance measures began to emerge along with professional organizations interested in standards setting and ongoing training, although there would be an occasional minor inconsistency in their guidelines. Organizations such as the American Board of Medical Genetics (ABMG) and others began to require proper certification and ongoing education to be a must – especially with the boom in molecular genetics and genetic testing becoming commonplace. With more genetic research, there was a greater need for expert skill in the interpretation of tests so that patients could be correctly diagnosed. Overall, all these changes reflect an industry that keeps up with the needs of modern healthcare, all toward improved patient outcomes through more, more effective diagnostic approaches (Figure 1.4).

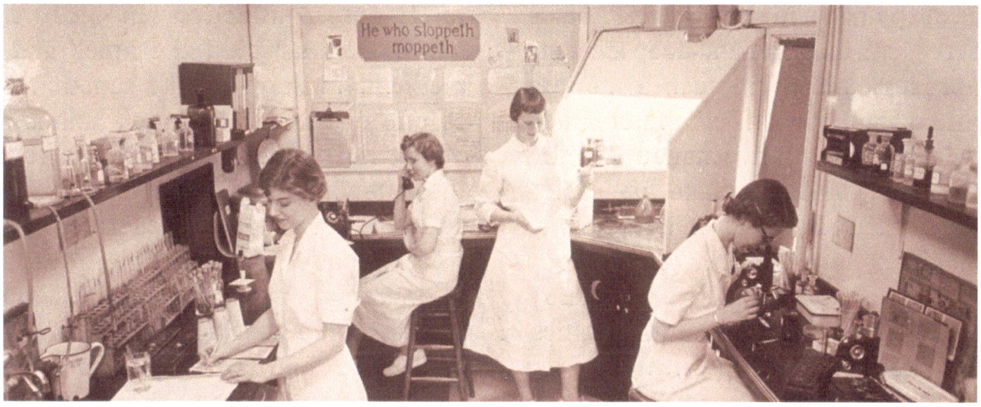

Figure 1.4. Early practices and the evolution of laboratory medicine.

Source: https://www.pharmacy.umn.edu/sites/pharmacy.umn.edu/files/2024-07/sloppeth-crop.jpg.

1.1.2. Key Figures in the History of Clinical Pathology

Visionary thinkers led clinical pathology where it is now. Let's consider Dr. Paul Ehrlich—a German physician and scientist of the late 1800s—who turned our strategy for diagnosing disease on its head. He invented a number of staining methods that allowed for easier identification of minute pathogens under a microscope, which in turn enabled physicians to diagnose diseases with more accuracy. Ehrlich's concept of employing a particular stain opened new fronts in immunology and serology, allowing us to select blood pathogens with greater ease. His lab still constitutes a significant portion of lab routines; even today, most methods trace their origins to his initial breakthroughs. There is Dr. Harvey Cushing, widely referred to as the "father of modern neurology," whose pre-1900s work dispensed with the distinctions between pathology and brain surgery. He devised new brain tumor surgery techniques and formulated diagnostic techniques that focused on an in-depth study of tissue samples. His research—painstakingly targeted at microscopic observations—did much to broaden our knowledge of neurological issues. In most cases, he promoted a systematic way of collecting patient data, one that increasingly became part of clinical research. His work not only improved surgical techniques but also highlighted the importance of pathology in identifying brain disorders correctly, revolutionizing patient care in the process. Another important contribution to clinical pathology was brought forth by Dr. Robert Koch. In the late 19th century, he formulated what we today refer to as Koch's postulates, rules that connect certain pathogens to specific diseases. His identification of the bacterium causing tuberculosis had far-reaching ripple effects—not merely for diagnostic use in the clinic but also for public health efforts at preventing disease before it was able to spread. Koch's fastidious methods for isolating and growing bacteria set the stage for much of the subsequent microbiology research. His firm and precise approach still resounds in modern practice, with present-day clinical pathology following to unfold on the grounds he established (Bray et al., 2024; Srivastava et al., 2020).

1.1.3. Milestones in the advancement of diagnostic techniques

Diagnostic techniques have made some wild leaps over the years, completely altering how we go about clinical practice. Imaging—radiology, if you will—started with X-rays and immediately turned into a means of spying inside our bodies. AI also joined the party, with machine and deep learning helping to process images in such a manner as to improve segmentation, computer-aided diagnosis and even pre-emptive maneuvers. Yes, all those intelligent systems make life easier, but they do run into roadblocks on data quality and ethics at times, so we keep having to keep perfecting things in most cases (Najjar, 2023). Another leapfrogging was molecular diagnostics, which really shook things up with the way we diagnose diseases at the genetic level. It began with polymerase chain reaction (PCR), an instrument that was capable of amplifying DNA to make our analysis a lot more accurate. Next came next-generation sequencing (NGS), quickly deciphering millions of pieces of DNA simultaneously. The technique provides rich information about genetic idiosyncrasies and even reveals variations in gene expression between cases—ranging from cancer genomics to detecting infection. In most cases, NGS has placed targeted therapies and precision medicine in the spotlight, sanctioning its place as one of the greatest innovations of modern diagnostics (Satam et al., 2023). Today, we see these technologies start to overlap with one another, creating an integrated approach to treating patients. Think about it: the marriage of imaging with molecular diagnostics and standard lab testing means early detection of disease, and more specific treatments for every person. Telemedicine is an added bonus that offers remote use of these tools, a nice added advantage. And as technology continues to develop, there is an awful lot of evidence that even more hybrid and adaptable diagnostic modalities lurk in the wings. Collectively, these milestones reflect our ongoing commitment to enhancing patient care—even if there are still some ethical and practical barriers to overcome (Satam et al., 2023).

Test Your Knowledge

1. How did the invention of the microscope contribute to the rise of clinical pathology as a discipline?
2. What were the major milestones in the development of laboratory-based diagnosis in the 19th and 20th centuries?

1.2. Role of Clinical Pathologists

Learning Outcome

- Responsibilities in laboratory management and oversight;
- Collaboration with other healthcare professionals;
- Contribution to patient care and treatment decisions.

Clinical pathology entails a range of responsibilities that influence how we diagnose, treat, and manage patients—though complicated, it actually boils down to meticulous lab work and good communication with physicians. A clinical pathologist is actually a doctor who spends most of his/her time reviewing laboratory tests; he/she examines fluids, tissues, and cells to find diseases. They act as a go-between for lab results and clinical conclusions, requiring tests to be done correctly and consistently—this extra vigilance decreases misdiagnoses and maintains patient safety at center stage. Over the past few years, specialties like infectious diseases and oncology have placed more importance on clinical pathologists. For example, in the field of oncology, as personalized medicine picks up speed, pathologists are being integrated into multidisciplinary teams to interpret complex molecular and genetic data in a way that ensures patients receive treatments that truly align with their needs (Dacic, 2024). They are also prominently involved in clinical trials, where they guarantee specimen handling and testing go through stringently stringent, sometimes iterative, quality control. This ongoing contribution naturally enables the creation of evolving treatment protocols, which overall leads to better patient outcomes. With healthcare continuing to evolve as a result of advances in technology, clinical pathologists' work is going to become even more different. Automated diagnostics and digital pathology are capable of speeding up diagnosis and enhancing precision.

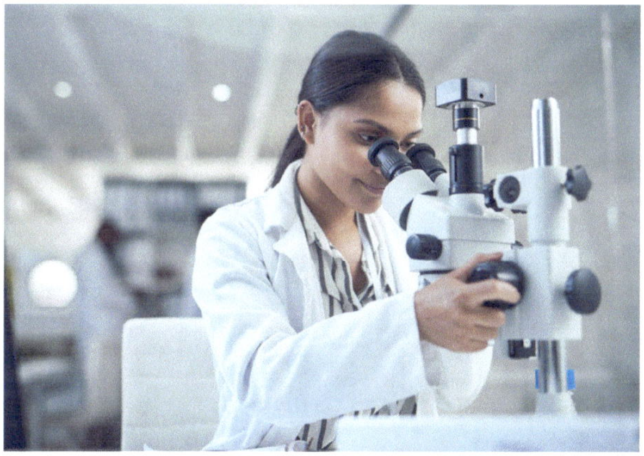

Figure 1.5. Role of clinical pathologists.

Source: https://external-content.duckduckgo.com/iu/?u=https%3A%2F%2Fmedical.rossu.edu%2Fmedia%2F14581%2Fpathology.jpg&f=1&nofb=1&ipt=6d22fd088a88b390eee87ac2eb174144cd5cc60c61892820d9048df62b79c9cd.

But most of the time, they still depend on the human element—a trained pathologist's knowledge—to actually make sense of the results. More recent studies even draw attention to their place in navigating the ethical side of emerging technologies, like AI diagnosis. Through their participation in these debates, they guarantee guidelines that serve the demands of patient care as well as the drive for innovation (Secora et al., 2025). As a health care environment which is always on the move, the services of skilled pathologists are still unequivocally essential (Figure 1.5).

1.2.1. Responsibilities in laboratory management and oversight

Good laboratory management is not about checking boxes; it is about juggling a set of challenges that put you squarely in compliance with regulations and focusing on patient safety and quality. Leaders of the laboratory, in most cases, realize that an agile quality management system (QMS) that closely adheres to FDA guidelines is absolutely essential. Rita D'Angelo's model, for instance, outlines such ideas as risk categorization, check-and-balance steps, and being well-sponsored by leadership—a mix that indeed enables a culture of compliance and ongoing improvement. With more labs foraying into the realm of generating in-house tests (LDT), managers must stay ahead of issues from regulation needs and process changes to deliver results that are not just dependable but also accurate. Generally, such a strategy not only protects patient outcomes but enhances laboratory flow as well. Besides adherence to rules, lab management also entails molding a harmonious team that stays razor sharp through ongoing training. Proper training sessions impart laboratory employees with competencies to navigate the rollercoaster of modern clinical pathology. When good leaders examine existing practices and interweave design controls, they establish a culture that values accountability and high performance—even if that means repeating the same concepts multiple times. Staff is kept up to speed on new technology and new methodologies through frequent workshops and seminars, creating a level of awareness that is key to reliable test results. These iterated and repeated attempts over the years are the foundation of a strong system of oversight based on quality management principles from. Shifting gears, leadership role changes in lab management set its own challenges and obligations that aren't always conveniently on a roadmap. Prior department chairs have indicated that exiting a managerial role can initiate meaningful changes in responsibilities and expectations. Planful transition becomes quite critical—it enables outgoing leaders to pass on their knowledge and positions their replacements approximately in line with the lab's set vision. This baton passing not only ensures continuity but also creates space for new thoughts and incremental innovation in how labs function. A well-prepared transition plan lessens leadership transition risk and keeps precious institutional memory alive. Ultimately, lab management is about balancing near-term management with long-range planning that reacts to the ever-changing world of clinical pathology so labs can meet both the challenges of today and tomorrow in healthcare delivery.

1.2.2. Collaboration with Other Healthcare Professionals

Collaboration with other health professionals is essential. In clinical pathology, collaborative work improves diagnostic accuracy and getting patients the right care—a point that is consistently emphasized. Pathologists, radiologists, nurses, and other specialists each contribute their own unique viewpoint, creating a kind of care ecosystem that takes into account the whole patient, rather than just symptoms.

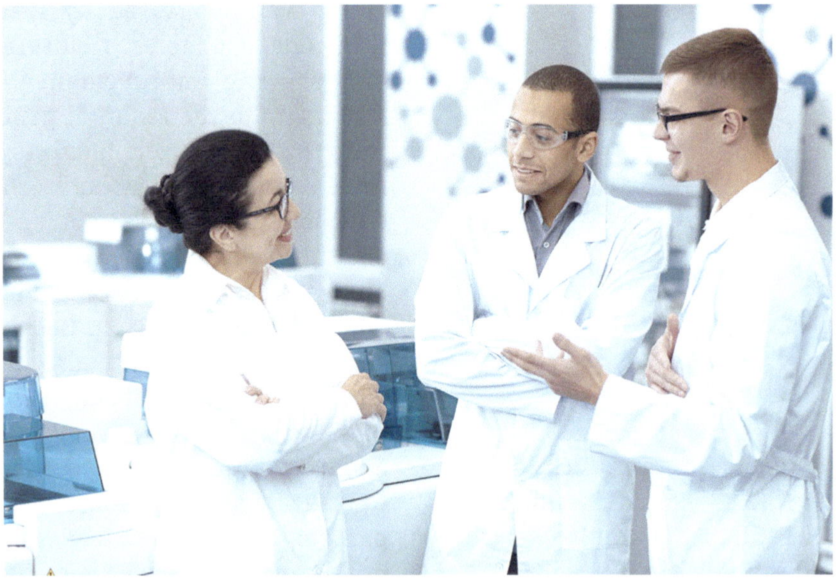

Figure 1.6. Collaboration with other healthcare professionals.

Source: https://external-content.duckduckgo.com/iu/?u=https%3A%2F%2Fwww.techno-path.com%2Fuk%2Fwp-content%2Fuploads%2F2019%2F12%2Fclinical-pathology-technopath.jpg&f=1&nofb=1&ipt=f3c266053c8749da266e86f0e9366f93babfebf9549ca22390ae96e248588792.

Recently, there has been a deluge of fresh data sets and observing tools coming into play, but in general, getting all these innovations implemented will rely on a good, interprofessional design. If professionals collaborate, they will be able to determine when to employ these new technological resources so that they fit with current practices rather than disrupting everything out of balance (Aranda et al., 2020). Briefly, collaboration does become the pillar of modern clinical practices with the process of learning about and treating patient conditions becoming smoother. Interprofessional education (IPE) has now emerged as a key driver of educating health professionals to shatter their silos. Reviews and studies evidence suggests that, in most cases, such learning experiences have the potential to create better communication and enhanced mutual respect between professions (Harthy et al., 2015). Working together side by side isn't just about acquiring facts; it's about believing deeply in one another's unique role and skills—no matter when sometimes the learning is a little messy. Working in IPE can hone diagnostic skills for clinical pathologists as well as cement the idea that it takes a team effort to solve complex problems. Such collaborative learning, flawed as it is, reiterates the sense that each contribution matters. Now, with digital health and other new technologies pushing the boundaries even wider, harmonious cooperation is more necessary than ever before. New technology provokes practitioners to think differently about dominant methods, and in fact, the implementation sometimes stalls because frontline specialists won't fully trust or even embrace the innovations. A form of collective architecture—a framework that has an unmistakable audit trail for emerging strategies—can help create that necessary trust among users (Aranda et al., 2020). In the end, this attitude of collaboration not only ensures that the new tools really fit their ultimate use, but also is a measure of the shared obligation to elevate the quality of patient care by well-trained, collaborative efforts (Figure 1.6).

1.2.3. Contribution to Patient Care and Treatment Decisions

Clinical pathology is a very gritty but crucial department that really dictates how patient care is figured out. It is a marriage of lab tests and diagnostic tests that gives physicians a snapshot of what is happening with disease so they can go pick up treatments. Consider diagnostic testing – getting quality lab results is really kind of the fulcrum for establishing the right treatment trajectory, and those numbers can influence clinical decisions more than you realize. The ASCP, for instance, still maintains that confirming skills on the merit of competency is most important; they insist that having BOC credentials enhances lab quality, which operates to keep patients safe. These credentials guarantee lab professionals have the know-how to deliver precise results – and since those results are integrated into about 70% of medical decisions, it speaks volumes of how inextricably clinical pathology, laboratory management, and better outcomes are linked (Baker et al., 2024). Even more advanced diagnostic tools are revolutionizing patient management. Look, in pediatric traumatic brain injury cases, physicians have to choose between running a CT scan and opting for an MRI, and that decision can actually make all the difference. CT scans are usually chosen because of their expediency in emergency situations, while MRIs have the capability to peck a little deeper to uncover the more subtle realities of brain injuries and other issues. This form of split decision-making depicts that the majority of the time, putting both together is the smart choice for the best results. Recent findings indicate that if clinicians select an imaging modality carefully, it can have a significant effect on treatment regimens and prognoses–essentially improving the quality of care in young patients (Abdulsalam et al., 2024). Remaining abreast of continuing professional education is, generally, essential to preventing standards from declining in clinical pathology. Programs like those run by the ASCP help create a workforce that isn't just competent but is also nimble enough to respond to shifting health needs. They are able to address problems like workforce shortages and also help improve diversity, equity, and access in the lab environment, making the whole healthcare system strong. With lab professionals continuously learning and refining their skills—even with occasional minor hiccups in their workflows—patient safety and diagnostic accuracy are enhanced. Essentially, having a well-trained lab team is significant since their feedback directly contributes to clinical decision-making and indirectly improves patient outcomes in our complex healthcare landscape (Baker et al., 2024).

Test Your Knowledge

1. What are the primary responsibilities of a clinical pathologist in modern healthcare systems?
2. How do clinical pathologists collaborate with other healthcare professionals in patient management?

1.3. Diagnostic Techniques in Clinical Pathology

Learning Outcome

1. Overview of laboratory tests and their purposes;
2. Emerging technologies in diagnostic pathology;
3. Importance of accuracy and reliability in test results.

There has been a great deal of turmoil in diagnostic methods in recent times, in fact revolutionizing clinical pathology. New techniques now help detect diseases much more accurately and dependably. Raman spectroscopy, for example, is now a good prospect for analyzing tissue samples. In the past, issues like not fully removing paraffin from samples slowed things down, but it turns out that using super mirror stainless steel slides can clear away pretty much all the paraffin, which in most cases makes Raman scatter work a lot better. This tweak not only makes immunohistochemical staining easier but also smooths out the whole diagnostic process. With superior staining coupled with trusted Raman imaging, the options for precise pathology readings grow—something pathologists can truly appreciate (Bell et al., 2019). In the meantime, a new wave rolls in as Computer-Aided Diagnosis (CAD) systems come into play. While CAD has been standard in radiology for a while now, bringing it into digital pathology has been a bit bumpy. Today's research now presents a protocol-based CAD viewer that has been specifically designed for breast cancer workups. Visual analytics are utilized by this system to refine image analysis after the Nottingham Histologic Grade, and through observing how pathologists examine tissue slides, the study recognizes areas that are going to take a little extra time. Early practice-based reviews suggest that the CAD viewer fulfills the diagnostic needs without compromising accuracy and minimizes manual labor, pointing to the vast potential of computer utilization in speeding up diagnostic accuracy (Corvo et al., 2018). All these advancements seem to bring us closer to precision medicine in pathology. As the technology advances, combining computerized systems with improved imaging may be able to provide care that is more suitable for every patient. Improved diagnostics enable doctors to intervene earlier and outcomes of treatment can be optimized. Further, these new methods are motivating labs to implement common protocols, thus enhancing overall quality in practice. The synergy between leading-edge imaging and computing technology is a sort of clinching moment for clinical pathology, leading the way to subsequent research and an unrelenting chain of diagnostic techniques that put precision and efficiency right at the fore (Figure 1.7).

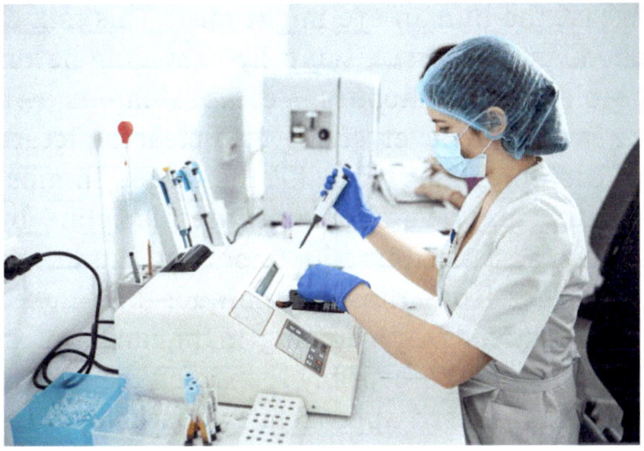

Figure 1.7. Diagnostic techniques in clinical pathology.

Source: https://cdn.flabs.in/webassets/919397855f803d31f1d4.png.

1.3.1. Overview of Laboratory Tests and Their Purposes

In clinical pathology, laboratory testing in fact paces the way that we are familiar with health. They are not routine procedures; they have become a crucial component of ascertaining disease, observing the health status of a patient, and even determining treatment. You might call them two kinds of tests. There's one kind that is applied to rule in or rule out a possible condition based on how somebody is feeling, and there's another kind that tracks the peaks and valleys of an illness and observes whether treatments are having an effect or not. All too frequently, the tests that are chosen is a function of the patient's symptoms, history, and even some unique biological markers that differ from patient to patient. When the right lab work gets incorporated into standard practice, it can make a diagnosis more accurate—and in many instances, allow practitioners to make better-informed decisions for improved patient outcomes. At the heart of a test's success is really a solid grasp of the biochemical principles behind it. In most cases, having the basic chemistry of these tests in hand accounts not only for the tests themselves but for the manner in which we're supposed to read the results. Blood tests, for instance, will give clues about anemia or infection issues, while other assays check out metabolic and organ functions to give a more general idea of health. And increasingly, molecular screening has turned the image on its head by being capable of detecting genetic mutations and even tiny infectious agents with some degree of specificity that was not there before. With improving techniques of testing, it becomes essential that professionals learn how to keep up with tech advancements and revised guidelines so they do not become victims of misreading tests. And then there is the problem of following accepted protocols. Standard practices – think about the ARRIVE guidelines – underscore how critical transparency and uniformity in reporting laboratory findings are. By complying with these standards, laboratories become progressively more repeatable and reproducible results, and this is as useful for decisions within clinical practice as it is for research activities (Percie et al., 2020). Guidelines of organizations which are engaged in the field of cardiovascular diagnostics (Ponikowski et al., 2016) also suggest that with a distinct, organized plan, clinicians are better able to select proper tests without any additional, redundant ones. Not only does this enhance diagnostic accuracy, but it also builds subsequent knowledge on what test results have in various populations of patients, eventually leading toward more individualized healthcare outcomes.

1.3.2. Emerging Technologies in Diagnostic Pathology

New technology has really shaken up diagnostic pathology. Digital pathology and AI have opened up new ways of imaging analysis not possible before. Rather than just looking at a microscope, slides can be scanned now – this allows remote consultations and for pathologists to collaborate with high-res images much more efficiently. When paired with AI programs, these computerized systems can pick up on subtle patterns that the human eye might miss. This mix of old and new not only improves diagnosis but also speeds up processes, typically providing better patient results and more efficient overall operations. Molecular diagnostics is establishing its own place in this new realm. It digs deep into genes at the molecular level, giving us a clearer picture of disease mechanisms and helping in the selection of therapies that really hit the target. In most cases, technologies like next-generation sequencing (NGS) are revolutionizing the discipline by delivering integrated genomic profiles. For conditions such as cancer, finding important mutations can mean treatments being much more targeted. Subtract from those techniques like liquid biopsy—though non-invasive—widening our scope diagnostically by catching malignancy in an early stage. In effect, these molecular advancements are almost imperceptibly reshaping the map of diagnostic pathology and nudging us toward a more precision-based approach. Telepathology ties the whole thing together by showing how technology will bridge distances. It allows pathologists to view and diagnose samples remotely, which reduces geographical constraints and even facilitates institutions to collaborate more easily. This not only speeds up access to expert know-how where it is most required, but also rationalizes laboratory workflows by reducing the reliance on physical slide shipping. Combined with ubiquitous data-sharing websites, telepathology provides an even more networked system—clinicians can directly access the diagnostic information essential to patient care. As these systems further develop, they seem set to rule the clinical pathology destiny, remembering that openness to alternative ways of doing things is essential for advancing diagnostics and patient care (Figure 1.8).

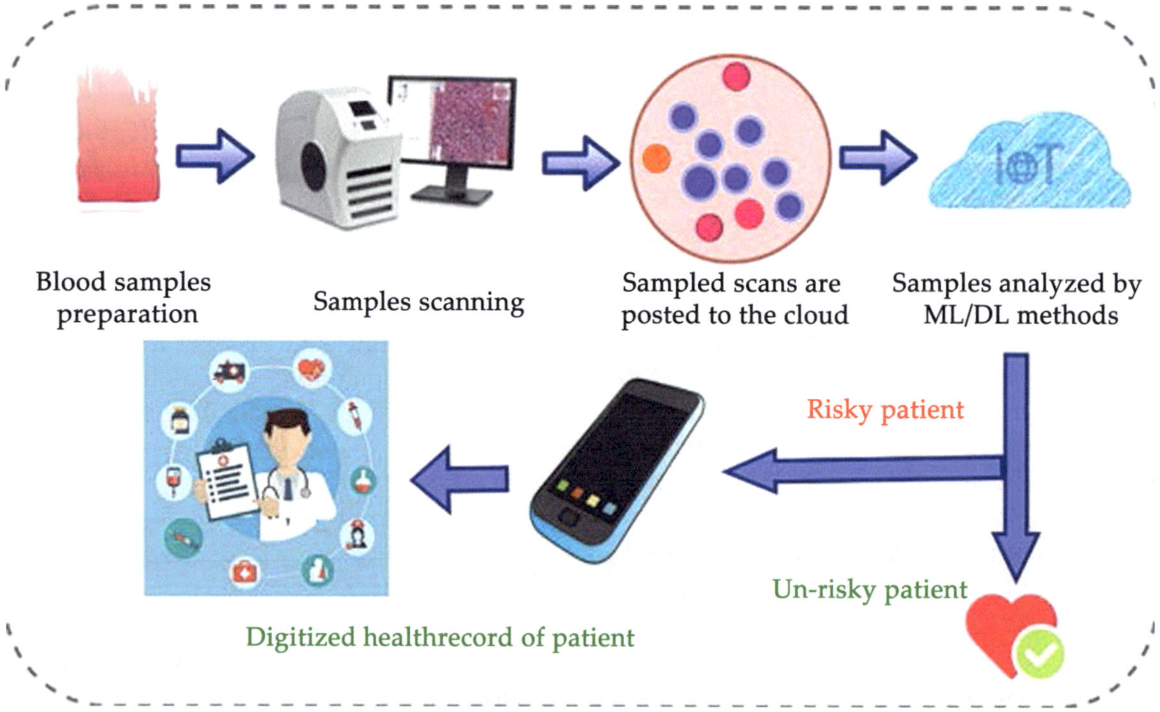

Figure 1.8. Emerging technologies in diagnostic pathology.

Source: https://ars.els-cdn.com/content/image/3-s2.0-B9780128214725000028-f20-02-9780128214725.jpg.

1.3.3. Importance of accuracy and reliability in test results

Clinical pathology laboratory test results really matter when making patient care decisions. They determine how diagnoses are made, treatments are chosen, and ultimately how safe patient care is. When tests are accurate, physicians obtain good data that enables them to respond quickly; when tests fail, however, misdiagnoses or even harmful treatments can exacerbate disease. Sometimes differences in the manner in which tests are carried out in varying environments undermine their consistency, and it's why it's such an important issue to keep a close eye on quality controls. Diagnostic equipment is continually improving—and you can see deep learning networks having a tangible impact here. On average, once a deep learning model has been adequately trained and audited, it can sift through complex data with remarkable accuracy, solving problems that get past the filters in traditional approaches. I recall one study that showed a deep learning algorithm attained up to 98% accuracy on digitized dermatopathology slides (Ayyagari et al., 2020). This kind of advance not only speeds up the whole diagnostic process but also builds a tremendous amount more confidence in results, being a valuable asset for pathologists working in everyday environments. Reproducibility in test results is another thing that you just can't overlook. The idea is very simple: tests have to yield the same result every time that there is variation in who gives them or what equipment is employed—even when, okay, there may be minuscule differences here and there. Look at the Lateral Scapular Slide Test: its validity is really doubtful when used on symptomatic groups (Bolooki et al., 2016). These minute inconsistencies can potentially mislead clinical decisions through the generation of conflicting interpretations of a patient's results. Finally, resolving the union of high accuracy with uniform, reproducible results is ultimately at the very heart of quality clinical pathology.

Test Your Knowledge

1. What are the major differences between biochemical, hematological, and microbiological diagnostic tests?
2. How are molecular diagnostic techniques, such as PCR, transforming clinical pathology?

1.4. Common Diseases Diagnosed Through Clinical Pathology

Learning Outcome

- Overview of hematological disorders;
- Role in diagnosing infectious diseases;
- Contribution to cancer diagnosis and management.

Clinical pathology plays a monstrous role in defining why people are ill, and things get rather grimy at times. You might find such issues like a loose anconeal process or fractured-up coronoid process, and doctors have a tendency to rely on high-tech examinations (e.g., elaborate X-rays and scans) to find these tiny misalignments of the joint that lead to a multifactorial mess. These issues are most commonly resolved, and in doing so, not only do they illuminate the diagnosis, but they also open up treatment avenues that are appropriate to the individuality of each patient, paving the way for a better prognosis for those suffering from elbow dysplasia (Gielen et al., 2011). Lung diseases, too, get their due share of innovation in clinical pathology. Cryobiopsy, for example, has just revolutionized pulmonary disease diagnosis. It is slightly unorthodox compared to standard biopsies—yielding bigger samples and more intense probing of the tissue—which can lead to diagnosing disease more accurately, specifically in patients with cancer or interstitial lung disease; sometimes it even avoids the frustrating artefacts that were present in previous techniques. Recent accounts indicate that this method may be on the verge of significantly enhancing pleural lesion diagnostic precision and becoming a valuable asset within a broad variety of settings (Griff et al., 2019). And then there is reality as it is experienced every day. Diabetes, coronary disease, and infection all depend very heavily upon laboratory testing to inform decision-making. Routine testing of blood for glucose or a lipid profile gives doctors a snapshot of an individual's metabolic health and can lead to earlier intervention. As disease grows more intricate, it becomes more valuable to correlate the laboratory test results with the way the patient is really doing. This integration of information not only informs diagnosis but also guides treatment pathways that can lead to better outcomes, illustrating just how critical clinical pathology is to present-day healthcare (Figure 1.9).

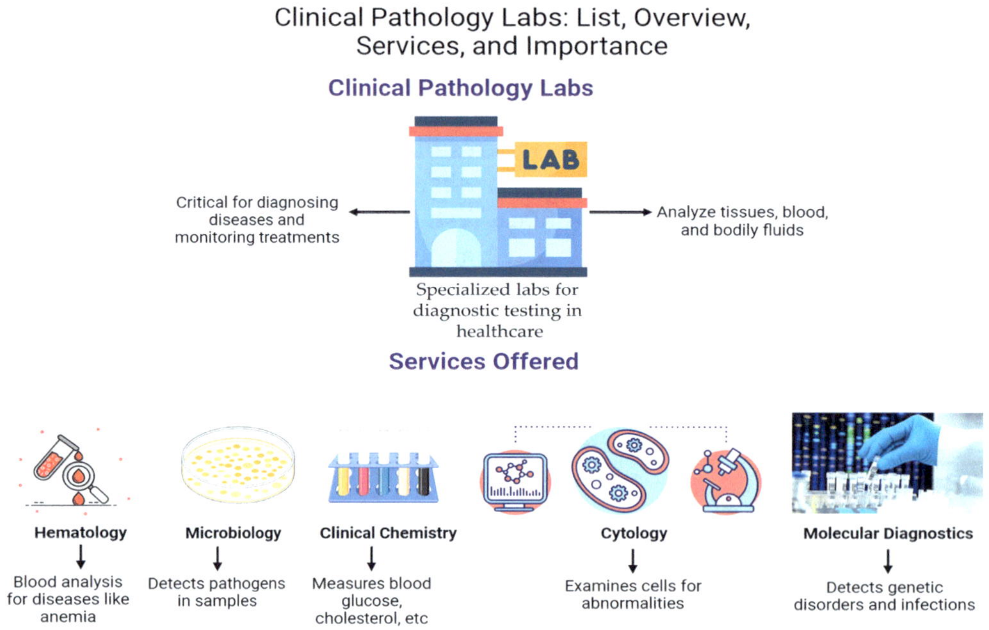

Figure 1.9. Common diseases diagnosed through clinical pathology.

Source: https://cdn11.bigcommerce.com/s-h68l9z2lnx/product_images/uploaded_images/zpb_32209054.png.

1.4.1. Overview of Hematological Disorders

Blood disorders occur in all shapes and sizes—it's a wild mirror image of just how intricate our blood actually is. Because, you see, disorders such as anemia, leukemia, and even clotting disorders occur with completely different causes and ways of acting within the body. Take, for example, sickle cell anemia or hereditary spherocytosis; in both of these, a genetic idiosyncrasy alters the structure and operation of red blood cells, at times causing an enlarged spleen and increased risk of infection. The way in which such structural idiosyncrasies are connected with the symptoms is what makes it really drive home the importance of getting to the bottom mechanisms at stake. Some studies, for instance, have further noted that in the context of sickle cell disease the spleen tissue has a lower density of lymphoid follicles from those that we have in hereditary spherocytosis

(Rita et al., 2016)—something that indicates quite distinct disease mechanisms. Generally, therefore, having a broad, general understanding of these conditions is desirable if we are to make correct diagnoses and direct clinical management accordingly. Other than the genetic part of it, inflammation itself becomes a critical player in the story of most blood diseases. Anemia of inflammation, which you usually happen upon in people who have long-standing chronic diseases, is usually defined by high levels of inflammatory markers like interleukin-6 (IL-6). This cytokine, overall, ends up controlling the production of hepcidin, the significant hormone that controls iron management—how much is on hand to produce new red blood cells. New approaches, such as therapy with bovine lactoferrin, are under study as ways of raising iron mobilization and maybe improving overall blood measures (Cutone et al., 2018). It's quite enlightening the way changing the balance between inflammation and blood cell production shows just how connected our body systems really are, encouraging doctors to consider treatments from multiple alternative angles. Stepping back after the initial diagnosis and treatment, long-term management of blood diseases becomes all the more relevant. Being aware of the small things that perpetuate every disease can allow for more specific, more individualized therapies. Where genetic conditions place patients at greater risk of complications, having a head start with early testing and some prophylactic measures can really be life-altering. In the meantime, the advances in molecular diagnostics and targeted therapies are transforming the way medicine tackles these issues, allowing for treatment of patients as individuals with customized care tuned to each disorder's unique characteristics. This steady evolution in what we understand and how we approach blood disorders is a reminder—though at times imperfectly—of the necessity to remain connected with the current research, especially in a medical landscape that seems to remake itself on a daily basis (Figure 1.10).

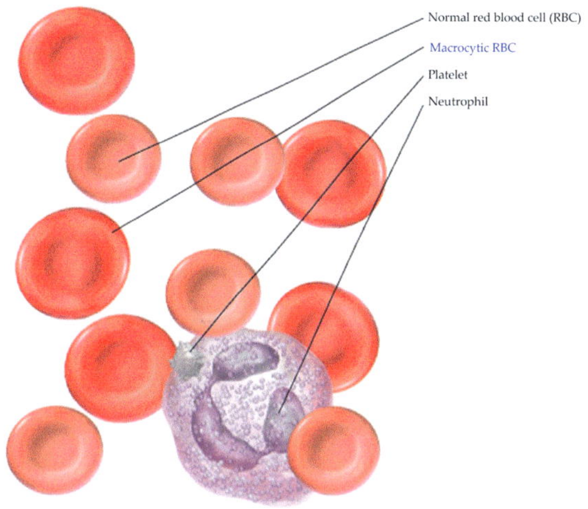

Figure 1.10. Hematologic disorders.

Source: https://i0.wp.com/basicmedicalkey.com/wp-content/uploads/2018/09/HEMATOLOGIC_DISORDERS-FF1.gif?w=960.

1.4.2. Role in Diagnosing Infectious Diseases

Infectious illnesses are also very sneaky, and discovering what's really going on typically involves a rapid, definitive diagnosis. Clinical pathology gets right to it with a mix of laboratory tests involving serology and culturing microbes through to molecular prestidigitation in the shape of PCR to find infections that might go undetected by a normal test. Occasionally, a germ can be carried over from one culture to refine treatment in just the right way, and when a molecular test is coupled with its quick results, it can be the difference between life and death in desperate cases. Most of the time, this isn't about making a spot diagnosis, though; it's about establishing the foundation for proper treatment, which is why clinical pathology is a cornerstone of modern health care. It's not all about finding pathogens, though. It. Clinically, the pathology occasionally gives us a glimpse of how a person's immune system responds. For instance, when laboratory reports show raised acute-phase proteins or specific antibodies, it can make it more precise to diagnose—especially if there is some overlap of the symptoms with other conditions. In immune-mediated necrotizing myopathy, for instance, further investigation through tissue specimens can clarify uncertainty between differing types of inflammation of the muscle or other potential infections. CT scans and other imaging devices also give an added dimension of data, showing just how widespread an infection can be, and these bits of data—when cross-referenced with lab tests—help doctors sort infectious from non-infectious problems. Clinical pathology even goes so far as to understand how disease works at a fundamental level. Take cases in the right lower quadrant: sophisticated imaging usually uncovers how the lymphatic network becomes engaged, suggesting whether an ailment is likely to be benign rather than malignant. Those typical patterns visible on tests can change the way a diagnosis and subsequent therapy are made. And when infection is the concern, a careful look at lymph nodes can light up not only what is responsible for the issue but also how it may arise. In general, the integration of imaging with lab data greatly enhances clinical decision-making, demonstrating the central position of clinical pathology in resolving complex infectious diseases and determining effective treatments (Figure 1.11).

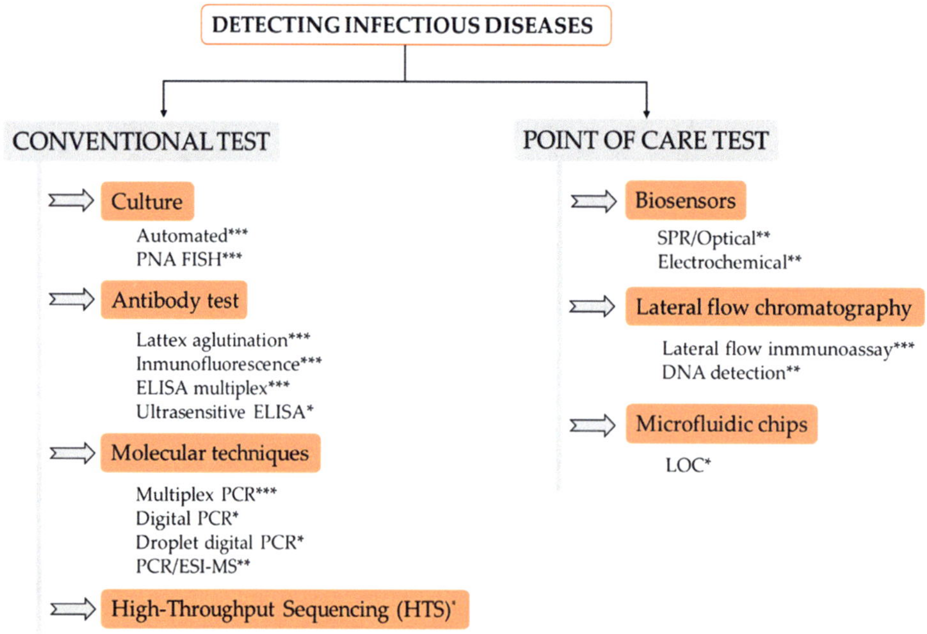

Figure 1.11. Role in diagnosing infectious diseases.

Source: https://www.mdpi.com/antibiotics/antibiotics-09-00916/article_deploy/html/images/antibiotics-09-00916-g001.png.

1.4.3. Contribution to Cancer Diagnosis and Management

Pathology and cancer diagnosis come together to drive innovation in patient care over the long term; digital pathology, for instance, is already breaking up the bad habits of how we diagnose. As more labs move towards digital systems, clinicians now can process tissue samples more rapidly—and, frankly, get answers much faster. Overall research shows that this new methods speed diagnosis while improving accuracy, which is key to successful outcomes, especially for common diseases like breast cancer. And it's not just a question of faster reactions—digital results also guide treatment protocols tailored specifically to individual patients, which ultimately enhances care and quality of life overall for patients battling cancer (El-Banna et al., 2025). Taking into account the cost implications of such advances is also important, particularly in limited-resource healthcare systems. A study among breast cancer patients suggested that digital pathology promises not only time but also cost savings and therefore optimizing the use of resources within the discipline. Even with high setup costs in the beginning, cost benefits over the long term make a strong case for integrating such technologies into core practice. Interestingly, the promise of more precise diagnostics extends beyond breast cancer; new technology would also redefine care pathways for other forms of cancer. However, with institutions going digital, keeping tight tabs on economic sustainability is paramount to ensure that pathology innovations actually yield tangible benefits to the healthcare system (El-Banna et al., 2025). Projections of digital pathology and molecular diagnostics are far from daily clinical use—there's an exponentially needed course for research that discussions of these topics predict. In studies of renal cancer, there has been debate over the combination of biobanking and digital technology, something that would potentially pave the way for increased scientific knowledge and improved clinical practice. At conferences, experts have emphasized that prioritizing digital pathology in renal cancer can spur international teamwork, helping to standardize research and diagnostic methods alike. Of course, hurdles like funding and training challenges still stand in the way, and these issues must be addressed if we're to tap into the full potential of these technologies. In summary, through thoughtful planning, we might see a quantum leap in the way cancer is diagnosed and treated across various fields (Figure 1.12).

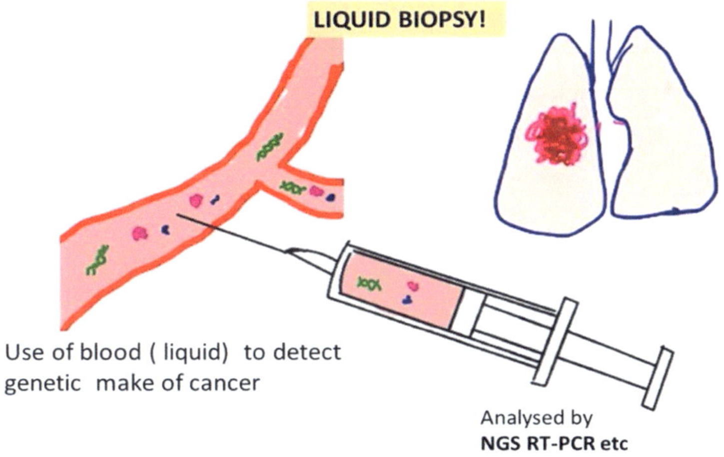

Figure 1.12. Lab diagnosis of cancer in pathology.

Source: https://ilovepathology.com/wp-content/uploads/2023/07/LAB-DIAGNOSIS-OF-CANCER-1024x576.jpg.

Test Your Knowledge

1. How is diabetes mellitus diagnosed and monitored using clinical pathology tests?
2. Which laboratory investigations are most useful for diagnosing hematological malignancies such as leukemia?

1.5. Quality Assurance in Clinical Pathology

Learning Outcome

- Importance of standard operating procedures;
- Role of accreditation and regulatory bodies;
- Continuous education and training for laboratory staff.

Quality assurance is crucial when it comes to guaranteeing diagnostic testing in clinical pathology is accurate and reliable. It's not just an issue of patient safety—when there are things like standardized protocols included, labs end up performing more predictably, and that boosts overall healthcare efficiency in most cases. For example, routine equipment calibration and compliance with specific regulations for specimen handling avoid errors in testing; such procedures, while being repeated or reworded from time to time, remain essential. Even the National Health Service has come to experience such procedures as the key to quality care in everyday laboratory work. Point-of-care testing, or POC testing, illustrates the intricacy of quality assurance in practice. Tests such as C-reactive protein (CRP) can potentially increase diagnostic accuracy and reduce inappropriate antibiotic use, but problems like reimbursement, quality control, and at times even practitioners' attitudes, can hinder progress. Much of the time, success with these tests appears to be dependent on intercommunication between regional care givers and central laboratory services, which ultimately benefits patients.

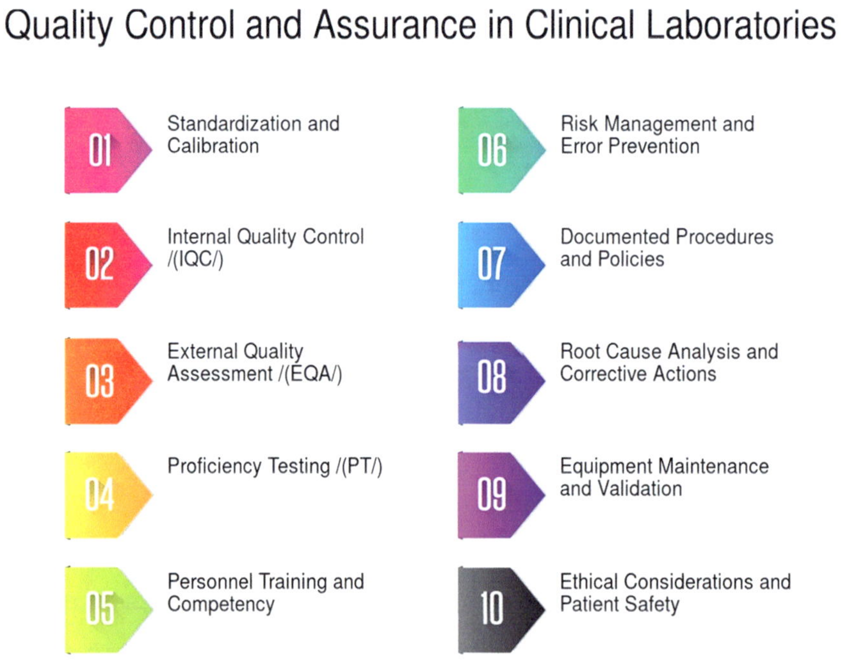

Figure 1.13. Ensuring quality control and assurance in clinical laboratory.

Source: https://fastercapital.co/i/Clinical-laboratory-quality-Improving-Clinical-Laboratory-Quality--Best-Practices-and-Strategies--Quality-Control-and-Assurance-in-Clinical-Laboratories.webp.

Sometimes they force stakeholders to remake strategies, all in the cause of creating a culture where quality is always at the forefront (Barlow et al., 2016). Alongside traditional laboratory work with conventional microscopes, advanced imaging techniques are also revolutionizing clinical pathology. Take high-frequency ultrasound, for instance; it is being shown some promise for detecting metastatic axillary lymph nodes in breast cancer patients—a timely reminder that new technology will have to augment established quality assurance measures. Of course, such technologies will need to be rigorously tested not just for their diagnostic performance but against quality measures like specificity and predictive value. When these technologies become certified, care providers generally can make better management decisions that improve patient outcomes. Ongoing studies and continuous quality-improvement processes in routine laboratory studies and these newer imaging technologies ultimately pave the way to a better level of care for patients (Clough et al., 2004) (Figure 1.13).

1.5.1. Importance of Standard Operating Procedures

Clinical pathology depends on keeping setting procedures—SOPs—if one is to get lab results that really hold up to accuracy and consistency. Laboratories rely on these guidelines so that tests will always be correlated, so physicians and nurses can trust what they see. Small differences in how a sample is handled can upset a diagnosis, so keeping to SOPs minimizes the level of human error. Take the case of early-stage mucinous ovarian carcinoma; in such a case, meticulous protocols are needed more so. Findings, like whether lymph nodes point to metastases, activate these routine procedures, making the processes even more accurate and guiding treatment regimens, which is just how much SOPs impact patient care (Buist et al., 2017). Today, the inclusion of molecular testing into routine lab procedures truly highlights why accurate, detailed SOPs matter so much. Mistakes at inception—i.e., at sample collection or transport—will disturb test reliability and, in the majority of cases, somehow end up affecting patient care. With the advent of molecular pathology, the challenge is only further compounded; more rigid guidelines are now imperative so that every step, from tissue fixation to extraction of DNA, is compliant with best practice guidelines. Internal validation, quality control, and regular audits seem like urgent control points that guarantee diagnostic trustworthiness. As labs build around these SOPs, they're better equipped to handle the curveballs and unexpected occurrences of molecular testing, leading to better results overall (Edsj et al., 2014). On another note, as clinical pathology keeps evolving, SOPs must be dynamic enough to keep pace with emerging technologies and techniques. In most instances, whenever new test procedures become available, traditional procedures must be reexamined and updated to accommodate the new scientific knowledge. Such adaptability does not just enhance diagnostic accuracy—it also puts laboratories in a position to address changing clinical requirements. And it is not just technical—it even allows medical personnel to convey vital information more effectively, which is crucial in deciding on treatments. In general, SOPs are not a convenience issue—rather, they are the cornerstone of clinical pathology and are of great value to patient safety and treatment success in almost any conceivable setting (Buist et al., 2017; Edsj et al., 2014).

1.5.2. Role of accreditation and regulatory bodies

Accreditation and regulation are at the heart of clinical pathology, keeping lab work in check and patients safe. They establish rules that go from the way the tests are conducted and the specimen managed to who is allowed to work in these laboratories. Their sometimes-draconian rules not only increase the validity of lab tests but also public trust in our health system. Accreditation labs show a genuine commitment to quality and best practices—which, in most cases, inspires confidence among physicians and patients alike. Every step, from initial sampling to ultimate report, is intended to meet the quality and ethical standards that patient care demands. Clinical pathology labs often lead the way in research that can change the practice of medicine and even influence policy. Generally speaking, following the rules and regulations of accrediting bodies does a lot towards upholding ethical standards, especially when the human subjects are in question. It is common practice for pathology teams to be the custodians of patient specimens, tasked with carrying out protocols that enhance participants' rights, safety, and welfare. Following through not only upholds the integrity of the data but also supports the validity of outcomes. Sometimes the results even presage important shifts in clinical practice or pave the way to authorization of novel medical devices and treatments, showing how much these safety nets are affecting (Panel et al., 2019). It is a balancing act, finding the right balance between stringent regulatory compliance and everyday lab operation. While some see rules as stifling creativity, they in fact form the cornerstone of effective and safe laboratory procedures. Through the incorporation of these standards into routine practices, laboratories create an environment which supports enhanced research and routine clinical service without detracting from their effectiveness of operation. Through emphasis on quality control and ethics, not only are clinical objectives attained but also labs are in a position to enhance medical knowledge. By accomplishing this, the accrediting and regulatory bodies keep clinical pathology consistent with the highest standards of care, consequently serving public health (Figure 1.14).

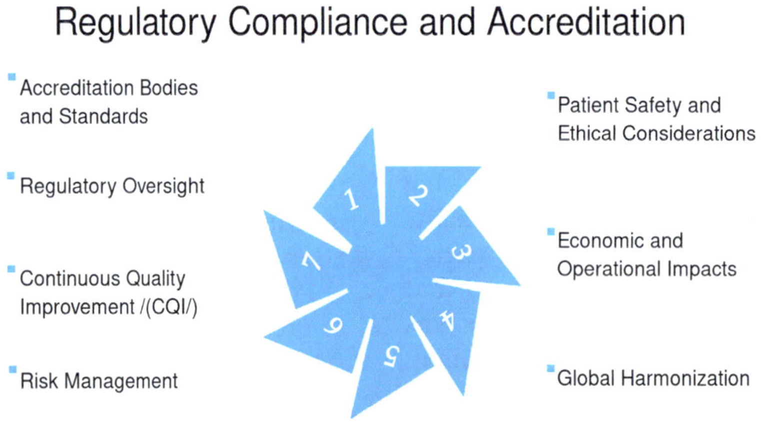

Figure 1.14. Role of accreditation and regulatory bodies.

Source: https://fastercapital.co/i/Clinical-laboratory-services--Quality-Assurance-in-Clinical-Laboratory-Services--Ensuring-Accurate-Results--Regulatory-Compliance-and-Accreditation.webp.

1.5.3. Continuous Education and Training for Laboratory Staff

Clinical pathology is racing ahead, and laboratory personnel truly need to keep learning on an ongoing basis—a fact it's hard to overstate. Training and education on an ongoing basis give personnel the ability to deal with new technology and evolving techniques. Lab methods updates, quality assurance protocols, and ever-changing rules create a kind of everyday excellence. Organizations like the Clinical Laboratory Standards Institute and the American Society for Veterinary Clinical Pathology also help by offering material that enhances competency and is of higher quality. As laboratories become more critiqued by accrediting agencies, staff are generally required to be sharp on federal regulations like those outlined in the Clinical Laboratory Improvement Amendments (CLIA) (Arnold et al., 2019). Competency checks, for instance, are similarly large when it comes to keeping the team on its toes. In the majority of cases, such assessments ensure that all staff have the necessary know-how to undertake complex diagnostics. Software such as practice simulations, casual but perceptive peer reviews, and ongoing quality-improvement projects all help in this direction. Tools. Creating a culture in which people feel at ease asking questions—albeit even revisiting fundamental principles—is one way to promote open conversation that, in itself, improves the day-to-day service of the lab. Blending formal sessions with informal, on-the-hoof education seems to enable the team to react more readily when clinical questions develop. Many of the expert suggestions, in return, point to the achievement that continuous emphasis on learning not only benefits the team but also eventually the patients (Wiegers et al., 2019). Another view is the appeal for training sessions specific to the varied needs of lab professionals serving in specialties. Those efforts should transcend technical competencies, ethical conduct, and even the sometimes-tricky aspect of communicating in healthcare on a daily basis. Workshops, web classes, and on-site training sessions ultimately cater to varied learning styles and busy schedules—no one-size-fits-all solution here. Sometimes a mentorship program, in which junior employees are assigned to work with old salts, fires up productive knowledge sharing (and might even help keep employees around longer). When well implemented, a system of continuous education equips laboratory teams to manage difficult situations and create innovative solutions within clinical pathology, further improving the quality of care given to patients (Arnold et al., 2019).

Test Your Knowledge

1. Why is quality control essential in clinical pathology laboratories?
2. What are the main components of an effective quality assurance program in pathology?

1.6. Future Trends in Clinical Pathology

Learning Outcome

- Impact of personalized medicine on pathology practices;
- Integration of artificial intelligence in diagnostics;
- Challenges and opportunities in the evolving field.

Technological development is transforming clinical pathology, with machine learning and AI enabling doctors to sift through tremendous amounts of data in ways that we had not seen before. AI helps detect aberrant behavior of cells in tissue samples—think of early cancer detection—and remember nearly 20 million new cases erupted in 2022 (Bray et al., 2024). Better testing devices are just a necessity. AI's role isn't just limited to quicker detection; it is also driving medicine toward more personalized approaches so that treatments can match each patient's unique tumor profile, which in most cases means better outcomes when precision matters. There's also a growing buzz about breaking down silos in healthcare. Clinical pathologists are increasingly teaming up with radiologists, oncologists, and other specialists, often in unexpected ways. This mixed approach combines different views on disease—from detection to managing follow-up care—and although one might argue that traditional pathology has its limitations, collaboration seems like a natural move (Livingston et al., 2020). It isn't always a neat process; sometimes the ideas repeat or overlap, but that's just how collaborative work evolves in a complex field like medicine. The focus on prevention is another big shift we're seeing. With an estimated cases of cancer projected to be around 35 million by 2050, pathologists are actually making a sincere effort to get into the prevention game (Bray et al., 2024). Screening on a regular basis, genetic testing, and assessing risk factors are becoming more and more routine aspects of the job. This transition represents the move from simply reacting to disease to really preventing it—empowering individuals to alter their lifestyles and, in the process, alleviating healthcare pressures in general (Figure 1.15).

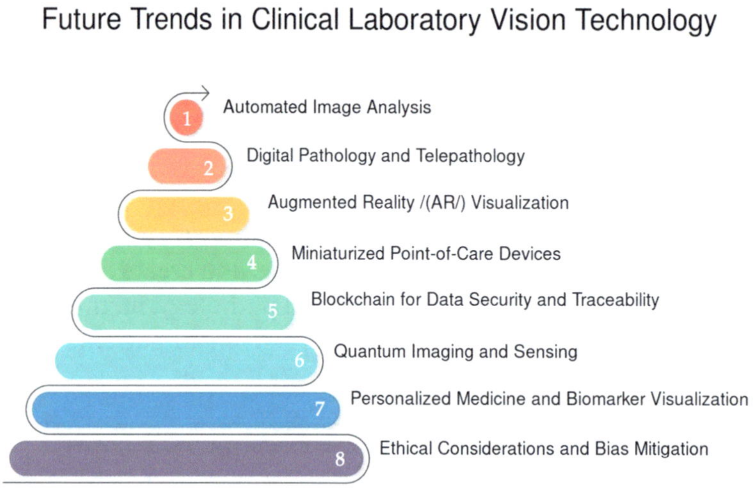

Figure 1.15. Future trends in clinical laboratory.

Source: https://fastercapital.co/i/Clinical-Laboratory-Vision-Advancements-in-Clinical-Laboratory-Vision-Technology--Future-Trends-in-Clinical-Laboratory-Vision-Technology.webp.

1.6.1. Impact of Personalized Medicine on Pathology Practices

Personalized medicine is revolutionizing the field of pathology. Rather than having one-size-fits-all, physicians are now moving towards individualized treatments—a revolution that's been spreading across much of pathology. Pathologists used to rely on fixed tests to select treatments in the past, but molecular methods now allow them to glimpse at genetic information. Today they integrate traditional methods with advanced genomic data to sharpen their diagnostics and more accurately tailor patient treatment plans. Overall, figuring out where lab medicine is headed isn't ever simple, and this continuous change demands pathology practices to reinvent themselves continuously (Fortina et al., 2015). All the commotion about biomarkers these days isn't hype—sample quality ultimately becomes quite critical in terms of tailoring treatments. The goal, of course, is to minimize those unpleasant side effects while making how effective treatments will be even better. Overnight, the pipes behind biobanks have become big business. The facilities now carefully collect, prepare, and store biological materials following preordained protocols so that nothing goes astray along the way. And with current technology, it's easy to trace samples and manage a mountain of data, facilitating sharing of material among research centers—a clean combination of old and new that sets the stage for future personalized medicine trials (Alessandroni et al., 2015). Technology aside, personalized medicine is revolutionizing professional roles and expectations in pathology. Pathologists are now more than ever working with multidisciplinary teams, often emerging as key players in discussions regarding precision treatment. Their experience of breaking open genomic data helps oncologists and other specialists make informed decisions on the best courses of treatment. This interaction enhances our understanding of why diseases manifest so differently in patients, making the pathologist a strategy advisor rather than a mere diagnostician. With the field always developing and changing, a small amount of ongoing retraining and learning aside is quite a must so that such specialists are kept current in the dynamic landscape of bespoke healthcare. In the end, the future of laboratory medicine quite literally does depend on flexibility, with a more specific and patient-oriented methodology in diagnosing and treating conditions (Fortina et al., 2015).

1.6.2. Integration of artificial intelligence in diagnostics

Nowadays, technology is so dominant in medicine – advanced techniques simply become the norm. Digital pathology is a leading example, setting the pace for daily diagnostics with image analysis in exacting detail. Take the Swiss Digital Pathology Consortium (SDiPath), for example; they've initiated a Delphi process (yep, that method of gathering expert opinions) to define best practices for clinical pathology digitization. They highlight scanners, quality checking, and digital workflows, all clearing the way for the inclusion of AI in our routine tests. Pathologists, trying to balance old-fashioned steps with new digital flair, see academic labs and private clinics becoming more and more wedded over the years. To a large extent, this future-looking move not only makes clinical processes more efficient but also meets ethical and operational requirements set out for clinical settings (Berezowska et al., 2023). There is also a significant push towards AI in diagnostics, driven by a greater need for enhanced accuracy and smoother reports.

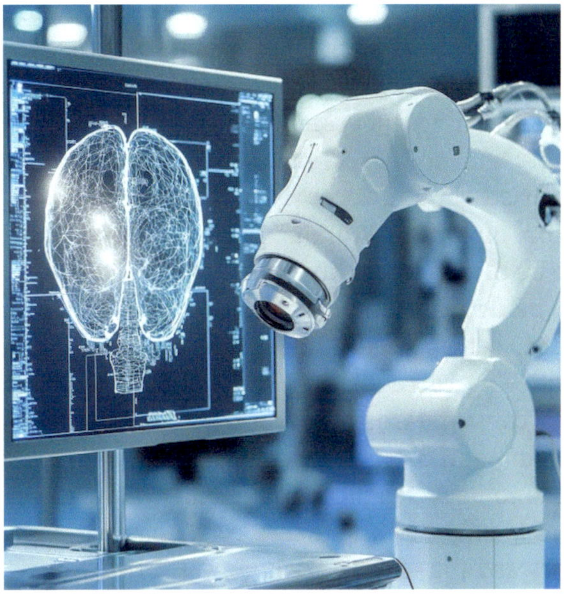

Figure 1.16. Integration of artificial intelligence in diagnostics.

Source: https://img.freepik.com/premium-photo/integration-artificial-intelligence-ai-biomedical-devices-enhanced-diagnostics_1314467-84942.jpg.

The growth of machine learning and imaging software is revolutionizing histopathology worldwide. For instance, the UK is undergoing a digital revolution that could help relieve workforce shortages while, on the whole, enhancing patient outcomes. Most surprisingly of all, perhaps, the NCRI Cellular Molecular Pathology (CM-Path) initiative and the British In Vitro Diagnostics Association (BIVDA) have been at the forefront. Their collaborative efforts are aimed at building, step by step, a model that not only enables the creation of AI tools but also lays the ground for their regulatory clearance. This agenda is a classic example of how interdisciplinarity partnerships—and, yes, repeated good practice—are required when bringing AI to diagnostics (Colling et al., 2019). Even with all of these promising innovations, integrating AI into diagnostics is not a hiccup-free process. A key component of integrating such sophisticated devices is to test them rigorously to guarantee they are reliable. Because computer image analysis is more and more used, standards for guaranteeing consistency and accuracy become progressively more important. Working pathologists, who need to be picked from diverse clinical settings, need to be deeply involved and share their expertise to direct such AI-based systems. In addition, adhering to regulatory regulations as well as ethical standards is categorically crucial in the acquisition of public trust. Scales of innovative technology with the responsibility of protecting the quality of patient care really chart the way forward for clinical pathology (Berezowska et al., 2023; Colling et al., 2019) (Figure 1.16).

1.6.3. Challenges and Opportunities in the Evolving Field

Technology has made clinical pathology a vastly different field over the past two years or so—tech innovations and more people examining their own health have really flipped things on their head. AI in pathology, for example, has a huge potential to improve diagnostic accuracy, but then there are the issues that come with it. AI can classify and predict illnesses like lymphoma (Shen et al., 2024) and, overall, they do this by speeding up what we already know of as diagnostic work, but they depend on having great, well-annotated data. If the data is not great or when there are inherent biases that come in, that can slow it down. It can even worsen health inequities that already exist. All in all, as the field evolves, it is important to balance having high-tech tools with having healthcare available for all. Making a decision about a treatment plan in clinical pathology really illustrates how complicated modern healthcare can be. After diagnosis, doctors have all sorts of hard questions to ask themselves—what treatment to employ and what dose would be optimal—too often relying on clinical trial data that, in most instances, doesn't perfectly fit into every patient's unique situation (Carini et al., 2024). The patients' reactions may be unpredictable, especially when therapies are administered in combination with each other, and these make the one-size-fits-all approach simply fail. In the midst of this, big data analytics and AI step in, offering a way of real-time adjusting treatments, if with a touch of doubt; these technologies aid clinicians in modifying care even where reactions in people wildly vary. Despite how alluring AI appears for improving clinical practice, there remain fairly many potholes along the path to optimum realization. Issues of data privacy, ethics, and calls for explicit regulations for using AI in medicine create some extremely difficult challenges. Toss in on top of that the expense and specialized talent needed to create these AI programs—something smaller health facilities might not always be able to afford (Carini et al., 2024). Even as the path ahead is quite complicated and sometimes a bit messy, the attraction of enhanced, more accurate diagnoses and enhanced patient benefits remains strong. For most cases, technologists, clinicians, and policy makers must be at the table in order to develop a means forward toward a future that includes innovative resources as part of a healthier, more equitable, and sustainable health care system.

Test Your Knowledge

1. How might artificial intelligence and machine learning impact diagnostic accuracy in clinical pathology?
2. What role will personalized medicine and genomics play in shaping the future of clinical pathology?

Summary

Clinical pathology isn't static; it keeps shifting as new medical research and tech roll in. The field forces us to dig into the reasons behind patient outcomes, sometimes in unexpected ways. Late fetal death cases, for example, often peel back layers of intricate problems—mixing the mother's health with her surroundings in ways that are hard to pin down. Chronic hypertension emerges as one of these variables, linking itself to subsequent pregnancy outcomes and reminding us of the regular check-ups and preventive interventions (Amaral et al., 2013). In the meantime, an unanticipated number of stillbirths remain unexplained, indicating that either genetic or social factors still evade our full comprehension, which in most cases invites us to question diagnostic approaches and care pathways. The surprise continues with conditions like frontotemporal dementia (FTD). Unusual protein patterns are sometimes seen and seem to go along with psychiatric symptoms which become inadvertent markers for the condition (Scarioni et al., 2023). Physicians increasingly blend more brain science into their practice, mixing up different ways of diagnosing and treating patients. This earthy, tiered approach not only helps to define FTD apart from other neurodegenerative mysteries, but it also illustrates how far clinical practices can be a messy, interlocked process. Placing atypical psychiatric symptoms on our checklists is an unmistakable sign that unravelling neurological sickness is not a single-minded pursuit—different experts have to work together, even if processes sometimes lead to a sequence of ad hoc moves. Looking at the big picture, the conversation of clinical pathology yields a muddle of causes, diagnoses, and patient outcomes. New studies on both maternal-fetal health and brain disease continuously raise questions that we must continue to develop our methods. Unexplained stillbirths and the difficult diagnosis of FTD are a reminder that constant study and new concepts are always necessary. And as we whirl with high-tech technologies and mix in degrees of data analysis, there's a greater potential to improve our diagnostic methods and improve patient care. Bottom line, the clinical pathology of the future seems on a path to more targeted medicine—although with a few bumpy roads and some unexpected detours to boot.

Patient care and clinical pathology go hand in hand. Laboratory diagnostics isn't simply numbers—it's the cutting edge of medicine today. Analyzing fluids and tissues to find disease supports treatment decisions in very real ways. With newer technologies like genetic testing and molecular diagnostics down the pipeline, doctors now married individualized options up to individual situations. This change, overall, enhances diagnostic accuracy while fewer trials and errors are required. And, in addition, there's rapid lab testing, wherein doctors can make therapy adjustments on the fly, which not only keeps complications from occurring but hastens recovery; it is an absolute game-changer for our healthcare system. Healthcare gets more and more complex by the day, and so does complexity, the relevance of clinical pathology starts to stand out. Consider the World Federation of Hemophilia (WFH) guidelines—they're not just dry reading; they demonstrate how laboratory findings inform treatment, particularly where cases such as hemophilia management are concerned. They are representative of a confluence of opinions from several experts who, in the vast majority of situations, convene to work out evidence-based strategies designed to improve patient care. They guide timely decisions and slot new innovations comfortably into day-to-day practice. In short, clinical pathology lays the groundwork for a holistic approach to caring by uniting hard science and clinical intuition. It's not solely about certain patients, but that. Laboratory information is also significant to public policy and health. Public policy is enhanced by seeing trends by grouping together disease and treatment outcome data that provide us with a larger picture of the shifts in our community's health patterns. Take the reporting of infectious outbreaks, for instance—the steady stream of laboratory findings can alert public health to action as well as the manner in which resources are allocated. With clinics and hospitals constantly vying to raise their standards, the function of clinical pathology in setting performance standards simply cannot be swept under the rug. Most within the field—reluctantly, yes, with some hiccups here and there—stress that sound laboratory practices train providers to meet new needs. In general, clinical pathology bridges the gap in the middle between lab medicine and integrative healthcare, powerfully influencing both medical practice and general public health policy.

KEY TERMS FROM THIS CHAPTER

Autoimmunity	Clinical chemistry	Clinical pathology
Complete blood count (CBC)	Cytology	Differential diagnosis
Hematology	Hemostasis	Histopathology
Immunohematology	Microbiology	Pathogen
Point-of-care testing (POCT)	Serology	Specimen collection
Tumor markers	Urinalysis	

Critical Thinking Questions

1. **What is the primary focus of clinical pathology?**
   a. Diagnosing mental disorders
   b. Studying disease through laboratory analysis of bodily fluids
   c. Performing surgical procedures
   d. Treating patients with antibiotics
2. **Which of the following is NOT a typical specimen used in clinical pathology?**
   a. Blood
   b. Urine
   c. Saliva
   d. Muscle biopsy
3. **What role does the clinical pathologist play in a healthcare setting?**
   a. Conducts physical examinations
   b. Manages laboratory testing and interprets lab results
   c. Prescribes medications directly
   d. Performs surgeries
4. **Which test is commonly used in clinical pathology to assess kidney function?**
   a. Complete blood count (CBC)
   b. Blood urea nitrogen (BUN)
   c. Liver function test
   d. Electrocardiogram (ECG)
5. **Hematology, clinical chemistry, and microbiology are branches of:**
   a. Clinical pathology
   b. Radiology
   c. Surgery
   d. Psychiatry

Answers to Critical Thinking Questions

1. (b); 2. (d); 3. (b); 4. (b); 5. (a)

Short answer Questions

1. What is clinical pathology, and how does it differ from anatomical pathology?
2. What are the main subspecialties included in clinical pathology?
3. How is specimen collection and handling important in clinical pathology?
4. What is the role of a clinical pathologist in patient diagnosis and treatment?
5. Name three common laboratory tests and the type of information they provide.

References

1. Al Harthy, S. N., Reñosa, M. D., Subhi, N. A., et al. (2015). A systematic review of the selected evidences on the effectiveness of inter-professional education (IPE) in developing interprofessional learning environment. https://media.neliti.com/media/publications/156082-EN-a-systematic-review-of-the-selected-evid.pdf (accessed on 1st July 2025).
2. Alaggio, R., Colombatti, R., De Vito, R., Fuligni, F., Gamba, P., Ichino, M., Pizzi, M., et al. (2016). Spleen histology in children with sickle cell disease and hereditary spherocytosis: Hints on the disease pathophysiology. https://core.ac.uk/download/80154258.pdf (accessed on 1st July 2025).
3. Aleid, A. M., Al Omireen, R. M., Enani, M. J., Alharbi, R., Alsubaie, O. F., Aljibreen, A. F., Aldehailan, M. S., et al. (2024). A review of imaging modalities in pediatric traumatic brain injury: Evaluating diagnostic accuracy and clinical outcomes: Cross sectional study. *Journal of Advanced Trends in Medical Research*. https://www.semanticscholar.org/paper/dcdebc46b9344dd18f98a485a51f76758dd18cb7 (accessed on 1st July 2025).
4. Alessandroni, J., D'Alessandro, R., Della Morte, D., et al. (2015). Ensuring sample quality for biomarker discovery studies–Use of ICT tools to trace bio sample life-cycle. https://core.ac.uk/download/98335415.pdf (accessed on 1st July 2025).
5. Amaral, N., Pedroso, C., Robalo, R., et al. (2013). Late stillbirth: A ten-year cohort study. https://core.ac.uk/download/71737385.pdf (accessed on 1st July 2025).
6. Aranda, C., Barreto, M., Coravos, A., et al. (2020). BioMeT and algorithm challenges: A proposed digital standardized evaluation framework. https://core.ac.uk/download/323307095.pdf (accessed on 1st July 2025).
7. Arnold, J. E., Camus, M. S., Freeman, K. P., Giori, L., Hooijberg, E. H., Jeffery, U., Korchia, J., et al. (2019). *ASVCP* Guidelines: Principles of quality assurance and standards for veterinary clinical pathology (version 3.0). *Veterinary Clinical Pathology, 48*, 542–618. https://doi.org/10.1111/vcp.12810 (accessed on 1st July 2025).
8. Ayyagari, D., Bonham, M. J., Chamarthi, R. V., Cockerell, et al. (2020). Tailored for real-world: A whole slide image classification system validated on uncrated multi-site data emulating the prospective pathology workload. https://core.ac.uk/download/288847206.pdf (accessed on 1st July 2025).
9. Bailey, D. N., Gorstein, F., Lipscomb, M. F., et al. (2016). Life after being a pathology department chair: Issues and opportunities. https://core.ac.uk/download/286729054.pdf (accessed on 1st July 2025).
10. Baker, J. B., & Spiczka, A. (2024). A-197 Enhancing patient safety and workforce sustainability through ASCP BOC credentials. *Clinical Chemistry*. https://www.semanticscholar.org/paper/9732446422096f054e9548f00c067df5fce029a5 (accessed on 1st July 2025).
11. Barlow, J., Hanna, G. B., Huddy, J. R., et al. (2016). Point-of-care C reactive protein for the diagnosis of lower respiratory tract infection in NHS primary care: A qualitative study of barriers and facilitators to adoption. https://core.ac.uk/download/77011336.pdf (accessed on 1st July 2025).
12. Bell, I., Brown, R., Caruana, D. J., et al. (2019). Rapid and complete paraffin removal from

human tissue sections delivers enhanced Raman spectroscopic and histopathological analysis. https://core.ac.uk/download/323200026.pdf (accessed on 1st July 2025).

13. Berezowska, S., Cathomas, G., Grobholz, R., et al. (2023). Digital image analysis and artificial intelligence in pathology diagnostics—the Swiss view. https://core.ac.uk/download/597777801.pdf (accessed on 1st July 2025).

14. Braak, H., Griffin, W. S. T., & Thal, D. R. (2008). Parenchymal and vascular Aβ-deposition and its effects on the degeneration of neurons and cognition in Alzheimer's disease. https://core.ac.uk/download/14527695.pdf (accessed on 1st July 2025).

15. Bray, F., Laversanne, M., Sung, H., Ferlay, J., Siegel, R. L., Soerjomataram, I., & Jemal, A. (2024). Global cancer statistics 2022: GLOBOCAN estimates of incidence and mortality worldwide for 36 cancers in 185 countries. *CA: A Cancer Journal for Clinicians, 74*, 229–263. https://doi.org/10.3322/caac.21834 (accessed on 1st July 2025).

16. Buist, M. R., Coffelt, S. B., Kenter, G. G., et al. (2017). Incidence of lymph node metastases in clinical early-stage mucinous and seromucinous ovarian carcinoma: A retrospective cohort study. https://core.ac.uk/download/80697087.pdf (accessed on 1st July 2025).

17. Cardriche, D., Chitty, A., & Matese, T. H. (2020). Gastric adenocarcinoma presenting as chronic back pain: A case report. https://core.ac.uk/download/305124169.pdf (accessed on 1st July 2025).

18. Carini, C., & Seyhan, A. (2024). Tribulations and future opportunities for artificial intelligence in precision medicine. *Journal of Translational Medicine, 22*. https://www.semanticscholar.org/paper/65d94b705d85169b37491f103664b00080c773c3a (accessed on 1st July 2025).

19. Clough, G. R., Haigh, L. I. G., & Truscott, J. (2004). Can high-frequency ultrasound predict metastatic lymph nodes in patients with invasive breast cancer? https://core.ac.uk/download/57890.pdf (accessed on 1st July 2025).

20. Colling, R., Macklin, P., Oien, K., et al. (2019). Artificial intelligence in digital pathology: A roadmap to routine use in clinical practice. https://core.ac.uk/download/275554119.pdf (accessed on 1st July 2025).

21. Corvo, A., van Driel, M. A., van Wijk, J. J., et al. (2018). Visual analytics in histopathology diagnostics: A protocol-based approach. https://core.ac.uk/download/577057342.pdf (accessed on 1st July 2025).

22. Cutone, A., Rosa, L., Conte, M. P., Lepanto, M. S., Valenti, P., & Paesano, R. (2018). Efficacy of lactoferrin oral administration in the treatment of anemia and anemia of inflammation in pregnant and non-pregnant women: An interventional study. https://core.ac.uk/download/188826915.pdf (accessed on 1st July 2025).

23. Dacic, S. (2024). Neoadjuvant therapy and lung cancer: Role of pathologists. *Archives of Pathology & Laboratory Medicine*. https://www.semanticscholar.org/paper/2b455c454d8a178be63f8c38211f0985afa47af9 (accessed on 1st July 2025).

24. D'Angelo, R. (2018). An agile quality management system for laboratory developed tests. https://core.ac.uk/download/212887868.pdf (accessed on 1st July 2025).

25. Driskell, O. J., Lee, J. L., Oien, K. A., et al. (2019). Pathology and regulation for research in the UK: An overview [version 2; peer review: 3 approved]. *F1000Research, 8*, 975. https://doi.org/10.12688/f1000research.19732.2 (accessed on 1st July 2025).

26. Edsjö, A., Baskovich, B., Cox, E., Schuuring, E., Dequeker, E., Thunnissen, E., et al. (2014). Guidance for laboratories performing molecular pathology for cancer patients. https://core.ac.uk/download/29190116.pdf (accessed on 1st July 2025).

27. El-Banna, A. (2025). Cost-effectiveness of innovations in pathology services in relation to cancer diagnosis and treatment management. https://core.ac.uk/download/305119668.pdf (accessed on 1st July 2025).

28. Fortina, P., Kricka, L. J., Park, J. Y., & Polsky, T. G. (2015). The future of laboratory medicine – A 2014 perspective. https://core.ac.uk/download/54509579.pdf (accessed on 1st July 2025).

29. Gielen, I., Samoy, Y., van Bree, H., et al. (2011). Dysplastic elbow diseases in dogs. https://core.ac.uk/download/55802068.pdf (accessed on 1st July 2025).

30. Griff, S. (2019). Einfluss der Art der Materialgewinnung auf die Diagnosefindung in der Lungenpathologie. https://core.ac.uk/download/222573993.pdf (accessed on 1st July 2025).

31. Heidari Bolooki, M., Jalaie, S., Morais, N., et al. (2016). Reliability, agreement, and diagnostic accuracy of the modified lateral scapular slide test. https://core.ac.uk/download/160796673.pdf (accessed on 1st July 2025).

32. Jones, J. L., Lee, J. L., Moore, D. A., Morris, et al. (2018). Time for change: A new training programmed for morpho-molecular pathologists? https://core.ac.uk/download/132211774.pdf (accessed on 1st July 2025).

33. Korf, B. R., Blitzer, M. G., Demmer, L., Feldman, G. L., & Watson, M. S. (2017). Report on the Banbury Summit Meeting on medical genetics training in the genomic era, 23–26 February 2014. *Genetics in Medicine, 19*, 1–6. https://doi.org/10.1038/gim.2017.38 (accessed on 1st July 2025).

34. Kung, T. H., Cheatham, M., Medenilla, A., Sillos, C., De Leon, L., Elepaño, C., Madriaga, M., et al. (2023). Performance of ChatGPT on USMLE: Potential for AI-assisted medical education using large language models. *PLOS Digital Health, 2*, e0000198–e0000198. https://doi.org/10.1371/journal.pdig.0000198 (accessed on 1st July 2025).

35. Lathiya, J., & Shah, D. A. (2021). MDCT evaluation of right iliac fossa pathologies with special emphasis on lymph nodal characteristics. *Indian Journal of Applied Basic Medical Sciences*. https://www.semanticscholar.org/paper/b6884640363d613d57a8c958ae4106a8a97119ce (accessed on 1st July 2025).

36. Livingston, G., Huntley, J., Sommerlad, A., Ames, D., Ballard, C., Banerjee, S., Brayne, C., et al. (2020). Dementia prevention, intervention, and care: 2020 report of the Lancet Commission. *The Lancet, 396*, 413–446. https://doi.org/10.1016/s0140-6736(20)30367-6 (accessed on 1st July 2025).

37. Murray, C. J. L., Ikuta, K. S., Sharara, F., Swetschinski, L. R., Robles Aguilar, G., Gray, A. P., Han, C., et al. (2022). Global burden of bacterial antimicrobial resistance in 2019: A systematic analysis. *The Lancet, 399*, 629–655. https://doi.org/10.1016/s0140-6736(21)02724-0 (accessed on 1st July 2025).

38. N/A. (2024). The current state of digital pathology, molecular diagnostics and biobanking in renal cancer: Kidney Cancer Association consensus statement. https://core.ac.uk/download/647985152.pdf (accessed on 1st July 2025).

39. Najjar, R. (2023). Redefining radiology: A review of artificial intelligence integration in

medical imaging. *Diagnostics, 13*, 2760–2760. https://doi.org/10.3390/diagnostics13172760 (accessed on 1st July 2025).

40. Panzironi, G., Pediconi, F., & Sardanelli, F. (2019). Nipple discharge: The state of the art. https://core.ac.uk/download/188829787.pdf (accessed on 1st July 2025).

41. Percie du Sert, N., Ahluwalia, A., Alam, S., Avey, M. T., Baker, M., Browne, W. J., Clark, A., et al. (2020). Reporting animal research: Explanation and elaboration for the ARRIVE guidelines 2.0. *PLOS Biology, 18*, e3000411–e3000411. https://doi.org/10.1371/journal.pbio.3000411 (accessed on 1st July 2025).

42. Perkins, R. B., Guido, R. S., Castle, P. E., Chelmow, D., Einstein, M. H., García, F., Huh, W. K., et al. (2020). 2019 ASCCP risk-based management consensus guidelines for abnormal cervical cancer screening tests and cancer precursors. *Journal of Lower Genital Tract Disease, 24*, 102–131. https://doi.org/10.1097/lgt.0000000000000525 (accessed on 1st July 2025).

43. Ponikowski, P., Voors, A. A., Anker, S. D., Bueno, H., Cleland, J. G. F., Coats, A. J. S., Falk, V., et al. (2016). 2016 ESC guidelines for the diagnosis and treatment of acute and chronic heart failure. *European Heart Journal, 37*, 2129–2200. https://doi.org/10.1093/eurheartj/ehw128 (accessed on 1st July 2025).

44. Satam, H., Joshi, K., Mangrolia, U., Waghoo, S., Zaidi, G., Rawool, S., Thakare, R. P., et al. (2023). Next-generation sequencing technology: Current trends and advancements. *Biology, 12*, 997–997. https://doi.org/10.3390/biology12070997 (accessed on 1st July 2025).

45. Scarioni, M. (2023). Clinicopathological correlations in frontotemporal dementia. https://core.ac.uk/download/587852976.pdf (accessed on 1st July 2025).

46. Secora, K., Lee, B., Smith, D., & Coppola, M. (2025). Expert consensus on the role of speech-language pathologists in working with deaf children who use American Sign Language in the United States: A classical e-Delphi study. *American Journal of Speech-Language Pathology*. https://www.semanticscholar.org/paper/9cffffe65bec4eb13922babfce7fa7684ccf16d1 (accessed on 1st July 2025).

47. Shaikh, S. M., Varma, A., Kumar, S., Acharya, S., & Patil, R. (2024). Navigating disease management: A comprehensive review of the De Ritis ratio in clinical medicine. *Cureus, 16*. https://www.semanticscholar.org/paper/e9fac30e65cb1ae35aafe3cf7e1c24d8f2dafc24 (accessed on 1st July 2025).

48. Shen, M., & Jiang, Z. (2024). Artificial intelligence applications in lymphoma diagnosis and management: Opportunities, challenges, and future directions. *Journal of Multidisciplinary Healthcare, 17*, 5329–5339. https://www.semanticscholar.org/paper/449f2376e360777ca43ee1fea2efa69ed5011b0b (accessed on 1st July 2025).

49. Srivastava, A., Santagostino, E., Dougall, A., Kitchen, S., Sutherland, M. L., Pipe, S. W., Carção, M., et al. (2020). *WFH Guidelines for The Management of Hemophilia*, 3rd edition. *Hemophilia, 26*, 1–158. https://doi.org/10.1111/hae.14046 (accessed on 1st July 2025).

50. Stoop, T. F., Seelen, L., van 't Land, F. R., van der Hout, A. C., Scheepens, J. C., Ali, M., Stiggelbout, A. M., et al. (2025). Nationwide implementation of the international multidisciplinary best-practice for locally advanced pancreatic cancer (PREOPANC-4): Study protocol. *BMC Cancer, 25*. https://www.semanticscholar.org/paper/dacc795afa2d561e0cf3b972ba6684cc75006c8b (accessed on 1st July 2025).

51. Trandafir, A., Bonjincă, V. C., Tulbă, D., & Onose, G. (2023). An odd case of immune-mediated necrotizing myopathy, complicated with sagittal, transverse and sigmoid sinus thrombosis. *Balneo and PRM Research Journal.* https://www.semanticscholar.org/paper/152af52bfbc8fa5a4212e1554c341f3d199d18f1 (accessed on 1st July 2025).

52. Wiegers, S. E., Ryan, T., Arrighi, J. A., Brown, S. M., Canaday, B., Damp, J. B., Díaz-Gómez, J. L., et al. (2019). 2019 ACC/AHA/ASE advanced training statement on echocardiography (revision of the 2003 ACC/AHA clinical competence statement on echocardiography). *Catheterization and Cardiovascular Interventions, 94*, 481–505. https://doi.org/10.1002/ccd.28313 (accessed on 1st July 2025).

CLINICAL LABORATORY TECHNIQUES AND INSTRUMENTS

2

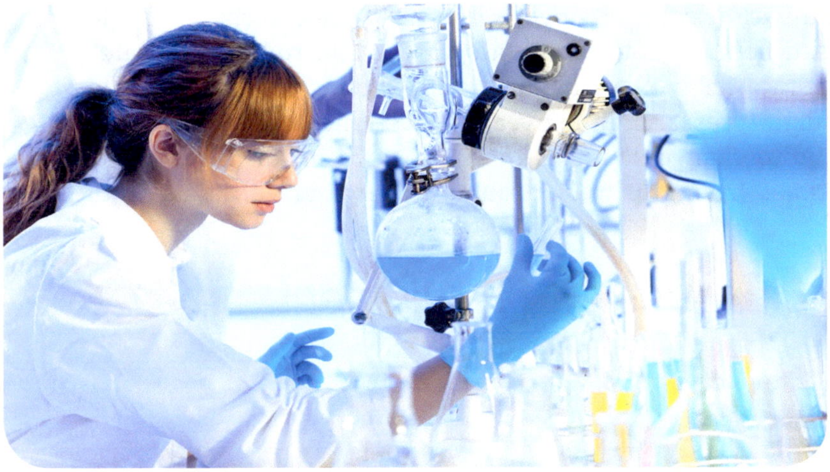

LEARNING OBJECTIVES

After studying this chapter, you will be able to:

1. List the types of clinical laboratory techniques;
2. Explain the common laboratory instruments;
3. Describe quality control in clinical laboratories;
4. Focus on the safety protocols in the laboratory;
5. Explore the emerging technologies in clinical laboratories;
6. List the challenges in clinical laboratory practices.

Introduction

Clinical laboratory methods have taken some pretty big leaps in the past few years—opening the doors to more accurate diagnoses and better patient care. Laboratories are now center stage in healthcare today because good testing is no longer an add-on; it is the impetus for effective treatments. For instance, liquid chromatography tandem mass spectrometry (LCTMS) has come a long way. This tool, on which so many are now reliant, can screen a variety of compounds, and that kind of ability enhances what labs can learn. These technologies not only enable labs to run more tests each day but also reduce the amount of human labor, reducing the possibility of simple errors. As patient needs to grow, it is clear that everyone in healthcare must stay on top of these methods—learning and adapting as new tech rolls in (Re et al., 2003). Another shift we're seeing is in genetics, which is reshaping the scene in ways that aren't always easy to predict. Genetics is now at the center of the concept of personalized medicine; physicians can now more accurately develop treatments to suit a patient's own individual genetic profile, in the majority of instances. As our understanding of which genetic variations actually do anything continues to grow, so too does the demand for speedy, high-throughput testing capable of keeping up with all this new data accurately—and truly, that is significant. Big mutation detection methods are promising, especially in areas like pharmacogenomics, in which knowing how a person might react to a drug is a game-changer. It all comes down to the reality that getting these tests to work requires a focus on both the machinery and deciphering the results—a challenge that's breaking ground for revolutionary improvements in patient care management (Schrijver et al., 2011). All these innovations—new testing technologies and new approaches—are converging in ways that are both exciting and a bit unsettling. The convergence of tools like LCTMS with evolving genetic tests is propelling us into an era of precision medicine; patients can receive treatments that literally fit their unique health profiles. Yes, and with it comes its own set of headaches, including having to sort through all the complex data and being able to easily integrate it into routine laboratory protocols. This is the only way that laboratories will be able to live up to their potential, increase patient results, and continue to drive further research in the years ahead. Ultimately, the way that lab equipment and procedures continue to change supports the need for constant research and a willingness to change—albeit sometimes having to work around a couple of quirks along the way (Figure 2.1).

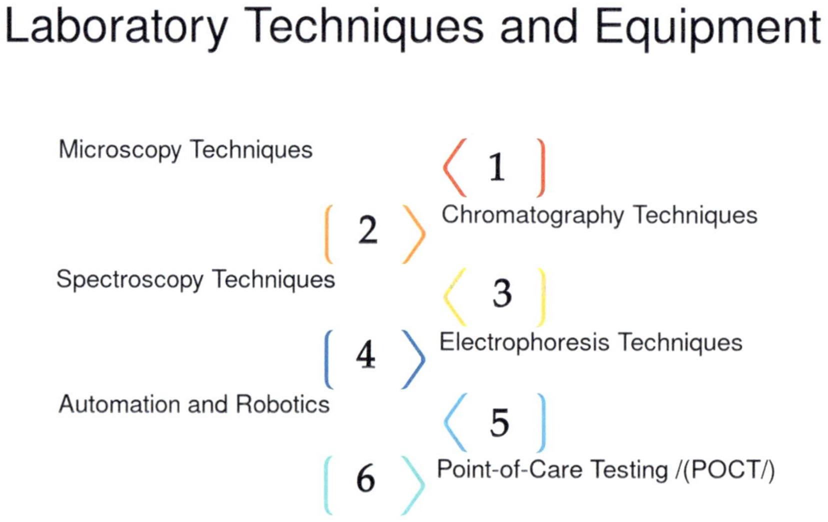

Figure 2.1. Clinical laboratory techniques and equipment.

Source: https://fastercapital.co/i/Clinical-laboratory-biochemistry-Understanding-the-Role-of-Clinical-Laboratory-Biochemistry-in-Disease-Diagnosis--Laboratory-Techniques-and-Equipment.webp.

Definition of Clinical Laboratory Techniques

Clinical laboratory methods come in many forms that aid in diagnosing problems and treating patients. Many techniques—oftentimes based on advanced machinery and strict protocols—are utilized to study samples like blood, urine, and tissues. Accuracy and reliability are crucial; usually, laboratories follow set procedures and advanced apparatus to ensure count results. Each test is optimized for its specific diagnostic application so that doctors can select key hints about a patient's disease. As laboratories acquire new technology and analytic techniques, they're enhancing their capacity to find diseases and track how effectively treatments are working. This step-by-step change is indicative of a broader trend toward precision medicine, where patient-specific data really drives decisions and quality control is always top-of-mind. Automation and digital technology are transforming laboratory diagnostics today; new equipment is equipped with functionalities that make sense of work, eliminate human errors, and accelerate result output. Automated analyzers and robotics are not flashy add-ons—these enable higher throughput while, oftentimes, ensuring quality. As such devices are embraced in the laboratory, the role of lab personnel is transformed and they have to learn new skills for handling and interpreting lab results generated by these machines. Statistical thinking and machine learning integration in the majority of instances lead to a deeper analysis of results, inclining to yield improved patient outcomes. Research into psychomotor skills on operations like laparoscopy (Chmarra et al., 2011) even prescribes how technology can enhance surgical competency—and, in the end, patient safety. Lab procedures are not limited to traditional approaches; it now encompasses the field of advanced monitoring systems that give real-time feedback on states of being. Biosensors and other detecting instruments are being investigated as potential monitors of biological activity in challenging environments like space stations, in which precision is essential (Arendale et al., 2025). These new instruments are a true attempt to continue raising the stakes in diagnosis, ensnaring pathogens or specific biochemical markers with an unprecedented sensitivity. As clinical laboratories continue to evolve, the introduction of diverse monitoring techniques into everyday practice seems more important than ever. By embracing these developments, laboratories play a pivotal role in integrated patient care, stressing the necessity of ongoing research and the willingness to grow in this essential field.

Importance of Laboratory Instruments in Healthcare

Lab technology has advanced leaps and bounds in recent years, completely revolutionizing the way we diagnose illness. Clinical labs now depend on high-tech devices like molecular analyzers and automated analyzers to enhance test accuracy while minimizing turnaround time for results. Getting infections early really counts—especially when every second matters to catch a pathogen. For example, nanobiosensors have shown an impressive capacity to detect signs of diseases such as dengue virus at an early stage, guiding clinicians towards timely interventions (Rajaei et al., 2025). Decreased delay allows doctors to provide goal-directed therapy immediately, which improves patient outcomes and lessens the overall burden of infectious diseases. One such development becoming popular is Laboratory-on-a-Chip (LOC) technology. Short and sweet, these little chips can run several tests at once, saving time and money in a manner that traditional techniques are simply incapable of replicating. Not only is this technique faster than older diagnostic tools, however, but it is also significantly more portable—a worthwhile benefit when time is of the essence. There are numerous success stories wherein devices like these have made lab workflows streamlined, increased the accuracy, and provided real-time results, all of which are quintessential to running patient care efficiently (Carlos, 2025). For the most part, with the advancement in healthcare, incorporating LOC and other such advanced devices is at the forefront of addressing current disease complications and enhancing treatment protocols. Lab equipment is not simply about generating diagnoses; it plays a truly crucial role in quality control, making test results consistent. Calibrators and advanced quality control systems collaborate to make every result as solid as it needs to be—safely critical because even slight errors can place doctors on the road to misdiagnosis and the wrong course of treatment. Additionally, ongoing training for lab staff in the proper handling of these machines is still required for keeping up with our standard of excellence. Worldwide, as medical infrastructure pushes towards better diagnostics and better patient safety, these machines remain a cornerstone of modern clinical practice—even though, every now and then, the tiny glitch slips through (Figure 2.2).

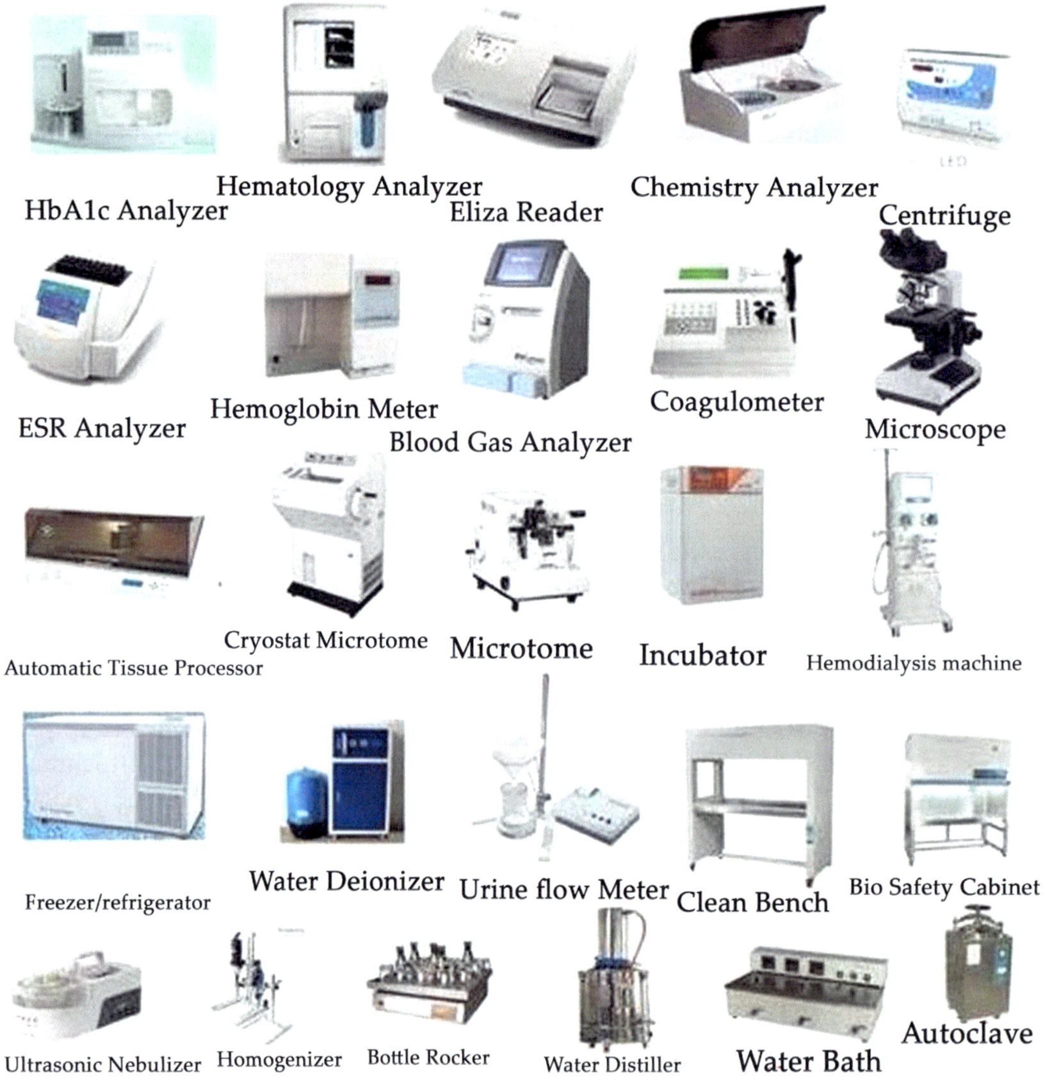

Figure 2.2. Laboratory instruments.

Source: https://external-content.duckduckgo.com/iu/?u=https%3A%2F%2F5.imimg.com%2Fdata5%2FSELLER%2FDefault%2F2021%2F2%2FXH%2FHD%2FHO%2F96155770%2Flab-instrument-500x500.jpg&f=1&nofb=1&ipt=7cab2de23932fa99b01b43a0cc6109bd38518fa08c66cd66fa8828e1e1bdb43c.

2.1. Types of Clinical Laboratory Techniques

Learning Outcome

- Hematology techniques;
- Microbiology techniques;
- Biochemistry techniques.

Clinical lab tests have come a long way, combining technological breakthroughs with more complex diagnostic needs. Immunoassays, for example, are catching a lot of attention because they can spot tiny amounts of biomarkers. They use antibodies to flag certain substances found in samples—a method that's pretty valuable whether you're looking at an infection or an autoimmune issue. Probes such as ELISA and western blotting all act as excellent reminders of how versatile these methods can be in both clinic and research applications. They yield results quickly and even assist in monitoring how diseases are evolving and whether or not treatments function as they are supposed to. Generally speaking, we can anticipate further improvements in immunoassay methods to continue to disrupt the detection of diseases, as hinted at in earlier laboratory medicine predictions (Fortina et al., 2015). Molecular diagnostics is another colossal component of the clinical laboratory puzzle. The field centers around the analysis of genetic material, and it's really transformed the way we understand and manage disease at the very root of the issue. Technologies such as PCR and next-gen sequencing spot that shift nicely, moving us further in towards more individualized medicine. In most cases, they enable clinicians to review specific nucleic acid sequences, which may then inform treatment strategies to accommodate individual genetic profiles. These newer methodologies continue to emerge and are set to advance prevention and treatment practices. It is increasingly clear that the merging of modern technology with traditional methods is necessary to enhance patient care and enhance diagnostic performance, as some writings on future trends in the lab have indicated (Fortina et al., 2015). Biophotonics now represent a new frontier of laboratory science that utilizes light-based processes to pursue deeper diagnostics. There is something magical about photons' action in the vicinity of tissues—providing clean peeks into cell functions and structures, and at times providing us with the possibility of non-invasive testing. Technology like optical coherence tomography and fluorescence imaging portrays a scenario in which light is a key player in diagnosing illness, especially cancer and pathology. A recent workshop sponsored by the National Institute of Standards and Technology even went as far as to point out that we need to have improved biophotonic tools in order to keep up with needs today. As a whole, with these light-based methods continuing to evolve, they'll influence the way we carry out diagnostics, from single interventions to public health approaches in general.

2.1.1. Hematology Techniques

Techniques and equipment in hematology have come a long way, paralleling broader trends in the operation of clinical laboratories. In days gone by, blood testing was synonymous with tedious manual drudgery—making smears and cell counting using hemocytometers. While these techniques laid the groundwork, they were often time-consuming and, honestly, prone to errors. Then came automatic counters, which drove analysis to lightning speed so that blood samples could be analyzed dozens of times faster and more precisely. In most laboratories today, fancy machines analyze several parameters in one pass, so they can check a variety of cell types simultaneously. That shift toward automation not only keeps work rolling along but also builds confidence in diagnoses, which pays off in improved patient care. Now, how automation has been implemented in laboratory practice truly brings into focus how crucial tech advancement is to keeping healthcare at its peak. Hematology's methods in recent years have been redefined behind the scenes by new technology, as if there has been a steady dialogue between researchers and clinicians on the front line. Research from thousands of studies has helped push the knowledge of blood diseases forward, and technologies like sophisticated imaging, molecular diagnostics, and even computer smarts now place layers on what was once simply simple cell counts. Often, you'll find the brilliant and innovative use of these systems—sometimes even in the unconventional—welcomes comprehension way beyond the norm. They would all agree that they have led to faster, more targeted therapies in oncology and chronic disease treatment—a fact that speaks volumes about the dynamic evolution of new technologies in the laboratory. The future, for many experts, is highly promising for hematology, to be combined with a combination of excellence, novel ideas, and interdisciplinary cooperation. In recent publications (Fortina et al., 2015), buzz has been generated around merging new reagents with new electronics to make the quantification of cell properties better. Point-of-care devices, for instance, promise to take us out of centralized labs—a relief for rural populations or settings where resources are limited. Meanwhile, fresh technology is now focusing on rare forms of cells, lighting up some of the dark alleys of blood diseases that were always in the shadows. With the technology advancing further, talk of ethics, quality control, and regulation is becoming equally important to ensure standards. Generally, this evolution not only pays homage to past achievements but also reinforces a continued focus on enhancing patient care through innovation (Fortina et al., 2015) (Figure 2.3).

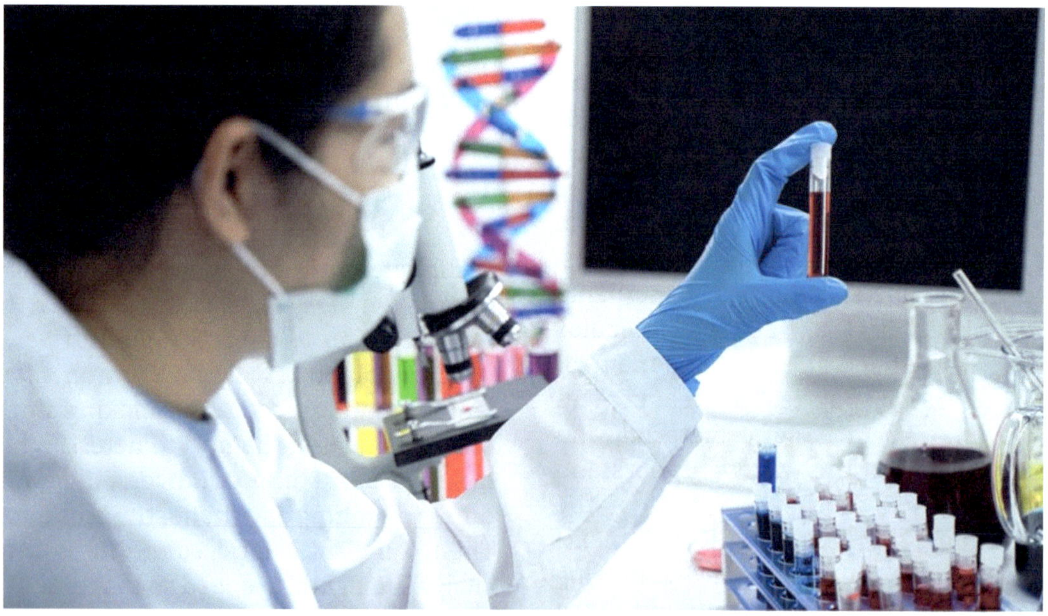

Figure 2.3. Hematology techniques.

Source: https://external-content.duckduckgo.com/iu/?u=https%3A%2F%2Fi0.wp.com%2Fpost.medicalnewstoday.com%2Fwp-content%2Fuploads%2Fsites%2F3%2F2020%2F01%2FGettyImages-1183390789_hero-1024x575.jpg%3Fw%3D1155%26h%3D1528&f=1&nofb=1&ipt=f2b328f8aadda05f0987e9b3d457d886a7b4f9ee4c1e7b052902f833d313a905.

2.1.2. Microbiology Techniques

Microbe identification in the clinic is crucial for proper diagnosis and treatment. Culture techniques—while still widely used—can sometimes be deplorably slow, causing patient care to slow down. You can see techniques like Gram stain or basic biochemical tests yield initial indications about the pathogen, but they take a few days before yielding a clear answer. All in all, modern molecular techniques such as 16S rRNA sequencing give more data, and there is MALDI-TOF mass spectrometry, which can detect microbial species within minutes; the innovation speeds up the workflow and even improves outcomes (Pyne et al., 2023). Microbiological techniques do more than simply signpost the bug; they also inform treatment decisions. Take dental care, for example—diagnosing and treating oral disease often relies upon what the lab finds. In reality, techniques like microscopy, culturing, and even molecular testing help reveal the content within dental biofilms and infections. This type of repeated microbe-checking allows practitioners to select certain antimicrobial agents according to the case at hand. In most cases, when a root canal is proven culture-negative, there is greater possibility of long-term success and lesser risk of secondary infection (Claesson et al., 2022). Introducing advanced microbiology into labs isn't merely a question of better patient care—it's also a means of making smart investments in equipment. Comparing technologies like MALDI-TOF MS, laboratories typically look at options like MBT Sirius IVD vs VITEK-MS, with regard to accuracy, fundamental technology differences, and real-world operating conditions. Such sharp cost estimations and tech comparisons allow laboratory managers to make a selection of tools that meet clinical needs as well as financial constraints. This forward step toward novel strategies mirrors the greater movement in precision medicine where identification of microbial causes and alteration of treatment choice are hand-in-hand (Pyne et al., 2023) (Figure 2.4).

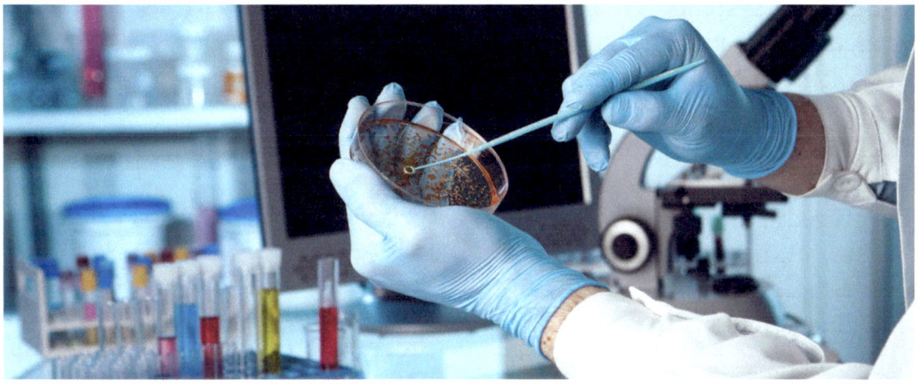

Figure 2.4. Microbiology techniques.

Source: https://external-content.duckduckgo.com/iu/?u=https%3A%2F%2Fttk.elte.hu%2Fmedia%2F53%2Fb5%2F6b934960a73e5bc202f2aaea3ef53f3170658a2d5a4a65e20a4a64d4850d%2Fmicrobiology-tojpeg-1493806871478-x2.jpg&f=1&nofb=1&ipt=6212be95867b961d8a4e837049acaf9478cb99fc796f7e10c6e8b09ca340fafe.

2.1.3. Biochemistry Techniques

New developments in biochemistry have, in fact, altered the manner in which labs perform tests; scientists can now examine central molecules with accuracies previously unimaginable. ELISA and PCR, for example, are now preferred tests—essentially daily staples within these labs—to sort out ailments quickly and accurately. These methods, you see, assist in the detection of biomarkers as well as track the development of diseases and how successful treatments are in taking hold. Sensitivity and specificity of assay are further cranked up, so laboratory tests become more accurate and enable doctors to take more accurate decisions from the biochemical data. Moreover, emerging technology fueled by ongoing research will further fine-tune these methods, with a future vision where diagnosis can keep pace with growing focus on personalized medicine (Fortina et al., 2015). Marriage of aged biochemistry techniques with new-generation devices has enabled analysis choices that once were too distant a reality. Mass spectrometry and NMR spectroscopy, for instance, illustrate how such advanced technologies can peel back layers of metabolic pathways and reveal the molecule's structure. They not only provide a good overview but also give hard numbers, which is essential to untangle the complicated interactions at play in healthy and diseased systems. Think about how analyzing metabolites in body fluids can reveal vital physiological changes, facilitating diagnoses from endocrinology to oncology. Increasingly, high-throughput technology coupled with data analysis is transforming conventional lab procedures, streamlining them and, in most cases, taking patient care to a whole new level (Bradley et al., 2016). Where labs explore how biochemistry intersects with disease pathways, their capabilities truly get a boost. Analysis of such variables as protein interactions, enzyme kinetic analysis, and genetic variations paints a more comprehensive picture of disease mechanisms. This, in a large number of instances, is behind the pressure for certain treatments—specifically, for long-term conditions like obesity and diabetes, in which basic biochemical processes have an enormous impact. Finding out how adiponectin levels correlate with complications of obesity is but one example of how important these tests are to managing complicated disease. By ironing out these links, clinical laboratories not only aid basic research but also move closer to uniting laboratory breakthroughs and real patient care (Fortina et al., 2015) (Figure 2.5).

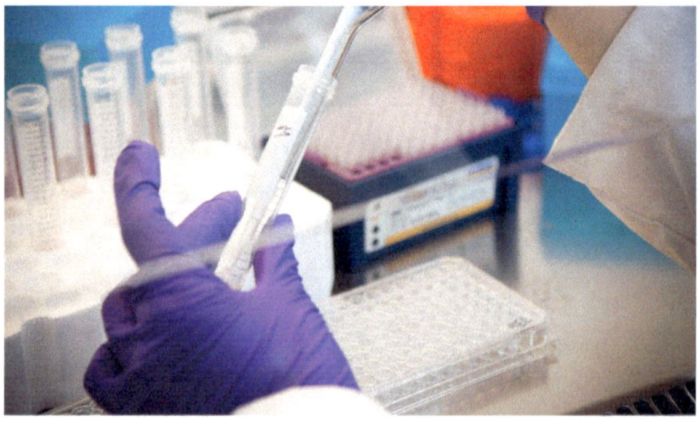

Figure 2.5. Biochemistry techniques.

Source: https://external-content.duckduckgo.com/iu/?u=https%3A%2F%2Fpioneer4ss.com%2Fwp-content%2Fuploads%2F2022%2F09%2FMedical-Biochemistry-Clincial-Biochemistry.jpg&f=1&nofb=1&ipt=fac5d48db0161b6df274a9552c46e5d0e3a0603ba49bee26e8939908953344ad.

Test Your Knowledge

1. How do biochemical assays differ from hematological techniques in clinical diagnostics?
2. What is the role of microbiological techniques in identifying infectious diseases?

2.2. Common Laboratory Instruments

Learning Outcome

- Microscopes;
- Centrifuges;
- Spectrophotometers.

Clinical labs use a mix of standard gear to test and break down biological specimens—each in its own way. A spectrophotometer, for instance, really leaves its mark by examining how chemicals absorb light in a sample. It's just a trick of the hand that enables scientists to measure amounts of proteins, nucleic acids, and metabolites, which is really significant for diagnosis and research. At the same time, techniques like mass spectrometry (MS) are emerging more often, especially when dealing with omics studies. Broadly speaking, MS offers high sensitivity and selectivity and is beneficial in the identification and quantification of complex molecules that have a tendency to signify disease and open the doors for personal medicine (Ferreira et al., 2024). By utilizing this, including these tools in laboratory procedures allows professionals to track health conditions and develop better treatment plans. Another must-have in any laboratory, the centrifuge rotates samples to separate their parts according to density.

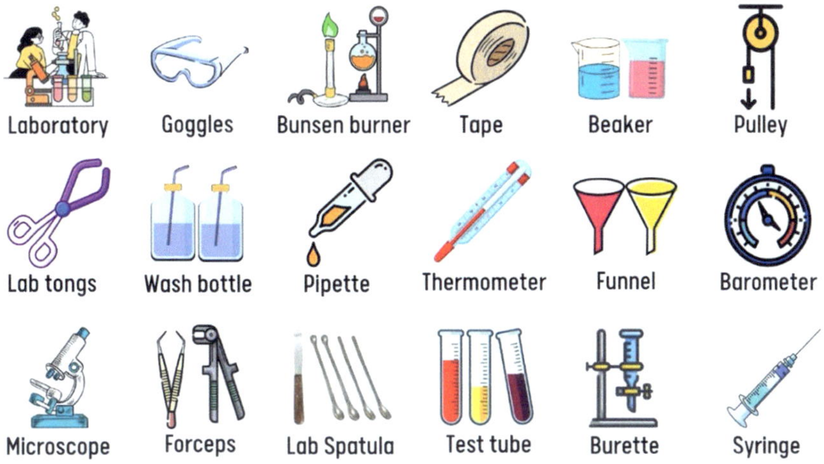

Figure 2.6. Laboratory equipment.

Source: https://external-content.duckduckgo.com/iu/?u=https%3A%2F%2Fi.ytimg.com%2Fvi%2F80Ov4EgBVS0%2Fmaxresdefault.jpg&f=1&nofb=1&ipt=a40466ce97fab0c57f2c24d6fbf51b63d6e49b76826203788d30b69f77cfefba.

This is important for many procedures, such as in blood testing, where plasma and cells need to be separated out for further examination. Since centrifugation is so efficient, laboratories can analyze samples quicker, accelerating overall. In addition, advances in this technology have added ultracentrifuges that can distinguish subcellular fragments and heavier molecules for further study; such findings give a closer look at cellular functions and how different parts interact, findings that are often of central significance in the understanding of disease causation. Combined with other diagnostic methods, centrifugation rounds out the laboratory cycle and provides healthcare professionals with fast, accurate information (Almuhaidb et al., 2021). And then there are the advanced imaging systems, a relatively new feature in the modern laboratory, that enable technologists to see literally cellular arrangements and pathology. Techniques like immunohistochemistry and fluorescence microscopy help reveal where antigens are situated and place cellular activity in the spotlight—enhancing diagnostic accuracy and shedding light on how disease arises and responds to treatment. As laboratories increasingly combine imaging with genomic and proteomic methods, they're better able to unravel disease mechanisms. The increased sensitivity and specificity of contemporary imaging modalities also help ensure that issues are simpler to identify early on, thus allowing enhanced patient outcomes ultimately. Generally, it is crucial to keep a constant interest in seeing laboratory equipment being updated if clinical practice is to keep up with the diagnostic needs of today (Ferreira et al., 2024) (Figure 2.6).

2.2.1. Microscopes

Clinical laboratories have really evolved in the diagnosis of diseases—microscopy is now at center stage in ways that were simply not achievable before. Having the ability to visualize cells and small microorganisms in detail has made it easier to diagnose difficult health issues, which in most cases means that patients receive improved care. Remember, microscopes were rudimentary appliances in the past; today, they are appliances that reveal to us even tiny molecular structures. The structure and shape of cells are important to study in order to effectively diagnose all sorts of ailments, from cancers to chronic infections. Most specialists will usually say that ongoing development in microscopic technology usually reflects changes that occur across clinical chemistry and molecular pathology (Fortina et al., 2015).

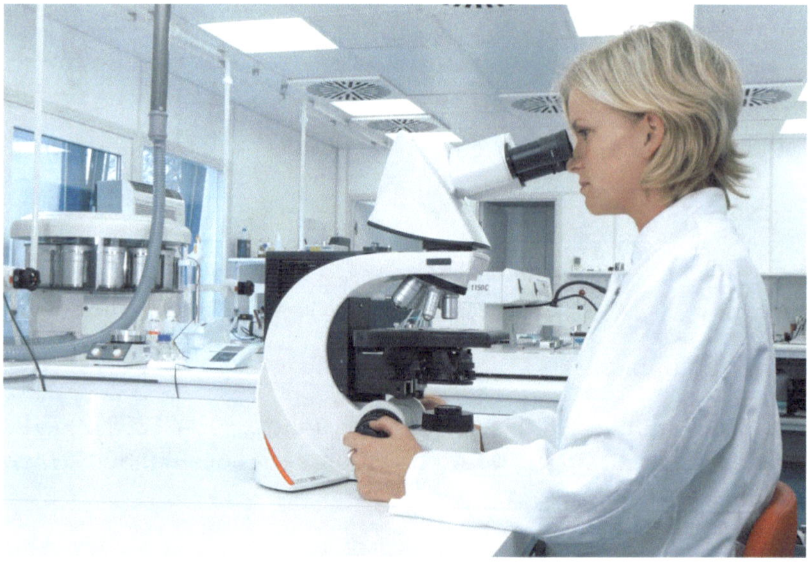

Figure 2.7. Microscopes.

Source: https://external-content.duckduckgo.com/iu/?u=https%3A%2F%2Fwww.leica-microsystems.com%2Ffileadmin%2F_processed_%2F2%2F1%2Fcsm_Laboratory_Clinical_microscope_DM2000_8a5ba0091c.jpg&f=1&nofb=1&ipt=057cc345ea3ef9e95fc1c5cb9cbebd113157235f21c84db7add08ebbab794545.

Biophotonics with microscopy is another monumental step for laboratory diagnostics, expanding the limits of what we can measure. By playing around with the behavior of light and biology, these methods have managed to simplify the whole diagnostic process, offering real-time imaging and analysis at the cellular level – it's pretty much a game changer. Workshops like those offered by the National Institute of Standards and Technology call attention to the significant significance of new measurement instruments, emphasizing the mounting significance of biophotonic diagnostics in labs today. Such a measurement discourse even indicates the contours of what future advances in technology will look like. As the field keeps moving, these advanced microscopy techniques are becoming essential for not just pathfinder research but also improving standard laboratories' routine clinical diagnoses (Brownstein et al., 2007). Looking back, the past of microscopy in laboratories really chronicles technology and medicine being dependent on each other. As increasingly more labs start using cutting-edge imaging technology, the potential to detect disease just continues to get better showing a fairly direct correlation between technological progress and better health outcomes. This continued cycle of development leads practitioners and researchers to come back and look over their shoulders at old methodologies, so they can squeeze as much benefit as possible out of contemporary microscopic techniques. While technology advances at a breakneck rate, it is necessary for laboratories to stay flexible and visionary. This approach not only prepares them for the challenges of diagnostics in the present day but also for the changes which are inevitable in the future while still maintaining the microscope as an essential part of current clinical practices (Fortina et al., 2015) (Figure 2.7).

2.2.2. Centrifuges

Separating the parts of biological samples has really hastened clinical diagnoses and research. It's not always easy to work with these types of samples, which is why centrifuges—those spinning machines—have become so essential in laboratories. They work by utilizing centrifugal force to separate material based on weight; think about how blood separates into serum, plasma, or different cellular layers. These separated materials eventually prove to be precious to future testing and treatment. Laboratories today use all sorts of centrifuges—from small microcentrifuges to more powerful ultracentrifuges—each modeled for its particular class of task, which in most cases adds speed and accuracy into the equation. It is not an exaggeration to say that with increasingly refined centrifuge technology, so too do laboratory operations become more and more streamlined, eventually leading to patient care and propelling medical research ahead. Centrifuges aren't just for plain-vanilla separations, either; they've been making waves in other fields of science. For instance, when scientists examine life sciences in space, they have utilized enhanced centrifuge technology to observe how biology acts in the presence of microgravity. In many instances, research has indicated that the insights gleaned through these missions regarding gravity's influence on cells and general physiological responses may revolutionize our fundamental understanding of them. Such advancements don't merely present a new sandbox upon which to perform their tests, but introduce entirely new ways in which one is able to perform lab procedures—showing that centrifuges are far more than devices for separation. And then of course, there is the educational benefit. Centrifuges are used as an active learning tool when teaching students everything from the basics of sedimentation to the mechanics behind how these devices work. A proper knowledge of centrifugation is very basic to laboratory technicians because it controls the way they handle and prepare samples. Due to the importance this holds in medical diagnosis, intensive knowledge of centrifuge technology helps improve the larger picture of laboratory results. With the evolution of how well centrifuges work (and, come on, there's always a little something more that can be done), it appears these devices will only continue to have a bigger and bigger effect on classroom learning as well as on everyday lab protocols (Nicogossian et al., 2025) (Figure 2.8).

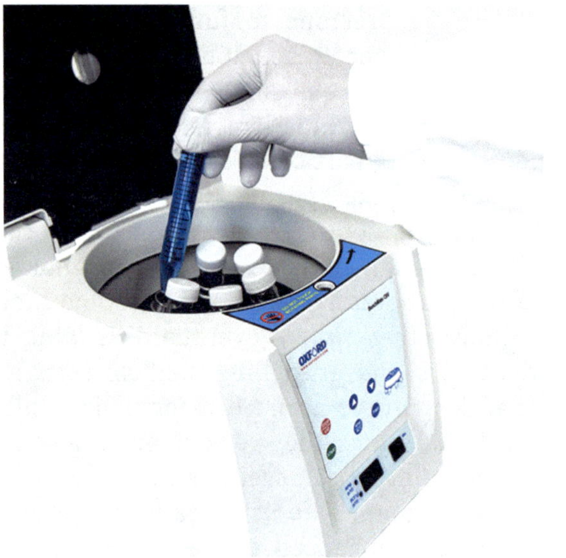

Figure 2.8. Clinical centrifuge.

Source: https://external-content.duckduckgo.com/iu/?u=https%3A%2F%2Fwww.oxfordlp.com%2Fwp-content%2Fuploads%2F2022%2F04%2FOxord-Lab-Products-Clinical-Centrifuges.png&f=1&nofb=1&ipt=bca25b18d6a1e27495e52a41fcb9f1e484556e3ba29f7f8cb943118ccff7222a.

2.2.3. Spectrophotometers

Spectrophotometers have actually transformed the way laboratories function today. These devices measure the light a sample absorbs at specific wavelengths, so you don't go roundabout on this. You just get an idea of the biochemical reactions involved. They're used to measure the concentration of biomolecules like glucose and proteins in a sample—which is really helpful in detecting diseases early. Their extremely high sensitivity and real-time measurements guarantee that decisions at clinics can be made quickly, something that is extremely crucial when every second matters. With the evolving times and the progress in clinical diagnostics, these machines keep evolving by always striving to deliver accuracy and reliability. It's not just about numbers, however.

In science, there's another side where spectrophotometers help us uncover more complex biochemical interactions. By interfacing with microfluidic technology, researchers have created tiny analytical devices that cut reagent use and wastage to a minimum while enhancing efficiency. This kind of approach really does bring medicine down to a personal level, where treatments are tailored in relation to precise biomarker levels.

You see, studies on adjusting measurement techniques and even merging these tools with other bio-analytical techniques reveal just how able they are—measuring from proteins right down to nucleic acids and bridging the gap between clinical observation and a broader biological understanding. There are, of course, some drawbacks too. You need sensitive calibration, and complex biological samples can sometimes lead to results being disrupted by matrix effects.

Typically, resolving such challenges entails the introduction of cutting-edge methodology—like fiber-based bio-analytical devices highlighted in recent literature (Hosseini et al., 2017)—which not only detect a variety of analytes but are also easier to use and more cost-effective. Small design and operational tweaks may further enhance detection limits and selectivity, and that would be a significant boon for clinical diagnostics. As lab procedures continue to expand and develop, spectrophotometers remain versatile and vital in the ongoing process of creating better healthcare solutions (Figure 2.9).

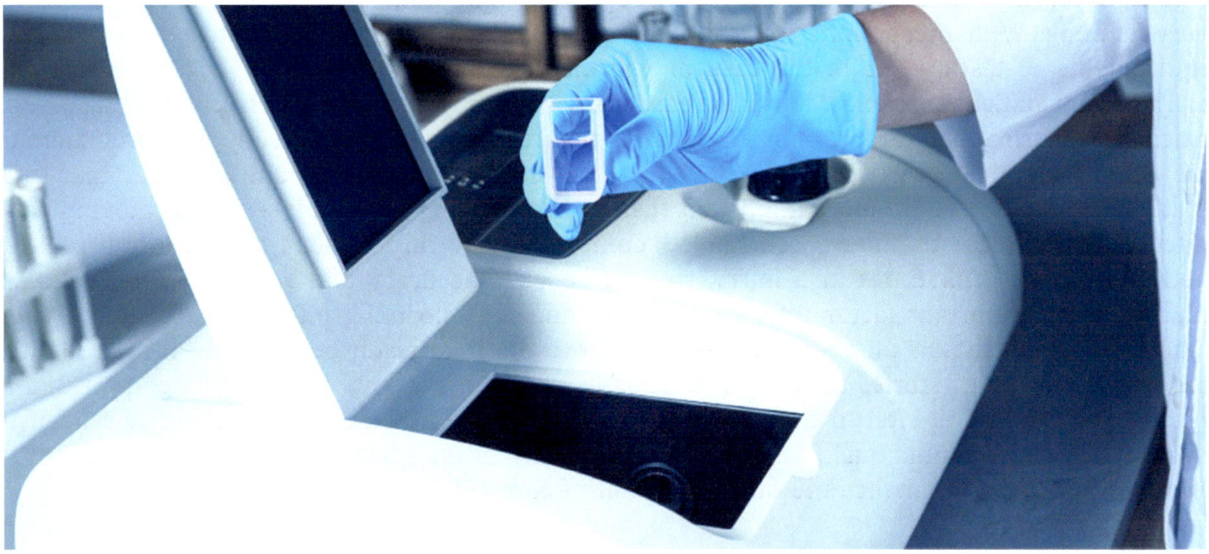

Figure 2.9. Spectrophotometers.

Source: https://external-content.duckduckgo.com/iu/?u=https%3A%2F%2Flabdepotinc.com%2Fmedia%2Fwysiwyg%2FArticles%2FTLD_Blog_2024_Sept_1_Banner.jpg&f=1&nofb=1&ipt=01ae9ac4d6ec83eeec2050b66d05d65946f8a65429c807df9a926db065aa3fb4.

Test Your Knowledge

1. What are the functions of a spectrophotometer in clinical testing?
2.. How does an automated hematology analyzer improve the accuracy of blood investigations?

2.3. Quality Control in Clinical Laboratories

Learning Outcome

- Importance of quality control;
- Methods of quality assurance;
- Role of standard operating procedures.

Test results have to be precise to the dot in our labs, especially since technology is constantly disrupting how we define things. Next-gen sequencing is becoming a go-to instrument for determining genetic quirks, so having hands-on quality tests in place is imperative. This new sequencing method has really made waves as a fast, high-throughput way of changing molecular genetics—but it's not all sunshine. There are still hitch-ups with handling the instruments, keeping the chemicals in a stable state, and filtering through the data. It is for this reason that building stable quality standards tailored to NGS is imperative for its inclusion in regular clinical application (Adey et al., 2012). In brief, quality maintenance ensures not only patients' health but also confidence in molecular testing overall. Genetic testing in labs is getting more advanced, which only raises the bar for quality control. We're learning more about genetic variants every day, which pressures labs to use fast, high-output methods that still deliver solid results. Sure, it is now possible to check thousands of genetic markers at once, but reading through that mountain of information can be pretty overwhelming. With these shifts, quality checks need to respond to the unique cost and care requirements of testing like in the case of pharmacogenomics. When error occurs, errors can easily disrupt patient therapies. For this reason, support of sound quality assurance measures is critical to ensuring labs do not only produce precise results but also correctly interpret them in true clinical practice (Schrijver et al., 2011). Clinical needs shift as well, and it's clear that total quality control systems are more important than ever. Emerging lab trends—such as moving from large, centralized labs to more decentralized, point-of-care settings—mean that quality processes need to keep up, sometimes in a hurry, to provide both accuracy and reliability. Reproducible results are an important factor for patient safety and for informing physician decisions. When labs perform robust tests along the way—sampling to the final result being read—labs are better able to handle the mysteries of today's diagnostics. Let's not forget, providing ongoing training for lab professionals is vital to the adherence to these standards. In general, there is a need to have flexible and dynamic quality measures for not only to maintain people's trust in laboratory reports but to overall enhance the quality of clinical care (Figure 2.10).

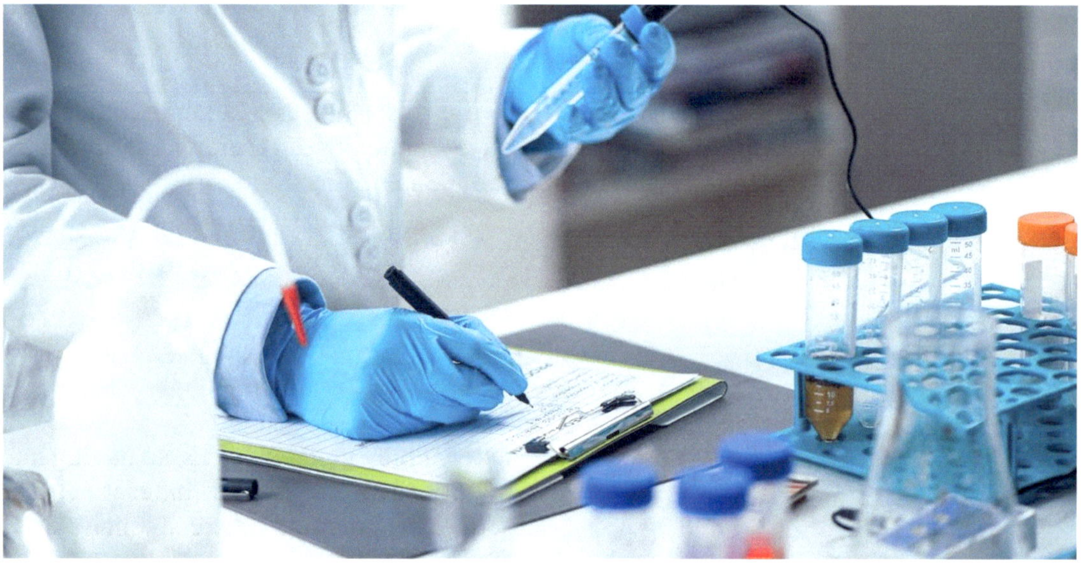

Figure 2.10. Quality control in clinical laboratories.

Source: https://cdn.labmanager.com/assets/articleNo/27442/aImg/50021/lab-quality-assurance-l.jpg.

2.3.1. Importance of Quality Control

In work in the clinical laboratory, getting the correct results just can't be negotiated. New technology such as next-generation sequencing (NGS) has significantly transformed the field, enabling researchers to probe genetic details that were previously out of reach. But this incredible high-throughput capability is effective only if robust, log-scalable quality controls are in place. Recent publications suggest that the incorporation of NGS into routine diagnostics requires laboratories to adopt standard quality protocols, rendering each test reproducible as well as clinically relevant. These practices not only make genetic tests more credible but also build confidence among patients and physicians, even more so strengthening laboratory services in general (Adey et al., 2012). As laboratory equipment grows more adaptable, so does the demand for similarly adaptive quality controls. Substandard quality control isn't a small speed bump; it has the potential to cascade and cause misdiagnoses and even treatment problems that hit the economy and society hard. A systematic but adaptable approach assists labs in coping with the problematic aspects of new machinery and data analysis. By closely observing every step of the process-even when at times observation isn't quite consistent—mismatches can be detected and corrected early, keeping diagnostic results integrity on target. Scrutiny is especially needed when new technology, with all its uncertain idiosyncrasies, comes into play (Fortina et al., 2015).

And then, naturally, there's the lively realm of lab medicine itself, which emphatically requires a quality-first, anticipatory mindset. Broadly speaking, as new and developing methods continue to redefine the science, projections about laboratory practices need to be accompanied by an unwavering commitment to quality assurance. Take a glance back at the history of laboratory medicine, and you can realize that even in the midst of all this speculation, quality has always been the name of the game. Building a genuine culture of quality control not only gets labs ready to handle the sophistication of evolving technology and evolving regulations, but it also earns the confidence of all stakeholders involved. Where technology and standards are constantly on the go, quality control is the solid ground upon which innovations of the future are built (Fortina et al., 2015).

2.3.2. Methods of quality assurance

Good clinical lab results start with basics – quality assurance is critical right from the start. Labs do not operate on a single step, but rather have a process which starts when a sample is collected and goes right up to data analysis. One critical aspect here is having clear, simple guidelines—generally called SOPs—that are available to everyone. These SOPs overall need to be constantly re-evaluated and amended as new scientific information and novel technologies emerge. The staff in the labs also needs training sessions; it refines skills and ensures everyone is adhering to the procedures that safeguard quality. Internal and external quality controls ensure an additional layer of assurance, so there is a greater likelihood of the results being reliable (Kang et al., 2020). Clinical laboratories such as metabolomics can be highly sophisticated. There are many steps of the process that can introduce minute errors that add up over time. An effective quality assurance strategy should ideally encompass the pre-analytical, analytical, and post-analytical phases, and address the operational realities of logistics and data processing. For example, the proper sampling methodology and equipment calibration being flawless are most critical to data integrity. In most cases, applying machine learning algorithms to identify errors and clean data can further improve the solidity of a study. Scientists at the cutting edge of metabolomics normally advocate for rigorous quality testing in order to keep data valid and reliable (Kang et al., 2020). Fluorescence methods also need to be treated with a light hand in terms of quality. Good measurements here depend on the identification and elimination of instrumental artifacts, which is key to coordinating fluorescence data from various methods such as microarrays and flow cytometers. It comes a long way when labs invest time to create good fluorescence standards—standards that, in addition to confirming how well equipment is performing, also facilitate quantitative analysis scientists depend on. Whether spectral responses or intensity ranges are in need of being checked, such standards are the key to high-quality clinical information. Lastly, sustaining these tight yet reasonable quality standards is needed in order to assist the discipline in progressing and establishing authentic trust in the findings (Figure 2.11).

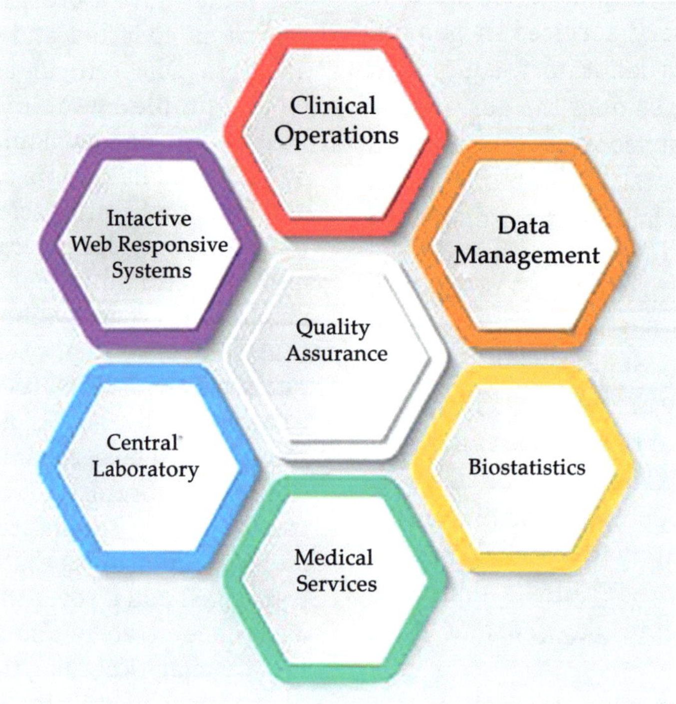

Figure 2.11. Methods of quality assurance.

Source: https://diagnosearch.com/userfiles/images/quality.png.

2.3.3. Role of Standard Operating Procedures

Clinical labs are based on accurate, routine regulations that keep all the wheels turning. SOPs – that's what everyone uses for standard operating procedures – are not checklists; they ensure work is consistent, accurate, and always on target. They spell out nearly every step in daily routines, from handling samples, running tests, or even the upkeep of equipment. When labs follow these steps, errors fall and results are sounder – which is, overall, important for arriving at the proper diagnosis and treatment. Furthermore, with these steps in place, there is greater accountability as everyone clearly understands what needs to be done, and they are a handy guide for orienting new employees. Aside from helping ensure smooth operation, these steps further improve the convenience of compliance with various regulations and accreditation standards. The labs need to adhere to established regulations by organizations such as the Clinical Laboratory Improvement Amendments (CLIA) and the College of American Pathologists (CAP). The accurate, written SOPs play an important role in proving compliance in case of audits and inspections to maintain the accreditation. Often than not, a clear set of operating procedures prepares labs to address the evolving requirements of healthcare quality assurance more successfully. And when issues do occur, by keeping these processes in place, labs are able to quickly institute correctives – which serves to uphold the confidence of healthcare professionals and patients alike. Regular examination and update keeps these procedures current with current lab technology best practices as well. SOPs even force labs to seek continuous quality improvement and drive innovation. They provide a framework for auditing existing practices, detecting inefficiencies, and finding areas requiring change – even to the extent of having labs refine techniques or implement new equipment. For example, with the advent of fresh developments like automated systems or machine learning software, the lab can make procedural changes to include these developments in addition to established procedures, bringing them into synergy with lab goals and patient care procedures. Recording each procedural update offers an extra layer of accountability and builds a sort of cumulative repository of best practices in different settings. Lastly, the diligent execution of SOPs not only contributes to improved daily performance but also has a decisive influence on improved patient outcomes, further pointing to their indispensable role in our healthcare system.

Test Your Knowledge

1. Why is internal and external quality control important in laboratory operations?
2. How are control samples used to maintain accuracy and reliability of test results?

2.4. Safety Protocols in the Laboratory

Learning Outcome

- Personal protective equipment (PPE);
- Chemical safety measures;
- Biological hazard management.

Laboratory safety protocols go far beyond box-ticking—they create a culture of true accountability and watchfulness on behalf of everyone. You can see that following these procedures not only keeps the team safe but also keeps test results and samples stable. There's training, proper equipment usage, and even clearly defined emergency protocols all combined; these processes aid people in the lab with dealing when unexpected things happen when harm is imminent. Occasionally labs perform safety audits and update training documents so everybody is aware of the most current on procedures, which generally foster ongoing improvement. Biological contamination is a large issue that can destroy both worker safety as well as real accuracy of research findings. Lab cells, those precious organisms, are more prone to contamination and mix-up, and stringently following safety protocols minimizes such risks to a great extent. Standard rules regulating the treatment of cell cultures address significant facets such as establishing cell identity, valid cryopreservation, and preventing microbial contamination—all essential measures in avoiding common errors that jeopardize research. In the majority of instances, having these protocols in place not only increases confidence in the data but also aligns with the ethical requirements our scientific practice must satisfy, things oversight groups are always on the lookout for. And then there is the legal and ethical aspect, which can't be simply dismissed. Every lab struggles with a maze of regulations on the use of animal and human tissues; therefore, maintaining good, effective procedures is essentially imperative. You'll find laboratory procedure guidelines don't only tell you how to choose and keep equipment around—refined ones will also help guide you through common troubleshooting issues. These guidelines, indirectly, give safety more strength and determine legal requirements, allowing labs to function within ethical guidelines. Overall, having these protocols in place from the beginning sets the stage for a more secure laboratory environment, which ultimately promotes scientific progress and increases public trust in clinical research (Bonica et al., 2017; Capes-Davis et al., 2014) (Figure 2.12).

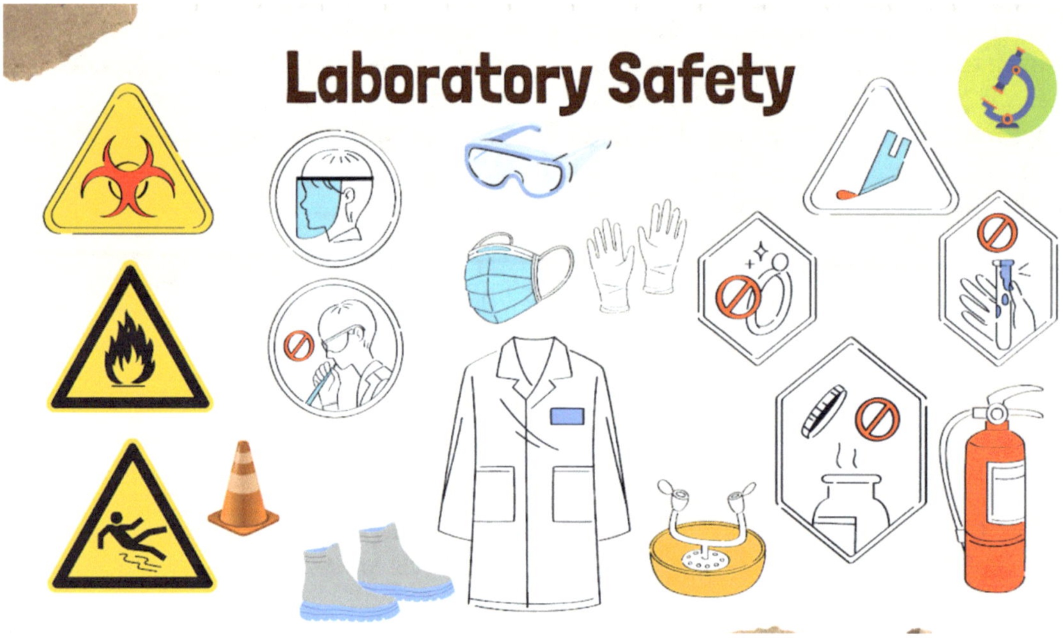

Figure 2.12. Safety protocols in the laboratory.

Source: https://blogger.googleusercontent.com/img/b/R29vZ2xl/AVvXsEhnP7_ev4kc8gjmCH5ajEsTX2uGE0930At-k097bKrxXPOGDRh7QKx-BiPObfNazGvHny5c1eGi84kZU5dkJhH04kVQsM_8lnBrqUiVnGTP9fAiTO_XzyORsZQKbfd-VXLHP1hyphenhyphenbhROK3zohUYQpZ_-nWmQz6vdIp6JU8Cwqb_OtZqNc8xbKpta88hkDDF2/w1200-h630-p-k-no-nu/lab%20safety.png.

2.4.1. Personal Protective Equipment (PPE)

Safety in clinical labs is paramount—a fact that cannot be overlooked. PPE, or personal protective gear, is a barrier between lab workers and harm that may be biological, chemical, or even physical. The majority of studies primarily suggest that proper use of PPE isn't all about ticking compliance boxes; it helps foster a culture where safety is at the top. Proper use of PPE minimizes exposures to infectious agents and harmful substances, thereby enhancing both workplace safety and overall efficiency. Creating clear instructions for PPE use is a critical step. The instructions typically cover the right equipment to choose, the right way to put it on, and the right way to dispose of it. The literature (Oosthuysen et al., 2015) notes that ongoing training is required for health professionals to remain abreast with these practices. Interestingly, compliance can vary considerably from center to center, implying training should be adjusted in some way to accommodate different settings. Researchers even propose to use simple audit-feedback tools to check PPE usage in real-time—giving a more immediate view of infection control practice. In the majority of regions where healthcare resources are limited, it is even more difficult to remain within guidelines for PPE. There are typical gaps around the world: developed countries have enough resources and well-defined policies, but most developing countries are restricted by material deficiency and lack of training (Fossey et al., 2014). In addition to increasing the risk for healthcare workers, this compromises patient safety. Therefore, innovative solutions have to be created to increase the supply of PPE and enhance proper utilization across the board. Most of the time, the innovative solutions allow every clinical laboratory to adopt high infection prevention standards even though the journey is not entirely smooth (Figure 2.13).

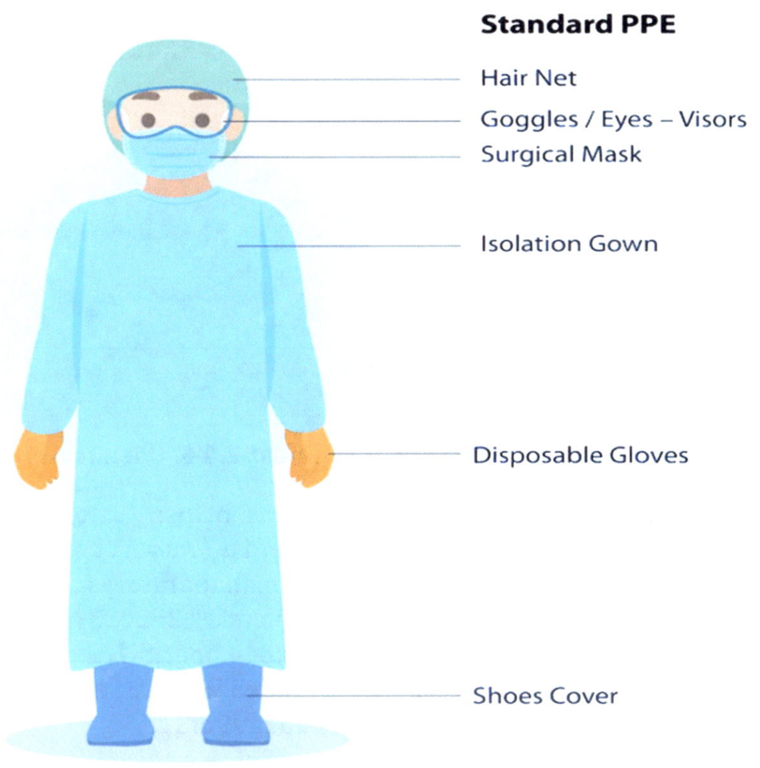

Figure 2.13. Personal protective equipment (PPE).

Source: https://external-content.duckduckgo.com/iu/?u=https%3A%2F%2Fcdn.shopify.com%2Fs%2Ffiles%2F1%2F0278%2F4860%2F5809%2Ffiles%2FPPE-Full-ShutterStock_large.jpg%3Fv%3D1595338239&f=1&nofb=1&ipt=ab4533ad75ab19f62e1308a9f6d7ed92a2e66b4a059b21952cff8b9eef9de9e3.

2.4.2. Chemical safety measures

To be a clinical lab worker is to never be free from being aware of safety, especially when dealing with dangerous chemicals in the production process. Laboratory workers are typically taught hands-on, so they really do know what they're doing—this is where they go through those Material

Safety Data Sheets (MSDS) that outline what a chemical is, how you should be able to handle it, and what to do when something goes wrong. Correct labelling and storage of chemicals is not just a matter of box-ticking; it's a simple step that prevents spontaneous exposures or unwanted reactions. And ready availability of protective items like gloves, masks, and eye shields gives an extra layer of protection. Studies have shown, on the whole, that these kinds of practice minimize risks of accidents with chemical work and are, therefore, a necessity in laboratories today. Basic training is only half the solution. Routine reviews and updating of safety procedures are equally important. Laboratories need to go over their own procedures on a regular basis and make sure what they do complies with the latest guidelines and rules from groups like OSHA and the CDC. Regular audits—even when they're sometimes tedious—get risks early before they become big problems and offer a means to correct them in a hurry. This constant cycle of verify and reverify not only minimizes risks but also, little by little, builds a mindset in which safety seems like part of the teams daily routine. In most contexts, complying with these shifting rules is sufficient so that labs operate smoothly and keep everyone's well-being in plain sight. Chemical safety protocols have to address outside hazards as well, such as microbial contamination, which can have significant impacts on the success of laboratory results. Bizarrely enough, cell line contamination or even contamination alone can get horribly out of control with critically undermining an experiment's validity. Keeping track of authenticating and managing cell cultures is the best approach towards being able to properly deal with such risks. Most labs nowadays hybridize straightforward, solid protocols for the acquisition, authentication, and even cryopreservation of cell lines; these processes guarantee nothing can go wrong. Labs can also protect themselves not only from chemical issues but even biological ones with proper contamination controls. Finally, integration of chemical and biological safety controls raises research quality as well as honors ethics in compliance with what modern laboratory practice is all about, some literature on guidelines and standards for laboratories suggests (Capes-Davis et al., 2014; Mody et al., 1994) (Figure 2.14).

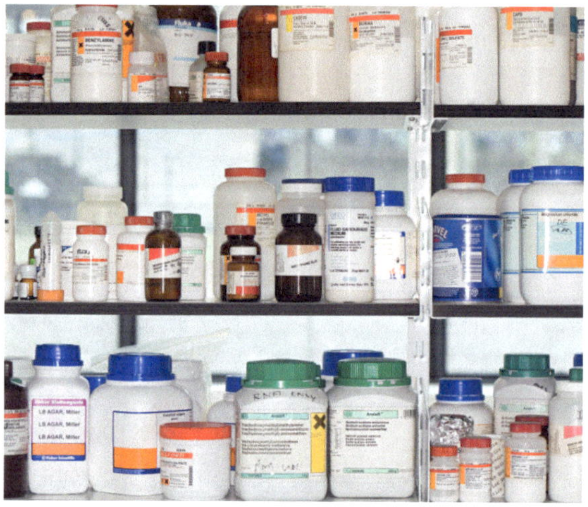

Figure 2.14. Chemical safety in laboratories.

Source: https://external-content.duckduckgo.com/iu/?u=https%3A%2F%2Fwww.nationallaboratorysales.com%2Fwp-content%2Fuploads%2F2023%2F04%2FChemical-Shelf-768x644.png&f=1&nofb=1&ipt=c3941fccbee7381ed5e555f64037a1dc29e1939d4c4d3517880c83a1a99df215.

2.4.3. Biological hazard management

Clinical laboratory work is not all about operating tests—it is where science interfaces with the everyday practice of safety, and biological hazard management is critical. Laboratory personnel and the broader community at large rely on staying current, even if a small mistake such as cross-contamination of cultured cells can drastically lessen results. At times, even the smallest mistake might render an entire research endeavor useless. To avoid contamination and deter unwanted microbial intruders, guidelines have been established to confirm and preserve cell cultures appropriately. This spread of knowledge across enables laboratories to steer clear of pitfalls without compromising on quality in bioethics and biosafety (Capes-Davis et al., 2014). It is also advantageous to take proactive steps. Hands-on training reminds people regularly of the dangers associated with biological materials—this is not a question of rule enforcement, it is a question of creating an actual safety culture. Try to think of it in terms such as this: knowing how to properly utilize PPE and taking care when handling, storing, and disposing of these materials is just as important as the implementation of any new equipment. More often than not, new technologies and new laboratory procedures not only improve precision of data but also the speed of controlling hazards. Through constant updating of training procedures, laboratories can stay ahead of surprise threats and new regulations (Nicogossian et al., 2025). Cooperation is also what makes a difference. Institutions need to cooperate with regulators in order to comply with national and international standards. This is not all about adhering to established protocols; it is about talking openly about what is going well, debating best practice, and even exploring potential biosafety concerns. Exchanging tales from the trenches – the triumphs and the disasters – proves to be a valuable investment in improving daily practice. By and large, this blend of ongoing collaboration and education works to help labs navigate the high-stakes field of biological hazards, so that pursuing the sciences isn't in pursuit of safety (Capes-Davis et al., 2014; Nicogossian et al., 2025) (Figure 2.15).

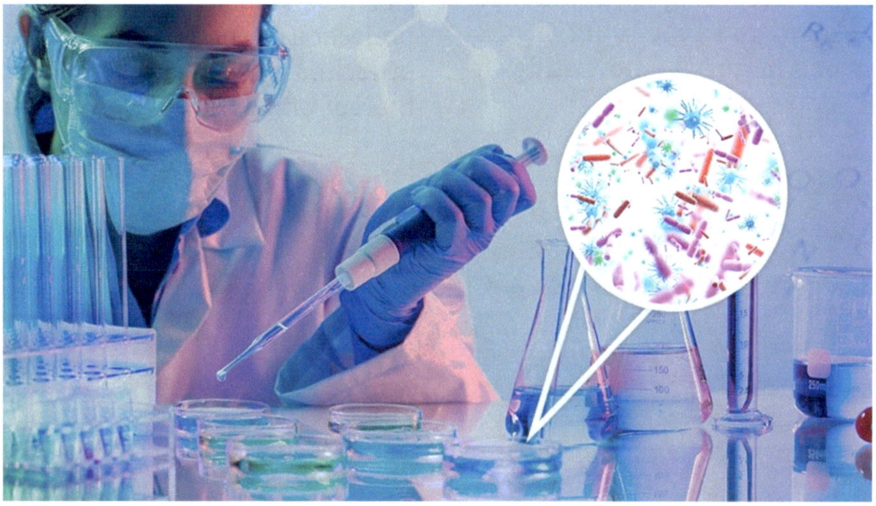

Figure 2.15. Biological hazards.

Source: https://external-content.duckduckgo.com/iu/?u=https%3A%2F%2Fhsseworld.com%2Fwp-content%2Fuploads%2F2019%2F10%2Fbilogical-hazards.jpg&f=1&nofb=1&ipt=955147772303f67448d49d5724006dabc6839bb0e8a2d26911d94296d71f3298.

Test Your Knowledge

1. What personal protective equipment (PPE) is essential in a clinical laboratory?
2. How should hazardous chemical spills be managed to ensure laboratory safety?

2.5. Emerging Technologies in Clinical Laboratories

Learning Outcome

- Automation in laboratory processes;
- Point-of-care testing devices;
- Molecular diagnostics advancements.

Genetic testing technology has improved in ways that scarcely even sound conceivable today—it completely redefines medical labs by enabling them to handle huge amounts of information at one time, something formerly deemed unthinkable. Labs can now test thousands of genetic changes at the same time, so doctors can tailor therapies according to a patient's own genetic makeup. You read a lot in the literature about pharmacogenomic testing; it is a great example, and it is very promising but in its own way gives puzzles. Detection of genetic variants has certainly improved a lot, but it remains a messy process to figure out what they actually mean. This mix of advance and complexity necessarily makes one ask about how genomic information should be incorporated into patient care plans. In most cases, they need to be managed—especially as the wave of personalized medicine grows and greater and more detailed genetic information has to be interpreted and used in everyday clinical practice (Schrijver et al., 2011). The future for clinical laboratories is not solely about new technology, though; economic factors and shifting priorities in terms of resources also play a large part. Changing economic circumstances typically force the purveyors of medical care to wonder whether complex diagnosis technology can be of use. Surprisingly enough, earlier projections were too gloomy concerning the pace of technological advance and the implications thereof on health care (Fortina et al., 2015).

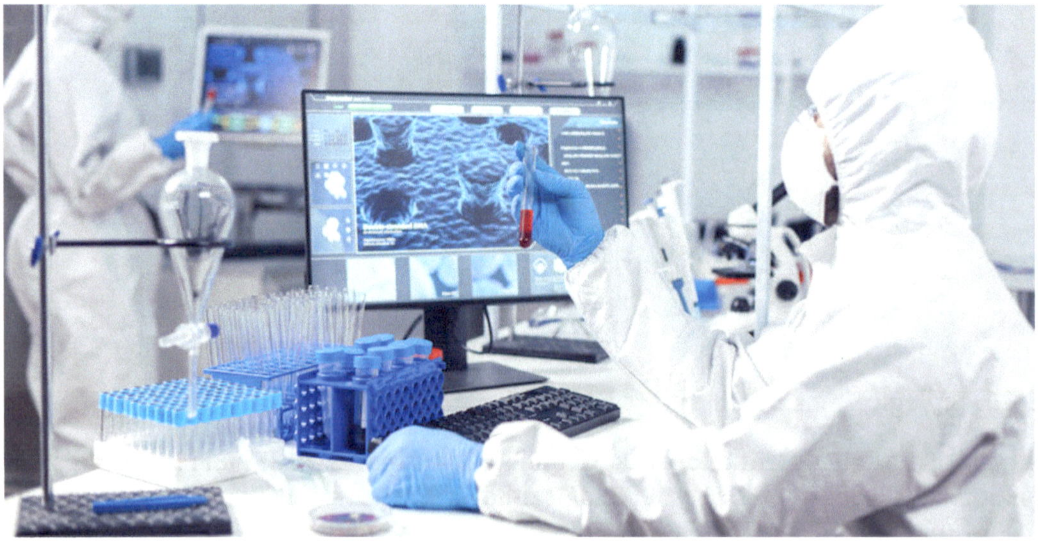

Figure 2.16. Emerging technologies in clinical laboratories.

Source: https://external-content.duckduckgo.com/iu/?u=https%3A%2F%2Fcairoscan.com.eg%2FEn%2Fimages%2FLabs%2Fgeneral.jpg&f=1&nofb=1&ipt=87e42cee6ee5f995764a3c71a5d1c423c8c6443328732f83dd043262684dbac7.

Therefore, all those interested—policy makers to laboratory assistants—should have ears to the ground and be ready to adapt. Overall, an open and flexible strategy that connects innovation to economic reality may well liberate smarter methods of applying new laboratory methods into daily practice without losing accessibility or affordability. Aside from the revolutions in genetic analysis, innovations like AI and automation are shaking up daily life in laboratories. Computer algorithms, for instance, tend to make for more accurate diagnoses and streamline workflows—which, in the process, helps minimize human error and fight backlogs, well, for the most part. Automation steps in to do those repetitive tasks, freeing up laboratory staff to focus on more problematic, more advanced analyses and interpretations. As these technologies start to communicate with each other, labs are at a place where higher throughput can co-exist with higher accuracy. This shifting landscape with lightning pace shows that labs will need to continue to transform to harness the full potential of these emerging tools. Eventually, as labs incorporate more of these advancements, they'll be much better positioned to meet the rising challenges and demands of healthcare today (Figure 2.16).

2.5.1. Automation in Laboratory Processes

Lab processes have really evolved considerably over the years, thanks in large measure to advances in technology and automation. Earlier, lab technicians would perform all the tasks manually, which typically meant results might be variable or subject to human error. With automated systems entering the picture these days, clinical labs generally see enhanced reliability and less trouble. These automated setups help alleviate the time spent on redundant work and keeping test results more consistent. Automation speeds up, enabling laboratories to sort through high numbers of samples in high-density settings. Future research even expects that this overlap between automation will continue to evolve further, driven by emerging technology and ever-evolving socio-economic circumstances (Fortina et al., 2015). There are some technical shortcuts, as well, that are causing a ruckus in how labs measure things like creatinine levels. Take the old Jaffé reaction test, for example—ubiquitous but often thwarted by interfering substances which could distort the final values. Conversely, newer methods such as capillary zone electrophoresis separate nicely between creatinine and other substances. This change leads to greater precision levels and less manual handling, limiting possible errors. These developments improve the quality of diagnoses and enable laboratories to handle samples more efficiently, something that is greatly appreciated in present-day clinical settings (Guo et al., 1998). The future of laboratory automation is very bright, with ongoing innovation on the horizon to revolutionize clinical diagnostics. Automation software continues evolving, sometimes incorporating artificial intelligence or machine learning to recognize patterns and adjust operations. Overall, these technologies are capable of handling vast quantities of data, making diagnoses quicker and very accurate, with a recommendation of what resources will be needed next. In the majority of cases, historical projections show a clear trend: laboratories are moving towards technology that delivers rapid, high-quality results with reduced cost and resource preservation (Fortina et al., 2015). Overall, embracing automation not only highlights what laboratories are already able to accomplish but also provides a glimpse of the approaching wave of clinical instruments and techniques that will further improve patient care and operational efficiency.

2.5.2. Point-of-Care Testing Devices

Laboratory medicine's been a rollercoaster ride

of late—there's always something new, and one of the more glamorous ones is POCT (point-of-care testing). These devices spew out answers by the patient's side, so you don't have to wait on some far-off lab to gear up. They're constructed in such a manner that even a person who doesn't have a lot of lab experience can operate them with minimal fuss. With medicine increasingly shifting towards a patient-focused setup, POCT not being readily accessible isn't merely a nice added perk, but flat-out imperative for timely decisions. But if you think that trying to predict where lab medicine is headed is a lock, history has other plans—long-term usefulness and reliability remain sketchy propositions (Fortina et al., 2015). There is also enough evidence to prove that POCT actually improves patient management—especially with chronic illness or acquiring infectious disease before they can establish themselves. Where there are not many central labs due to infrastructure or logistics issues, these simpler tests can really relieve the pressure. Expense generally plays an important part too; fewer complications mean tests are cheap and safe. You might have heard news regarding such developments like dried blood spots or pooled sample testing; such new ideas have made viral load monitoring very easily (Bartlett et al., 2012). Sometimes the same fact is repeated: making the tests more precise not just gives more precise diagnoses but also convinces patients to comply with their regimen, hence saving healthcare in the long term. Down the road, POCT devices seem ready for an overhauling based on new technology breakthroughs and policy reforms that will keep things moving. Streamlining testing procedures – and providing a little friendly competition among manufacturers – might really make it more accessible and affordable. As it turns out, when governments, health practitioners, and tech designers work together to create guidelines (especially where resources are scarce), all involved gain. Along with the quick diagnostic payoff, mainstreaming POCT into overall healthcare planning might help reduce public health problems, enhance national health outcomes, and lay the groundwork for a more coordinated, more accessible system of care (Bartlett et al., 2012) (Figure 2.17).

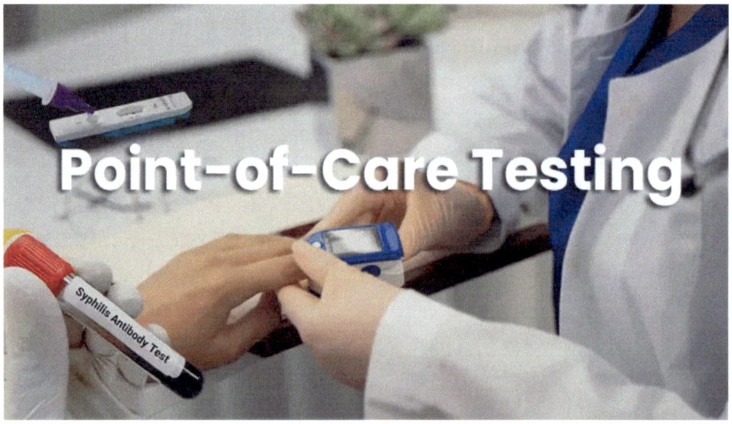

Figure 2.17. Point of care testing.

Source: https://external-content.duckduckgo.com/iu/?u=https%3A%2F%2Fwww.wissenresearch.com%2Fwp-content%2Fuploads%2F2022%2F10%2FPoint-of-Care-Testing.webp&f=1&nofb=1&ipt=362d1e34024f0e53415be3b3f7087f478c755ef77040e7c1511653140fde0149.

2.5.3. Molecular Diagnostics Advancements

Molecular diagnostics have really transformed medicine. PCR and NGS, for example, now speed up tests and narrow our ability to sense disease – and, on top of that, permit us to investigate more deeply into gene change and fine points of pathogen features. This makes it possible to shape treatments for each individual based on their unique genetic profile, which, in most cases, is good for patients—especially those coping with hard challenges like cancer or stubborn infections. Labs keep pressing for still more sensitive tests, and it's almost like every new discovery drives us closer to an entire diagnostic revolution, even if occasionally the ride is a bit bumpy. Biosensing technology is emerging into the spotlight as well. Take the single-particle interferometric reflectance imaging sensor (SP-IRIS), for instance; it measures biological nanoparticles with sensitivity levels that approach the impossible. Electronic biosensors, by the counting of specific biomolecules, can minimize detection limits – which more likely than not leads to earlier, more accurate diagnoses. Generally, such innovations have far-reaching consequences for clinics, most notably in the detection of early indicators of disease and pathogens. These practices, though applied at times a little irregularly, are intended to elude false positives and negatives, giving practitioners the information they need (Avci et al., 2017). AI is another frontier that's revolutionizing molecular diagnostics. Machine learning now navigates soiled, messy data, linking symptoms to genetic hints and generally enhancing diagnostic precision. As we drift away from subjective, pre-Fangorn judgments to the world of hard facts, medical education has to play catch-up – future doctors will have to marry digital savvy with sound clinical judgment. While the potential of AI is immense, there are ethical subtleties and occasional biases that we just can't turn a blind eye to (Galdames et al., 2024). Ongoing research, often with a hint of unpredictability, reveals that a multidisciplinary approach is crucial for fully leveraging AI's potential without compromising patient care.

Test Your Knowledge

1. How is next-generation sequencing (NGS) transforming clinical diagnostics?
2. What role does automation and robotics play in modern clinical laboratories?

2.6. Challenges in Clinical Laboratory Practices

Learning Outcome

- Staffing and training issues;
- Regulatory compliance;
- Technological integration.

Clinical labs are in rapid evolution with newer automated instrumentation and new methods of diagnosis waiting in the wings. Tests are done more accurately and more quickly, but everything is not hunky-dory. Labs will order too many tests at times and not enough on others—both of which mess with resources and may end up costing a small fortune while possibly injuring patients. It is a complex situation that essentially invites laboratories to modify their game plan and allocation of resources. Review of outdated methods in the majority of cases could be the key to providing assurance that costs are matched with the need to maintain quality care (Devis et al., 2024). Management and education of the laboratory also are not meeting the needs of available technology. Most assert that the aged, nearly "indoctrination"-type of instruction just isn't working anymore for aspiring lab experts. The day-to-day functions in most labs also have a somewhat disorganized feel to them, lacking the discipline required in this rapidly evolving field. A marriage of on-going improvement and an expanded range of pedagogies—combined with a little judicious government support, like the creation of regional inspection facilities—can go a long way to preparing lab personnel to meet modern challenges (Zhou et al., 2023). And then there is the subtle tango between laboratory practice, financial limitations, and environmental stewardship. Balancing people, planet, and profit forces labs to break out of the business of performing unnecessary tests. Cutting the fat in testing unloads financial costs and reduces environmental waste—win-win. By eliminating the fat from testing, labs can save money and reduce their environmental impact without sacrificing patient safety. All this truly highlights that smart, sustainable governance is more essential than ever for an improved, more efficient system (Devis et al., 2024) (Figure 2.18).

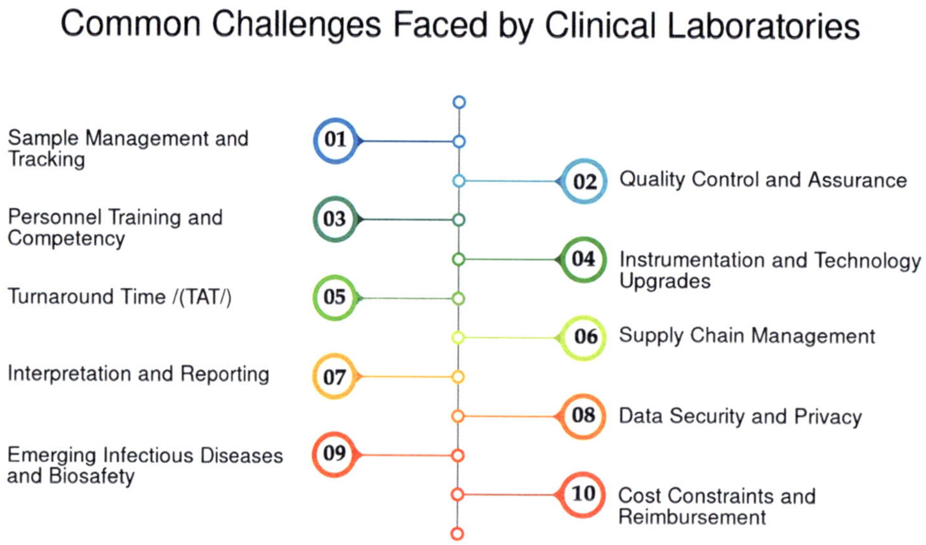

Figure 2.18. Clinical laboratory challenge.

Source: https://encrypted-tbn0.gstatic.com/images?q=tbn:ANd9GcQQlMqfOrbofu0RHfJe0NPmJTUqSwVugllEYQ&s.

2.6.1. Staffing and Training Issues

It's not the techniques or the tools that do the trick, it's the individuals who labor in the clinical labs. Whether a given technique or device works or not generally depends on the humans themselves – their skill, training, and even their interpersonal relationships. To work in a laboratory requires high standards of precision, so one can't just get some warm body on the job; one needs to pick and choose one's staff well and train them well. Training is more than technical know-how – a great deal of it focuses on the need for teamwork and open communication. When frontline individuals feel valued and included, they will contribute spontaneously but extremely valuable, which helps the lab get through day-to-day operations as well as those more challenging ones. Manpower management goes far beyond filling empty slots. Overall, it is about forward thinking and looking ahead to what the lab will need in the future. Recruitment techniques should not just be geared towards individuals who possess the right technical skill, but also individuals possessing the soft skills required to function in an efficient team. This balanced approach, blending hard skills with personal insight, tends to enhance effectiveness and patient outcome. In general, a skilled and assured staff can accommodate rapid changes in clinical practices and equipment by continuous training and professional growth. Training and staffing have significant linkage with problems related to labor relations and organizational administration. For instance, unions will usually battle for lab workers by advocating for better working conditions and making sure training sessions actually benefit the employees. There is some truth to when management and unions collaborate – it usually creates an open, communicative work environment, which in turn fuels morale and retention rates. As explained by Figueroa et al. (2012), such collaborative setups provide employees with a stake in decision-making for their work although, at times, it weakens the team with some extra back-and-forth. Generally, such involvement has the impact of enhancing training outcomes and reinforces a laboratory's operation integrity and eventually affects patient care and general clinical effectiveness in the long term.

2.6.2. Regulatory Compliance

Regulation compliance is necessary in the operations of clinical labs, into which different techniques and machines are thrown. Labs conduct from genetic sampling to stem cell research, so they deal with a mysterious labyrinth of local, national, and even international regulations. Safety and effectiveness in these ever-evolving disciplines depend on these regulations, even when at times the new regulations seem to clash with new ideas.

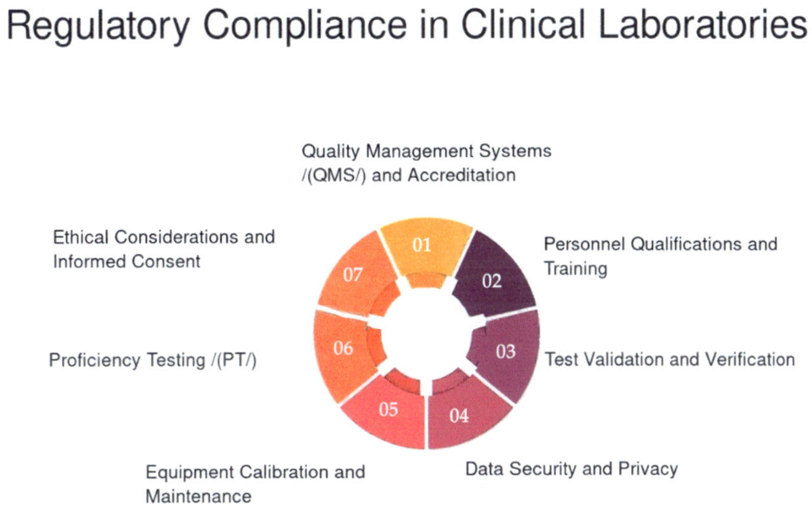

Figure 2.19. Regulatory compliance in clinical laboratory.

Source: https://fastercapital.co/i/Clinical-laboratory-segment--Navigating-the-Clinical-Laboratory-Landscape--A-Comprehensive-Guide--Regulatory-Compliance-in-Clinical-Laboratories.webp.

For the most part, these rules neatly keep patient care in top form and the results of research sound—though that balance is frequently a tug-of-war of sorts. When labs become global, though, matters are more complex. Clinical trials in stem cell medicine, for example, reveal stark differences between regulations country to country, and such patchwork is apt to make it hard to level practices worldwide. Scientists adapt to the local setting, and at times, take on procedures that are different from what is accepted internationally. Often, such deviations mix in new configurations that force local and international procedures to influence each other, driving the whole discipline to innovate (Rosemann et al., 2014). It's a situation that is as complex as it is interesting. Beyond the lab bench, regulation's effects spill over into ethical and economic spheres. Lab groups often have to spend a lot of money on training and new equipment, which can be obstacles for smaller groups-even while it is complying with the regulations that generates patient trust, regulator trust, and trust from funding organizations. A strong compliance history can build a lab's reputation and even create more collaborative arrangements and financial rewards. Yes, the journey is rocky and full of hurdles, yet the process can also lead to new best practices that move science and ethics forward together (Pearson et al., 1998) (Figure 2.19).

2.6.3. Technological Integration

The rapid pace of technology advancements is revolutionizing clinical labs in ways you might not expect. Labs nowadays are mixing high-end equipment with streamlined, if somewhat improvised, methods that enhance speed and reliability in testing. Computerized systems—robot sample handlers and leading-edge analyzers—are performing advanced tests with fewer human errors. This pairing of technology generally brings down turnaround times and has a tendency to deliver more accurate results. Labs have even started utilizing computer software to direct data, and when integrated with electronic health records (EHRs), test results and patient data appear almost instantly. Generally, these technologies bring care quality and workflow to a new level, even though the process sometimes seems a bit unorganized. Tech integration also reorients clinicians' measurement of patient conditions. New imaging technology like OCT now facilitates high-resolution images for formerly challenging conditions to assess properly. Agreement on how to identify entities like lamellar macular holes and epiretinal membrane foveoschisis (Bottoni et al., 2020) means specialists are able to reach a consensus, in most cases once finer details are made apparent through more advanced imaging. With these new technologies, labs can more precisely differentiate conditions that once seemed nearly impossible to tell apart, lowering misdiagnosis and holding out hope of treatments tailored to a patient's condition. This impact goes beyond the patient—it's slowly changing routine clinical practices too. On the treatment side of the ledger, developments like gene therapy and stem cell therapies promise an entire new era of lab medicine. New hope for recalcitrant retinal disease is a practically revolutionary shift, showing how novel laboratory technologies can lead to revolutionary treatments (Sarwate et al., 2023). With gene therapy to correct genetic issues, laboratories are already rewriting what we used to think could not be cured; and with stem cell therapies toward the restoration of retinal tissue, there is actually a coming together of laboratory innovation and patient wellness. Yes, there are still ethical concerns and delivery mechanisms to sort out, but overall, these developments not only make more accurate diagnostics and treatments available, but also propel medicine toward a more human-centered and personalized future.

Test Your Knowledge

1. What are the major challenges in maintaining accuracy and reliability in laboratory testing?
2. How do clinical laboratories cope with limited resources and high patient demand?

Summary

Clinical laboratory practice and technology are ever-changing, and change drives more efficient healthcare diagnosis and treatment. New methods don't only sharpen test data—but accelerate the whole system and allow it to run more efficiently. Medical education, as an instance, must move away from outdated, cookie-cutter models and test out newer, more varied approaches that truly create hands-on competence and build genuine critical thinking for next-generation lab professionals. Several studies, including those on the ways that laboratory work in China is evolving, suggest that these kinds of changes in education expose students to the real issues that exist in modern-day clinics. When schools, hospitals, and equipment firms work together, they end up with a labor force that can handle grimy, complex lab setups, ultimately resulting in improved patient care (Zhou et al., 2023). The labs now are more and more dependent on technology, and techniques like machine learning and deep learning are a huge deal here. They are really good at going through EHRs to find out early signs of disease and handle patient care in a shorter time. Through the mining of enormous databases of health data, clinicians can dig up patterns that were not there before— paving the way for earlier interventions and treatments specifically suited to every patient. Some studies on the way that EHRs interface with machine learning allude to how such systems improve the manner in which we diagnose diseases, thereby improving patient outcomes. Incorporating these intelligent, data-driven technologies into daily lab procedures isn't a nicety; it's rather necessary in today's rapidly evolving medical landscape (Swinckels et al., 2023). Technology innovation and day-to-day clinical practice have become irrevocable, demonstrating that continued research in lab instruments and techniques is the norm. Everyone—from governments and schools to hospitals—must contribute to push innovations that enhance lab work and diagnostics. It's obvious that research expenditure, or the measured construction and constant adjustment of advanced equipment, has a large role to play in creating laboratory settings that are both effective and consistent. And by upholding good lab management practices and quality control, we're able to ensure these new methods perform well with clinical needs. In general, the literature suggests that innovation space is crucial in propelling labs towards excellence, which ultimately results in patient care and quality healthcare improvement (Zhou et al., 2023).

Clinical laboratory methods have come a long, long way—diagnostics are more accurate and reliable these days. LCTMS is a case in point; it essentially wedded two mass spectrometers to conduct large-scale analyses with minimal hand labor, far removed from the old chromatographic techniques. Yes, LCTMS does have a cost and it is confusing, but its build quality and overall usefulness more than make up for it. Being able to test a broader range of compounds is something that most labs are already using, and experts even say that it could potentially replace items such as HPLC and GCMS in most scenarios (Re et al., 2003). Apart from propelling analytical techniques, incorporating laboratory equipment into research has thrown new light on the secrets of biology. For instance, experimentation on platforms such as the U.S. Polar Platform provides clues about gravitational biology and life support idiosyncrasies. There is a bizarre interaction between space research and earth-based biology that tends to promote multi-disciplinary approaches overall, enabling us to understand how life accommodates different gravitational forces. In these missions, equipment not only gathers orbiting data but also captures vital insights on planetary and cosmic events—even if occasionally the data come through a bit kinked. Such vast research unavoidably extends beyond clinical application, as advances in space have a tendency to ripple back and affect health and biotech on Earth. Lab techniques are not all high-end analysis today; they are converging with innovative tech that is focused on better patient care. Equipment capable of monitoring biological markers in real time is paving the way for personalized medicine, really revolutionizing treatment in new ways. High-throughput machines such as next-generation sequencing make diagnoses finer while detecting disease at an early stage and deciding on targeted therapies. As these tools become more user-friendly and ubiquitous, they might well alter the manner in which clinicians develop treatment plans. Together, these breakthroughs attest to the extent to which clinical labs are central to delivering technology into healthcare—to ultimately yield better patient outcomes as well as an optimized system.

KEY TERMS FROM THIS CHAPTER

Analyzer	Autoclave	Blood gas analyzer
Calibration	Centrifuge	Culture media
Electrophoresis	Hemocytometer	Incubator
Microscope	PCR (polymerase chain reaction)	Pipette
Quality control (QC)	Reagent	Specimen labeling
Spectrophotometer	Staining	

Critical Thinking Questions

1. **Which instrument is commonly used to measure the concentration of substances in a solution based on light absorbance?**
   a. Centrifuge
   b. Spectrophotometer
   c. Incubator
   d. Microscope
2. **What is the purpose of a centrifuge in a clinical laboratory?**
   a. To count blood cells
   b. To separate components of a fluid by spinning
   c. To magnify microorganisms
   d. To store reagents
3. **Which technique is used to detect the presence of specific proteins or antibodies in a sample?**
   a. Gram staining
   b. Electrophoresis
   c. ELISA (Enzyme-Linked Immunosorbent Assay)
   d. Western blotting
4. **What is the function of an autoclave in the clinical lab?**
   a. To cool down reagents
   b. To sterilize equipment using steam under pressure
   c. To measure pH
   d. To analyze urine
5. **Which of the following instruments is used to manually count blood cells?**
   a. Hemocytometer
   b. Centrifuge
   c. pH meter
   d. Incubator

Answers to Critical Thinking Questions

1. (b); 2. (b); 3. (c); 4. (b); 5. (a)

Short Answer Questions

1. What is the principle behind spectrophotometry, and what is it commonly used for in clinical labs?
2. How does centrifugation assist in preparing samples for analysis?
3. Describe the difference between manual and automated laboratory techniques.
4. What is microscopy used for in clinical pathology, and what are the common types of microscopes used?
5. Explain the purpose of electrophoresis in laboratory diagnostics.

References

1. Adey, A., Gehring, A., Benet-Pagès, A., Bainbridge, M., Bentley, D., Bergmann, C., Clark, A., et al. (2012). Diagnostic applications of next generation sequencing: Working towards quality standards. https://core.ac.uk/download/19418347.pdf (accessed on 1st July 2025).
2. Almuhaidb, A., Olson, D., & Aadam, A. (2021). Advancements in endoscopic biliary interventions by gastroenterology. *Seminars in Interventional Radiology, 38*, 280–290. https://www.semanticscholar.org/paper/92e4a8106989cec2cd736cc45b7541219c1f7976 (accessed on 1st July 2025).
3. Ardila, C. M. (2025). Advancing healthcare through laboratory on a chip technology: Transforming microorganism identification and diagnostics. *World Journal of Clinical Cases, 13*. https://www.semanticscholar.org/paper/851feb461807fffbe5add9837f6eb474cdc49250 (accessed on 1st July 2025).
4. Arendale, W. F., Kilgore, M. V., & Zahorchak, R. J. (2025). Definition of a near real time microbiological monitor for space vehicles. https://core.ac.uk/download/pdf/42821826.pdf (accessed on 1st July 2025).
5. Avci, O., Connor, J. H., Sevenler, D., Trueb, P., et al. (2017). Robust visualization and discrimination of nanoparticles by interferometric imaging. https://open.bu.edu/bitstream/2144/40114/4/Final_JSTQE_070116.pdf (accessed on 1st July 2025).
6. Bartlett, J. G., Department of Health and Human Services, Fajardo, E., Hamers, R. L., Bygrave, H., Jani, I., et al. (2012). Challenges and opportunities for the implementation of virological testing in resource-limited settings. https://core.ac.uk/download/pdf/10674424.pdf (accessed on 1st July 2025).
7. Bonica, M., Students of Health Management 721.01, & University of New Hampshire. (2017). *Healthcare Management Primer*. https://core.ac.uk/download/215509297.pdf (accessed on 1st July 2025).
8. Bottoni, F., Chang, S., Figueroa, M. S., Gaudric, A., et al. (2020). Optical coherence tomography-based consensus definition for lamellar macular hole. https://core.ac.uk/download/288432554.pdf (accessed on 1st July 2025).
9. Bradley, J. L. (2016). Obesity and asthma: Adiponectin receptor 1 (Adipo R1) and adiponectin receptor 2 (Adipo R2) are expressed by normal human bronchial epithelial (NHBE) cells at air-liquid interface (ALI) and expression changes with IL-13 stimulation. https://core.ac.uk/download/79819852.pdf (accessed on 1st July 2025).
10. Brownstein, M., Dowell, M. L., Gaigalas, A. K., Hoffman, R., et al. (2007). Biphotonic tools in cell and tissue diagnostics. https://core.ac.uk/download/323070689.pdf (accessed on 1st July 2025).
11. Capes-Davis, A., Davis, J. M., Downward, J., Freshney, R. I., et al. (2014). Guidelines for the use of cell lines in biomedical research. https://core.ac.uk/download/42355834.pdf (accessed on 1st July 2025).
12. Chmarra, M. K., Gómez Aguilera, E. J., Lamata de la Orden, P., Oropesa García, J. L., et al. (2011). Methods and tools for objective assessment of psychomotor skills in laparoscopic surgery. https://core.ac.uk/download/148661114.pdf (accessed on 1st July 2025).
13. Claesson, R., Johansson, A., & Belibasakis, G. (2022). Clinical laboratory diagnostics in

dentistry: Application of microbiological methods. *Frontiers in Oral Health, 3*. https://www.semanticscholar.org/paper/22627647de0a29ff4488839356c34bd6d817247a (accessed on 1st July 2025).

14. Devis, L., Closset, M., Degosserie, J., Lessire, S., Modrie, P., Gruson, D., Favaloro, E., et al. (2024). Revisiting the environmental impact of inappropriate clinical laboratory testing: A comprehensive overview of sustainability, economic, and quality of care outcomes. *The Journal of Applied Laboratory Medicine*. https://www.semanticscholar.org/paper/5490a62088303eddf9671d06439e8679e84b6627 (accessed on 1st July 2025).
15. d'Onofrio, G. (2021). Full-field hemocytometry. Forty years of progress seen through *Clinical and Laboratory Hematology* and *The International Journal of Laboratory Hematology*. https://core.ac.uk/download/604623263.pdf (accessed on 1st July 2025).
16. Ebert, P., Engel, A., Hoffmann, K., Macdonald, H. R., et al. (2005). *Journal of Fluorescence*. https://core.ac.uk/download/210638942.pdf (accessed on 1st July 2025).
17. Ferreira, C., Lima Gomes, P. C. F., Robison, K., Cooper, B. R., & Shannahan, J. H. (2024). Implementation of multiomic mass spectrometry approaches for the evaluation of human health following environmental exposure. *Molecular Omics, 20*, 296–321. https://www.semanticscholar.org/paper/3a28a33921b608f1f59cf7b37585dd5e4fb873b2 (accessed on 1st July 2025).
18. Figueroa, M., Katz, L., & Lazes, P. M. (2012). How labor-management partnerships improve patient care, cost control, and labor relations: Case studies of Fletcher Allen Health Care, Kaiser Permanente, and Montefiore Medical Center's Care Management Corporation. https://core.ac.uk/download/33611597.pdf (accessed on 1st July 2025).
19. Ford, R. E., Kushnir, M. M., Muck, W., Murdter, T. E., Rashed, M. S., Streit, F., et al. (2003). Liquid chromatography-tandem mass spectrometry–Application in the clinical laboratory. https://core.ac.uk/download/19418476.pdf (accessed on 1st July 2025).
20. Fortina, P., Kricka, L. J., Park, J. Y., & Polsky, T. G. (2015). The future of laboratory medicine–A 2014 perspective. https://core.ac.uk/download/54509579.pdf (accessed on 1st July 2025).
21. Fossey, A., Oosthuysen, J., & Potgieter, E. (2014). Compliance with infection prevention and control in oral health-care facilities: A global perspective. https://core.ac.uk/download/222967688.pdf (accessed on 1st July 2025).
22. Guo, H. (1998). Determination of creatinine and creatine by capillary electrophoresis: A thesis presented in partial fulfilment of the requirements for the degree of Master of Science in Chemistry at Massey University. https://core.ac.uk/download/148645066.pdf (accessed on 1st July 2025).
23. Hosseini, S., Martínez-Chapa, S. O., & Vázquez-Villegas, P. (2017). Paper and fiber-based bio-diagnostic platforms: Current challenges and future needs. https://core.ac.uk/download/157613422.pdf (accessed on 1st July 2025).
24. Kang, Y. P., Kim, H. M., Kwon, S. W., NGHI, T., et al. (2020). Toward a standardized strategy of clinical metabolomics for the advancement of precision medicine. https://core.ac.uk/download/288117835.pdf (accessed on 1st July 2025).
25. Lee, A. C. H. (2009). Ergonomics of the operative field in pediatric minimal access surgery. https://core.ac.uk/download/1591398.pdf (accessed on 1st July 2025).

26. Mody, K. A. (1994). Managing occupational hazards confronting healthcare workers. https://core.ac.uk/download/232278107.pdf (accessed on 1st July 2025).

27. Nicogossian, A. E. (2025). Space life sciences strategic plan. https://core.ac.uk/download/pdf/42811984.pdf (accessed on 1st July 2025).

28. Oosthuysen, J. (2015). Infection prevention and control audit-feedback instrument for oral health care in South Africa. https://core.ac.uk/download/222966850.pdf (accessed on 1st July 2025).

29. Pearson, G. S. (1998). Article X: Pharmaceutical building blocks. https://core.ac.uk/download/135047.pdf (accessed on 1st July 2025).

30. Pyne, A., & Bhattacharya, S. (2023). Option appraisal of matrix-assisted laser desorption ionization time of flight systems for a diagnostic microbiology laboratory. *Journal of The Academy of Clinical Microbiologists, 25*, 8–15. https://www.semanticscholar.org/paper/1495cfc39d8e4af446b296b29f8e18d3ae85ec55 (accessed on 1st July 2025).

31. Rajaei, S. N., Darvish, M., Zare, A., Abdollahi, H., Alivirdiloo, V., Hajiabbasi, M., Ghazi, F., et al. (2025). Advances in nano biosensors for rapid and sensitive detection of dengue virus biomarkers by using clinical laboratory. *Journal of Clinical Laboratory Analysis, 39*. https://www.semanticscholar.org/paper/8eeea37228f80e1347cfc606cbc06bba2c707ef9 (accessed on 1st July 2025).

32. Rosemann, A., Bharadwaj, B., Birch, B., Boeije, H., Brhlikova, P., Brunsson, N., et al. (2014). Standardization as situation-specific achievement: Regulatory diversity and the production of value in intercontinental collaborations in stem cell medicine. https://core.ac.uk/download/30609220.pdf (accessed on 1st July 2025).

33. Sarwate, R., Kundap, R., Gadre, G. A., Patil, P., & Shirke, D. B. (2023). Emerging therapies in retinal diseases: From gene therapy to stem cell interventions. https://core.ac.uk/download/596247487.pdf (accessed on 1st July 2025).

34. Schrijver, I., & Wiita, A. P. (2011). Clinical application of high throughput molecular screening techniques for pharmacogenomics. https://core.ac.uk/download/323063319.pdf (accessed on 1st July 2025).

35. Seaman, W., & Whitehouse, J. H. (2001). Florida marine biotechnology: Research, development and training capabilities to advance science and commerce. https://core.ac.uk/download/11016354.pdf (accessed on 1st July 2025).

36. Suazo Galdames, I. (2024). De la anatomía al algoritmo: Alcance de las competencias diagnósticas asistidas por inteligencia artificial en la educación en ciencias de la salud. https://core.ac.uk/download/630469681.pdf (accessed on 1st July 2025).

37. Swinckels, L., Bennis, F., Ziesemer, K. A., Scheerman, J., Bijwaard, H., de Keijzer, A., & Bruers, J. (2023). The use of deep learning and machine learning on longitudinal electronic health records for the early detection and prevention of diseases: Scoping review. *Journal of Medical Internet Research, 26*. https://www.semanticscholar.org/paper/bbb3bd1ff203e5707eb29234cb5666cb68c0a264 (accessed on 1st July 2025).

38. Zhou, M., Yao, Y., & Wu, G. (2023). Improvements in clinical laboratory techniques, technologies, and practices with a focus on the equipment and personnel: A consolidated review. *Journal of Clinical Medicine: Current Research*. https://www.semanticscholar.org/paper/8f1fb6805eb5bdc19e32ed4f82d3c30291297589 (accessed on 1st July 2025).

COMPOSITION AND FUNCTION OF BLOOD

3

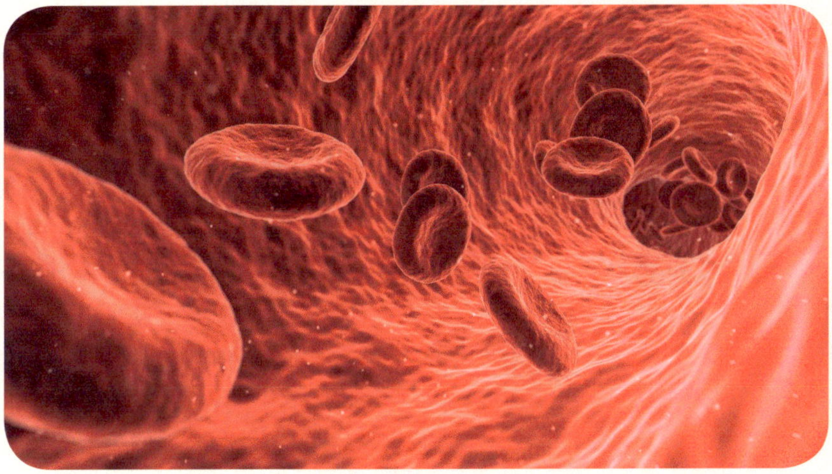

LEARNING OBJECTIVES

After studying this chapter, you will be able to:

1. Explore the components of blood;
2. Define plasma composition;
3. Discuss about red blood cells;
4. Describe white blood cells;
5. Explain platelets and coagulation;
6. Illustrate the blood typing and transfusions.

Introduction

Blood is not just some other fluid in the body; it is the hub of how our systems keep running, for the most part being a lifeline. Tissues and organs get their vitamins, oxygen, hormones, and even trash cleaned out by blood, which carries these essentials without complaint. Take a closer glance, though, and you'll see blood isn't a one-note drink—it's red cells that bring oxygen, white cells that fight off invaders, plasma, and a bit here and there that all in combination keep us going. All those layers, piled up again and again on each journey to the lab, have made blood a natural magnet for research. By and large, when you get to study the makeup of blood, you're peeling away layers of intricacy that are way deep within body function and overall health-even when the picture occasionally appears sort of blurry. Aside from just what makes up blood, its role reverberates into other corners of our physiology. It's not only delivering us the good stuff like nutrients and oxygen, but blood also maintains our body temperature and pH. Others prefer to think of it as a busy messenger, carrying messages between systems that might not even look connected at first glance. New research even suggests the annoying little critters that make our mouths their home can fine-tune blood pressure regulation—thanks to a domino cascade of dietary nitrates and nitric oxide generation (Barth et al., 2019). Overall, these results remind us of that individual-by-individual decisions and nanosecond-by-nanosecond interactions between bodily molecules can have a scandalous impact on heart health, even if it all looks more complicated than it would be neat to unravel. Looking inside the blood a little more carefully gives us hints not only about our own health but also about broad public health secrets. You can come to realize that differences in blood, related to age, gender, or ethnicity, at times dictate the form and administration of treatments for different people. It's interesting—nearly surprising—to discover that technology like GPS is used in sport medicine, whereby scientists correlate blood characteristics with sports performance (Van der Merwe et al., 2018). This combination of sports science, everyday nutrition, and blood science indicates a future beyond that will see medicine personalized, treating individuals to their unique requirements based on the idiosyncrasies of their blood. In the end, understanding the twists and curves of blood composition and function quite often is key to enhancing health outcomes for large numbers of people even if that endeavor is never direct (Figure 3.1).

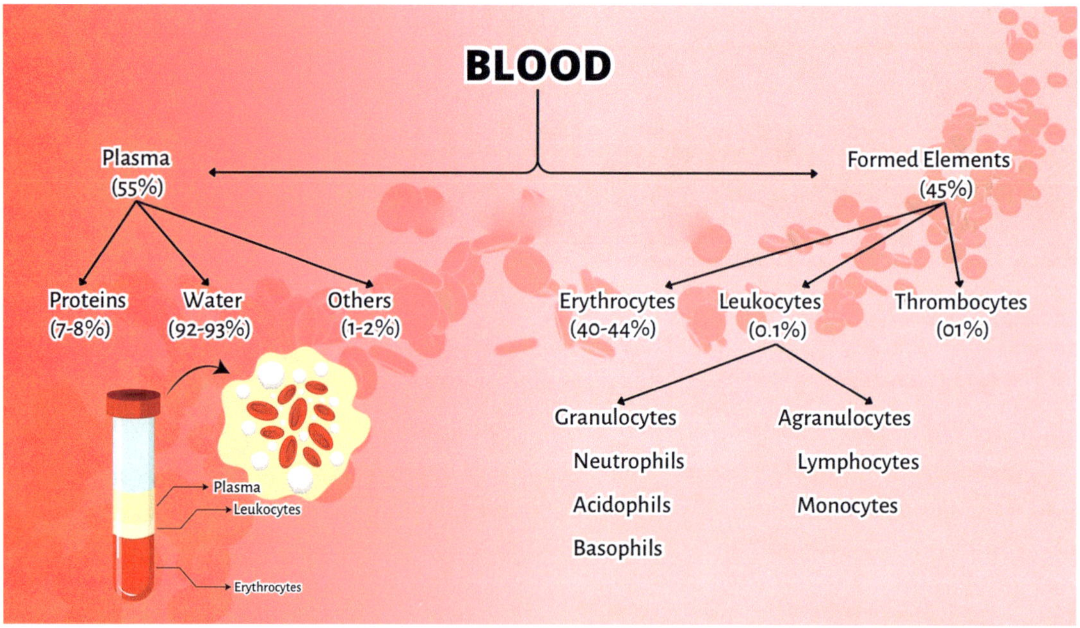

Figure 3.1. Blood and its composition.

Source: https://blogger.googleusercontent.com/img/b/R29vZ2xl/AVvXsEi-TTIsTR4w4oEjQEpKy618G4miyBvrYoXGrLTYIRtHFAabzPG_SzMbrRqCilRSsK24apAYH8Sr-JxFl3D4EU6J8e5n45hIxTCus1Yp4c_eOdKZAs_4j7nX_zIi0ufO-C-MmprFo0QSYaoftrsQIlNP_iSWMFyCVWwGeflJBwE_WG_kioOn11YkM7TANA/s1920/9D658056-AC28-409A-A8AA-1A3F816204B8.jpeg.

Definition of Blood

Blood is not just a liquid flowing through our veins—it's a living system that does so many things all at once. Your blood is made up mostly of plasma, red and white blood cells, and platelets in your body, and it doesn't just carry oxygen and nutrients around; it carries the waste away too. Various parts have different functions, rather like a multitasker that not only carries important stuff around but also protects against infections (white blood cells are like little soldiers) and assists in closing up wounds with necessary proteins. It's absolutely vital to know what blood all is really about if you would like to understand its many tasks in keeping our body in balance and secure. If you listen closely, blood is approximately 55% plasma and 45% what I call cellular material. Plasma—the water-pale yellow liquid filled with water, electrolytes, proteins, hormones, and nutrients—is a speedy freeway for the delivery of many different elements to where they're needed. Red blood cells, filled with hemoglobin, are the oxygen-transport heroes. And whereas white blood cells are less numerous, they're just as vital in sensing and destroying unwelcome intruders. And don't forget platelets; the minute units quickly come together to form clumps which stop bleeding, even though they're the smallest fraction. This mixture, all functioning in its own capricious way, is responsible for a lot of our health and can warn us if things go wrong. Blood is not only for the delivery of gases, nutrients, and wastes—it also keeps us balanced overall. It regulates temperature, pH, and even fluid volume outside cells, as well as delivering hormones that coordinate functions in different parts of the body. In the majority of cases, even small changes in its composition can signal diabetes or heart disease. Some clinical research is suggesting that a more detailed analysis of blood's physical and biochemical properties might reveal disease precursors (Abt et al., 2012; Antonopoulos et al., 2019). In general, it would appear that unlocking blood's many secrets is the secret to understanding how the human body works, and is the subject of much current medical investigation—even if its complexity at times appears to be a little overwhelming.

Importance of Studying Blood

Blood is significant. It plays a large role in advancing medicine and keeping one in normal everyday health. Similar to a clogged road system, it carries around nutrients, hormones, and waste within the body - all for equilibrium, in most cases. More often than not, scrutinizing its makeup close up yields minuscule information regarding one's health, even indicating potential infections or illness. Researchers have, by and large, studied the low numbers of microbes connected with many diseases and found that blood samples can at times provide indications of underlying problems. For example, some studies have shown that traits within gut flora are linked with Crohn's disease and show just how synchronized blood material can be with overall bodily function. These findings emphasize the value of further blood research, which can help us uncover the mysteries of disease processes and improve treatments (Bertz et al., 2017). Blood testing offers a glimpse into broad public health challenges - think about heart issues, for instance. Decades-long investigations of cardiovascular and stroke conditions have ironically resulted in a plethora of major breakthroughs. In all but a few cases, when blood testing is combined with other indicators like cholesterol and glucose levels, it is clear that early warning signs capture are very significant. Not only does such research enhance individual care, but it also guides community programs to decrease the number of heart disease and stroke occurrences (Buxton et al., 2011). At times, these revelations even come from the most unlikely sources, proving that our circulatory system contains more secrets than one would imagine. Peering into blood tells us more than mere medical diagnostics; it tells us a tale about how our body is really working. This liquid contains hints on how efficiently organs are functioning, what the immune system is doing, and—even the rate of metabolism overall. Labs that check the levels of substances like red and white blood cells and platelets generally give doctors a snapshot of disease ranging from infection to clotting disorders or anemia. In most cases, the information informs more precise treatments and encourages prevention too. When you think about it, discovering blood isn't so much an intellectual exercise—it's a steppingstone to improving healthcare and improving lives in general (Bertz et al., 2017).

Overview of Blood Composition and Functions

Red blood cells are fascinating. They're not just little oxygen-delivery units; they absorb oxygen in the lungs and transport it to tissues, and then—they even help deliver carbon dioxide back so you can breathe it out. Recently, groundbreaking proteomic analysis studies have actually peeled back the layers on the erythrocyte membrane to show that such cells have a remarkably rich inner life that goes far beyond simple gas exchange.

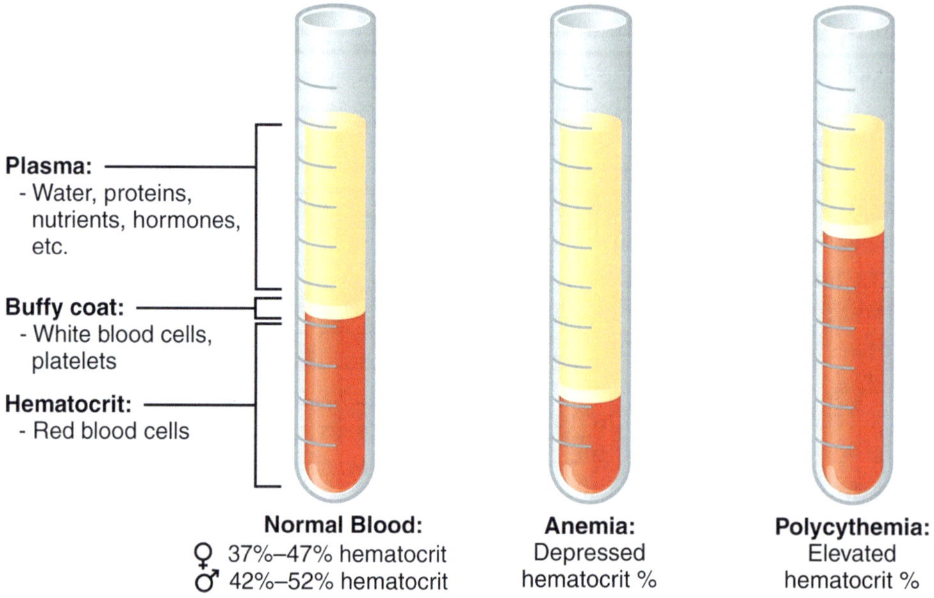

Figure 3.2. Blood composition and functions.

Source: https://pressbooks.bccampus.ca/pathology/wp-content/uploads/sites/1260/2022/12/composition-of-blood.jpg.

Even in most cases, such cells betray adhesion molecules similar to other cell types, indicating they have roles in cellular interactions and immune function (Oliveira et al., 2010). A lot is going on in blood, too. Plasma, which makes up approximately 55% of the volume of blood, is no sedate fluid; it's a harried delivery vehicle for metabolites, hormones, and waste products of metabolism. It's also packed with proteins that regulate everything from blood clotting to immunity. White blood cells, or leukocytes, are all shapes and sizes, like lymphocytes and neutrophils, and they're all co-operating (sometimes in cooperating combinations) to fend off invaders. If you take the time to think about it, all these different elements of blood are all part of keeping our bodies in balance and fending off infection (Berger et al., 2016). Blood's role is so much more far-reaching, far more than just carrying gases around. It keeps pH levels steady and keeps body temperature from running amok, so to speak, like a natural buffering against external variations. Hemostasis, the clotting mechanism that keeps us from bleeding when we're hurt, is another example of how blood functions to protect us. Additionally, the interaction between different cells and plasma proteins encourages healing of wounds and recovery from infection. In general, blood is not merely a transport medium, but rather an active, multifunctional participant in virtually every aspect of our overall physiology (Oliveira et al., 2010) (Figure 3.2).

3.1. Components of Blood

Learning Outcome

- Plasma;
- Red blood cells (erythrocytes);
- White blood cells (leukocytes).

Blood is not a liquid; it's a jumble of ingredients that work together in some pretty odd combinations to keep our bodies running at their best. Take plasma, for example—it makes up approximately 55% of our blood and basically acts as the transportation belt for nutrients, hormones, and waste. Mostly water, plasma also carries electrolytes, proteins, and a variety of organic and inorganic bits that help our metabolic processes run as they should. You've got proteins like albumin, globulins, and fibrinogen in there too, which generally help maintain the right balance in pressure, defend against invaders, and ensure proper clotting. And, in a sort of reserve capacity, plasma carries other factors that adjust blood thickness and flow, influencing how well our blood circulates.

Most of the time, this shifting set isn't simply a matter of juggling around—it's an active part of the adjustment that keeps us healthy and alive. Red blood cells, being the most common cell type in our circulation, have an important role to play in oxygen delivery. These biconcave, hemoglobin-containing cells are tailored to trap oxygen and deposit it where it's headed, energizing our tissues for aerobic work.

Their elastic cell membranes and absence of a nucleus enable them to pass through even the tiny capillaries, providing them with all that much-loved surface area for gas exchange. When there are not enough of them—a condition that we call anemia—it truly says a lot about just how important their job is in keeping our body's oxygen supply. Hormone messages, especially erythropoietin, always regulate both their development and their longevity, modulating based on what the body requires. In all, if these cells are not at maximum capacity, tissues might not get the oxygen to perform at their best, a reminder of how they work diligently for our overall health.

Platelets might be quantitatively less than red cells, but in the management of bleeding, they are completely irreplaceable. These tiny fragments, which are the product of megakaryocytes in bone marrow, spring into action when a blood vessel is injured. Almost like emergency responders, platelets quickly coalesce to form a temporary plug that closes off the bleeding and gives subsequent healing tissue a crude scaffolding. It's not a one-act show, either—the whole clotting process is a series of signals, clotting factors, and pathways, with the platelet being the star of the show. When something goes awry with their function, it can lead to complications like runaway bleeding or even unwanted clotting.

Some studies actually propose a role for platelets in regulating inflammatory and immune responses. Anyway, knowing all these varied things does serve to put in perspective how blood comes in not just to transport things but also to heal and keep our internal balance intact (Figure 3.3).

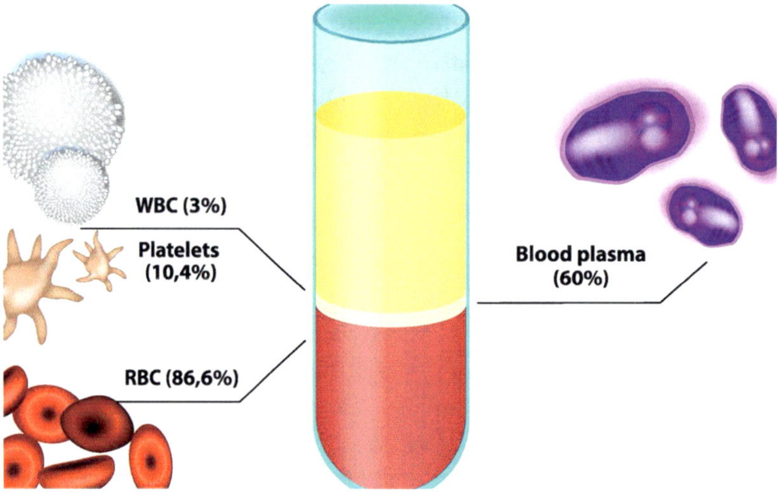

Figure 3.3. Components of blood.

Source: https://external-content.duckduckgo.com/iu/?u=https%3A%2F%2Fwww.lifeservebloodcenter.org%2Fwebres%2FImage%2Fblood-components-header.jpg&f=1&nofb=1&ipt=c876c1432d49818e9ce82a61e9695f4f0651e75a6c4d06e2723b2e414bf1c2da.

3.1.1. Plasma

Plasma is one of the most essential pieces of the blood jigsaw. It makes up approximately 55% of our blood and is the pale yellowish liquid—mostly water mixed with proteins, electrolytes, nutrients, and even some waste products. For most occasions, albumin is the protein that keeps osmotic pressure stable while globulins help with immune processes, and then there is fibrinogen, which comes in to form clots in the event of injury. This cocktail of diversity is not just reorganizing cells; it's keeping our emotional equilibrium intact by giving the tissues what they need so that life-sustaining functions go on uninterrupted even when conditions change. Plasma not only serves as a delivery system but also acts to moderate the responses of our bodies. When you're in motion or change your diet, plasma can flow in unforeseen directions. For instance, once you have a bout of exercise under way, the body will discharge tiny packages called microvesicles (MVs) into the blood. These little messengers carry bioactive molecules that make the cells "talk" to one another, driving the heart and blood vessels toward quick reactions and even long-term adaptations. Most often, the changes point out just how malleable our circulatory system is, although you may not realize so simply from the work that it does hauling stuff. Apart from the delivery of nutrients and messages, plasma also plays an important role in immune protection and inflammation. The suspended immunoglobulins are around the clock to identify and destroy the intruders like bacteria and viruses by binding to them and tagging them for other immune cells to kill. Plasma is also a storage complex facility—it transports various signaling substances, such as cytokines, which control our immune reactions. Sometimes, in inflammatory responses, cell-derived microvesicle production seems to enable cells to communicate in a way that is not so linear (Mourot et al., 2018). In general, plasma is not a passive substance; its dynamic transport, control, and protective functions make it an integral part of how our bodies establish health, even if its functioning at times seems a bit capricious (Figure 3.4).

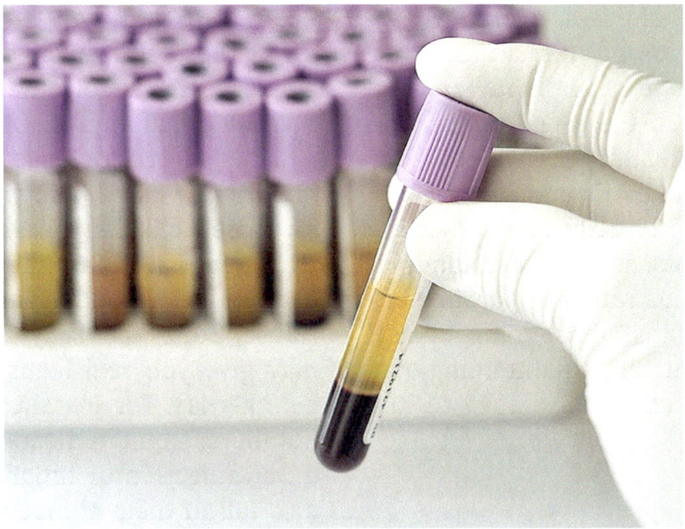

Figure 3.4. Plasma.

Source: https://external-content.duckduckgo.com/iu/?u=https%3A%2F%2Fimg.medscape.com%2Fnews%2F2014%2Fts_140729_blood_test_tube_laboratory_800x600.jpg&f=1&nofb=1&ipt=3eba22f8d8b1fa8e54f90cc01e19378fcd998446db45720e80129f98fa66ac57.

3.1.2. Red Blood Cells (Erythrocytes)

Blood works to a large degree because of its cells – specifically red blood cells, or erythrocytes. These biconcave small workers transport oxygen from our lungs to tissues and back to the lungs as carbon dioxide. Their shape, which provides them with a huge surface area compared to volume, allows for gas exchange. New methods, including laser interference microscopy and Raman spectroscopy, have shed some light in the last few years on how the actual shape of these cells influences their work. In most cases, patients with cardiac problems exhibit abnormalities in the shape and composition of their red blood cells, thereby disrupting oxygen delivery. Thus, the methods of increasing oxygen supply need to aim not only at conventional treatments but also at improving how hemoglobin works in O_2 transport (Gromova et al., 2016). Focusing more on details, the ultrastructure of erythrocyte membranes has been coming into focus—mostly because it is applicable for both normal body functions and disease cases. Proteomic analyses have, in a very fascinating manner, shown us that such membranes are not just a gas-transport shell. They do possess a collection of stick-in molecules which could regulate the way that cells talk. This finding prompts us to challenge the long-held assumption that red blood cells merely serve as passive messengers; they could be doing a more active role in keeping our vessels healthy. Some scientists think that by modifying these factors of adhesion, we might be able to open up potentially entirely novel ways of curing disease where red blood cell function goes awry. By examining the dynamic performance of those membranes, researchers are gradually piecing together how structural differences in their composition can affect both oxygen transport and blood function overall (Oliveira et al., 2010). If you take a step back and examine what red blood cells do, their function is more than simply transferring gases; they're a key to general body health and in the processes, we use to fight off disease. Studies of erythrocytes in different states of illness – cardiovascular disease is a particularly good example – have noted profound changes in membrane lipids and even in the slight viscosity differences that hinder normal passage of gases. Overall, these advances suggest that it's not just a matter of symptom treatment – we need therapies that address the subtleties of the cells themselves. Continued research is leading the way toward early diagnosis techniques that may catch on to these subtleties, potentially leading us to more effective treatments. As our understanding slowly builds, it becomes rather apparent that red blood cells are not just about transporting oxygen; they're also critical in maintaining our circulatory system in check (Gromova et al., 2016) (Figure 3.5).

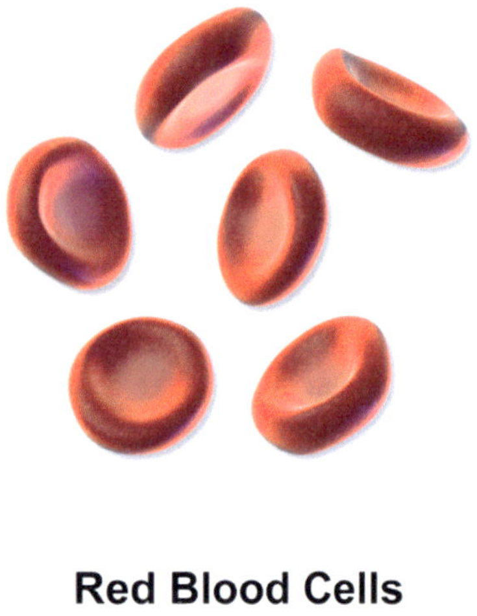

Figure 3.5. Red blood cell.

Source: https://upload.wikimedia.org/wikipedia/commons/3/39/Blausen_0761_RedBloodCells.png.

3.1.3. White Blood Cells (Leukocytes)

White blood cells are the unsung heroes that the immune system relies on. They have the entire network of proteins and cells wrapping around these leukocytes, which are the most critical for killing infections and unwelcome guests. They mostly come from the bone marrow, where stem cells split into different types – like neutrophils, lymphocytes, and monocytes. All of these classes, on the other hand, target bacteria, viruses, or other pesky intruders. The division of function enables the body to develop a highly specific defense against disease. In the majority of cases, knowledge of the functions of these cells helps researchers create new treatments since alterations in their numbers usually reflect underlying medical conditions (Musa, 2022). Leukocyte counts in your blood may give you real leads on what is going on health-wise. For instance, a big spike in their numbers might indicate your body's fighting off an infection or inflammation of some sort, or a fall in their numbers might indicate bone marrow difficulties or even drug reactions. Doctors make diagnoses ranging from allergies to more serious infections based on such leads. The number of these white blood cells, which segments them into different groups, informs us even further about how your body reacts to stress. Generally speaking, this close review shows that these cells are not sitting on the sidelines; in fact, they have an active role in evening things out. A tight handle on how they function opens doors to more refined diagnostic and treatment strategies (Drake-Holland et al., 2018). Leukocytes do not just push germs away—these cells play a big role in repairing tissues and controlling inflammation too. When things get tense, these cells rush headlong into the trouble spot, signaling for additional immune reinforcements to repair the location. Sometimes that involves phagocytosis when some of these cells actually digest the trash to start repairs. Their findings with the vascular glycocalyx also demonstrate how extremely intertwined the immune system and cardiovascular health are. If these processes come to a halt, it can result in chronic inflammation or a whole host of issues, so it makes a pretty clear point that getting deep into the mechanisms of leukocytes is important to help decipher many diseases (Musa, 2022) (Figure 3.6).

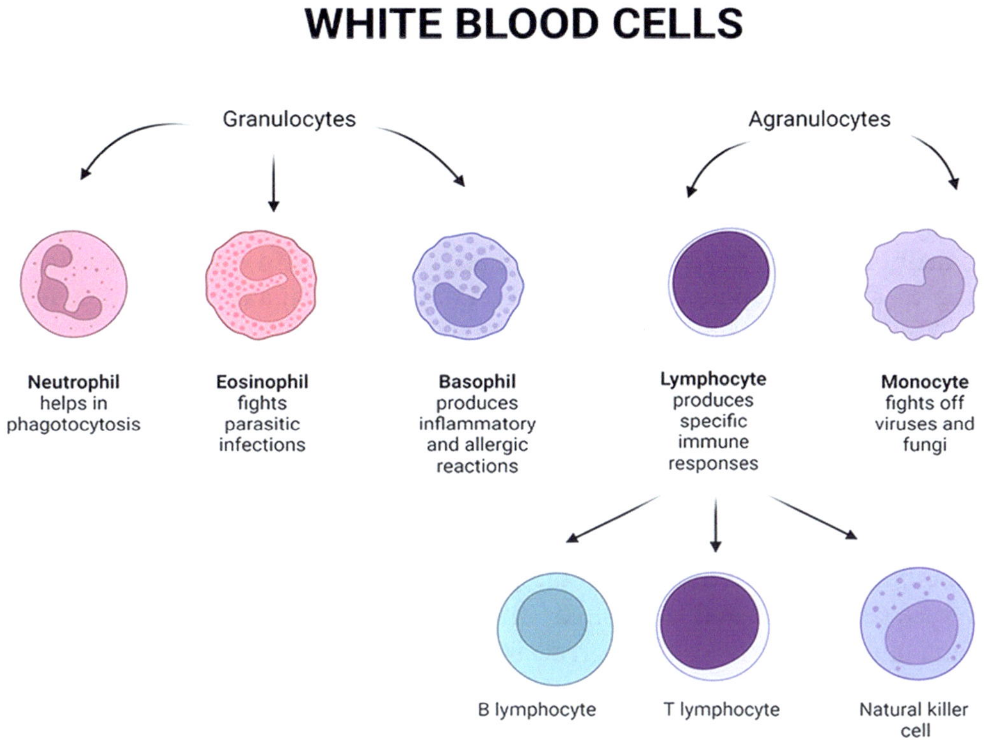

Figure 3.6. White blood cells (leukocytes).

Source: https://encrypted-tbn0.gstatic.com/images?q=tbn:ANd9GcTPcv0bvClRkW_Rx253rD6GicMiQy9U9pxvkg&s.

Test Your Knowledge

1. What are the four main components of blood and their primary functions?
2. How does the cellular portion of blood differ from the plasma portion?

3.2. Plasma Composition

Learning Outcome

- Water content;
- Proteins in plasma;
- Electrolytes and nutrients.

Blood is a wild mixture of things that keeps our body in operating condition and stimulates metabolism. The liquid part, plasma, makes up about 55% of blood composition and carries water, proteins, electrolytes, nutrients, hormones, and even waste. Mostly, plasma is about 90% water – functioning more like a solvent that is used to drive these molecules around in our blood. Albumin, globulins, and fibrinogen are just a few examples of proteins that are important not only for maintaining water levels within the body and keeping our immune system on its toes; they also serve to clot the blood when a clot is necessary. As it happens, getting a sense of how these elements bump around and balance out can truly serve to measure overall health, as even modest changes in plasma composition may suggest underlying issues. Scientists have been studying small bubbles in plasma called extracellular vesicles (EVs)—small messengers that are made up of exosomes and microvesicles. These vesicles carry proteins, lipids, and fragments of genetic material between cells in surprising and at times enigmatic manners. Current research has confirmed that these small messengers have a large role to play in our everyday lives, as well as addressing issues such as cancer and inflammation. As we learn more about them, there has been a trend— in most cases—toward open approaches to studying them, leading to the development of guidelines known as Minimal Information for Studies of Extracellular Vesicles 2018 (MISEV2018).

These guidelines, although detailed, exist primarily to ensure research integrity by requiring proper documentation of extracellular vesicle (EV) functions in relation to overall blood composition and body health (Théry et al., 2018). Studying the interaction between plasma components and muscle effort reveals new perspectives regarding how body function is determined by blood composition. The subtle cues of calcium, in the view of some studies, are said to regulate muscle gene expression, linking nerve function to the properties of our blood. Free calcium, balanced by electrolytes such as sodium and potassium, directly affects slow-twitch and fast-twitch muscle fibers. Calcium fluctuations in cells, spurred in part by the way in which motor neurons fire, regulate muscle-specific gene expression. Not only does this illustrate a rather intricate relationship between plasma composition and muscle physiology but it is also one that points to plasma as more than a delivery system—it's a participant in cellular signaling mechanisms (Damm et al., 2014) (Figure 3.7).

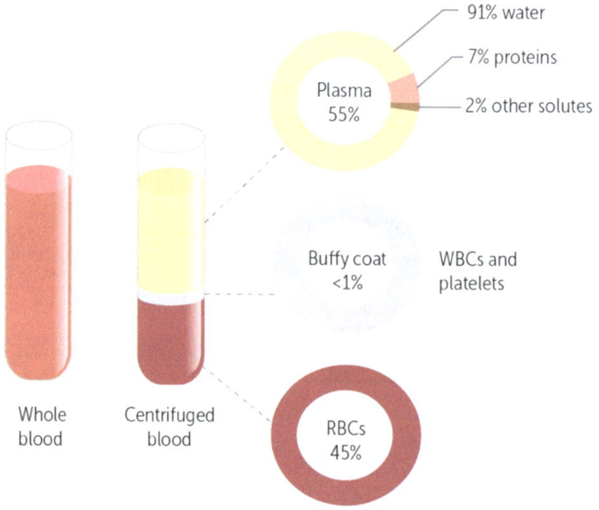

Figure 3.7. Plasma composition.

Source: https://external-content.duckduckgo.com/iu/?u=https%3A%2F%2Fusmle-rx.com%2Fwp-content%2Fuploads%2F2021%2F02%2FPlasma-Composition.png&f=1&nofb=1&ipt=068c8c3d0aabd4c16331b3543537909ef5d054d85fe629eba1d23d2711e9c69e.

3.2.1. Water content

Blood is an active mix of materials that indicates all the work that it performs in our body. Take water – it makes up about 90% of blood plasma and isn't just filler. It pushes through nutrients, hormones, and waste, ensuring some cells get what they need. Water also plays the role of keeping blood volume and pressure within limits, and, in general, if its quantities get too away from usual, the fluidity and flow of the blood may be affected. Water's work does not stop here. It also keeps our body temperature steady. With its great ability to absorb and distribute heat, water cools the body every time it becomes too hot—whether from the environment or physical activity. This cooling function is instrumental in situations involving physical activity and changing environments. Moreover, by helping eliminate waste through sweating and urination, water seals into a system that relies on proper hydration, even if at times it might seem a bit convoluted. Another aspect is how our diet is a part of this whole equation. Some studies have shown that what we eat—such as iodine-enriched feed or sea algae additives—can alter blood composition and even fluctuate enzyme and protein levels (Shadrin et al., 2024). Since most cases are focused on added hydration, this actually activates other metabolic activities. By calmly increasing water content through our intake, we may well be improving blood function as well as general health. Ultimately, understanding the function of water in blood reminds us that nutrition and hydration complement each other in balancing the body to perfection.

3.2.2. Proteins in Plasma

Proteins in our blood don't do nothing—instead, they work in most surprising ways to keep everything under control. Albumin, for instance, is everywhere and plays more than one role. It keeps fluid levels steady even while transporting hormones and fatty acids around. Other proteins like globulins and fibrinogen play roles too. One assists immune defenses and the other springs into action when clots are produced. If you look at how the proteins substitute and complement each other, you can see how even small alterations can result in diseases; that's why many clinicians keep their concentrations under very close observation. Plasma proteins do not play a spectator role; they play an active role in a wide range of biochemical reactions that are essential to our everyday requirements.

Fibrinogen, for instance, changes into fibrin during injury in a perfectly timed course that halts the bleeding. Scientists have even documented how variations in protein composition can influence how our bodies heal. One study compared platelet-rich plasma with hyperacute serum and determined that, even with identical preparation methods, differences in cytokines and growth factors (Bánáti et al., 2019) can really make the difference in healing. This blend of protein amounts and physiological responses emphasizes the importance of protein analysis in diagnostics and treatments. On a larger level, proteins collaborate in ways that go far beyond what each does individually. Generally speaking, high molecular weight kininogen (HMWK) at times helps to dislodge other proteins—fibrinogen, for instance—from cell surfaces, revealing a rather intricate style of teamwork (Beugeling et al., 1996). In other words, plasma proteins not only carry nutrients, but also regulate immune responses and the body's reaction to damage and inflammation. Studying these interactions can give clues as to why certain diseases occur and could even result in new therapeutic opportunities. Overall, understanding how these molecules interact is key to building our basic science knowledge and clinical practices in hematology (Figure 3.8).

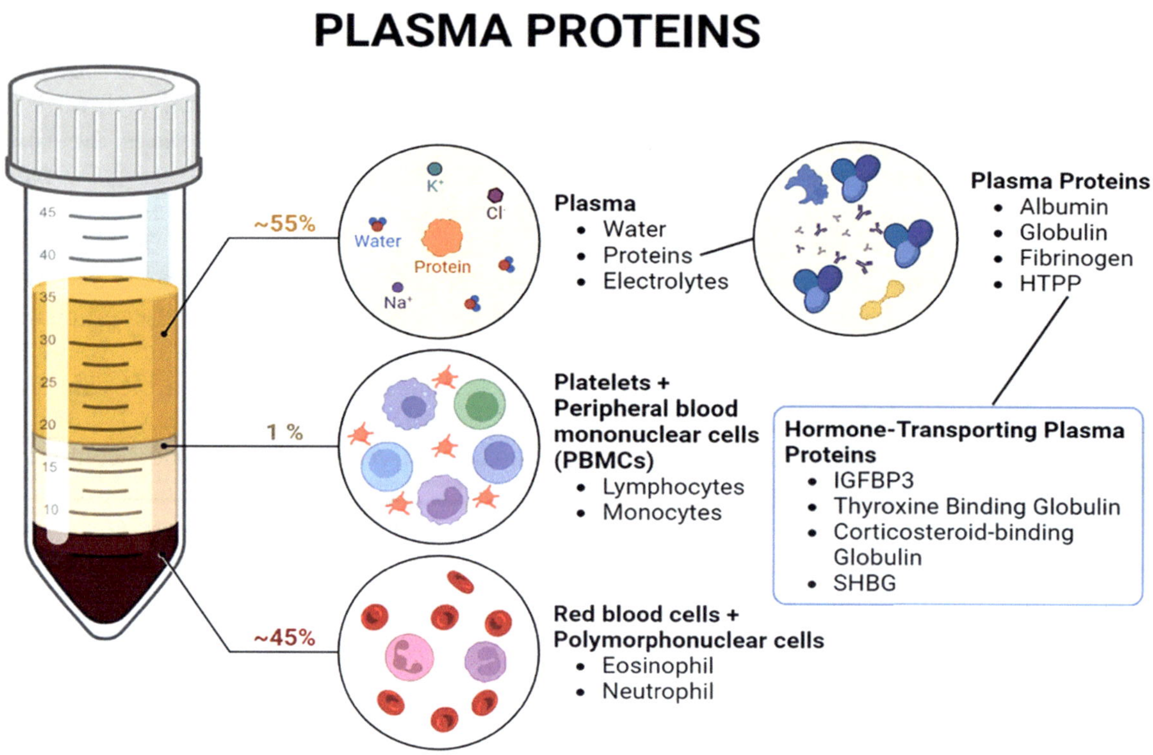

Figure 3.8. Proteins in plasma.

Source: https://external-content.duckduckgo.com/iu/?u=https%3A%2F%2Fendoconsult.b-cdn.net%2Fwp-content%2Fuploads%2Fplasma-proteins-768x538.png&f=1&nofb=1&ipt=decc46f99328043e64270fb5cbab4303e42e0fd9ed1a2b257b88e1a30fa91c2b.

3.2.3. Electrolytes and nutrients

Electrolyte balance is essential to our overall well-being—it's one of those that we never actually do think about, but do actually need for maintaining blood in top condition. Sodium, potassium, calcium, and chloride, just to mention a few, all have their own little tasks: sodium maintains fluid status and osmotic pressure just so (sodium controls osmotic pressure, for example, while potassium—essential—allows heartbeats and muscle contractions). In the vast majority of situations, when these levels are off, there are severe consequences for one's health. Even in unphysiological conditions, such as space travel, where metabolic needs are greater, it is clear that an understanding of the functions and the sources of these electrolytes is crucial. As the LSRO report most commonly indicates, making sure you get the right mix of these vital ingredients is no small thing, especially where your body needs differ in microgravity environments (Altman et al., 1986). Along with electrolytes, nutrients—like vitamins and trace minerals—aid in keeping blood in proper working condition. Take iron, for example; it's absolutely crucial to hemoglobin development, which is what enables red blood cells to deliver oxygen to the body. And last but not least, there are minerals like zinc and copper that, believe it or not, are highly associated with enzyme activity and in fact play a part in antioxidant defense. The body needs a constant supply of these nutrients because the lack of them results in anemia and weakened immunity. In the majority of cases, there is a kind of back-and-forth exchange between electrolytes and such nutrients that fuels core functions like energy production and cell regeneration. Science, including science on astronauts suffering from metabolic challenges, showcases the importance of eating sensibly with balanced meals and balancing nutrients (Kalmar et al., 2009). Balancing electrolytes and nutrients is not a complicated matter reserved for radical situations—it applies to all of us. Nowadays, however, so many diets depend on processed foods, high in sodium, but with extremely minimal nutrients, and that is sure to throw your body's equilibrium into turmoil. Eat whole nutrient foods to prevent deficiencies and assure best blood functioning. Public health education campaigns that inform people about the importance of doing these correctly can have a lasting influence. Understand how electrolytes and nutrients function together to help create sound nutritional advice. This is not just daily well-being; it also helps us better deal with nutritional needs when in extremely challenging, high-risk situations (Altman et al., 1986; Kalmar et al., 2009).

Test Your Knowledge

1. What are the major proteins found in plasma, and what roles do they play?
2. How does plasma help in maintaining osmotic balance and pH stability?

3.3. Red Blood Cells

Learning Outcome

- Structure and function;
- Hemoglobin and oxygen transport;
- Lifespan and recycling of red blood cells.

The composition of blood at the microscopic level holds numerous secrets about its varied work within the body. Red blood cells, or RBCs, are responsible for a significant amount of oxygen transport. Take erythrocytes, for instance—these have a biconcave shape that is not simply for show but gives them ample surface area to improve gas exchange. They absorb oxygen in the lungs and distribute it to tissues, and they help carry carbon dioxide the opposite way. Recently, new protein discoveries have enabled us to look inside and observe what drives these cells, down to the organization of their membrane packed with adhesion molecules that might be doing more than pumping gases, potentially even enabling some cell-to-cell communication in the blood (Oliveira et al., 2010). It's no one-trick pony, either. Red cells, along with platelets and leukocytes, mix things up in ways that can affect clot formation—most significantly in diseases such as cardiovascular disease. Clotting (thrombosis) sometimes engages these cells directly. A clot in most cases is not merely a tidy package of red cells; it is a disorganized agglomeration of RBCs, platelets, fibrin, and leukocytes. Briefly, RBCs appear to initiate the clot to form and then remain to maintain it stable. Understanding this patchwork is key to appreciating treatments that might prevent those fatal clogs from occurring that cause less blood to flow (Alkarithi et al., 2021). RBCs don't just carry gases throughout our system, either—helping to maintain things balanced. They serve a sort of repository function for nitric oxide, which is quite important to maintaining relaxed blood vessels and healthy functioning. That dual role, carrying oxygen and storing nitric oxide, would be consistent with some new studies suggesting that adhesion molecules on such cells might enable them to communicate directly with other cells in our vessels. In addition, as the composition of these cells is changing, it could indicate larger body changes, such as response to low oxygen or inflammation; these, in turn, will become useful adjuncts to clinical examination. And as more and more becomes known about the function of red blood cells, the prospect of new treatment—especially in cardiovascular disease—is both alive and promising (Oliveira et al., 2010) (Figure 3.9).

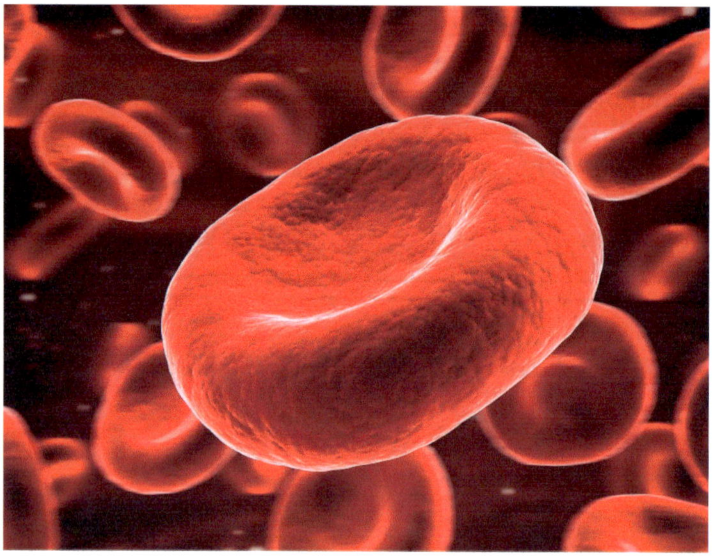

Figure 3.9. Red blood cells.

Source: https://external-content.duckduckgo.com/iu/?u=https%3A%2F%2Fhealthjade.com%2Fwp-content%2Fuploads%2F2017%2F09%2Fred-blood-cells.jpg&f=1&nofb=1&ipt=7d4495dbfe396e619090e848044778f66371cc62e12ef9a3f726e4e131f86b72.

3.3.1. Structure and Function

Blood components combine with one another in patterns that determine the strength and nature of our circulatory system. You observe it when a clot—by which physicians refer to a thrombus—develops, as cells and other fragments come together in surprising combinations to create something hard. When observed more closely, one discovers fibrin, red blood cells, platelets, leukocytes, and even neutrophil extracellular traps all knotted up together. They all have a part to play, so fibrin is crucial in maintaining things firm, while platelets start the clotting. From time to time, when something like a heart attack or acute ischemic stroke occurs, the constitution of these clots becomes altered, just proving how adaptable blood is. Overall, this seemingly disorganized but purposeful mix not only shows that structure and function are intertwined, but also reflects new ways of approaching thrombotic complications (Alkarithi et al., 2021). Blood does more than coagulate—it also drives many necessary operations that keep our systems in balance. Consider red blood cells, for example: their biconcave, nearly vintage shape puts them in excellent condition for most gas exchange by providing additional surface area and reduced distance for oxygen travel. Their membranes, bearing varying charges and lipid compositions, then become involved in the manner such cells interact with the blood stream. For example, a more negatively charged vessel lining has been found to control what gets through, even in areas that are narrowed, such as the blood-brain barrier (BBB). Fundamentally, how some drugs get past these barriers relates to the specific architecture of our blood cells and also points to the relationship between design, the manner in which things are carried around the body, and even how drugs interact with us once inside (Castanho et al., 2012). The structure of blood also springs into action in immune reactions and inflammation. Leukocytes, heterogeneous in form and size, highlight the body's responsive nature in the face of different challenges. In a clot, the mixture under the control of these white blood cells exhibits an image of a multidimensional rapid response to injury—cells not only help build the clot but also discharge chemicals that drive inflammation. This frequent realignment and interaction between the components, particularly during disease states, illustrates vividly that a little bit of structural heterogeneity may contribute to significant functional variation. Understanding most of these little changes in most instances is quite crucial in developing improved treatments for diseases such as thrombosis. And as ongoing studies peer into these relationships, it becomes only clearer that both the fine details and the master plan of our blood have an important part to play in keeping us healthy (Alkarithi et al., 2021) (Figure 3.10).

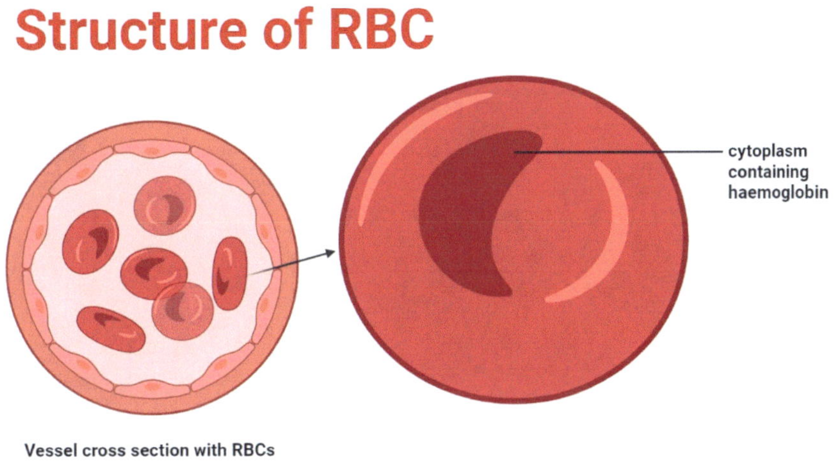

Figure 3.10. Structure of red blood cells.

Source: https://microbenotes.com/wp-content/uploads/2024/04/Structure-of-Red-Blood-Cells-RBCs.jpeg.

3.3.2. Hemoglobin and oxygen transport

Oxygen moves around our bodies in a way that completely depends on hemoglobin—a special protein found in red blood cells. The protein has four parts, with each part having its own heme group that can hold an oxygen molecule. Once one heme molecule binds to oxygen, it appears to get the others to hold oxygen with less effort. That is, in the lungs, the hemoglobin picks up oxygen seamlessly and then deposits it where it's needed in the tissues. The way hemoglobin oxygenates is not set; it depends on things like pH, carbon dioxide, and even temperature—things that, in most cases, mirror what's occurring metabolically in different parts of the body. Aside from the mere carriage of oxygen, hemoglobin has another important function: it helps in the elimination of carbon dioxide, a byproduct of the metabolism of our cells. In tissues, not only does it pick up oxygen, but it also seizes carbon dioxide and carries it back to the lungs, which we breathe out. This two-fold job is necessary in order to sustain our breathing and acid–base balance. The Bohr effect, for instance, is the fact that when carbon dioxide levels rise and the environment is slightly more acidic (lower pH), hemoglobin releases oxygen more readily. And thus, when we are stressed—exercising, for instance—this trait has a clear effect on delivering oxygen precisely when it is required. In the last few years, we have learned more about how changes in hemoglobin function can influence our health. Diseases such as thalassemia and sickle cell anemia, for instance, exist because hemoglobin is constructed incorrectly, which disrupts its function to carry oxygen. These illnesses highlight just how critical the design of the protein is in making us healthy. And that's not all: conditions such as type 2 diabetes mellitus (T2DM) have been associated with hemoglobin level and function alteration, which may interfere with oxygen delivery and even enhance the risk for cardiac complications (Galicia-Garc et al., 2020). While scientists remain to find new treatments, how hemoglobin handles carbon dioxide and oxygen remains an important piece of the puzzle for future clinical advances (André et al., 2019) (Figure 3.11).

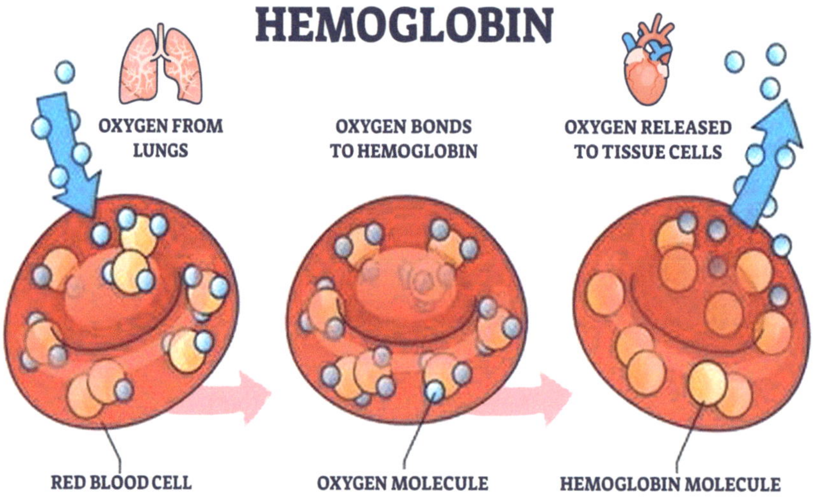

Figure 3.11. Hemoglobin and oxygen transport.

Source: https://www.shutterstock.com/image-vector/hemoglobin-oxygen-gas-transportation-mechanism-260nw-2386001795.jpg.

3.3.3. Lifespan and Recycling of Red Blood Cells

Red blood cells do have a natural lifespan. They start in the marrow and spend about 120 days circulating throughout our bloodstream in unrest before they finally die. With the passage of time, as they age, they tend to change in tiny but crucial ways, so that the spleen is forced to keep an eye out, eliminating those spent cells. Once tagged, the cells are broken into fragments so that useful pieces like hemoglobin and iron are released and can be reused to form new cells—a recycling mechanism that efficiently keeps the body's balance of key resources from overwhelming the system. Inside the body, the cells undergo both internal stress as well as oxidative stress. When red blood cells are pushed through narrow capillaries, mechanical strain and shifting microenvironments summate and sometimes result in damage. Most frequently, after their about 120-day duration is complete, such damaged cells undergo lysis in hemolysis, and macrophages scavenge the resultant detritus. The freed iron, now being unbound, is not wasted; it is required to synthesize new blood cells and power many metabolic processes. This ongoing cycle, in turn, reveals the surprising relationship between the cells' ability to function and the organism's health. This connection keeps scientists working especially in the context of aging populations. Recent studies have begun to uncover mechanisms that control red blood cell longevity. Oxidative stress, a bit of genomic instability, and plain old aging itself all seem to chip away at these cells, perhaps being connected with diseases like anemia and even heart disease. Mostly, this work is part of bigger studies on mechanisms of aging—autophagy, for instance, the process of naturally breaking down old parts of cells. Therefore, gaining better insight into the aging and recycling of these cells enhances our knowledge of blood health and also emphasizes the need to integrate outcomes of research into aging to address age-related disorders more effectively (Daniel et al., 2021; Guo et al., 2022).

Test Your Knowledge

1. How does the biconcave shape of red blood cells enhance their function?
2. What role does hemoglobin play in oxygen and carbon dioxide transport?

3.4. White Blood Cells

Learning Outcome

- Types of white blood cells;
- Role in the immune system;
- Mechanisms of action against pathogens.

Our health depends in large part on our ability to fend off invaders, and white blood cells—or leukocytes, as they're more widely known—are the secret to this task. They are a kind of elite corps of defense, descending upon infection, invading pathogens, and other violators. Neutrophils, for example, will be first to arrive, rapidly engulfing and consuming germs through phagocytosis. And then there are the lymphocytes, like T cells and B cells, that generally become adept at recognizing specific antigens and building long-term defenses. Most of the time, coordination between these cells and the rest of the immune system creates a delicate balance that supports and maintains our overall health. White blood cells do more than they destroy invaders—also organize the body's overall immune response and control inflammation. Macrophages, which sometimes develop from monocytes, have a unique function since they search for infectious agents and clear cellular debris. Macrophages release chemical messengers called cytokines that recruit more immune cells and amplify protective responses. This cascade of inflammation is needed to stop infections but, if uncontrolled, can lead to tissue damage. For the most part, finding the right balance is the key; an overactive response could provoke chronic inflammatory diseases, while an underactive one may expose the body to harm. The combination of white blood cells in our bloodstream is constantly changing and provides insight into our overall well-being. Although their numbers typically remain within a certain window, changes can be cause for alarm. For instance, an excessively high count—leukocytosis—can indicate that infection, inflammation, or even leukemia is at work, and an extremely low count, leukopenia, indicates that the immune system is impaired.

Latest studies have, in general, identified specific populations of leukocytes as having particular functions in the course of a disease. For instance, in cancer immunotherapy, the augmentation of T cell function can typically lead to improved treatment results. It is not just the number of cells; the way the cells behave in interaction with other blood constituents—such as platelets and plasma proteins—actually determines our body's defense topology (Joel et al., 2020; Ou et al., 2023) (Figure 3.12).

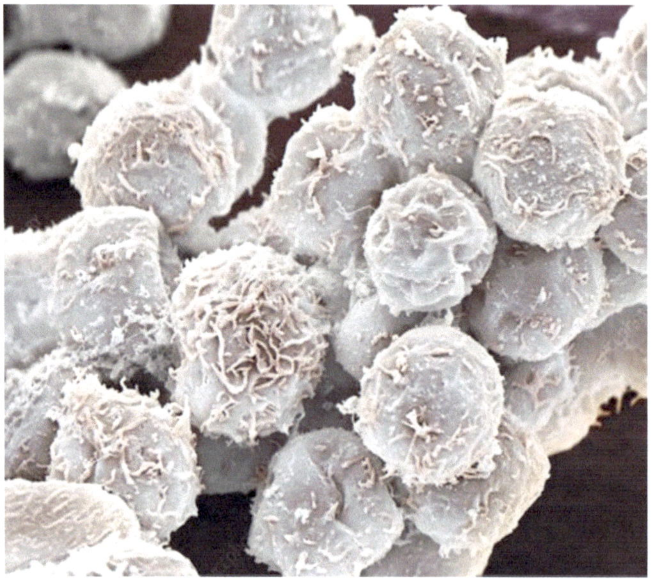

Figure 3.12. White blood cells.

Source: https://external-content.duckduckgo.com/iu/?u=https%3A%2F%2Ftse1.mm.bing.net%2Fth%3Fid%3DOIP.kSDg6V9TTvEckTC2hcQBlAHaGY%26pid%3DApi&f= 1&ipt=9ef157a70ade31c127e7a0d327660c524d116ead49b58438eb29aa5847460bd0.

3.4.1. Types of white blood cells

White blood cells are indispensable members of our immune system – they come in all sorts of varieties, including lymphocytes, neutrophils, monocytes, eosinophils, and basophils, each developing from bone marrow stem cells. Lymphocytes, for instance, develop into B cells and T cells that actually drive adaptive immunity, while neutrophils, the most common in the group, usually get there first when inflammation occurs. Monocytes, the largest of the group, eventually become macrophages or dendritic cells, which are responsible for engulfing and presenting foreign particles to initiate further protection. Take a closer look at those lymphocytes. B cells, for the most part, secrete antibodies that tag and impair pathogens, basically paving the way for them to be destroyed. But then again, T cells come in different flavors – helper T cells and cytotoxic T cells – that coordinate and execute immune responses, with some overlap in their roles. It is amazing how these cells even possess a memory of past invaders, enabling the immune system to devise a faster response when the same miscreant returns. This memory effect, in most instances, is the reason why immunizations are so effective and why our defenses are so wonderfully coordinated. And then there are the granular leukocytes, eosinophils and basophils, which have specialized roles against allergies and parasites.

Eosinophils mobilize in response to large, multicellular parasites and regulate allergic reactions by releasing inflammatory signals; basophils, though less numerous, help initiate inflammation by spilling out histamine and other mediators (a bit erratically, usually). Their work reveals not only the many different types of white blood cells but the natural, almost spontaneous collaboration in protecting the body's defenses – one that propels ongoing advancements in immunology and the search for better treatments to fight autoimmune disease.

3.4.2. Role in the Immune System

Structure of blood is critical to our body's defense, a mix of cells coming together in peculiar combinations. White blood cells (leukocytes) take center stage as the first line of defense against germs, but are not the same. See, you have lymphocytes, monocytes, and granulocytes – all adding their own role to making things go along. Unexpectedly, immune cells cluster not just in the central locations like primary hematopoietic locations, but also manifest in other tissues all over the body to form a network that helps with localizing and maturing defense response.

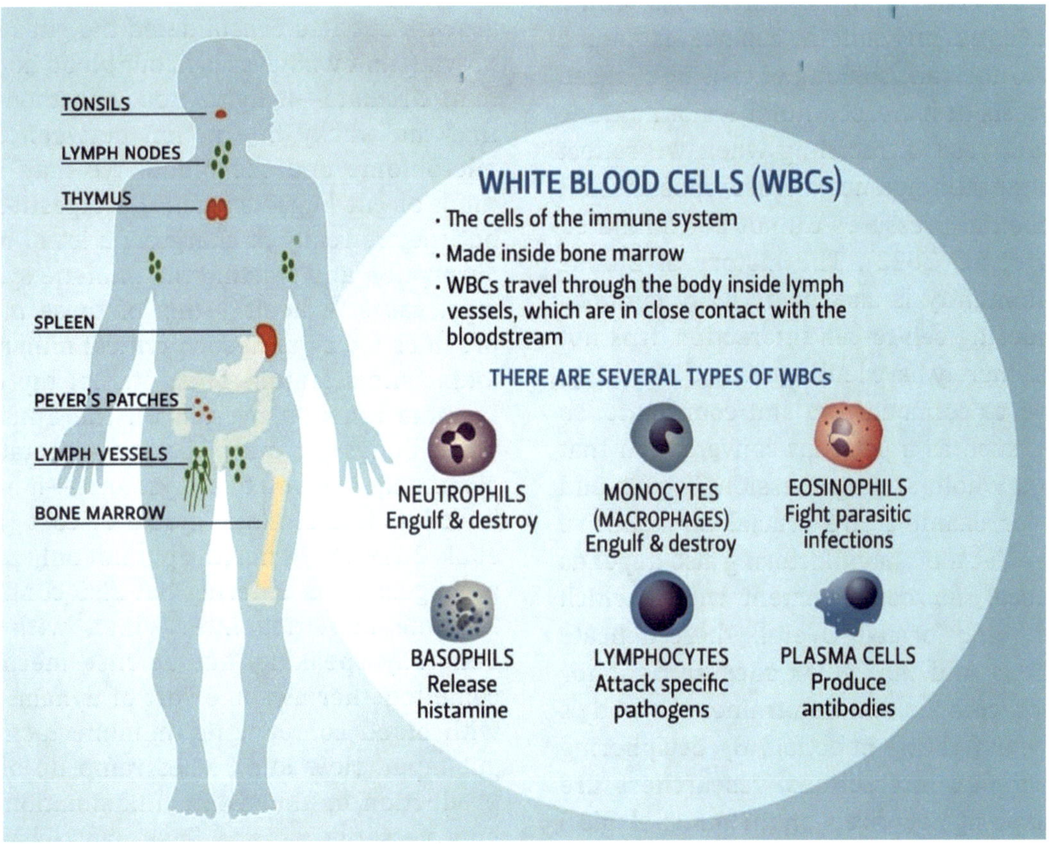

Figure 3.13. Role in the immune system.

Source: https://external-content.duckduckgo.com/iu/?u=http%3A%2F%2Flpi.oregonstate.edu%2Fsites%2Flpi.oregonstate.edu%2Ffiles%2Fimmune-system.png&f=1&nofb=1&ipt=27777d83f341a0e02ebeeea757efec05775c331c76d367ed527915cd7f9dd215.

In most cases, current evidence (Suo et al., 2022) suggests that lymphoid and myeloid subsets acquire their full immune functions somewhat later, a fact of utmost significance for successful host defense in normal and pathological situations. In addition, external influences play a prominent role in the behavior of these cells. For instance, chronic stress such as overpopulated housing conditions can subtly but indeed influence immune reactions. Studies on dromedary camels indicate that under restricted mobility, these camels have alterations of the white blood cell count – recording indicators such as leukocytosis and even shifts in the manner the cells clump together. This would mean that stress may shift the balance of immune function to aberrant, sometimes causing reduced phagocytosis at increased numbers of immune cells. It's a case of recalling when we reflect on immune competence across species that environmental pressures cannot be eliminated (Hussen et al., 2022). The history of bloods role in immunity is also made more complex by considering cell-to-cell interaction. It is not enough to merely have leukocytes in the vicinity; they have to communicate and coordinate, so to speak, such as a pleasant conversation that leads to a whole strategy session. T cells and B cells, for example, are crucial for adaptive immunity, but their manufacturing also depends on the local microenvironment within which they are being formed. Overall, these delicate interactions and molecular cues account for why blood composition determines the body's capacity for fighting infection. By deciphering these complex interactions, researchers are slowly mapping new directions in immunological disease therapy and regenerative medicine, as previewed by discoveries in early human immune development (Suo et al., 2022) (Figure 3.13).

3.4.3. Mechanisms of Action Against Pathogens

Our body also fights invaders in a rather bewildered fashion, with blood playing a large role in the fray. Immunoglobulins, or simply Igs, are like frontline soldiers that latch onto nasty bacteria, viruses, and other baddies. They can disable these aggressors on their own or call upon reinforcements from other immune cells. More frequently than not, it has been discovered that purified Igs given orally (even though derived from, for instance, ovine serum) seem to calm the immune system in animal models (Balan et al., 2019). Not only does this kind of immunity boost help the host with enhanced growth, but also consolidated the gut's barrier, proving that whatever is in our blood does more than circulate—it fights, too. And then add to that the wacky interaction between the gut microbiome and the blood. We may tend to think of gut bugs as plain old digestive aides, but they're really in charge of a lot of nutrient absorption and starting the immune system in most cases. A healthy mix of these microbes provides a way to absorb critical minerals like iodine and selenium, both vital for thyroid and immune function overall. On the other hand, when things get out of balance—a state most commonly referred to as dysbiosis—it has been linked to autoimmune thyroid disease (Eöhlich et al., 2019). So, a healthy gut not only prevents pathogens from entering but also controls the immune activities intertwined with blood. Generally speaking, our defense mechanisms come together as some sort of dynamic dance with blood components, immune tactics, and gut input. How our bodies ramp up antibody production or downshift inflammation shows how versatile we are. Take short-chain fatty acids produced by gut microbes, for example; these tiny substances power intestinal cells and help keep the gut lining healthy. And microbial impacts can even reset how factors in the blood, like those managing thyroid hormones, operate (Balan et al., 2019; Eöhlich et al., 2019).

Understanding all these loosely connected, sometimes messy interactions is key to coming up with novel therapies that exploit the makeup of the blood along with the immune system and the microbiome-even if the process isn't completely clean.

Test Your Knowledge

1. What are the major types of white blood cells and their functions in immunity?
2. How do WBCs differ in their response to bacterial versus viral infections?

3.5. Platelets and Coagulation

Learning Outcome

- Structure and function of platelets;
- The coagulation process;
- Disorders related to blood clotting.

Platelets are activated when blood vessels are injured. They are some of the first to stick to the inner, open layer and are quick in their activation and discharging of granules full of clotting material. That immediate response—providing an initial seal—is the basis for allowing fibrinogen to be converted into fibrin, which then holds the clot in place. What surface the blood comes into contact with is curiously significant. Some materials will cause fibrinogen to be drawn towards them and stick more, and some that trap proteins like albumin can even prevent it (Bantjes et al., 1972). Medical science continues to challenge us to research stored platelets more vigorously. Storage at room temperature, for example, makes them degrade over time, so more research has concentrated its efforts on preservation methods like cryopreservation. With dimethyl sulfoxide as a cryoprotectant, it has been discovered that the platelets are kept at about –80°C for long periods—though this freezing does affect their shape and normal behavior. In the majority of cases, the frozen platelets do seem to trigger clotting factors sooner, thrombin and fibrin being produced earlier than room-temperature-stored ones. In general, while cryopreservation holds much promise, especially in the event of an emergency, its broader impact on platelet function is yet to be profoundly examined (Compernolle et al., 2020). In clinical situations such as transfusion medicine, it becomes even more complex. Cryopreserved platelets are more likely to clear faster from circulation and to branch out into several subpopulations. Even small changes in major receptors, such as GPIbα, may be the explanation for these platelets' predisposition to clotting and reduced rate of recovery after transfusion.

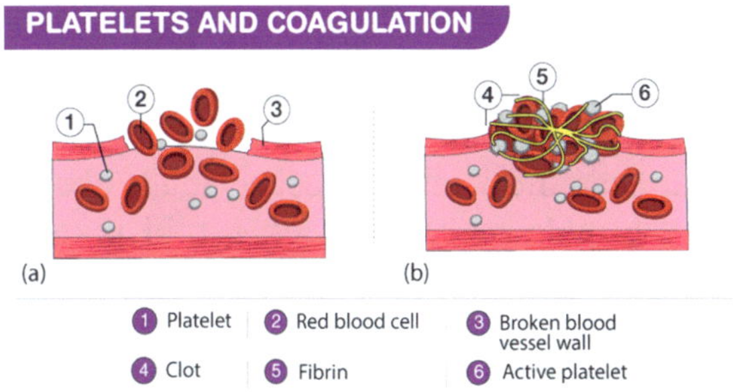

Figure 3.14. Platelets and coagulation.

Source: https://external-content.duckduckgo.com/iu/?u=https%3A%2F%2Fcdn1.byjus.com%2Fwp-content%2Fuploads%2F2019%2F01%2FPlatelets-and-Coagulation.png&f=1&nofb=1&ipt=e554bc40ac5292fe7bb6f8168573e56a8b491f2e91ea8d2a7b4c772892bc39a2.

This delicate balancing act—trying to achieve effective clotting without inducing unwanted thrombus, particularly in the setting of trauma or massive bleeding—is delicate work. In the majority of cases, further thorough research is needed to fully understand these dynamics and optimize the use of cryopreserved platelets for a variety of medical conditions (Compernolle et al., 2020) (Figure 3.14).

3.5.1. Structure and function of platelets

Platelets sit at the very heart of blood clotting—a messy but essential process where myriad elements within our bloodstream work together to halt bleeding. Born from megakaryocytes in bone marrow, these small, nucleus-free fragments are packed with granules of clotting factors and signaling particles. When a vessel is damaged, these granules spill into the surrounding space and let loose a chain of activity that eventually leads to clotting. Usually, when stimulated, platelets undergo a dramatic change: they stretch out, become clumped, and release chemicals that further enhance clotting. Looking closer at what triggers this stimulation—like granule fusion with the outer cell membrane (process directed by SNARE proteins)—shows us precisely how critical platelets are to keeping our blood vessels intact and controlling bleeding (Joshi et al., 2018). If you examine it more closely, you'll observe that the makeup of granules within platelets is far more than evenly balanced. There are at least two types—alpha granules and dense granules—and each type contains its own set of proteins with various functions. This is not a random quirk of their being; it's a critical part that involves their response to losing blood. For example, protein stability of VAMP-7 and VAMP-8 has the ability to significantly impact the release of granules. Capping granule release, as per some research, particularly in genetically modified characteristics from mice, is found to minimize procoagulant activity but maintain the clotting mechanism relatively intact (Joshi et al., 2018). This degree of fine balance is necessary to avoid arrest of bleeding without leaning too far in the direction of causative clot formation. Platelet activation also drifts along a range of signal pathways—take the RAP GTPase family, for instance, which helps activate integrins and cause platelets to bind together. Knocking out certain RAP variants in experiments was found to not only interfere with platelet function but also to uncover backup routes to integrin activation. Notably, RAP1B has been shown to have a pronounced impact on releasing contents from alpha granules and on activating RAC1, a regulator of the cell skeleton that is required to play a significant role in clot structure. Notably, while these signals are of very significant importance in thrombus formation, they seem less significant when ensuring that blood vessels are stable during growth or inflammation. This two-sided task really highlights the complex, sometimes moody, nature of how platelets control clotting and inflammation in our bloodstream (Figure 3.15).

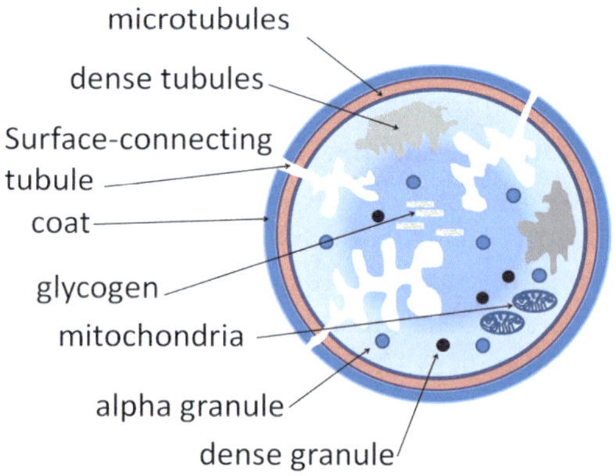

Figure 3.15. Structure and function of platelets.

Source: https://encrypted-tbn0.gstatic.com/images?q=tbn:ANd9GcRgEGM5borJzINpRuGM6JbZm_Rblbfr046bmA&s.

3.5.2. The coagulation process

Clotting in the blood is dependent on a strange set of blood factors that behave in an unintuitive way. When a vessel is damaged, the lining cells get broken down—previously hidden players like collagen and tissue factor come into the forefront. This release leads to a chain reaction where clotting proteins and enzymes interact and finally result in thrombin. You literally can't overstate how important it is that there is enough of these proteins in the system; small variations can cause the system to tip in favor of inducing either bleeding side effects or fatal clots. In the majority of cases, research shows that levels of such crucial proteins may vary quite broadly within their normal ranges, so individual differences make a huge difference (Caruso et al., 2009). It's also of importance that the true surface blood has a huge impact on the whole clotting story. Based on whether or not a material is attracted to water (hydrophilic) or not (hydrophobic), blood compatibility will differ—leading to how good platelets stick together and triggering the intrinsic pathway of clotting. For example, surfaces that are likely to bind with fibrinogen will promote platelet clumping, while surfaces favoring albumin may even retard this stickiness. Researchers have, over the years, developed sophisticated materials such as synthetic heparinoids and hydrogels that will reduce platelet adhesion and prevent excess clotting in some environments. These developments not only improve medical devices' safety but also illuminate for us how the properties of a material can alter our body's clotting response (Bantjes et al., 1972). But mechanical failures are not the entire tale; our genes and what we do day-to-day also play a role in how our blood clots. Heredity or even something as prosaic as what we eat may affect clotting protein concentration. Some new data even suggest that a nutrient-rich diet actually keeps these levels in healthy ranges, thus lowering cardiovascular risk. It's extremely fascinating to observe how the dynamic interaction between life-style choices and genetic predispositions can cause persons with identical genetic descriptions to have extremely divergent tendencies for clotting. Appreciation of this intricate vignette is crucial in the design of particular treatments and diagnostic techniques that would substantially improve patient care. Briefly, internal processes of our biology and external environment converge in determining the clotting process, with significant outcomes for clinical practice (Caruso et al., 2009).

3.5.3. Disorders related to blood clotting

Hemostasis keeps our blood vessels in check, and when that balance is disrupted, it can really get out of control. Take hemophilia—some kind of genetic defect where there just aren't enough clotting factors available, so the body's purpose of being able to keep bleeding at bay gets screwed up. Even small cuts or scratches become gushing bleeding episodes that drag on, sometimes serving up joint problems as a side effect. In most cases, the unpredictability and regularity of these bleeds render factor replacement therapies necessary, a testament to the fact that those coagulation proteins are essentially the behind-the-scenes workhorses of successful clot formation and general vessel health (Becker et al., 2003). And then there is thrombosis, which essentially flips the script around. Here, instead of clotting too little, the body clots too strongly—at times in spots where it just shouldn't. These rogue clots can do damage by cutting off circulation, and in the most extreme scenario, leading to strokes or heart attacks. Often, something like long periods of inactivity, other illnesses, or even our own genetic predispositions triggers the system to go into hyperdrive. Overall, this hypercoagulability is a complex problem that doctors attempt to manage with anticoagulants, hoping to walk the fine line of coagulation (Ritson et al., 2007). If you examine closely the interaction of blood components, it is obvious how crucial it is to be aware of clotting disorders. Abnormalities such as thrombocytopenia, say, lead to a low platelet count impairing the body's ability to clot—resulting in an episode of easy bruising or bleeding that just won't quit. Some patients are faced with regular monitoring and treatment to boost platelet levels or simply ward off the protracted bleeds. It all serves to illustrate that each part—platelets to clotting factors—is on its own making a crucial contribution to hemostasis. In most cases, the wide range of coagulation disorders requires individualized diagnostics and customized treatments, reflecting our ongoing quest to better understand these mechanisms and improve patient outcomes (Becker et al., 2003) (Figure 3.16).

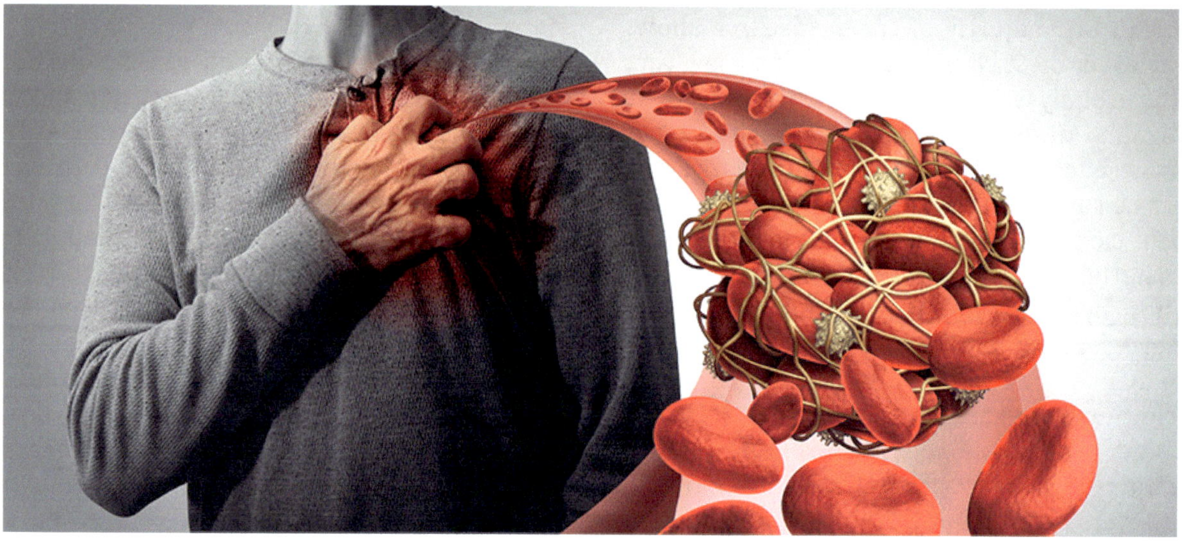

Figure 3.16. Blood clotting disorders.

Source: https://www.metropolisindia.com/upgrade/blog/upload/2022/08/Blood-Clotting-Metropolis-healthcare-limited.png.

Test Your Knowledge

1. What role do platelets play in the blood clotting process?
2. How does the coagulation cascade function to stop bleeding?

3.6. Blood Typing and Transfusions

Learning Outcome

- ABO and Rh blood group systems;
- Importance of compatibility in transfusions;
- Risks and benefits of blood transfusions.

Blood is an extremely complex fluid that keeps our bodies in balance and provides oxygen where it's required. Its composition isn't all about the foundation elements—blood also exhibits a variety of types, primarily categorized under the ABO and Rh groups. Compatible blood is absolutely required since a mismatch may occasionally lead to damaging immune battles—a reaction that results when the recipient's antibodies target strange antigens in the blood being transfused. When demand for transfusions rises, especially in areas where resources are scarce, getting down to specifics about what makes up blood is overall crucial to further improving treatment outcomes and safeguarding patients (Margaret et al., 2018). Sound blood typing simply can't be overemphasized, particularly in chaotic emergency settings. Having a patient's blood type on hand also makes it easier for medical personnel to decide the transfusion to be given, with a built-in guard against hemolytic reactions in many cases. The blood is typically mixed with anti-A and anti-B antibodies to monitor clumping behavior that will indicate the presence of certain antigens. If the patient cannot inform one of their blood groups—possibly because they are already unconscious or ill—universal donor blood (O type) is usually used as a temporary measure, reflecting the challenge of weighing transfusion protocols against the urgency of instant, life-saving needs (Eldridge et al., 2016). Blood donation logistics are inextricably intertwined with public efforts in giving blood. There should be sufficient blood supplies not only for routine operations but also for the treatment of trauma and diseases like hemophilia or anemia.

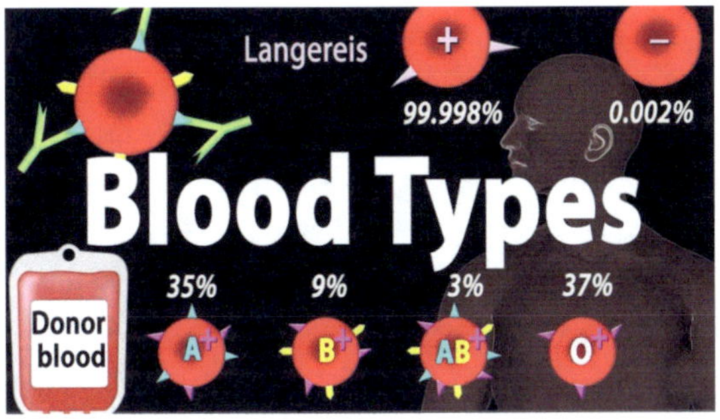

Figure 3.17. Blood types.

Source: https://external-content.duckduckgo.com/iu/?u=https%3A%2F%2Fi.ytimg.com%2Fvi%2FcKnEdvrmHK4%2Fmaxresdefault.jpg&f=1&nofb=1&ipt=01094575367883c2dd6b2ade9dddfb51e5c4b9fcb727783c4e5af119fc51c992.

Blood banks, being the focal points of this system, work assiduously to ensure that every contribution is screened, typed, and stored with safety in mind for future use. Public awareness campaigns (which, in most cases, do actually have an effect) can encourage more people to donate blood by underlining the benefit of having access to a supply that reflects the population's genetic diversity. Ultimately, instilling a culture of voluntary donation helps to reinforce fairness and accessibility in transfusion medicine—a basis upon which effective delivery of healthcare is constructed (Margaret et al., 2018) (Figure 3.17).

3.6.1. ABO and Rh Blood Group Systems

Blood is a messy, messy world. You can't help but question how well we're doing without these microscopic biochemical details. Consider the ABO system, for instance—it's not just a categorization of transfusions and transplants; it's something else. In plain terms, red blood cells carry A or B tags (or perhaps neither) nor that's it because our genes decide it. Each person's blood type shows these markers, which are there because enzymes put them there by adding sugar molecules in what seems to be a random fashion. In recent years, research into biochemistry has helped the world understand how these antigens are constructed and can be linked to various health dangers, and maybe more significantly, that ABO could have an even larger impact on susceptibility to disease and nutritional issues than it was first thought (Ewald et al., 2016). And then there's the Rh system, which kind of works together with ABO but does its own thing. It's identified by the RhD antigen—this tiny marker has some major issues, especially pregnancy. In most cases, if a woman who is Rh-negative has a Rh-positive baby, things can get complicated. The mother's antibodies will actually destroy her baby's red blood cells, sometimes causing hemolytic disease of the newborn that can cause life-threatening anemia or even jaundice. Understanding how Rh operates not only helps with transfusions and prenatal testing, but also makes clinicians aware of its role in immunity and other health factors (Ewald et al., 2016). The ABO and Rh systems transcend the clinic into the general terrain of health and society. Researchers have discovered—in a number of studies—that your blood group can be linked with the risks for diseases like gestational diabetes mellitus (GDM). For example, one prospective pregnancy study found that individuals with non-AB groups had a higher risk of contracting GDM compared to their AB counterparts, so certain antigens might even have a protective effect. These discoveries bring to mind the role played by blood group systems in reproductive health and uncover promising avenues for individualized medical strategies. Further research into this area is gradually painting in a fuller picture about exactly how our blood types influence overall health, at times in the most unexpected ways (Figure 3.18).

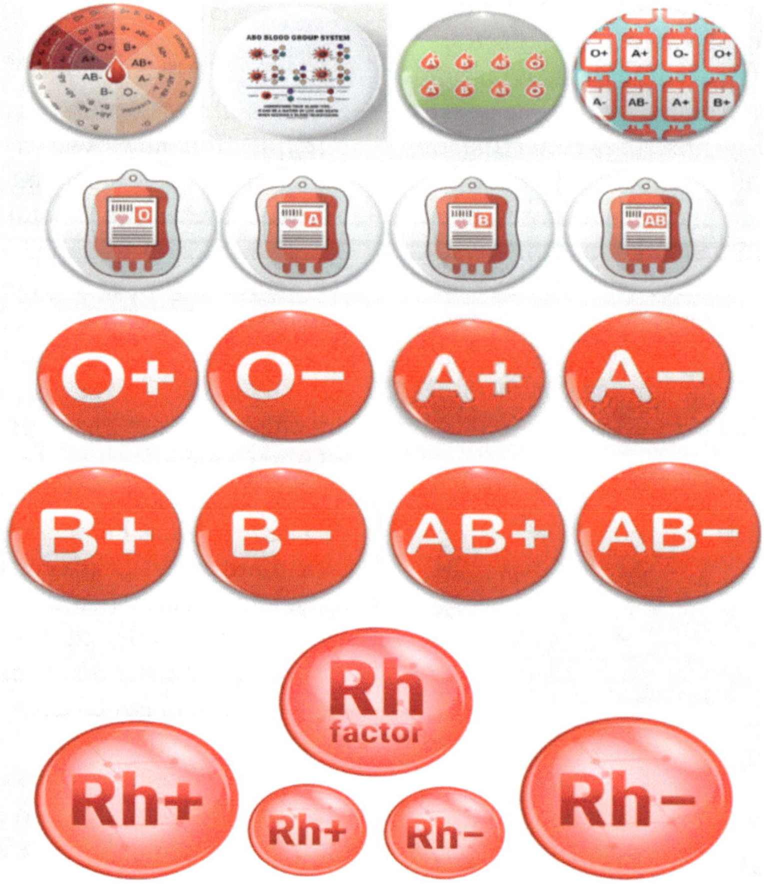

Figure 3.18. ABO and Rh blood group systems.

Source: https://www.mediresonline.org/uploads/articles/1720785659image.png.

3.6.2. Importance of Compatibility in Transfusions

Blood transfusions rely on a good match between the donor and recipient. It's not a routine—making the donor red blood cells wear unfamiliar markers, the recipient immune system will likely react, sometimes violently. Patients who have built up antibodies, such as from past transfusions or even pregnancy, will more likely experience these reactions. For the most part, even a small mistake in cross-matching can escalate into life-threatening hemolytic reactions; leaving these tests out is a risk not worth taking. In fact, problems with mismatched blood do really highlight why accurate typing and careful screening have become so integral standard procedures for guaranteeing patients' safety. Animal medicine is not an exception. Worldwide, it is still necessary to make sure that animal blood is still compatible – although the practice varies slightly, sometimes significantly. Blood banking research shows that most veterinarians opt not to use compatibility testing before a transfusion, which can be a recipe for disaster and actually raise the mortality rate. In a majority of instances, a good check for compatibility would all be in the end, reducing risks and enhancing results for animal patients in a manner that resonates with the imperative for safe, effective transfusions. On another battlefield, science is exploring new ground by reconsidering conventional blood products. A concept that is receiving some consideration is the creation of red blood cells grown in the laboratory. This could be a game changer, especially for patients with rare blood types who struggle to receive a match. Such technologies can alleviate pressure on donor stockpiles while simultaneously improving issues related to immune incompatibilities. Research is ongoing confirming that such artificial cells do not induce unwanted alloimmune responses. In short, transfusion medicine is now a combination of old-school compatibility testing and cutting-edge cell manufacturing technique—a move that demonstrates our ongoing commitment to advancing patient care with science, good testing, and a healthy dose of innovation (Figure 3.19).

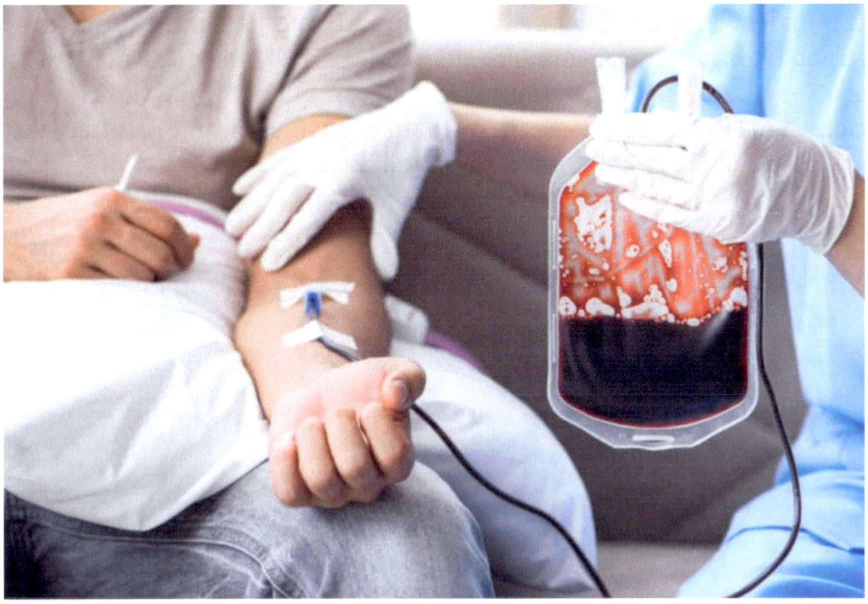

Figure 3.19. Blood compatibility.

Source: https://cdn.hellodoctor.com.ph/wp-content/uploads/2021/05/blood-compatibility-chart.jpg?w=750&q=100.

3.6.3. Risks and benefits of blood transfusions

Transfusions these days are something of a mixed bag—on the one hand, a lifesaver, and on the other hand, with their own bag of problems. Oftentimes, when a patient experiences uncontrolled blood loss as a result of an accident or surgery, transfusions step in by providing the essential ingredients—red cells, plasma, and platelets—to deliver oxygen and trigger clotting. This isn't entirely about emergency treatment; such treatments also go a long way for individuals who have chronic anemia or individuals who witness their counts get dented by aggressive treatments like chemotherapy. Hospitals, generally, must adhere to strict safety regulations to achieve the best outcomes while minimizing risks (Margaret et al., 2018). Naturally, remember that there is no absolutely risk-free medical treatment. Occasionally, transfusions provoke reactions as simple as fevers and allergies or as dire as acute hemolytic incidents. Even with precautions in place, and with blood screened cautiously, there's always a nagging concern that infections will be transferred – think HIV or Hepatitis B and C – that forces medical staff to be that much more careful. And then there is the intriguing complication of alloimmunization, when the body starts to treat donor blood as a foreign body, making future transfusions more complicated and even requiring further interventions. It all equates to medical personnel having to balance very carefully the potential benefits on each individual basis against these risks (Eldridge et al., 2016). Taking into account everything, latest developments and the most up-to-date practices are finally starting to shift how we handle blood transfusions. Improvements like improved screening and even the possibility of examining alternatives—like drugs that get the body to produce additional blood cells—are gradually reducing our intense reliance on the traditional transfusions. The rising tide of precision medicine also means treatments can be more finely tailored to the requirements of an individual patient, and that is an agreeable development. Integrated into a functioning health care system, these new approaches are part of the process of creating safer environments and better patient outcomes. Lastly, better insight into the composition of blood and constant, careful surveillance of its use provide doctors with the instruments they require to handle the complex problems of transfusions more effectively (Margaret et al., 2018).

Test Your Knowledge

1. What are the differences between the ABO and Rh blood group systems?
2. Why is blood type compatibility important in transfusions?

Summary

Blood isn't just a liquid that carries things around; it's a living blend of red cells, white cells, and plasma that mainly keeps us in balance. You may imagine these elements merely carry around the nutrients, but in fact, they have a much more extensive function in keeping our bodies in balance-even when something goes wrong. Take, for example, illnesses like myotonic dystrophy type 2. In such a condition, a variation from the usual level of blood can inform us a great deal about our metabolism. Bioelectrical impedance analysis readings tend to pick up on variations in the body composition, indicating muscle wasting and other changes in metabolism. These fine-tuning signals, or how effectively our muscles function, mean that small abnormalities on blood tests actually can be evidence of underlying illness (Frezza et al., 2024). Meanwhile, blood demonstrates a remarkable ability to adapt—especially after we get in shape. Other things being equal, the more we get in shape, the healthier blood readings such as the hematocrit index are. In the majority of cases, the sports like soccer players undergoing regular, organized training experience notable elevation of red cell concentration and oxygen supply. It is not just a question of being aesthetically pleasing on paper; the alterations can find expression in enhanced overall well-being and sports performance. Little wonder that sports scientists are finding blood composition data increasingly valuable for tracking both health and sporting performance (Chen et al., 2022). Finally, learning how blood works, both in its day-to-day function and in reacting to stressors, opens up an entire universe of information. In most cases, integrating work on blood parameters along with current biomedical advances helps to delineate how we can diagnose issues and even optimize physical capability. The connections you see between composition, metabolism, and bodily ability mean the need for further research. Both clinics and sports programs now depend on ongoing blood testing to guide treatment and maximize performance. This coupling of athletic and clinical knowledge not only deepens our underlying knowledge of blood's multifaceted roles—it sets the stage for new, out-of-the-box approaches to training and disease management (Chen et al., 2022; Frezza et al., 2024).

Blood is really amazing—it's not just a simple liquid but an interactive mix that keeps our bodies moving. Red blood cells (or erythrocytes) take charge of delivering oxygen by using hemoglobin to capture oxygen directly from the lungs and transport it to where it is needed; while white blood cells (leukocytes) arrive to destroy unwanted microbes. And then plasma, which makes up around 55% of blood and is a type of multi-purpose highway to carry nutrients, hormones, and even waste products. Platelets, too, play a part in the process, helping to activate clotting when injuries occur. In a way, this blend makes blood a multipurpose transporter that helps not only to deliver but to protect. Blood is not only about moving stuff around, though—its role to provide internal stability is important too. Overall, it regulates our body temperature by getting rid of the heat created during metabolism and keeps things from getting too out of whack. It harmlessly carries electrolytes, proteins, and hormones that regulate the pH values of our tissues, which helps with the acid-base balance required for cellular function. It's interesting to know that even within these regulatory roles, platelets are involved in ensuring proper hemostasis (preventing excessive bleeding) following an injury, proving that blood's dual purpose is transport and regulation in one dynamic system. If you examine closely, the function and structure of blood are established through a mix of factors like genetics, diet, and environment. For instance, sufficient iron is crucial as it is required to produce hemoglobin in red blood cells—a lack of which causes anemia, with the blood being unable to transport oxygen so well. Meanwhile, the bone marrow is very resilient, dedicated to the body's requirements by augmenting the number of white blood cells when the body is infected. These adaptive functions illustrate the complexity of blood constitution in disease and health. In most circumstances, knowledge of these layers helps to confirm our knowledge of blood as a liquid but also its central significance to the maintenance of our internal equilibrium.

KEY TERMS FROM THIS CHAPTER

Albumin	Antibodies	Antigens
Blood typing	Buffy coat	Coagulation
Erythropoiesis	Fibrinogen	Globulins
Hematocrit	Hemoglobin	Hemostasis
Oxyhemoglobin	Phagocytosis	Plasma
Platelets (thrombocytes)	Red blood cells (erythrocytes)	Rh factor
Serum	White blood cells (leukocytes)	

Critical Thinking Questions

1. What is the primary function of red blood cells (RBCs)?

a. Fight infections

b. Transport oxygen

c. Produce antibodies

d. Regulate body temperature

2. Which component of blood is responsible for clotting?

a. White blood cells

b. Plasma

c. Platelets

d. Red blood cells

3. What is the fluid portion of blood called?

a. Serum

b. Plasma

c. Lymph

d. Hemoglobin

4. Which blood cells are involved in defending the body against infections?

a. Red blood cells

b. Platelets

c. White blood cells

d. Plasma proteins

5. Which protein in red blood cells carries oxygen?

a. Albumin

b. Fibrinogen

c. Hemoglobin

d. Globulin

Answers to Critical Thinking Questions

1. (b); 2. (c); 3. (b); 4. (c); 5. (c)

Short Answer Questions

1. What are the main components of blood, and what percentage does each make up?
2. What is plasma, and what are its primary constituents?
3. Name the three main types of blood cells and describe their basic functions.
4. What is the role of hemoglobin, and which type of blood cell contains it?
5. Describe how blood contributes to immune defense mechanisms.
6. In what ways does blood help regulate body temperature and pH?

References

1. Abd Wahab, M. B. A., Mahmood, S., Mohamad Rus, M. A., Mustar, S., et al. (2020). Quality control improvement at Jana DCS Sdn. Bhd. https://core.ac.uk/download/12007130.pdf (accessed on 1st July 2025).
2. Abt, J. P., Allison, K. F., Crawford, K., Lephart, S., et al. (2012). The relationship between musculoskeletal strength, physiological characteristics, and knee kinesthesia following fatiguing exercise. https://core.ac.uk/download/12212102.pdf (accessed on 1st July 2025).
3. Alfarano, C., Calise, D., Ceccaldi, C., Cussac, D., et al. (2012). Alginate scaffolds for mesenchymal stem cell cardiac therapy: Influence of alginate composition. https://core.ac.uk/download/16754759.pdf (accessed on 1st July 2025).
4. Alkarithi, G., Ariëns, R. A. S., Duval, C., Macrae, F. L., et al. (2021). Thrombus structural composition in cardiovascular disease. https://core.ac.uk/download/459166924.pdf (accessed on 1st July 2025).
5. Altman, P. L., & Fisher, K. D. (1986). Research opportunities in nutrition and metabolism in space. https://core.ac.uk/download/pdf/10458014.pdf (accessed on 1st July 2025).
6. Antonopoulos, D., Armitage, G., AVA, Singapore, Azad, T., Bäckhed, F., Schneeman, B. O., et al. (2019). Establishing what constitutes a healthy human gut microbiome: State of the science, regulatory considerations, and future directions. https://core.ac.uk/download/323068488.pdf (accessed on 1st July 2025).
7. Balan, P., Han, K. S., & Moughan, P. J. (2019). Impact of oral immunoglobulins on animal health—A review. *Animal Science Journal, 90*, 1099–1110. https://doi.org/10.1111/asj.13258 (accessed on 1st July 2025).
8. Bánáti, F., Cseh, D., Hinsenkamp, A., Holczer, T., et al. (2019). The composition of hyperacute serum and platelet-rich plasma is markedly different despite the similar production method. https://core.ac.uk/download/322920657.pdf (accessed on 1st July 2025).
9. Bantjes, A. (1972). Clotting phenomena at the blood-polymer interface and development of blood compatible polymeric surfaces. https://core.ac.uk/download/pdf/11474222.pdf (accessed on 1st July 2025).
10. Barth, B., Bennett, B., Bryan, M., Cantera, R., Chen, X., et al. (2019). Frequency of tongue cleaning impacts the human tongue microbiome composition and enter salivary circulation of nitrate. https://core.ac.uk/download/323382019.pdf (accessed on 1st July 2025).
11. Becker, J., Bergmeier, W., Bermejo, D. A., Bertozzi, C. R., Bokoch, G. M., Bos, J. L., et al. (2018). Functional redundancy between RAP1 isoforms in murine platelet production and function. https://core.ac.uk/download/160811950.pdf (accessed on 1st July 2025).
12. Becker, R. C., Blanco, A., Blomback, B., Cambas, E., Chantarangkul, V., Chitolie, A., et al. (2003). Guidelines on fibrinogen assays. https://core.ac.uk/download/9349786.pdf (accessed on 1st July 2025).
13. Benavides Damm, T., & Egli, M. (2014). Calcium's role in mechanotransduction during muscle development. *Cellular Physiology and Biochemistry, 33*, 249–272. https://doi.org/10.1159/000356667 (accessed on 1st July 2025).
14. Berger, N. (2016). Identification of biomarkers of colitis to monitor effects of dietary omega-3

polyunsaturated fatty acids in the interleukin-10 gene-deficient mouse model of inflammatory bowel diseases: A thesis presented in partial fulfilment of the requirements for the degree of Doctor of Philosophy in Nutritional Science at Massey University, Manawatū, New Zealand. https://core.ac.uk/download/148643310.pdf (accessed on 1st July 2025).

15. Bertz, M., Calus, S. T., Edwards, C. A., Gaya, D. R., et al. (2017). The distinct features of microbial 'dysbiosis' of Crohn's disease do not occur to the same extent in their unaffected, genetically linked kindred. https://core.ac.uk/download/77601080.pdf (accessed on 1st July 2025).

16. Beugeling, T., Poot, A. A., & Turbill, P. (1996). Proteins involved in the Vroman effect during exposure of human blood plasma to glass and polyethylene. https://core.ac.uk/download/pdf/11452553.pdf (accessed on 1st July 2025).

17. Brodkorb, A., Egger, L., Alminger, M., Alvito, P., Assunção, R., Ballance, S., Bohn, T., et al. (2019). INFOGEST static *in vitro* simulation of gastrointestinal food digestion. *Nature Protocols, 14*, 991–1014. https://doi.org/10.1038/s41596-018-0119-1 (accessed on 1st July 2025).

18. Buxton, M. J., Grant, J., Hanney, S., Pollitt, A., et al. (2011). Project Retro sight: Understanding the returns from cardiovascular and stroke research: Case studies. https://core.ac.uk/download/6113193.pdf (accessed on 1st July 2025).

19. Caruso, P. (2009). Molecular bases of the modulation of coagulation factor levels. https://core.ac.uk/download/11822454.pdf (accessed on 1st July 2025).

20. Castanho, M. A. R. B., Domingues, M. M., Freire, J. M., Ribeiro, C., et al. (2012). Translocating the blood-brain barrier using electrostatics. https://core.ac.uk/download/12426979.pdf (accessed on 1st July 2025).

21. Chen, X., & Zhang, H. (2022). Soccer player's physical training for physical function improvement. *Revita Brasileira de Medicina do Esporte*. https://www.semanticscholar.org/paper/de6b0d4f8731c229612bc8225629e8c1c152bed4 (accessed on 1st July 2025).

22. Compernolle, V., Feys, H., & Six, K. (2020). Platelet biochemistry and morphology after cryopreservation. https://core.ac.uk/download/287941861.pdf (accessed on 1st July 2025).

23. Drake-Holland, A., & Noble, M. (2018). Development of the damaged glycocalyx hypothesis–A review. *3*. https://www.semanticscholar.org/paper/ed4aeaf95ed8b14660559b8e2b6127bcea406b73 (accessed on 1st July 2025).

24. Eldridge, S., Chan, C., Campbell, M. J., Bond, C., Hopewell, S., Thabane, L., & Lancaster, G. (2016). CONSORT 2010 statement: Extension to randomized pilot and feasibility trials. *BMJ*. https://doi.org/10.1136/bmj.i5239 (accessed on 1st July 2025).

25. Ewald, D. R., & Sumner, S. (2016). Blood type biochemistry and human disease. *WIREs Systems Biology and Medicine, 8*, 517–535. https://doi.org/10.1002/wsbm.1355 (accessed on 1st July 2025).

26. Frezza, E., Merra, G., Greco, G., Goglia, M., Seraceno, S., Boffa, L., Mercuri, N. B., et al. (2024). Changes in body composition revealed by bioelectrical impedance analysis reflect strength and motor performance in myotonic dystrophy type 2. *Frontiers in Neurology, 15*. https://www.semanticscholar.org/paper/8df911e7de6aa94ffc2cde7e310b0d0860941936 (accessed on 1st July 2025).

27. Fröhlich, E., & Wahl, R. (2019). Microbiota and thyroid interaction in health and disease. *Trends in Endocrinology and Metabolism, 30*, 479–490. https://doi.org/10.1016/j.tem.2019.05.008 (accessed on 1st July 2025).

28. Galicia-García, U., Benito-Vicente, A., Jebari, S., Larrea-Sebal, A., Siddiqi, H., Uribe, K. B., Ostolaza, H., et al. (2020). Pathophysiology of type 2 diabetes mellitus. *International Journal of Molecular Sciences, 21*, 6275–6275. https://doi.org/10.3390/ijms21176275 (accessed on 1st July 2025).

29. Gromova, N. V., Imarova, O. G., Martynova, M. I., Revin, V. V., et al. (2016). Role of membrane lipids in the regulation of erythrocytic oxygen-transport function in cardiovascular diseases. https://core.ac.uk/download/228177833.pdf (accessed on 1st July 2025).

30. Guo, J., Huang, X., Dou, L., Yan, M., Shen, T., Tang, W., & Li, J. (2022). Aging and aging-related diseases: From molecular mechanisms to interventions and treatments. *Signal Transduction and Targeted Therapy, 7*. https://doi.org/10.1038/s41392-022-01251-0 (accessed on 1st July 2025).

31. Hussen, J., & Al-Sukruwah, M. A. (2022). The impact of the animal housing system on immune cell composition and function in the blood of dromedary camels. *Animals, 12*, 317–317. https://doi.org/10.3390/ani12030317 (accessed on 1st July 2025).

32. Joshi, S. (2018). Controlling platelet secretion to modulate hemostasis and thrombosis. https://core.ac.uk/download/232583826.pdf (accessed on 1st July 2025).

33. Kalmar, I. D., Verstegen, M. W. A., Maenner, K., Zentek, J., et al. (2009). Tolerance and safety evaluation of N,N-dimethylglycine, a naturally occurring organic compound, as a feed additive in broiler diets. https://core.ac.uk/download/pdf/29229191.pdf (accessed on 1st July 2025).

34. Kibitkina, A., Vasilevskaya, E., Tolmacheva, G., Kotenkova, E., Polishchuk, E., Pchelkina, V., Karabanov, S., et al. (2025). Tryptophan-induced effects on the behavior and physiology of aging in tryptophan hydroxylase-2 heterozygous mice C57BL/6N. *Veterinary World, 18*, 296–310. https://www.semanticscholar.org/paper/e0aa9066de653bb1f1ab3582bf6138603ef91c43 (accessed on 1st July 2025).

35. Klionsky, D. J., Petroni, G., Amaravadi, R. K., Baehrecke, E. H., Ballabio, A., Boya, P., Bravo-San Pedro, J. M., et al. (2021). Autophagy in major human diseases. *The EMBO Journal, 40*. https://doi.org/10.15252/embj.2021108863 (accessed on 1st July 2025).

36. Kruk, M. E., Gage, A., Arsenault, C., Jordan, K., Leslie, H. H., Roder-DeWan, S., Adeyi, O., et al. (2018). High-quality health systems in the Sustainable Development Goals era: Time for a revolution. *The Lancet Global Health, 6*, e1196–e1252. https://doi.org/10.1016/s2214-109x(18)30386-3 (accessed on 1st July 2025).

37. Leiz, J., & Schmitt-Ott, K. M. (2019). Claudins in the renal collecting duct. https://core.ac.uk/download/286097290.pdf (accessed on 1st July 2025).

38. Mourot, L., Rakobowchuk, M., & Wilhelm, E. N. (2018). Exercise-derived micro vesicles: A review of the literature. https://core.ac.uk/download/288430488.pdf (accessed on 1st July 2025).

39. Musa, M. (2022). Blood count of patients of the dialysis ward in Mitrovica. *Technium BioChemMed*. https://www.semanticscholar.org/paper/860b0dd6dc767b1c11e9d5e89dc941a01dd1930e (accessed on 1st July 2025).

40. N/A. (2025). *Aerospace Medicine and Biology: A Continuing Bibliography (Supplement 231)*. https://core.ac.uk/download/pdf/42856677.pdf (accessed on 1st July 2025).

41. N/A. (2025). *Aerospace Medicine and Biology: A Continuing Bibliography with Indexes.* https://core.ac.uk/download/pdf/42846226.pdf (accessed on 1st July 2025).

42. Nagy, S. (2020). Global players with local impact: Novel biomarkers for fertility. https://core.ac.uk/download/345434102.pdf (accessed on 1st July 2025).

43. Oliveira, S. de, & Saldanha, C. (2010). An overview about erythrocyte membrane. https://core.ac.uk/download/12426151.pdf (accessed on 1st July 2025).

44. Ou, X., Wang, H., Tie, H., Liao, J., Luo, Y., Huang, W., Yu, R., et al. (2023). Novel plant-derived exosome-like nanovesicles from *Catharanthus roseus*: Preparation, characterization, and immunostimulatory effect via TNF-α/NF-κB/PU.1 axis. *Journal of Nanobiotechnology, 21.* https://doi.org/10.1186/s12951-023-01919-x (accessed on 1st July 2025).

45. Patel, H. H., & Zuniga-Hertz, J. P. (2019). The evolution of cholesterol-rich membrane in oxygen adaption: The respiratory system as a model. https://core.ac.uk/download/323066198.pdf (accessed on 1st July 2025).

46. Pellegrin, S., Severn, C. E., & Toye, A. M. (2021). Towards manufactured red blood cells for the treatment of inherited anemia. https://core.ac.uk/download/459190713.pdf (accessed on 1st July 2025).

47. Poh, D. (2020). Blood banking in small animal medicine: A survey of current practices and assessment of a technique to prevent transfusion-related complications. https://core.ac.uk/download/395062516.pdf (accessed on 1st July 2025).

48. Riley, J. S., & Tait, S. W. G. (2020). Mitochondrial DNA in inflammation and immunity. *EMBO Reports, 21.* https://doi.org/10.15252/embr.201949799 (accessed on 1st July 2025).

49. Ritson, C. G., & Welch, P. H. (2007). A process-oriented architecture for complex system modelling. https://core.ac.uk/download/64232.pdf (accessed on 1st July 2025).

50. Shadrin, N. V., Ostapchuk, P., Kuevda, T., Prazukin, A., Firsov, Y. K., Gassiev, D. D., Zubochenko, D., et al. (2024). The effect of adding filamentous green algae *Cladophora* to the diet of rabbits on their blood parameters. *Agricultural Science Euro-North-East.* https://www.semanticscholar.org/paper/df726ecd21c0b55361f4b869a396b58d47ff6ce7 (accessed on 1st July 2025).

51. Suo, C., Dann, E., Goh, I., Jardine, L., Kleshchevnikov, V., Park, J. E., Botting, R. A., et al. (2022). Mapping the developing human immune system across organs. *Science, 376.* https://doi.org/10.1126/science.abo0510 (accessed on 1st July 2025).

52. Théry, C., Witwer, K. W., Aïkawa, E., Alcaraz, M. J., Anderson, J. D., Andriantsitohaina, R., Antoniou, A., et al. (2018). Minimal information for studies of extracellular vesicles 2018 (MISEV2018): A position statement of the International Society for Extracellular Vesicles and update of the MISEV2014 guidelines. *Journal of Extracellular Vesicles, 7.* https://doi.org/10.1080/20013078.2018.1535750 (accessed on 1st July 2025).

53. Van der Merwe, F. H. (2018). GPS analysis of a team competing at a national Under 18 field hockey tournaments. https://core.ac.uk/download/187724717.pdf (accessed on 1st July 2025).

54. Zhang, C., Li, Y., Wang, L., Sun, S., Liu, G., Leng, J., Guo, J., et al. (2015). Blood group AB is protective factor for gestational diabetes mellitus: A prospective population-based study in Tianjin, China. *Diabetes/Metabolism Research and Reviews, 31*, 627–637. https://doi.org/10.1002/dmrr.2650 (accessed on 1st July 2025).

COMPLETE BLOOD COUNT (CBC) AND PERIPHERAL SMEAR

4

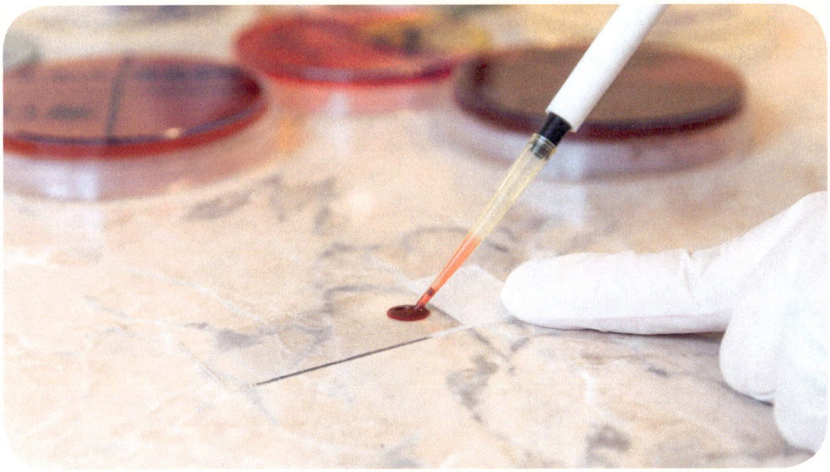

LEARNING OBJECTIVES

After studying this chapter, you will be able to:

1. Give components of a complete blood count;
2. Discuss the interpretation of CBC results;
3. Define the role of peripheral smear;
4. Describe correlation between CBC and peripheral smear;
5. Explain clinical applications of CBC and peripheral smear;
6. Focus on the limitations of CBC and peripheral smear.

Introduction

Hematology exams usually start when someone actually looks at the blood itself—starting, maybe, with a count from a complete blood count (CBC) and what a peripheral smear (PBS) can tell you. A CBC tells you directly how many red cells, white cells, and platelets you have, and it can tell you about problems from fairly common, everyday ones to more sinister ones like malignancies. But in most cases, that initial screening isn't enough; if anything is amiss, a PBS is written to double-check and probe further. Combining both methods at the same time enables practitioners to catch the fine details in a patient's condition, and on balance, this combination has a tendency to set up treatment options for the individual that seem a bit more tailored to the individual. Even with the most recent automated CBC machines of today, several labs continue to utilize a good, old-fashioned PBS. Blood smear examination by hand can also pick up minute cell shape changes that machines can't. For example, observing uncommon cell shapes can signal diseases like leukemia or anemia—so the pathologist's judgment (with all their expertise) can be critical in such cases. It's interesting that, despite newer technology being on hand, more and more physicians keep on ordering PBS tests, a practice that has generated controversy as to whether such smears provide useful added information over that which is already provided by the CBC (Lal et al., 2024). In most cases, a good knowledge of what each test has to offer can be the deciding factor. On the question of ordering which tests to order, being smart about ordering is essential. Telling the healthcare staff when a PBS is actually needed appears to get things going along fairly well. Inter-department communication and improved electronic record systems have also proven effective at eliminating unnecessary smear orders, and research now indicates that this approach works (Jazi et al., 2024). Finally, reevaluation of the function of the PBS in combination with the CBC maximizes utilization of valuable resources, better serves the patient, minimizes the added load on lab staff, and overall facilitates healthcare to carry on more effectively—albeit perhaps accepting a little bit of suboptimal imperfection in the process (Figure 4.1).

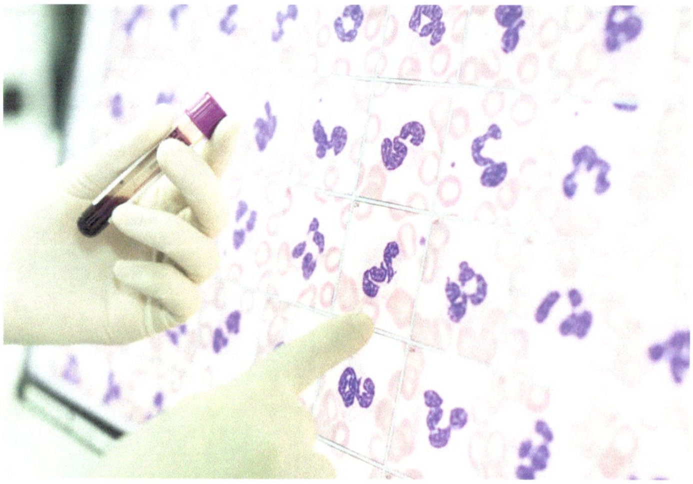

Figure 4.1. Complete blood count (CBC) and peripheral blood smear.

Source: https://noul.com/app/uploads/2024/12/shutterstock_784647403-1024x683.jpg.

Definition of Complete Blood Count

A complete blood count (CBC) is not just a set of numbers—it's really a snapshot of an individual's blood health. It tells us about different kinds of cells like red blood cells, white blood cells, and platelets, all of which come into play when testing for issues ranging from infections to blood conditions. Robotic devices spit out these numbers quickly, but for all the technological progress, a quick eyeball scan at a peripheral blood smear (PBS) still picks up on subtleties that are beyond a computer eye. For most cases, knowledge of how a CBC works speeds on-the-spot screening for sickness problems, and the traditional smear fills in the gaps when there is minute cell change present (Lal et al., 2024). The CBC will typically initiate a doctor's exam, establishing initial standards that can guide subsequent specialty tests. It's a rapid standard test done at routine checkups or when patients mention that they are overwhelmingly tired, look pale, or have undergone spontaneous bleeding. The Sysmex platform and other equipment are designed to minimize human mistakes and speed up the process. Nevertheless, peripheral blood smear still holds its significance—it explores physical cell composition in ways the simple figures might not. When the initial CBC suggests something more profound, a manual inspection can prove to be a deciding factor in the understanding of the complete picture, and thus more rationalized decisions on the doctors' part (Kumari et al., 2024). Current blood work now couples CBC and peripheral smear analysis, an indication of how our practice of hematology has evolved. As the CBC blasts out numbers to determine potential issues, the smear offers a richer, more qualitative view of what the cells are really doing. Over time, hospitals have discovered that efficiency and full testing need not be mutually exclusive—that they have adjusted test-ordering practices accordingly. For instance, some educational programs have even cut back on unwarranted smear requests without shutting down the diagnostic process. When the clinicians realize when to rely on each tool, the care for patients is improved and lab operations are smoother. In general, the use of CBC and PBS together not only saves time lost but also enhances the quality of care in treating blood disorders (Lal et al., 2024).

Importance of CBC in Medical Diagnostics

Diagnostic workups are a huge deal in routine healthcare, and the CBC is no exception. The CBC gives doctors a quick glance at someone's blood – red cell count, white cell count, platelet count – and rattling out data that might otherwise pass by unremarked. A hemoglobin decrease might implicate anemia while atypical white cell counts can represent infection or even leukemia and lymphoma; at times a quick glance at a blood smear provides the added information on cell shape and function, which comes in very handy when things are not right, as in the case of certain types of hairy cell leukemia (Zatsepina et al., 2024). The CBC is not merely a question of nailing down a diagnosis; it is also an excellent instrument for tracking how a patient is doing. Repeated CBCs enable clinical teams to track drug response, adjust meds, and identify side effects before they become a significant problem. For instance, in the treatment of a disease like malaria, traditional microscopy can fall victim to issues with smear quality or the knowledge level of the observer. In most cases, the addition of malaria antigen or antibody tests to complement the results of the CBC has a major impact (Park et al., 2006). The combination of CBC, blood smear analyses, and ancillary tests serves to emphasize the inherent flexibility of the CBC in patient care. As much as medicine continues to change, the CBC remains a reliable member of the bag of tricks. It works well as a quick screen and as a more elaborate work of the diagnostic puzzle – something especially true for rural or resource-limited settings. Its utilitarian simplicity enables it to be applied widely in an effort to raise alarms for health issues on a timely note, often speeding up care when every second matters. Finally, by combining CBC results with a review of blood smears, clinicians are provided with a balanced picture to guide them in handling complex cases and ultimately improve patient outcomes (Figure 4.2).

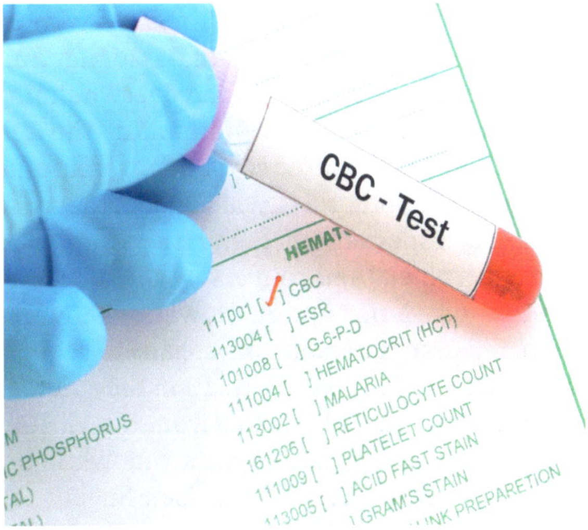

Figure 4.2. CBC in medical diagnostics.

Source: https://ayushmandiagnostics.com/blog/wp-content/uploads/2023/11/CBC-Blood-test.jpg.

Overview of Peripheral Smear and Its Relevance

Peripheral blood smears are one of the main diagnostic tools, alongside the complete blood count (CBC). Specialized machines print out tons of numbers, but if you really want to know what is happening with the cells in the blood, a brief peek at a smear will tell you more about their shape and size. In a way, these slides are helpful in identifying anemias, leukemias, and such low-platelet disorders that tend to slip through the cracks. Many studies have, for the most part, indicated that a well-prepared and confirmed smear will expose peculiarities that the systems will miss (Randive et al., 2025). If doctors correlate data from both the CBC and microscopic observation, they're much better equipped to make knowledge-based decisions about patient care. Even if otherwise normal CBC, surprise can lie in the smear. Pathologists, on detailed scrutiny, can identify clues which indicate blood disorders, e.g., hemoglobinopathies. For instance, it was discovered in one study that significant numbers of pregnant women were carrying abnormal hemoglobin even though they had normal CBC and primary smears—women were often carriers of beta-thalassemia trait (Randive et al., 2025). So, in the overwhelming number of cases, that second look at the cell data is a useful insurance policy, reminding physicians of subtle clues which may otherwise be missed, especially in high-risk groups like pregnant women. And conversely, one does not wish to overuse this option. Nowadays, there is increasing practice among physicians to request these smears, but extra information they yield is sometimes minimal. Evidence from the various hospitals overall appears to show that while the number of smears orders has risen hugely, the new information they provide is relatively tiny, and it is causing the hospitals to discuss more closely when in fact to order a smear (Lal et al., 2024). As this process is adapted to maximize efficiency, achieving peripheral smears on target can conserve precious lab time and resources and enhance patient outcomes. It remains a vital goal in the practice of hematology to this day to have this kind of balance between efficiency and correct diagnosis.

4.1. Components of a Complete Blood Count

Learning Outcome

- Red blood cell (RBC) count;
- White blood cell (WBC) count;
- Platelet count.

A CBC is more of a quick snapshot of how efficiently a body is functioning overall rather than a laboratory test. Hemoglobin saturation gives us a pretty good sense of oxygen delivery, and hematocrit levels basically inform us about how much of the blood is made up of red cells. Then you've got the red blood cell indices like Mean Corpuscular Volume (MCV) and Mean Corpuscular Hemoglobin Concentration (MCHC) that dig deeper into issues with cell size or color; generally speaking, when MCV readings stray from the norm, microcytic anemia might be at play, perhaps signaling an iron shortage. Looking at all these pieces very closely not only notifies one of anemia, but also leads one to search for the causes of it — which, in most cases, actually make a considerable difference in how a patient is treated. White blood cell counts also show up as a prominent item on the CBC, providing one with a general idea what the immune system is up to. Leukocytes—our body's natural protectors—increase at times of acute infection or inflammation, yet drop when diseases like bone marrow disease or autoimmune disorders arise. The differential count that classifies the white blood cells on the basis of type also gives us more information; for example, an excess of neutrophils can indicate a hot spot for bacteria, while an increase in lymphocytes may signal a hot spot for viruses. Overall, understanding these cell dynamics will probably sharpen diagnostic accuracy and aid clinicians in creating more discriminating treatment protocols (Jakovljević et al., 2010). Platelets round out the picture with their role in blood coagulation and wound repair. Their numbers can vary in ways that are significant—a low platelet count (thrombocytopenia) can be due to inhibition of the bone marrow or even increased destruction secondary to autoimmune disease. High platelets (thrombocytosis) can indicate infection or inflammatory diseases. These variations are enough to mandate a review of platelets, as they will tend to reflect what an actual patient is currently experiencing. Where anemia is seen with the coexistence of blood cancers, e.g., the platelet story might uncover underlying pathology not even anticipated at the time (Tuli et al., 2017).

4.1.1. Red Blood Cell (RBC) Count

Medical professionals know that the tracking of red blood cell (RBC) counts is a serious issue—it is important when it comes to deciding how well someone is. Doctors check these counts to see if the blood is delivering oxygen like it is meant to, and from that easy reading, they can realize that a patient's got anemia or polycythemia.

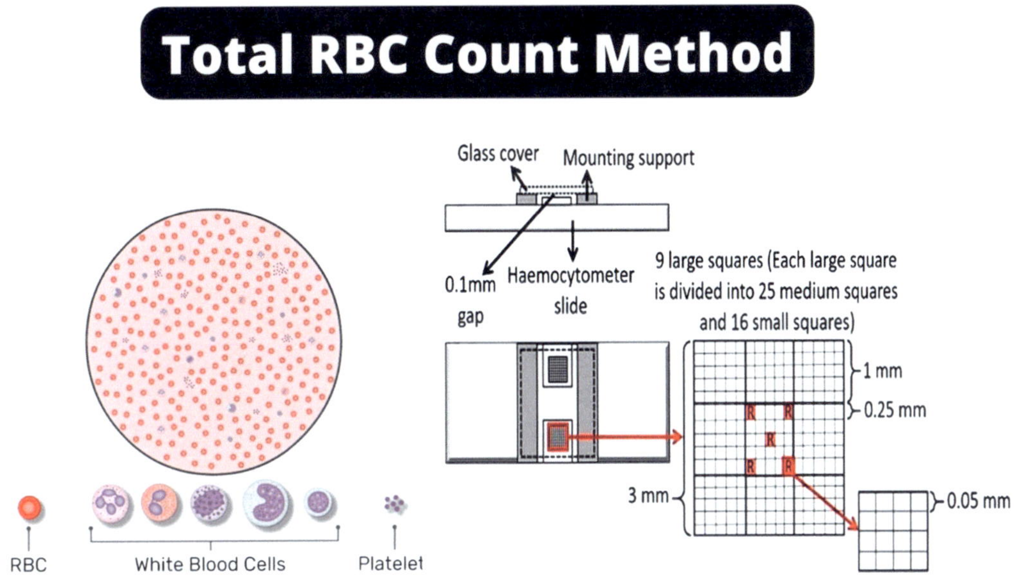

Figure 4.3. Total red blood cell (RBC) count.

Source: https://external-content.duckduckgo.com/iu/?u=https%3A%2F%2Fbiologynotesonline.com%2Fwp-content%2Fuploads%2F2022%2F07%2FTotal-RBC-Count-Method.jpg&f=1&nofb=1&ipt=43e25f4b09b80472822cf750778ddf22225c8e4132fca614bf6e5d013e9cbac2.

You may recall that during the COVID-19 pandemic, RBC counts began to fluctuate irregularly, and even one study showed that men had higher RBC counts than women, so gender-based ranges became important (Salem, 2024). It's interesting to think about how altering this single count can reflect issues not just with overall health, but with how well treatments can work. The RBC count is a basic component of the complete blood count (CBC) picture, giving a broad picture of overall blood status. Values like Mean Corpuscular Volume (MCV) and Mean Corpuscular Hemoglobin Concentration (MCHC) give doctors clues about the nature of these cells; if abnormality shows up, then it could indicate lack of fundamentals like vitamin B12 or iron, or even suggest more complicated, genetic conditions. For instance, research at high altitude has seen such counts be far off from the baseline that national standards would have been expected to shift, suggesting there can be instances where local standards are better (Yuan et al., 2024). Overall, this illustrates how much our surroundings can influence blood characteristics, and why health plans have to be adjustable enough to account for this. Tracking RBC count fluctuations is the best means of observing how various diseases progress. With acute infections or severe disease, as occurred during those sudden surges of the COVID-19 pandemic, big RBC number differences can be the initial signs of something being wrong, especially when increased red cell distribution width tends to be matched with more adverse consequences. One study described RBC counts in patients as being significantly reduced from non-infected controls, implying that these values are not merely diagnostic but also treatment-guiding. In most cases, this means tracking RBCs as more than a box-ticking exercise but as an essential part of patient management and prognosis in current medical practice (Figure 4.3).

4.1.2. White Blood Cell (WBC) Count

Diagnosis of blood disorders is started with a critical review of white blood cell counts in a normal complete blood test (CBC). Counts of WBC are a good sign of whether the immune system is healthy or not – they can even hint at underlying issues. An abnormal count can indicate anything from infection to some cancers. For instance, when WBC is higher than normal, it will most likely suggest leukocytosis, a symptom that is very prevalent in leukemia patients, as suggested by some current research. In research, the necessity to monitor not only WBC but also peripheral blasts in leukemia patients was highlighted, even going so far as to report predictive values for non-graying scattergrams (Lismayanti et al., 2024). All of this does seem to be in favor of why it's so crucial to investigate WBC counts. In the case of chronic inflammatory diseases, such as chronic obstructive pulmonary disease (COPD), higher WBC counts at times can serve as a pre-signal of flare-ups. Overall, evidence does seem to suggest that higher baseline counts – including neutrophils – are usually associated with a higher risk of acute attacks in the long run. One long-term study revealed that patients with elevated WBC levels had noticeably more severe COPD events (Yoon et al., 2024). This suggests that WBC counts are not only convenient for establishing a diagnosis; they also inform us on how a disease is likely to develop. In this sense, such counts serve both as a diagnostic indicator and an advance indication of what is to follow, and this allows medical professionals to inform their treatment plans accordingly. Peeking beyond diagnosis, WBC counts monitored give clues regarding the effectiveness of treatments and even a patient's upcoming progress. Regular monitoring can show whether a treatment is on track or not, especially for patients waiting for therapies in blood cancer or chronic illnesses. Fluctuations in these numbers over time can suggest that the changes must be acted upon or that more interventions can be of benefit – like when a sudden rise in neutrophils is a sign of an ongoing inflammatory or infectious process and needs immediate response. An unambiguous understanding of how these changes relate to other clinical information lays the groundwork for a more targeted response to care. By and large, the outcome of a CBC is more than merely a figure, but instead is an important component in patient management decision-making, indicative of its true daily practical relevance (Figure 4.4).

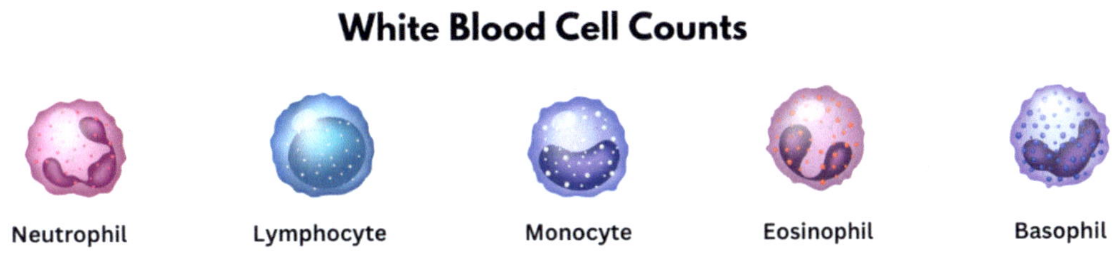

	Cytosis	Cytopenia
Total WBC	> 11,000	< 4,400
Neutrophils	>7,700	<1,500
Lymphocytes	>3,500	<1,500
Monocytes	>800	<200
Eosinophils	>350	<40
Basophils	>100	<10

Numbers expressed per ul; divide by 1,000 to convert to x 10^9/L

Figure 4.4. White blood cell counts.

Source: https://external-content.duckduckgo.com/iu/?u=https%3A%2F%2Fwww.thebloodproject.com%2Fwp-content%2Fuploads%2F2023%2F03%2FCheat-sheet-122.png&f=1&nofb=1&ipt=27c70ec48e7b050f495969ab636bd07335933f95fcdab683b730b3c6f74a85cd.

4.1.3. Platelet Count

Good diagnosis is rooted in accurate lab work, and this is especially true with hematology. Take the CBC – platelet count tells you a lot about the ability of the blood to clot; when platelet counts decrease, bleeding disorders are often on the horizon. Thrombocytopenia – low platelets, plain and simple – actually sounds the warning bells, as it can ultimately appear as bleeding disorders. But though automated hematology analyzers are now universally employed, they do not always reveal the truth to you. Most frequently, they actually end up displaying spuriously low platelet counts as a result of platelet clumping—a phenomenon that in most instances needs to be double-checked with a peripheral smear. In totality, valuing the quirks of the platelet count is an absolute requirement for doctors who want to pin down the right diagnosis and deliver proper care (Meena et al., 2023). Facing these challenges head-on, it is only logical to use advanced analytical techniques to distinguish true thrombocytopenia from the imposter known as pseudothrombocytopenia. Current research tends to indicate that taking a close look at the platelet histogram is important – it provides both visual and good numbers regarding any clumped platelets. When physicians combine CBC information with a reading of the peripheral smear, they can actually increase their accuracy of diagnosis. Overall, with sensitivity lying roughly at about 73.60% and specificity lying roughly at about 93.60%, such histogram flags are a huge deal in current clinical practice. This approach comes some way in cutting down on the large amount of uncertainty both to clinicians and patients (Meena et al., 2023). New computerized systems like the Abbott Alinity h-series are further altering the way platelet counts are acquired and interpreted, to new levels of efficiency and precision. These high-speed analyzers process specimens at an incredible rate, which is a very welcome advantage for high-volume testing. Compared to tests between computerized slide preparation and antiquated manual techniques, the new techniques are shown to offer results nearly as good as the antiquated techniques. However, peripheral smears by hand remain a useful standby when something unusual crops up on the automated reports. As hematology continues to progress, by marrying the new strengths of newer technology with tried and tested, traditional techniques is the best means of achieving the optimal result for patients (Figure 4.5).

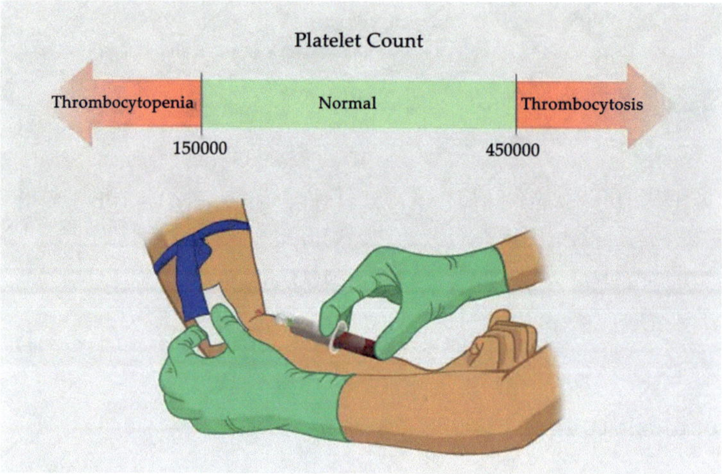

Figure 4.5. Platelet count.

Source: https://external-content.duckduckgo.com/iu/?u=https%3A%2F%2Fimage.myupchar.com%2F4776%2Foriginal%2Fplatelet-count-in-hindi.png&f=1&nofb=1&ipt=1bf3dce48649cdc6398ae0901d3bdb3438dd5ea8a91953f14e362d2c80e3fcb1.

Test Your Knowledge

1. What are the key parameters measured in a complete blood count?
2. How does CBC differentiate between red blood cell, white blood cell, and platelet counts?

4.2. Interpretation of CBC Results

Learning Outcome

- Normal ranges for CBC components;
- Common abnormalities and their implications;
- Factors affecting CBC results.

A CBC is absolutely essential in everyday clinical practice. It's one of those first things physicians think about when trying to diagnose blood issues. The numbers – white blood cell count, hemoglobin, and platelets – can mean anything from infections, anemias, to even leukemia. Once in a while, a peculiar scattergram is noticed on a CBC with the implication that platelets are being phagocytosed by other cells, and this can misleadingly represent thrombocytopenia. A case of an 85-year-old patient (Eloísa et al., 2022) showed how these false impressions can be made as in a patient who is receiving treatment for monoclonal gammopathy. This case highlights how valuable it is to examine both the raw values and the generated scattergrams;

recognizing these quirks not only improves the diagnosis but also saves patients from unwanted, sometimes dangerous, tests. It makes a tremendous difference to see the big picture behind those figures as well. Age, gender, history, and even ongoing treatment can subtly modify the CBC findings. For example, in the evaluation of neonates with suspected hereditary spherocytosis, the resulting elevated mean corpuscular hemoglobin concentration (MCHC) should be weighed against symptoms like jaundice and anemia. In broad terms, diagnostic steps like the HS index tend to tidy up the procedure – albeit, in most cases, their sensitivity and specificity will depend on which group is in question (Patrick, 2021). That is why physicians need to be judicious, integrating the computer results with real-world judgment and the judicious use of periodic additional tests. Incorporating a peripheral blood smear with CBC data can make the difference in just how accurate a diagnosis can be. CBCs give you numbers, but a blood smear gives you a peek at the actual cells – from detecting spherocytes to an abnormal white cell pattern. In that above illustration with the 85-year-old patient, the smear indicated such as phagocytosed platelets and neutrophil satellitism (Eloísa et al., 2022), which clarified just what was occurring. Combining these two approaches together not only confirms the automated findings but also makes it possible to distinguish between disorders that could share the same CBC values. In short, merging the hard data with the qualitative analysis gives a more stable platform for professionals to better enjoy and react to the rich richness of blood disorders (Figure 4.6).

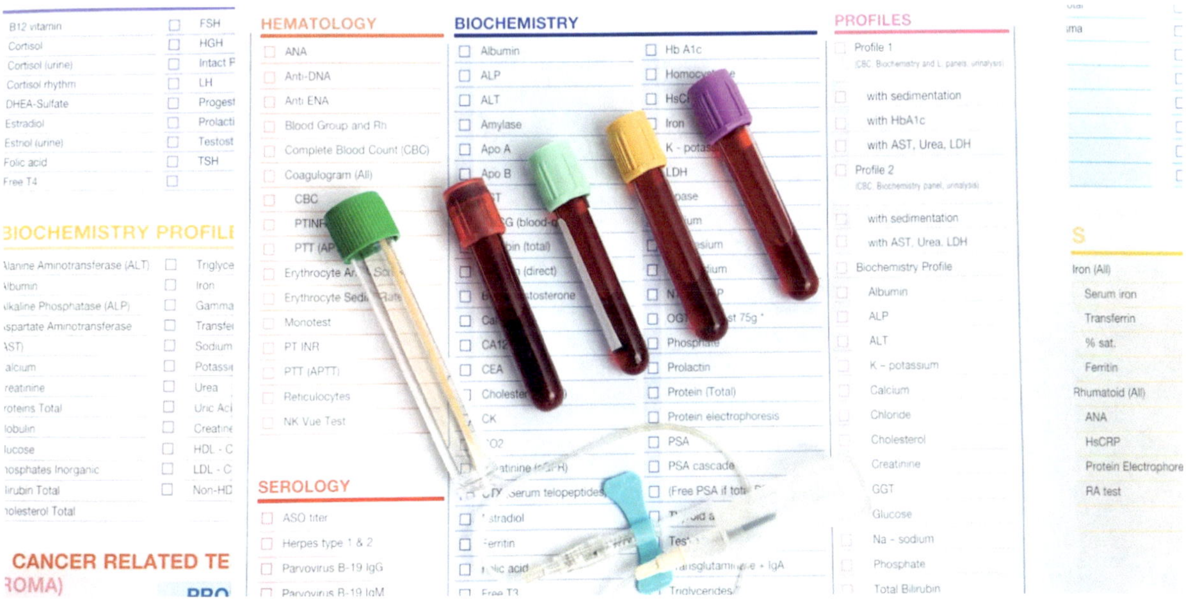

Figure 4.6. Interpretation of CBC results.

Source: https://images.theconversation.com/files/570974/original/file-20240123-19-h34bd4.jpg?ixlib=rb-4.1.0&rect=0%2C107%2C2120%2C1060&q=45&auto=format&w=1356&h=668&fit=crop.

4.2.1. Normal Ranges for Complete Blood Count Components

Knowing what's typical on a CBC the key to a healthy blood test is really. For most individuals, establishing these normal values—such as the number of red blood cells—are important in determining health and detecting disease. For instance, for an average adult man, red blood cells usually are between 4.5 and 5.9 million for every microliter, and for women, they have around 4.1 to 5.5 million. Hemoglobin also has its own range, generally 13.5 to 17.5 grams per deciliter in men and roughly 12.0 to 15.5 in women. If the test results deviate from these ballpark figures, it may be a clue—maybe anemia or polycythemia—that exploration is in order. White blood cells add another level to the combination, generally ranging between 4500 and 11,000 per microliter. An amount greater than that (leukocytosis) can be indicative of infection or inflammation, and less than that (leukopenia) might be due to suppressed immunity or bone marrow dysfunction. Neutrophils, the vital class of white cells, protect our immune defense. Generally, a normal body releases more than 1×10^9 neutrophils per kilogram of body weight a day from the bone marrow, a balance achieved by balancing cell manufacture with removal of aging cells (Hong et al., 2011). From time to time, such normal variation tells us more about how well our body is having its immune system prepared to respond. In addition to the red and white cells, platelets are also key in the prevention of bleeding. Normally, there are 150,000 to 450,000 platelets per microliter. If these values deviate—low platelets increasing the risk of bleeding (thrombocytopenia) or elevated numbers causing clot concerns (thrombocytosis)—then there's usually more to investigate. Less common disorders, like SDS, will also distort these numbers, highlighting the value of being familiar with all these ranges. In most patients, observation of the set of platelets along with other constituents in total is helpful to doctors in making a more comprehensive image, especially for atypical blood disorders (Dror et al., 2011). As a whole, keeping these normal values in mind actually increases our ability to sense, study, and address blood-related issues effectively (Figure 4.7).

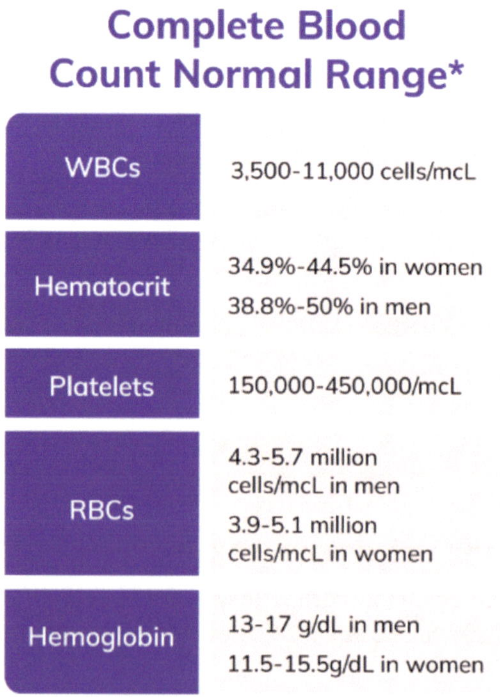

Figure 4.7. Normal ranges for CBC components.

Source: https://wordpresscmsprodstor.blob.core.windows.net/wp-cms/2021/11/99-1.webp.

4.2.2. Common Abnormalities and Their Implications

White blood cell counts give a glimpse of what is occurring within a body. A rise in the cells at times could indicate an infection or possibly an attack of inflammation, whereas falling counts can hint at bone marrow issues or an impaired immune system. Distinguishing, say, SIRS from sepsis typically depends on segmented neutrophil and lymphocyte counts – that most studies in dogs typically find that the septic animals will have reduced median numbers of segmented neutrophils compared with the SIRS animals (Gori et al., 2020). It helps to show that tracking these white blood cell alterations is very important in the clinic. Red blood cells also have their own set of leads. Anemia – characterized by low red blood cell count or hemoglobin level – can occur due to chronic disease, nutritional deficiencies, or even cancers. In the majority of cases, unscrambling the cause of these red blood cell changes not only helps to diagnose blood diseases but also helps to shed light on a patient's overall state and his or her reaction to therapy. Platelets put it all together in a CBC. Low platelet level may be a consequence of overutilization within clots like disseminated intravascular coagulation, or as a decrease in production following bone marrow issues. In contrast, being in excess of platelets may occasionally reflect on inflammation or even malignancy. It isn't a case of substituting figures for a diagnosis; abnormal counts for plates also play a contribution to surgical risks, treatment regimens, and a long-term prognosis. In one research effort, researchers discovered that certain platelet ratios in dogs with broad inflammatory reactions seemed to correlate with survival outcomes after a sepsis diagnosis (Gori et al., 2020). All told, each component of the CBC puzzle adds richness, perhaps some roughness, to a patient's picture.

4.2.3. Factors affecting Complete Blood Count results

CBC values can vary in any number of ways depending on what's going on in the body at the time that the test is taken. How hydrated you are, how much exercise you've been doing, even your usual daily rhythms—all of these can make the numbers that are read change. If you're dry, for example, the blood will be more concentrated so hemoglobin and hematocrit can appear artificially high. A short bout of intense exercise can temporarily raise your white cell level. Age and sex also add a complicating factor; they subtly recalibrate what is "normal." Generally, a peripheral smear can provide more information on the makeup of the bloods (Patra et al., 2021). Medications also do their own way of altering these tests. Most of the common drugs—blood thinners, chemotherapy drugs, steroids—have the ability to change things around. Blood thinners, for instance, can extend bleeding time and interfere with platelet counts, while chemotherapy can reduce cell counts by suppressing bone marrow production. Some medications will even change white blood cell counts, indicating a changed immune function on occasion. This mix of drug effects means doctors need to comb through a patient's medication history carefully; it's essential for figuring out if what you're seeing is drug-induced or something else entirely. Pairing this info with a peripheral blood smear can really round out the picture (You et al., 2015). Health issues add another layer of complexity to CBC outcomes. Disease like chronic infection, persistent inflammation, or malignancies can disrupt the formation of blood cells such that red cells, white cells, and platelets go beyond their normal levels. Take COVID-19, for example—it can lead to an unusual immune response that manifests as typical alterations in blood cells, which would be picked up by a smear. Increased neutrophil-to-lymphocyte ratio in extreme infections in most instances gives doctors a clue about the prognosis. In general, these changes are a reminder that the seemingly simple figures cover up a complex ballet of physiological activities (Patra et al., 2021) (Figure 4.8).

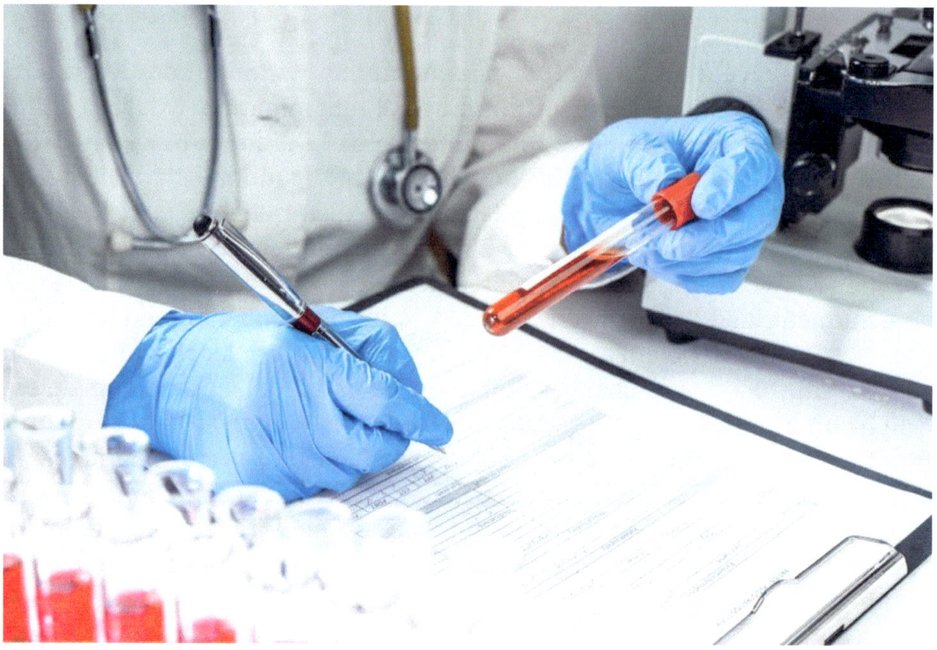

Figure 4.8. Complete blood count (CBC) results.

Source: https://sa1s3optim.patientpop.com/assets/images/provider/photos/2569921.jpeg.

Test Your Knowledge

1. How does anemia present in CBC results, and which indices are most useful in classification?
2. What does leukocytosis or leukopenia indicate in clinical practice?

4.3. The Role of Peripheral Smear

Learning Outcome

- Definition and purpose of peripheral smear;
- Procedure for obtaining a peripheral smear;
- Key features analyzed in a peripheral smear.

Peripherals leap in after an initial CBC hint at something being amiss. They provide a quick look at our blood's cells – red cells, white cells, and platelets – allowing us to eyeball such things as cell size, shape, and color without all the additional ado. Unusual shapes or color? That can suggest conditions such as anemia or even leukemias of several types. Every now and again you might even spot aberrant lymphocytes, which leads clinicians to look more closely into lymphocyte conditions—a type of portent of more investigation and finding out what's really going on. These smears are not solely for detecting abnormalities; they're a first option for tracking the course of established conditions and the effectiveness of treatments. For chemotherapy patients or those with chronic blood disorders, regular checking of a smear is able to find even minor variations in the levels of blood cells. This test, which monitors the overall composition as well as individual cell features, gives clues regarding the working ability of the bone marrow and provides some of the patient's prognosis. In diseases like T cell large granular lymphocytic leukemia (T-LGLL) (Philipp et al., 2016), the smear may even suggest potential mutations alongside commenting on overall marrow health, giving clinicians a better-rounded diagnostic picture. With all the current methods like flow cytometry and molecular diagnostics being in the limelight, the convenience and pervasiveness of peripheral smears guarantee they continue to be part of the forefront in practice. For the most part, though, an optimally prepared smear can supplement other advanced tests directly, providing a better overall view of a patient's blood status. A little experience with smear interpretation does not hurt, either, so that healthcare providers can catch on to such things as immune-related adverse events—particularly in patients treated with immune checkpoint inhibitors (Bryan et al., 2021)—a bit earlier. In total, by merging these traditional methods with ones that are new, one finally has a truer, more integrated picture of a patient's condition on which to base timely and proper care decisions (Figure 4.9).

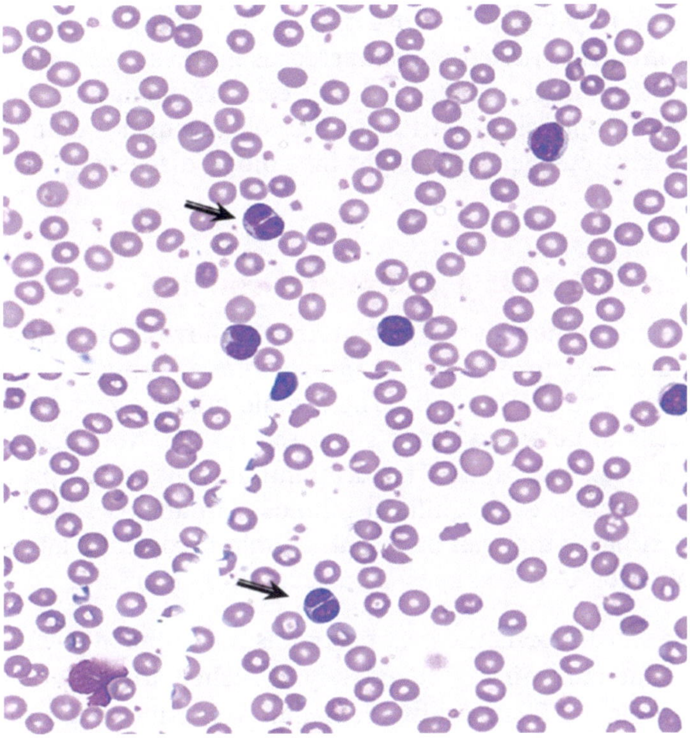

Figure 4.9. Role of peripheral blood smear.

Source: https://external-content.duckduckgo.com/iu/?u=https%3A%2F%2Fimages.journals.lww.com%2Fdshmj%2FSocialThumb.02275336-202406010-00005.F1.jpeg&f=1&nofb=1&ipt=7c6c39433b87f5e5f2029c493a43ff95528a3e37ba12b5bf6b4275612a61d01b.

4.3.1. Definition and Purpose of Peripheral Smear

A blood smear is more than a complete blood count. It gives you a window into the internal mechanisms of blood cells. A tiny sample of blood is pulled out thinly on a slide and stained so that its tiny components are visible under a microscope. This enables doctors to see the shape and appearance of red cells, white cells, and platelets. Counts in a CBC tell you how many, but the smear tells you what they actually look like crucial when screening for such conditions as anemia, leukemia, or other blood idiosyncrasies. In most cases, these visual cues provide a full picture of a patient's hematological health and dictate treatment options as unique as the patients themselves. The test is no one-and-done thing either. Repeating the smear can show cell appearance changes that can indicate whether or not treatment is on the right track, or something else is happening. For example, if the makeup of white blood cells is beginning to alter, it can be a sign of an impending infection or that the marrow is not producing as it should. Occasionally, especially in patients undergoing treatments such as immune checkpoint inhibitors (Bryan et al., 2021), the smear even picks up records of immune-related side effects. By tracking such data over the long term, professionals are able to modify therapy options, hopefully enhancing patient outcomes while remaining complication-free. Apart from diagnosis and ongoing monitoring, these smears also contribute to education and research. These give an idea of what is happening down at the cellular and molecular level. Many doctors, particularly those who are passionately committed to hematology, use smear reviews to improve their diagnostic skills and find new methods of approaching treatment methods. Research conducted using these tests can even indicate shifting patterns of disease, e.g., those that happen in CAR T-cell treatment responses (Santomasso et al., 2021). By and large, this simple slide - with its occasional novelty details - not only enhances diagnostic accuracy but also our general insight into blood diseases in the clinical and teaching setting.

4.3.2. Procedure for obtaining a peripheral smear

Making a peripheral smear is not merely a matter of following a recipe—it requires precise, hands-on effort. A healthcare provider first draws blood, typically with a needle, into an ethylenediaminetetraacetic acid (EDTA) tube. The sample must be processed quickly because any delay could allow the cells to deteriorate and cloud the results. Now that the blood is in hand, a small droplet is put on a clean glass slide. This drop initiates the smear procedure, and it's crucial that it spreads along the slide in even, uniform thinness. An angled slide is employed to pull the drop into a tidy single cell layer that can be examined microscopically later—this is an important step for eventual examination of cell shapes, as discussed by Florea et al. (2012).

Having achieved the smear down, the next portion is not as much technique and more keeping what's been done. The slide must air-dry completely; if rushed, the cells can become depopulated during staining. Upon drying, a fixative like methanol is usually added to act to keep the cells in place. This step is significant in that it holds the cells together, maintaining their forms for a genuine appearance. Routine stains—like Wright's or Giemsa—are applied next so the different cell components truly stand out. These stains reveal the different cell types better, which is critical when detecting disorders ranging from anemia to leukemias, the literature documents (Amarasinghe et al., 2021). Finally, the prepared slide is closely inspected microscopically. Here, professionals look at the stained cells at high power, noting variations in size, shape, and distribution. They check all closely to determine abnormalities and verify automated results double—the manual review can identify unexpected observations which are worth careful examination. In addition, white blood cell counting by hand helps build a deeper image of different populations of leukocytes and gives clues that can direct treatment, since all these processes make peripheral smears continue to be significant in today's blood analysis, as stressed by Florea et al. (2012) (Figure 4.10).

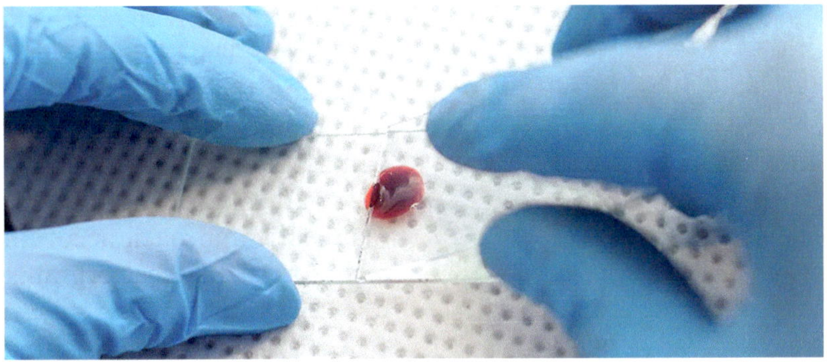

Figure 4.10. Procedure for obtaining a peripheral smear.

Source: https://todaysveterinarynurse.com/wp-content/uploads/sites/3/2025/03/Bellwood_BloodSmearReview_TVNSpring25_MainImage.png.

4.3.3. Key features analyzed in a peripheral smear

Examining a peripheral smear under the microscope enables doctors to pick up on things that a normal CBC just can't. It starts with red blood cells – their color, shape, and size is the tale of anemia or even hints at blood cancers. You notice small (microcytic) or unusually large (macrocytic) cells occasionally, which usually points to nutritional deficiencies or more severe bone marrow issues. Atypical cell distributions, like anisocytosis, add another layer of information about blood disorders. Computerized CBC equipment will give you more general, less specific answers, and the humble smear is still a uniquely necessary tool for this purpose. It is not only red cells, however. With a smear, you also get a look at white blood cells and platelets—key pieces of the hematological puzzle. Sudden increase or fall in white blood cells can reveal an infection, inflammation, or other process of the blood.

Detection of atypical lymphocytes or granulocytes in most cases can be premonitory signs of conditions such as leukemia. Alternatively, inspection of the characteristics of platelets in terms of size and granularity is significant in drawing attention to conditions such as thrombocytopenia or thrombocytopathy. These types of information, even repeated twice in one visit, ultimately result in more targeted therapies and better patient outcomes. Ultimately, that intimate, detailed review far surpasses a normal CBC; it gives a far more individualized profile. Having a chance to label anemia microcytic, normocytic, and macrocytic – typically, the crucial step – actually results in more assessment and treatment. Studies have shown, in most cases, the rampant occurrence of macrocytic anemia among specific populations, to which such tailored care should be directed. An example is that most nutritional deficiencies, as noted by Gani et al. (2020), will dramatically alter red blood cell features, and consequently an extensive smear analysis becomes practically inevitable. This suggests the contribution peripheral smears have, not just in diagnosis but also in guiding broader public health policy, as noted by Munguiko et al. (2020).

Test Your Knowledge

1. How does a peripheral smear help in identifying abnormal cell morphology?
2. What additional information can a peripheral smear provide that a CBC alone cannot?

4.4. Correlation Between Complete Blood Count and Peripheral Smear

Learning Outcome

- How CBC results guide peripheral smear analysis;
- Complementary information provided by both tests;
- Case studies illustrating the correlation.

Massive blood tests have indeed transformed diagnosis-making nowadays. CBC – Complete Blood Count – gives us raw numbers about red and white cells and hemoglobin levels, but the peripheral blood smear (PBS) explores what such numbers may even signify. Oftentimes, not the counts, but the smears tell us about slight changes in cell shapes and sizes. These tiny abnormalities are a sign of disorders ranging from benign to outright malignant, so follow-up on both tests is necessary. CBC and PBS kind of complement one another, giving a more accurate sign of hematologic health and having a tendency to signal red flags earlier before the issues get too far along. Separate. Recent application of automated hematology analyzers has introduced one additional dimension into the equation – scattergrams that pour out of the machines to help flag white blood cell disorders. By and large these scattergrams serve as neat, graphic screening tool, typically competing with or even surpassing old-school smear methods at 97–100% levels of accuracy (which is quite gracious, actually). They speed up the process by showing patterns of size, shape, and density of cells; these may be an early sign of the possibility of malignancies. A combination of these technologically enhanced results with conventional methods in most cases gives clinicians an edge in terms of early diagnosis, even though things sometimes become somewhat complicated in the process. Finally, one should not discount how the CBC and PBS complement each other. The CBC gives us direct quantitative data, and the PBS fills in qualitative gaps that might otherwise go unnoticed. Clinicians and hematopathologists alike are better served to be aware of this interaction and modify their diagnostic approach accordingly. With modern techniques like scattergrams part of the mix, diagnostic accuracy gets a noticeable boost. Overall, this evolving combination of traditional and automated methods isn't so much about discrete test results—it's reshaping the future of blood testing and patient care, keeping us all on our toes (Figure 4.11).

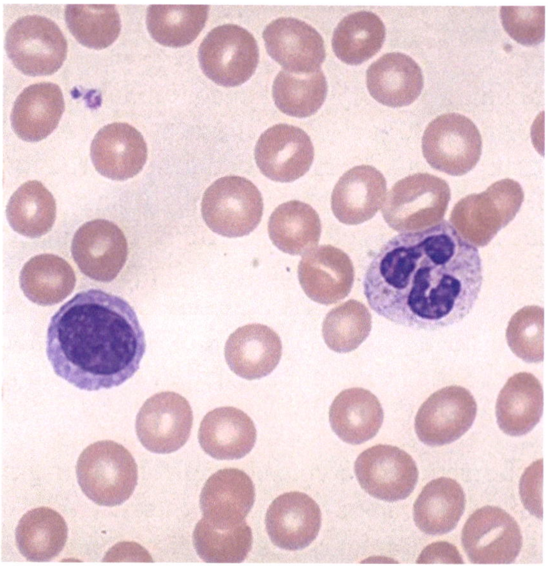

Figure 4.11. Correlation between CBC and peripheral smear.

Source: https://www.ganeshdiagnostic.com/admin/public/assets/images/product/1677931408-CBC%20with%20Peripheral%20Smear.webp.

4.4.1. How CBC Results Guide Peripheral Smear Analysis?

Complete Blood Count (CBC) tests combined with peripheral smear tests are really at the center of detecting blood-related issues. CBC testing starts by giving us figures like white cell counts, hemoglobin levels, and platelet counts. In most cases, these figures indicate that something is wrong. Consider the example of an abruptly elevated white blood cell count. It can signal an infection—perhaps even raise the specter of a malignancy of the blood—so, naturally, doctors set to work analyzing a peripheral smear. That smear, by showing what cells look like and behave like, fills in some of the blanks marked by the CBC. In general, this back-and-forth not only teaches us but also informs our overall sense of a patient's blood health. At times, glaring clues in the CBC can seriously narrow what to consider next in the smear. An elevated mean corpuscular volume (MCV) will point thought toward macrocytic anemia; a diagnosis often linked with vitamin B12 or even folate deficiencies. On the other hand, when hemoglobin is reduced, it can be suggestive of microcytic anemia and a test for conditions like iron deficiency or thalassemia. All these CBC trends act as a prod to prompt hematologists to seriously look for cell size asymmetry or cell asymmetry. In most cases, rather than being isolated numbers, CBC reports become the map that guides further exploration. Placing CBC findings alongside periphery smear observations only makes for a stronger clinical impression and better patient management. If abnormal cells—like blasts or dysplastic components—are seen in a smear, they tend to corroborate or illuminate what the CBC has suggested and typically steers the diagnosis towards something more specific. For instance, the occasional finding of atypical lymphocytes on the smear can be rationalized in the presence of high white cell counts, raising concern regarding potential lymphoproliferative disorder. In general, letting the CBC guide the reading of the smear is a clear indication of how modern hematology relies on combining these techniques with one another in order to enable clinicians to deliver care that's as accurate as it is timely.

4.4.2. Complementary information provided by both tests

Combining a CBC with a peripheral smear is actually very helpful when deciphering difficult blood problems. A CBC instantly reveals how many cells are in your blood, but sometimes it can be missing those minor details necessary to distinguish between similar disorders. For example, when a CBC would show an increase in platelets, a more detailed analysis by a peripheral smear reveals the subtle cell shapes that lead to diagnoses like myeloproliferative neoplasms (MPN). A recent study, in most cases, concluded that the integration of demographic data and CBC counts maximizes accuracy for MPN detection – i.e., the use of both tests can lead to quicker and more respectful decisions on further testing or referral (Jin et al., 2025). In real life it gets slightly more specific: computerized CBCs can report an abnormal count but easily miss some of the not-so-obvious abnormalities detectable by a close peripheral smear examination. Such closer analysis of cells not only sheds light on possible anemias or leukemias but also refines the CBC results. Sometimes, when a surprise finding is disclosed on a peripheral smear, it implies the need for more in-depth hematologic examination. In this way, the two tests complement each other to present a more vivid picture, guiding diagnosis and treatment options by combining plain numbers with detailed cellular findings (Lal et al., 2024). Recent attempts at standardizing the use of peripheral smears have shown some very promising results in practice. When they saw too many unnecessary peripheral smears being ordered, some laboratories included brief teaching sessions and altered the rules of ordering—resulting in fewer orders and higher diagnostic yield. As hospitals and clinics try to utilize resources better, understanding how CBCs and smears complement each other becomes increasingly important. They not only streamline clinical processes but also enable patient care by preventing important diagnostic opportunities from being overlooked and minimizing redundant testing (Lal et al., 2024) (Figure 4.12).

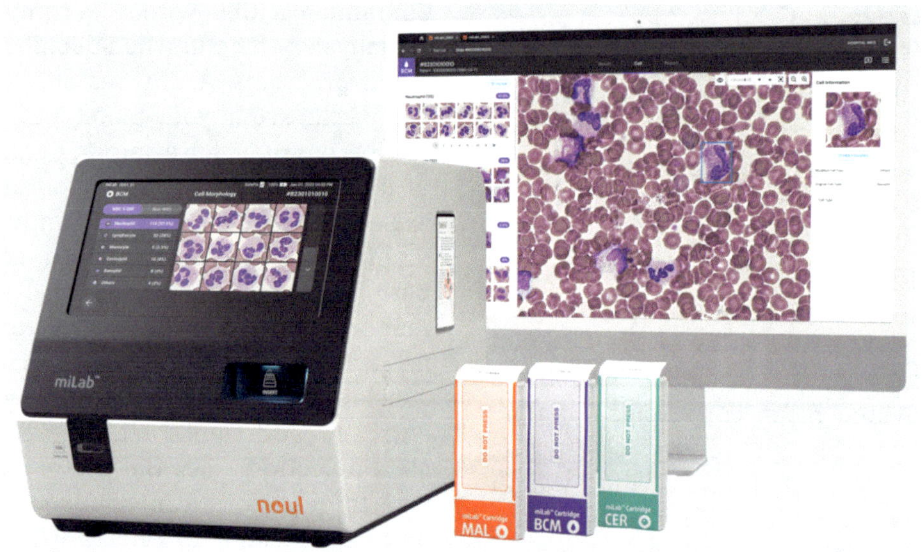

Figure 4.12. Complementary information provided by CBC and peripheral smear tests.

Source: https://noul.com/app/uploads/2024/11/milab_viewer_Cartridge_BCM-3-1024x609.png.

4.4.3. Case Studies Illustrating the Correlation

Hematological diagnosis reveals their subtleties when you go through real-life case examples. One study, which involved 200 clinician-ordered peripheral smears, reported – somewhat unexpectedly – that most of the results were essentially normal relative to the CBC results. In roughly one in every three cases, there just weren't any abnormalities present in the blood, which implies that the effort that goes into the production of these smears may at times yield meager additional information. Curiously, the lab's examination of the smears still caught all meaningful abnormalities, so one can ask whether each patient actually requires what amounts to redundant testing if the CBC is already perfectly accurate (Nagendra et al., 2024). Together, these arguments lead us to question how frequently and in what ways a peripheral smear is actually warranted in standard blood work. Hospital protocols also have an interesting story of adjusting protocol. One study found a persistent rise in the volume of peripheral blood smears ordered by doctors over a span of years—a growth that eventually forced administrators to reconsider their ways. A multidisciplinary panel finally got activated, offering a mix of provider education and new guidelines, and the result was pretty clear: even with an appreciably lower volume of smears, the overall clinical usefulness wasn't impacted—it even went up a bit. For most cases, the mix of prudence in ordering smears with computerized CBC testing appears to remove useful insight without wasting time or resources (Lal et al., 2024). A broader context, these results are larger than the individual cases themselves and look back on wider issues in healthcare. The series of case studies remind us that, despite improvements in automated blood results, a peripheral smear is still required when fine balancing is needed. As a whole, the same would also assume more focused training for medical practitioners such that they are in a place to judge better when a smear yields authentic added value. Clinicians can make better decisions on resource utilization and hopefully observe better results for their patients as they get more accustomed to the benefits—or sometimes limitations—of what these smears offer above CBCs (Lal et al., 2024).

Test Your Knowledge

1. Why is it important to correlate abnormal CBC values with peripheral smear findings?
2. How can a peripheral smear confirm or refine the interpretation of automated CBC results?

4.5. Clinical Applications of CBC and Peripheral Smear

Learning Outcome

- Diagnosis of hematological disorders;
- Monitoring treatment efficacy;
- Assessing overall health and detecting infections.

Blood smear and CBC tests give a real window to what is happening in one's blood. They are more than just numbers – these tests help warn of various issues like anemia, low white blood cells, or platelet problems by incorporating both numeric and visual warnings. For example, you might check for anemia by measuring hemoglobin and hematocrit, and looking at the smear gives a quick sense of red blood cell morphology straight away, indicating cells are oddly small or large. The pairing of tough facts and a bit of eyeballing aids in increasing diagnostic assurance, whether in ordinary check-ups or exploring specific blood problems. No wonder complications from blood disorders most often lead to more specific tests. Scrutinous analysis of white blood cells will oftentimes reveal traces of infection, inflammatory disease, or even cancer. Sometimes monitoring odd or abnormally appearing lymphocytes on a smear will be the initial indication of viral infection or as severe as acute lymphoblastic leukemia (ALL). In most cases, suggestions like those of the National Comprehensive Cancer Network (NCCN) (Patrick et al., 2021) suggest that adding the immunophenotyping with the CBC will provide the opportunity to refine risk stratification and therapy, adding some depth to the picture that will empower doctors to finish the puzzle. Outside the process of diagnosing a patient, these tests really find their application in monitoring for response to therapy and changes in disease." For example, in chemotherapy, regular CBC analysis can identify suppression of bone marrow, indicating that the treatment regimen might need to be altered. While platelet counts are generally reliable, they may at times be skewed by conditions such as EDTA-induced pseudothrombocytopenia – a minor glitch which, if undetected, could mislead interpretations (Véronique et al., 2020). Overall, the integration of CBC results with blood smear photographs gives doctors a fuller, occasionally imperfect but very human image of blood health, clearing the way for timely course correction and better results.

4.5.1. Diagnosis of Hematological Disorders

CBC and peripheral smear tests really take laboratory results back to the way we look at a patient's overall picture. The CBC can perhaps start by giving you quick returns of red cells, white cells, and platelets – all those figures that can presage a diagnosis of anything from anemia to leukemic change. Most commonly, when such findings crop up suddenly, doctors can decide which follow-up studies will be needed. Meanwhile, a peripheral smear inserts a quality control element of sorts—it identifies abnormal cell morphology that may not be captured by the CBC. Both tests used together give a kind of back-and-forth analysis that helps to identify blood disorders more specifically, although the process sometimes can seem somewhat unpredictable. It is not necessarily cut and dried either, since discriminating benign from malignant change in the blood is no simple task. Yes, the CBC will tell you the raw count, but it's that extra layer of understanding on the peripheral smear that creates a fuller picture. Take thrombocytopenia, for example – sometimes a lower-than-normal platelet count is due to bone marrow issues, and sometimes it's because the body is using up platelets faster than usual. Overall, integrating these kinds of diagnostic steps through evidence-based procedures can enhance decision-making (Azi et al., 2024).

Those systems integrating CBC data with real-time clinical cues can actually help general practitioners manage this complexity to make treatments not only timely but also on target. Hematology development, and illnesses such as COVID-19, have well brought to the fore the need for accurate blood analysis. Recent studies show that the type of complications that have occurred includes thrombocytopenia as well as venous thromboembolism and have even aggravated underlying blood conditions in some cases (Azi et al., 2024). As health care professionals steer through these issues, they're increasingly aware that studying the connection between infections and blood tests isn't abstract theory – it's a matter of life and death. Usually, this means ongoing upgrading and an openness to alter diagnostic approaches, integrating fresh therapeutic solutions appropriate for every patient's situation. Finally, when multidisciplinary teams work together and pool their experience with data obtained from the CBC and smear reports, patients do much better in managing their blood disorders (Figure 4.13).

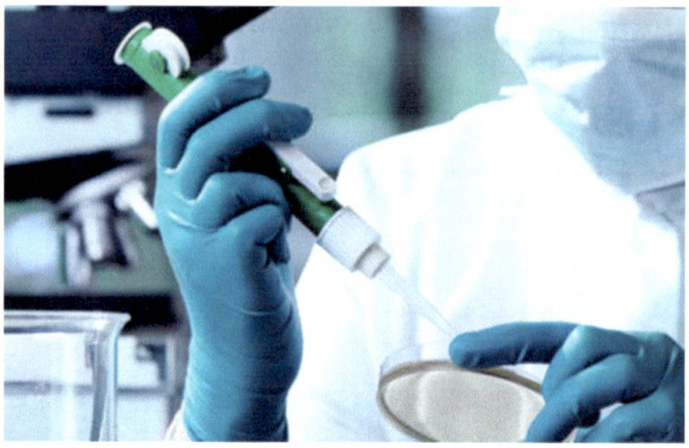

Figure 4.13. Laboratory diagnosis of hematological disorders.

Source: https://drmuralidaranhematologist.com/images/service/7.jpg.

4.5.2. Monitoring treatment efficacy

Watching how therapies affect blood disorders is almost a matter of having the right tests. The complete blood count (CBC) and a quick look at a peripheral smear are two workhorses that do much of the heavy work. In most cases, with the course of therapy, the CBC is showing changes in red blood cell counts, hemoglobin, and platelets – little tidbits that show whether things are going in the right direction. And then, of course, there is the peripheral exam, giving a microscopic view of cell shapes and identifying any abnormal changes that arise during treatment; these give information used to make clinical decisions. Constant monitoring of these parameters allows doctors to be able to determine whether a patient is responding as expected or whether the regimen must be adjusted; this makes monitoring on a consistent basis important in the treatment of patients (Vaishnavi et al., 2024). When anemias or blood cancers come into play, the combination of CBC results and what is seen on a peripheral smear becomes especially important. Red cell information on a CBC sometimes provides insight into why anemia is happening, and the smear reveals qualitative differences within cells that otherwise might go unnoticed. This mix of data provides a general impression of a patient's blood health, typically providing clues as to whether treatment is indeed on track. In the case of certain diseases, particularly hematological malignancies, looking at shifts in cell lineages from one test to the other can be the first sign of a worsening disease or relapse, which encourages physicians to act early. Generally, using these tests in combination simplifies clinicians' evaluation of therapy effectiveness and renders therapy more targeted to patient needs (Zatsepina et al., 2024). With increasingly complex treatment regimens, the need for the CBC and peripheral smear only grows – especially for chronic conditions. Even slight variation in blood test results has the ability to initiate early adjustment in a treatment plan, fine-tuning a patient's overall response. An example would be if hemoglobin is consistently low with ongoing treatment; it might prompt doctors to further investigate or modify medications to avoid complications. Linking lab results to clinical decision-making significantly increases the ability to care for patients ahead of time. In short, regular tests conducted with both smears and CBC not only quantitate the efficacy of therapy, but also make an integral practice more so by keeping treatments within the person's health profile (Vaishnavi et al., 2024).

4.5.3. Assessing Overall Health and Detecting Infections

Blood tests will teach you a lot about someone's overall health – sometimes the simplest test will tell you more than you can possibly guess. The CBC, for example, performs tests on red cells, white cells, platelets – and it does them all in one test – and it isn't presented in some neat checklist. Instead, it gives you a snapshot that might indicate underlying issues. A reduction of the red cells could point to anemia, and lowered counts of white cells (leukopenia) or platelets will raise an alarm, while a spike in white cells is usually a sign of the body's response to infection. Labs are usually following very strict protocols—good laboratory practices (GLP), if you want to be formal—to keep these results as accurate as possible, and that conservative approach is exactly why the CBC is such a valuable tool for catching problems early on (Abhijeet et al., 2025).

When it comes to chronic conditions, a CBC isn't always about diagnosing—something to check ongoing treatment and overall health. Take obesity, for instance. It's not just excess weight; it usually has higher lipid levels and inflammatory markers seen in the blood. In most cases, elevated white cells in a person who is obese can even make him more prone to infections or, worse, blood cancers like leukemia. Such a correlation is why monitoring CBC values is necessary, particularly for those with heightened risk.

Small tweaks, like altering your diet, sometimes lead to noticeable improvements in blood profiles, and, as many studies have confirmed, having a diet rich in nutrients can have real, positive effects on these numbers (Felemban et al., 2024). Doctors don't solely count on the CBC, though – they like to add a peripheral smear to the mix. By adding this extra step, blood cells are provided with the microscopic close-up; it shows things about shape and demeanor a routine test may not. Such abnormalities as atypical lymphocytes or subtle red cell shape changes only manifest themselves when you actually look at the cells.

With the two tools together, healthcare workers can assemble a more accurate picture—sometimes even detecting subtle changes hinting at a slow decline in health or signaling the need for a treatment modification. Tracking these from time to time can actually become a valuable part of keeping on top of overall health and detecting infections early (Abhijeet et al., 2025) (Figure 4.14).

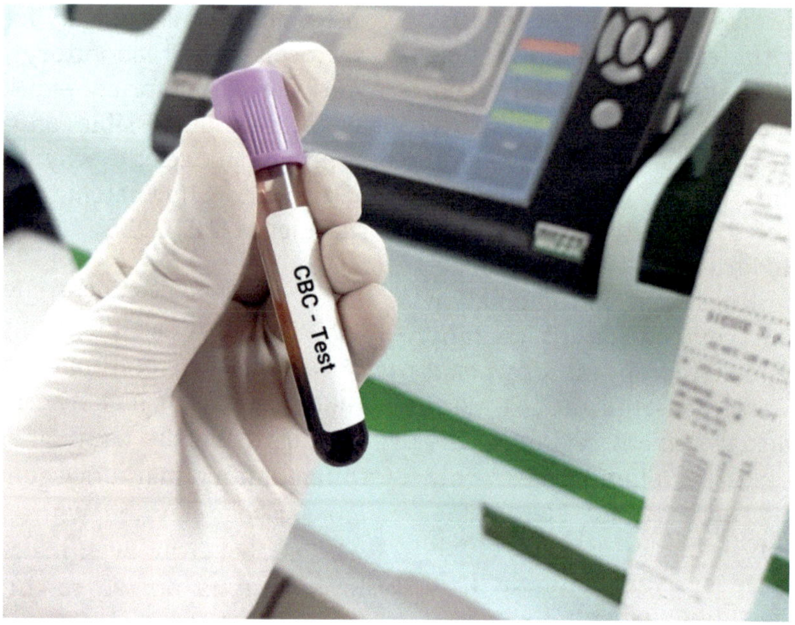

Figure 4.14. CBC test assessing overall health and detecting infections.

Source: https://www.advantagemedical.sg/wp-content/uploads/2024/04/51-1024x768.webp.

Test Your Knowledge

1. How are CBC and peripheral smear used in the diagnosis of different types of anemia?
2. In what ways do CBC and smear assist in monitoring infections and inflammatory conditions?

4.6. Limitations of CBC and Peripheral Smear

Learning Outcome

- Potential for false positives and negatives;
- Situations where results may be misleading;
- Need for additional tests for comprehensive diagnosis.

A CBC is simple to misread. The machines that run these tests are fast, but occasionally they make mistakes—registering false positives or negatives that mislead the clinical picture. They even demonstrated in one trial that, in certain cases, the proportion of false negatives surpassed safe limits (Comar et al., 2014). What this essentially means is that, though automated processes are easy, they can miss important blood abnormalities, thereby undermining patient safety. Reliance on these numbers alone can also involve ignoring some fine but significant things like certain blood disorders. In most cases, a CBC is an acceptable start, but it has to be supplemented; manual examinations and more specific clinical screening are usually needed. Peripheral smears looked at in finer detail can fill some gaps left by automation, although this technique is not free from problems. An expertly stained smear interpreted by someone who actually knows what they are doing can reveal subtleties that computer programs are prone to overlook (Florea et al.,

2012). Of course, the whole process depends significantly upon the ability of the technician and the care with which the sample was prepared. If an improperly done smear is conducted—maybe it was poorly prepared and stained—the risk of misinterpretation grows, and this serves only to exacerbate the challenges of dependence upon CBC results. Secondly, if laboratories become inundated with specimens, extra time and labor required for hand review can lead to delay. Overall, achieving a balance between fast automated screening and keen eyes of skilled personnel usually yields the best outcomes. Finally, the clinical environment under which CBC and smear reports are being interpreted also plays a huge role in making them reliable or not. Hemolysis, dehydration, or infection can bias CBC results, so much so that a subsequent test would be deemed warranted (Comar et al., 2014). Although peripheral smears can answer these queries, these too need to be viewed in light of the patient's background and the patient's state. For example, an extreme variation in white blood count might indicate very different possibilities depending on the history and symptoms of a patient—with those correlations often being highly critical. Overall, while both CBCs and smears are excellent assets in the arsenal of blood work, their weaknesses exist to remind us that there is no single test that tells the whole story, and a broader clinical assessment is usually required to render an accurate, useful diagnosis.

4.6.1. Potential for False Positives and Negatives

Hematological testing can be very problematic—false positives and negatives could actually alter patient management if not handled just so. In routine clinic practice, automated blood analyzers are relied upon to interpret CBC data, but, if they're not precisely calibrated, they could mislead. For instance, the International Consensus Group for Hematology Review established some guidelines to facilitate manual double-checking of results in order to reduce unnecessary peripheral blood smear (PBS) reviews. In general, it's important to keep both automated reports and manual tests under observation, since small differences can result in correctly normal conditions being reported falsely or, on the other hand, substantial pathologies being missed, which further jeopardizes patient safety (Bouwer et al., 2017). The need to integrate complicated algorithms into these machines has introduced some remarkable developments; however, the variability between dissimilar analyzers is a significant obstacle. In most cases, variable quality from automated devices necessitates standard operating procedures and prudent diagnostic regimens. A number of studies comparing various hematology analyzers stress that device-specific algorithms serve to improve the precision of clinical diagnostics and overall care of patients. If information from different sources does not agree, suspicion creeps into the diagnosis—too little specificity can lead to false positives, prompting clinicians to futile interventions, while low sensitivity will conceal significant health problems for which action is urgently needed (Brügel et al., 2021). Clearly, achieving the right balance between sensitivity and specificity in CBC and PBS tests is most crucial for improving laboratory reliability. It also becomes imperative, then, to regularly correct and optimize the algorithms used in laboratories. Close monitoring of false positive and negative ratios, especially when certain flags are triggered, can detect common errors in automated analysis, which sometimes lures laboratory personnel into altering their smear assessment criteria. This might even include, in some instances, sacrificing some flags for harmless conditions in order to improve the accuracy of the system output. Previous studies have in most cases suggested that recommendations by consensus could help lower the rate of false negatives in most lab environments. Overall, ongoing study and implemented changes to deal with the problem of false positives and negatives remain crucial for furthering diagnostic quality and facilitating better patient health outcomes (Bouwer et al., 2017) (Figure 4.15).

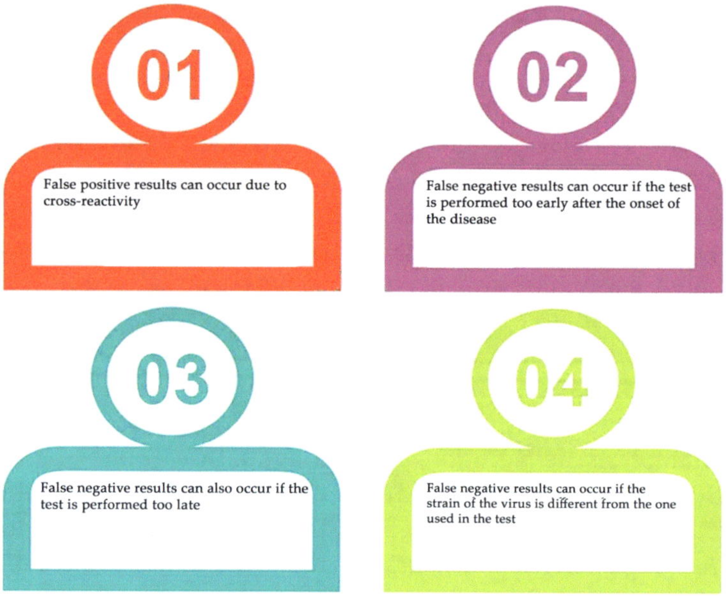

Figure 4.15. False positive and false negative results.

Source: https://fastercapital.co/i/Diagnosing-TBE--The-Science-of-Serology-Testing--False-Positive-and-False-Negative-Results.webp.

4.6.2. Situations where results may Be misleading

A Complete Blood Count (CBC) test and its peripheral smear sometimes send false signals—probably because there are so many variables that get into the test's accuracy. Automated analyzers, while quick and usually accurate, could possibly just overlook those small, easily overlooked blood abnormalities. In most cases, this fault does not manifest itself until a pathologist has to step in for a manual inspection of the smear. Relying too closely on these machine-derived statistics, without any further human expertise, can result in the critical hematological issues being overlooked (Lal et al., 2024). Ironically, even the sheer multitude of peripheral smears ordered by physicians have magnified these issues. Over the last few years, there's been an immense spike in such requests, leading to an overaging of tests that — honestly — really aren't providing much in the form of legitimate diagnostic return. A study showed that even when doctors' orders doubled, only an infinitesimal fraction of the tests even returned clinically significant issues. Overall, this over-reliance on peripheral smear investigation is so much so that physicians and laboratory staff need to revise their parameters for ordering such tests so that they avoid unnecessary investigations and laboratory fatigue (Lal et al., 2024). Taking another view, what the parameters of investigation of these smears can do is impact the diagnosis as a whole. For example, comparing standards from the International Council for Global Health Recommendations (ICGHR) with laboratory-specific guidelines at times produces obviously divergent results. When results are compared against these conflicting standards, it is obvious that changing standards can result in interpretations that don't quite fit. In most cases, while computerized CBCs do provide a good starting reference for screening, it is also necessary to have subsequent reviews that are both routine and properly attuned to the issue at hand—to ensure that clinicians are finally left with the right information they really need to integrate patient care (Kumari et al., 2024).

4.6.3. Need for additional tests for comprehensive diagnosis

New diagnostics. It's not exactly as straightforward as it would lead you to suppose. A cursory Complete Blood Count (CBC) or a quick peripheral smear glance at blood will give you a sense of blood health, but sometimes just doesn't paint the picture. You might have a CBC with only subtle hints that something is not right, but lurking beneath it can be a genetic spin—like an LPIN1 gene mutation—that only reveals itself if further tests, such as some antibody panels or genetic assays, are ordered (Bareja et al., 2025). The obvious sometimes just isn't obvious. We can't entirely depend on the CBC and smear, especially when the patient comes in with a mix of symptoms. Think about it: a patient who has fatigue or weakness in muscles might have a mild abnormality with their first batch of blood tests. And for diseases like rhabdomyolysis or myopathy, the standard results might come back close to normal adding to the uncertainty. Under these circumstances, doctors will often turn to more subtle measures, like whole-blood cytokine evaluation or a limited panel, which might reveal inflammatory markers not detectable by routine CBC (Yasuda et al., 2024). Contemporary attempts at individualized care make ancillary testing more unavoidable than ever. As medicine advances, it's not only discovering a problem that's important, but why it happens, too. Precision medicine, in broad terms, means that even a small gene mutation might change the treatment trajectory of a patient. For blood diseases and other disorders that are associated with them, the combination of genetic testing with the traditional ones gives an overall picture, wherein tiny details, which might otherwise go unnoticed, are examined, though the result sometimes arrives by way of rounded results (Figure 4.16).

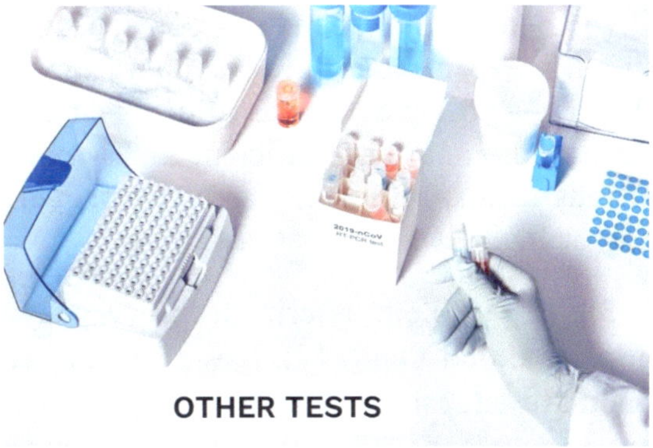

Figure 4.16. Other diagnostic tests.

Source: https://phoenixclinics.in/wp-content/uploads/2024/01/25-1-1024x683.jpg.

Test Your Knowledge

1. What are the common limitations of automated CBC in detecting abnormal cells?
2. Why might a peripheral smear sometimes fail to provide definitive diagnostic information?

Summary

Inter-departmental collaboration clearly works wonders when laboratories try to improve how they handle tests like the Complete Blood Count (CBC) and Peripheral Smear (PBS). Recent research shows that directed education interventions, in conjunction with changes to the rules on when to refer a PBS, can actually reduce unnecessary testing in healthcare settings. This one change not only saves valuable resources but also frees laboratory scientists and pathologists up to carry out other tasks, which in the majority of cases means that about 31.0–46.6 hours are saved each month (Lal et al., 2024). It is wonderful to observe how the minute shift of focus, especially where doctors are given more hands-on training, can make the whole process ever so slightly less complicated and more efficient. If you dig a little deeper, the numbers indicate that with a less complicated, more direct process, you can add to the clinical value of blood tests without sacrificing any of their diagnostic bite. After some rationalization, potential clinical value went up from approximately 3% to 4%, which means that fewer PBS reviews ordered by physicians can actually lead to more valuable results. Yes, auto-testing of blood is certainly timesaving, but some of that good old-fashioned PBS checking manually still detects the nuances that machines miss; a mix of both methods seems to be the key to keeping in balance (Kumari et al., 2024). This combination of technology and trained eye manual is usually sufficient to ensure nothing important slips through the net. Finally, reconsidering how we conduct CBC and PBS testing has implications for healthcare overall. Laboratories are always trying to find the ideal balance between automation and good old-fashioned manual consideration, and keeping up to date on testing rules and training seminars is paramount. The cooperation of hematopathologists, hematologists, and laboratory scientists—loosely at that as a team—show you how pooling together different observations can indeed make one more efficient and accurate in diagnosis. Evidently, the use of evidence-based methods means resources are being properly utilized, ultimately improving patient care but still being at high levels (Lal et al., 2024).

Biology of blood is critical in everyday clinical practice. Doctors often use lab work like the Complete Blood Count (CBC) – it quickly analyzes red cells, white cells, and platelets, giving an immediate snapshot of what's happening inside. The test is more than just numbers; it helps identify such conditions as anemia, infection, and other blood disorders. In the majority of cases, studies show that anemia is a significant worldwide issue, affecting close to one-third of the population. Clinicians therefore combine these laboratory findings with what they observe in patients to identify the underlying problems. This combination of information and observation not only detects anomalies but also provides avenues for further inquiry (Tuli et al., 2017). Then, of course, there is the peripheral smear, that one that goes a step further by examining blood cells through a microscope. In this case, details like a change in shape, size, or color of cells can lead towards certain conditions – for example, conditions like sickle cell disease or certain leukemias might be unraveled by simple such differences. In most cases, research has shown that acute white cell fluctuations even in asymptomatic people might represent an acute infection, a trend seen particularly during the COVID-19 era. I recall one study where a reduction of white cells, like mild leucopenia in childbearing-aged women, resulted in additional tests for possible SARS-CoV-2 infection. These minor, often underemphasized alterations definitely highlight the value of the peripheral smear in diagnosis (Gharib et al., 2021). As a whole, pairing the CBC with a peripheral smear simply is not feasible in today's medicine. These tests are more than just the detection of anemia or infection; they can track disease progression, quantify the response to treatment, and even warn of impending complications down the line. They complement each other to paint a wider clinical picture of a person's health, and they also provide pointers regarding larger public health patterns. Continued study continues to demonstrate that as our knowledge improves, these exams are changing—highlighting the reason why they continue to be a staple in standard clinical assessments (Gharib et al., 2021; Tuli et al., 2017).

KEY TERMS FROM THIS CHAPTER

- Anisocytosis
- Basophils
- Complete blood count (CBC)
- Differential leukocyte count
- Eosinophils
- Hematocrit (Hct)
- Hemoglobin (Hb)
- Lymphocytes
- Mean corpuscular hemoglobin (MCH)
- Mean corpuscular volume (MCV)
- Monocytes
- Neutrophils
- Peripheral blood smear
- Platelet count
- Poikilocytosis
- Red blood cell count (RBC)
- Red blood cell distribution width (RDW)
- Reticulocytes
- White blood cell count (WBC)

Critical Thinking Questions

1. **Which of the following parameters is NOT included in a standard Complete Blood Count (CBC)?**
   a. Hemoglobin (Hb)
   b. Blood urea nitrogen (BUN)
   c. White blood cell count (WBC)
   d. Platelet count
2. **What does a high white blood cell (WBC) count typically indicate?**
   a. Dehydration
   b. Infection or inflammation
   c. Anemia
   d. Liver failure
3. **In a peripheral blood smear, which cells are examined for abnormalities?**
   a. Only red blood cells
   b. Only white blood cells
   c. Only platelets
   d. Red cells, white cells, and platelets
4. **What condition is indicated by a low hemoglobin level on a CBC?**
   a. Leukemia
   b. Anemia
   c. Polycythemia
   d. Thrombocytosis
5. **What information can be obtained from the peripheral smear that a CBC cannot provide alone?**
   a. Hematocrit value
   b. Platelet count
   c. Cell morphology
   d. White blood cell total

Answers to Critical Thinking Questions

1. (b); 2. (b); 3. (d); 4. (b); 5. (c)

Short Answer Questions

1. What parameters are typically included in a Complete Blood Count (CBC) test?
2. What is the normal range for hemoglobin (Hb) in adults, and why is it important?
3. What is hematocrit (Hct), and what does a high or low value indicate?
4. What is a peripheral blood smear, and how is it prepared?
5. How can a peripheral smear help identify abnormalities in red blood cells, such as anisocytosis or poikilocytosis?
6. What types of white blood cell abnormalities might be detected on a peripheral smear?

References

1. Abd Wahab, M. B. A., Mahmood, S., Mohamad Rus, M. A., Mustar, S., et al. (2020). Quality control improvement at Jana DCS Sdn. Bhd. https://core.ac.uk/download/12007130.pdf (accessed on 1st July 2025).

2. Amarasinghe, R., Basnayake, B. A. D. J. C. K., Hettiarachchi, S. P., Melroy, D., et al. (2021). Review on photomicrography based full blood count (FBC) testing and recent advancements. https://core.ac.uk/download/577886377.pdf (accessed on 1st July 2025).

3. Antognoni, M. T., Cremonini, V., Gavazza, A., Miglio, A., et al. (2024). Hematological ratios and indices in canine large B-cell lymphoma. https://core.ac.uk/download/614101457.pdf (accessed on 1st July 2025).

4. Azi, C. I., Carsrud, N. D. V., Ezewudo, O., Flores, C., et al. (2024). Hematological conditions associated with COVID-19: Pathophysiology, clinical manifestations, and therapeutic approaches. https://core.ac.uk/download/621451769.pdf (accessed on 1st July 2025).

5. Baccini, V., Geneviève, F., Jacqmin, H., Châtelain, B., Girard, S., Wuillème, S., Védrenne, A., et al. (2020). Platelet counting: Ugly traps and good advice. Proposals from the French-speaking Cellular Hematology Group (GFHC). *Journal of Clinical Medicine, 9*, 808–808. https://doi.org/10.3390/jcm9030808 (accessed on 1st July 2025).

6. Bareja, N., Chionatos, R., Porto, C. V., Srinivasan, N., & Ghasemi, M. (2025). Adult-onset episodic rhabdomyolysis in a patient with a heterozygous Lipin 1 (LPIN1) mutation: A case report. *Cureus*. https://doi.org/10.7759/cureus.76772 (accessed on 1st July 2025).

7. Bouwer, N. (2017). Validation of hematology peripheral blood slide review rules at various tiers of diagnostic laboratories in South Africa. https://core.ac.uk/download/188771563.pdf (accessed on 1st July 2025).

8. Brown, P. A., Shah, B., Advani, A. S., Aoun, P., Boyer, M. W., Burke, P. W., DeAngelo, D. J., et al. (2021). Acute lymphoblastic leukemia, version 2.2021, NCCN clinical practice guidelines in oncology. *Journal of the National Comprehensive Cancer Network, 19*, 1079–1109. https://doi.org/10.6004/jnccn.2021.0042 (accessed on 1st July 2025).

9. Brügel, M. (2021). *Biomarker der Inflammation*. https://core.ac.uk/download/395059142.pdf (accessed on 1st July 2025).

10. Comar, S. R., Malvezzi, M., & Pasquini, R. (2014). Are the review criteria for automated complete blood counts of the International Society of Laboratory Hematology suitable for all hematology laboratories? https://core.ac.uk/download/pdf/82243955.pdf (accessed on 1st July 2025).

11. Dror, Y., Donadieu, J., Köglmeier, J., Dodge, J. A., Toiviainen-Salo, S., Mäkitie, O., Kerr, E. N., et al. (2011). Draft consensus guidelines for diagnosis and treatment of Schwachman-Diamond syndrome. *Annals of the New York Academy of Sciences, 1242*, 40–55. https://doi.org/10.1111/j.1749-6632.2011.06349.x (accessed on 1st July 2025).

12. Felemban, S., & Hamouda, A. (2024). A pilot study of diet lifestyle on complete blood picture, elements, and biological profile in females. *Trends in Immunotherapy*. https://www.semanticscholar.org/paper/ab1f5b88751b933e34274e2717afbb4aa17d1bd8 (accessed on 1st July 2025).

13. Florea, A. D., Gong, J., Gulati, G., Song, J., et al. (2012). Purpose and criteria for blood smear scan, blood smear examination, and blood smear review. https://core.ac.uk/download/46971873.pdf (accessed on 1st July 2025).

14. Gallagher, P. G. (2021). Difficulty in diagnosis of hereditary spherocytosis in the neonate. *Pediatrics, 148*. https://doi.org/10.1542/peds.2021-051100 (accessed on 1st July 2025).

15. Gani, M. U., Gupta, A., & Kumar, P. (2020). Macrocytosis is highly prevalent in Raebareli district, Uttar Pradesh, India. https://core.ac.uk/download/543136064.pdf (accessed on 1st July 2025).

16. Ganti, A. K., Loo, B. W., Bassetti, M., Blakely, C. M., Chiang, A. C., D'Amico, T. A., D'Avella, C., et al. (2021). Small cell lung cancer, version 2.2022, NCCN clinical practice guidelines in oncology. *Journal of the National Comprehensive Cancer Network, 19*, 1441–1464. https://doi.org/10.6004/jnccn.2021.0058 (accessed on 1st July 2025).

17. Gharib, W. F., Khamees, R. E., Nasser, H., Sobh, M., et al. (2021). COVID-19 related complete blood count changes among asymptomatic pregnant women. https://core.ac.uk/download/492945963.pdf (accessed on 1st July 2025).

18. Gori, E., Lippi, I., Lubas, G., Marchetti, V., & Pierini, A. (2020). Are leukocyte and platelet abnormalities and complete blood count ratios potential prognostic markers in canine sepsis? https://core.ac.uk/download/534224003.pdf (accessed on 1st July 2025).

19. Hong, C., Kidani, Y., A-González, N., Phung, T., Ito, A., Rong, X., Ericson, K., et al. (2011). Coordinate regulation of neutrophil homeostasis by liver X receptors in mice. *Journal of Clinical Investigation, 122*, 337–347. https://doi.org/10.1172/jci58393 (accessed on 1st July 2025).

20. Jagirdar, A., Jivani, T., Patel, S., Tailor, M., et al. (2024). Study of automated hematology analyzer's scatterplot patterns in white blood cell disorders. https://core.ac.uk/download/603896307.pdf (accessed on 1st July 2025).

21. Jakovljević, G., Kardum-Skelin, I., Krušlin, B., Mrsić-Davidović, M., et al. (2010). Pre-B-cell acute lymphoblastic leukemia with bulk extramedullary disease and chromosome 22 (EWSR1) rearrangement masquerading as Ewing sarcoma. https://core.ac.uk/download/11700102.pdf (accessed on 1st July 2025).

22. Jin, L., Li, L., Lu, Y., Cai, G., Lin, L., & Lin, J. (2025). Development and validation of a user-friendly predictive model using demographic and complete blood count data to facilitate early diagnosis on suspicion of myeloproliferative neoplasms. *International Journal of Laboratory Hematology*. https://www.semanticscholar.org/paper/acd5f643345bddeb7aad6cb278b1428bc4189fa4 (accessed on 1st July 2025).

23. Kumari, S., & Diwan, R. (2024). To study the effectiveness of International Consensus Group for Hematological Review (ICGHR) criteria for manual peripheral smear review. *International Journal of Scientific Research*. https://www.semanticscholar.org/paper/a2eff69f3890b5bd3d3841a3ce08f91255483c2b (accessed on 1st July 2025).

24. Kwak, M. S., Jeong, I. H., Cho, S. S., Woo, K., & Han, J. Y. (2022). Performance evaluation of the Abbott Alinity hs blood slide maker/stainer. *Annals of Laboratory Medicine, 42*, 482–484. https://www.semanticscholar.org/paper/c6f8bc6eb7616c592c35fbbb5355b55880ebb810 (accessed on 1st July 2025).

25. Lal, B. M., Wooldridge, J. T., Gaddam, M., Varma, A., Post, G. R., & Kumaran, M. V. (2024).

Strategies to optimize overutilization of provider-ordered peripheral blood smear review in a university hospital setting. *Blood*. https://www.semanticscholar.org/paper/367c8647e178c42c075f7ef3b33ba089e0e2e7f5 (accessed on 1st July 2025).

26. Lismayanti, L., & Arif, M. (2024). White blood cell and peripheral blast counts in leukemia patients with non-graying WBC-diff scattergram. *Indonesian Journal of Clinical Pathology and Medical Laboratory*. https://www.semanticscholar.org/paper/679a448f709d42d926d90f7c8c096be23edc0554 (accessed on 1st July 2025).
27. Meena, H., Sutrakar, S. K., Usmani, R. Q., Jain, R., Guru, A., Gupta, R., Shakya, V. K., et al. (2023). Utility of automated cell counter histogram in diagnosis of thrombocytopenia and pseudo thrombocytopenia. *Asian Journal of Medical Sciences*. https://www.semanticscholar.org/paper/0fd9b433b549e7ea187aeb6c980bd3c7d3a48672 (accessed on 1st July 2025).
28. Mohammadi Jazi, B., Nematollahy, P., & Maktoobian, N. (2024). Evaluation of the frequency of benign reactive lymphocytosis and lymphoproliferative disorders by flow cytometry in patients with persistent lymphocytosis in peripheral blood. *Journal of Renal Endocrinology*. https://www.semanticscholar.org/paper/4ff35a7e4f96b868f1d4aabc3e6b41e51057ae4e (accessed on 1st July 2025).
29. Munguiko, C., Mushabe, D., & Mwesige, S. (2020). Comparative assessment of red blood cell morphology in anemic children. https://core.ac.uk/download/387567179.pdf (accessed on 1st July 2025).
30. Nagendra, S., Mongillo, J., Dodge, K., Ranjitkar, P., Burns, B., & Allen, L. (2024). Clinician-ordered peripheral smear review by a pathologist has low clinical utility–A reference laboratory perspective. *The Journal of Applied Laboratory Medicine*. https://www.semanticscholar.org/paper/7074f9fd13b0a414db7090779a6de7605a347ea0 (accessed on 1st July 2025).
31. Park, T., Kim, J. H., Kang, C., Lee, B. H., Jeon, B., Lee, S., Chang, C. L., et al. (2006). [Diagnostic usefulness of SD malaria antigen and antibody kits for differential diagnosis of *vivax* malaria in patients with fever of unknown origin]. *The Korean Journal of Laboratory Medicine, 26*(4), 241–245. https://www.semanticscholar.org/paper/fc9ea864254d116b6db933eb58805c5957ee4029 (accessed on 1st July 2025).
32. Patra, M., Mohapatra, C., Kar, P., Prusty, N., & Nath, P. K. (2021). Multilineage hematologic pattern involvement in COVID-19–Evaluation from peripheral blood elements. *National Journal of Laboratory Medicine*. https://www.semanticscholar.org/paper/f12a6c88043cc5dafd9bf4dfc9123883da7aa1ab (accessed on 1st July 2025).
33. Pawar, A. B., Patil, A. M., Gaikwad, V. S., Purane, L. M., & Redasani, V. V. (2025). A review on: Interpretation and methodology of blood count. *International Journal of Pharmaceutical Research and Applications*. https://www.semanticscholar.org/paper/7ae75d01a9b8e715d81ba6054a2ce8f3e3100e94 (accessed on 1st July 2025).
34. Raess, P. W., Cascio, M. J., Fan, G., Press, R. D., Druker, B. J., Brewer, D., & Spurgeon, S. E. (2016). Concurrent STAT3, DNMT3A, and TET2 mutations in T-LGL leukemia with molecularly distinct clonal hematopoiesis of indeterminate potential. *American Journal of Hematology, 92*. https://doi.org/10.1002/ajh.24586 (accessed on 1st July 2025).
35. Rajurkar, V. D., & Chauhan, L. S. (2024). Comparison of red blood cell (RBC) histogram and indices on peripheral blood smears for the detection of anemia: A study protocol. *Cureus,*

16. https://www.semanticscholar.org/paper/ce5701b5d04aa8ae01a40d662f738bd53befab60 (accessed on 1st July 2025).

36. Randive, R., Sharma, S., Patwardhan, L., & Avhad, R. (2025). Is complete blood count sufficient to rule out hemoglobinopathy carrier state in females visiting antenatal care clinic: A study at one center. *Wadia Journal of Women and Child Health*. https://www.semanticscholar.org/paper/8b08d6cdc14b9850347b4c2f1239ec503a9c466e (accessed on 1st July 2025).

37. Salem, M. (2024). Complete blood count (CBC) and multivariate analysis as tools for predicting coronavirus (COVID-19) infectious. *Journal of Clinical Medicine of Kazakhstan*. https://www.semanticscholar.org/paper/3dbb3dda5c82c5b17a93133c0d4ac7cd3e6d0834 (accessed on 1st July 2025).

38. Santomasso, B., Nastoupil, L. J., Adkins, S., Lacchetti, C., Schneider, B. J., Anadkat, M. J., Atkins, M. B., et al. (2021). Management of immune-related adverse events in patients treated with chimeric antigen receptor T-cell therapy: ASCO guideline. *Journal of Clinical Oncology, 39*, 3978–3992. https://doi.org/10.1200/jco.21.01992 (accessed on 1st July 2025).

39. Schneider, B. J., Naidoo, J., Santomasso, B., Lacchetti, C., Adkins, S., Anadkat, M. J., Atkins, M. B., et al. (2021). Management of immune-related adverse events in patients treated with immune checkpoint inhibitor therapy: ASCO guideline update. *Journal of Clinical Oncology, 39*, 4073–4126. https://doi.org/10.1200/jco.21.01440 (accessed on 1st July 2025).

40. Tuli, A., & Yenilmez, E. D. (2017). Laboratory approach to anemia. https://core.ac.uk/download/322432622.pdf (accessed on 1st July 2025).

41. Urrechaga, E., & Fernández, M. (2022). Pseudo thrombocytopenia and leukocyte scattergrams: A case report. *Journal of Laboratory and Precision Medicine, 7*, 35–35. https://doi.org/10.21037/jlpm-22-42 (accessed on 1st July 2025).

42. Yasuda, I., Saludar, N. R., Sayo, A. R., Suzuki, S., Yokoyama, A., Ozeki, Y., Kobayashi, H., et al. (2024). Evaluation of cytokine profiles related to *Mycobacterium tuberculosis* latent antigens using a whole-blood assay in the Philippines. *Frontiers in Immunology, 15*. https://doi.org/10.3389/fimmu.2024.1330796 (accessed on 1st July 2025).

43. Yoon, E. C., Koo, S., Park, H. Y., Kim, H. C., Kim, W. J., Kim, K. U., Jung, K., et al. (2024). Predictive role of white blood cell differential count for the development of acute exacerbation in Korean chronic obstructive pulmonary disease. *International Journal of Chronic Obstructive Pulmonary Disease, 19*, 17–31. https://www.semanticscholar.org/paper/6e073d5bc8dedcdf524abd91a9ae280128c483ee (accessed on 1st July 2025).

44. You, E., Cho, S., Yang, J. J., Lee, H. J., Lee, W. I., Lee, J., Cho, K., et al. (2015). A novel case of extreme thrombocytosis in acute myeloid leukemia associated with isochromosome 17q and copy neutral loss of heterozygosity. *Annals of Laboratory Medicine, 35*, 366–369. https://www.semanticscholar.org/paper/34852a57b32aba56a8eab56e80ab7f48552fa3b4 (accessed on 1st July 2025).

45. Yuan, Z., & Jian, Z. (2024). Establishment and verification of reference intervals for blood cell analysis in extremely high altitude. *Frontiers in Physiology, 15*. https://www.semanticscholar.org/paper/ba3dd0cc7cc8ae9f16e3b0f99094fb190f4efaf0 (accessed on 1st July 2025).

46. Zatsepina, A., Peeke, S., & Xu, Y. (2024). Diagnostic challenges and treatment of hairy cell leukemia in a patient with sarcoidosis: A case report. *Blood*. https://www.semanticscholar.org/paper/23bd5661a139ce06f8b4b08da5319a18b64481e6 (accessed on 1st July 2025).

ANEMIA: CLASSIFICATION AND DIAGNOSIS

5

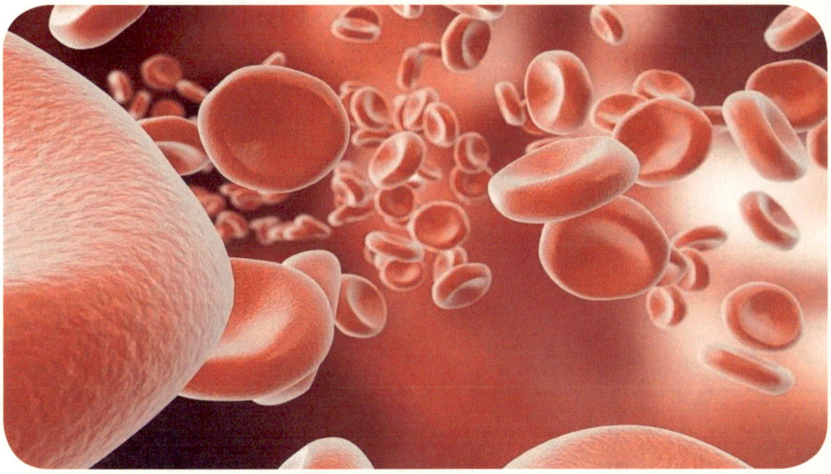

LEARNING OBJECTIVES

After studying this chapter, you will be able to:

1. Explain the types of anemia;
2. Describe the causes of anemia;
3. List the symptoms of anemia;
4. Explore the diagnostic methods;
5. Illustrate the laboratory tests;
6. Elaborate the treatment options.

Introduction

Anemia is a devious disease that forces doctors to get their methods both for diagnosis and classification wrong. It masquerades as low hemoglobin or simply low red cell count, and it exists in several varieties—each having some subliminal cause. Determination of these differences is, in most cases, essential to arriving at a correct diagnosis and creating the proper cure. The body consequences range from constant fatigue to even worse outcomes, including the failure of the heart, which completely devastate a patient's life. Since reasons for anemia can range from basic nutritional inadequacies to ongoing conditions, physicians end up screening an insane variety of factors—a mix that is at the core of recommendations now calling for a guarded, comprehensive work-up. Doctors tend to classify anemia into microcytic, macrocytic, and normocytic forms, each of which corresponds to different body conditions. In most cases, the microcytic form is due to iron deficiency or chronic disease that persists for a long time, and the macrocytic form is typically caused by a lack of vitamin B12 or folate (Brys et al., 2015). Normocytic cases, on the other hand, can alert to more generalized disease or perhaps even bone marrow errors. In reality, tools such as full blood counts and reticulocyte counts are depended on in order to determine the exact kind of anemia a patient has. Knowledge of these nuances helps clinicians tailor their treatment method to each patient's unique situation. Diagnosing anemia is much more complex than simply categorizing it. Physicians generally put together a full patient history, a physical exam, and directed lab work, all of which are part of a greater picture of what is actually occurring. Eating habits, chronic health issues, and even heredity are all part of the puzzle—variables that are at times duplicated and reassessed in the process of collecting a diagnosis. Recent work has delineated that in the case of atrophic gastritis – when there can be a potential overlap between issues of the stomach and abnormalities of the blood (Annibale et al., 2015) – long-term follow-ups can prove to be very real. Overall, these overlap points do reveal the need for a holistic approach that weaves together different strands of patient care in order to stretch for better all-around outcomes (Figure 5.1).

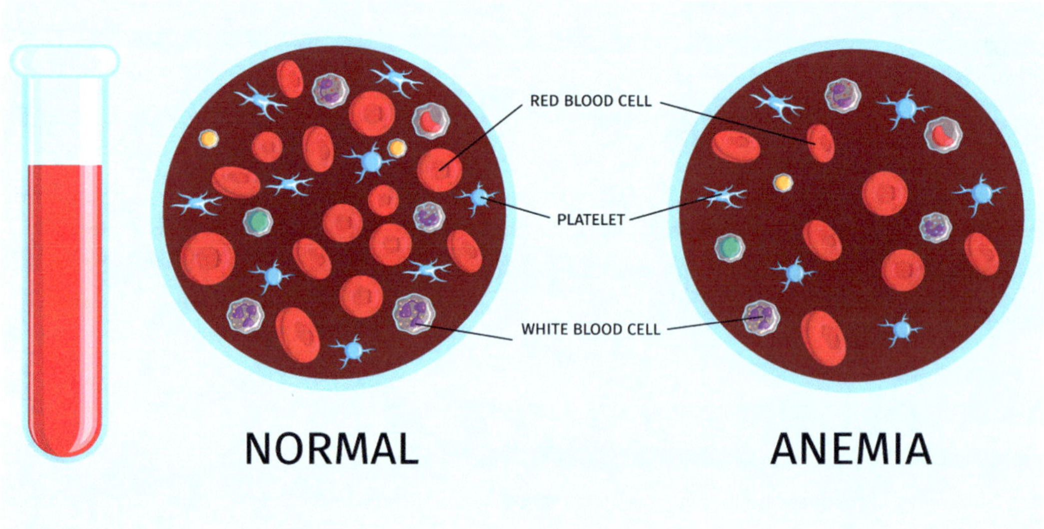

Figure 5.1. Anemia.

Source: https://www.yuktiherbs.com/wp-content/uploads/2022/08/anemia.jpg.

Definition of Anemia

Anemia is not all about low red cells—it's a collection of blood disorders where either amount or quality of RBCs is out of whack. Doctors will usually draw a complete blood count (CBC) to quantify, say, hemoglobin and hematocrit values, which in turn channel the condition into the mild, moderate, or severe categories. The numbers, certainly, but also watching the cells themselves; their size and shape give hints at what might actually be going on—everything from poor diet to chronic illness. This combination of data helps clinicians make treatment plans and track patients' courses over time. It helps to keep in mind causes of anemia are as varied as its presentation. You see, this condition can occur because of iron deficiencies or bone marrow conditions, and in most instances, red blood cells are classified as being in a number of categories—microcytic, macrocytic, or normocytic. Microcytic anemia, for example, typically presents with iron deficiency or thalassemia, while macrocytic cases typically suggest vitamin B12 or folate issues. Having these differences accurately matters because they impact diagnosis and treatment, and sometimes other less apparent problems complicate the situation. In recent times, there has been a great deal of debate about how inclusive we must be in the definition of anemia. Guidelines constantly get updated—often broadening the specs so more individuals are included, which makes it harder to distinguish genuine cases from false positives. This expansion of definitions can lead to over-hasty labeling and treatment where the dangers are not properly evaluated. In most cases, though, hitting just the right note is important, with advantages to be had from catching more cases not outweighing more harm than good—a debate that mirrors broader trends in healthcare (Bero et al., 2013; English et al., 2014) (Figure 5.2).

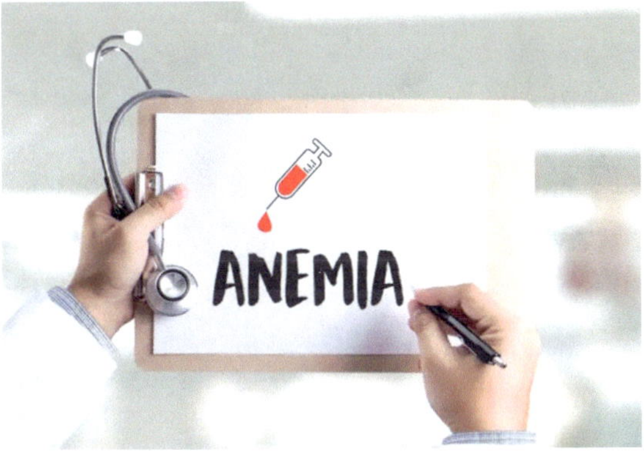

Figure 5.2. Understanding anemia.

Source: https://thumbnails.icloudhospital.com/tr:w-1536,f-webp,q-75/1-anemia-481b6c6e-4a56-42c7-ba0d-794939a5a859.webp.

Importance of Understanding Anemia

Anemia is not an isolated health issue—it has ripple effects on public health initiatives and routine medical care. It shows up particularly in vulnerable groups like kids and pregnant women, and the early detection usually prevents severe complications. Kids can get affected both physically and mentally and sometimes end up being subjected to challenges that limit how much they can do at school or in the workforce later on. The battle against anemia is more than just early detection and symptom relief; it also needs community efforts to spread information about its dangers and ways to prevent it. Including causes like nutritional deficiency or chronic illness in the computation makes you understand better why special interventions can actually have a major impact on global health outcomes (Bolt et al., 2015). Early detection of anemia saves money. New technology and methods are accelerating detection of the disease, so treatment can start sooner. Some of the latest models—even those that use machine learning to detect anemia in newborns—are living up to real promise by making some elements of the diagnosis more straightforward.

Such innovations can make fast-paced clinical workflows more efficient, lessen opportunities for error, and ultimately improve patient care. With stakes so high—untreated anemia in early life can have lasting negative impressions on health—it's crucial that we hop on the bandwagon of these technological developments (Cardenas et al., 2024). Embracing data-driven approaches, healthcare professionals will stand a better chance to tackle anemia in populations, paving the way for better outcomes. Understanding anemia means understanding it is not only about its direct symptoms but also how it interacts within the overall context of health. The condition tends to present itself with other long-term conditions in a manner that can complicate patient care. For instance, a diabetic patient may have a more difficult time if anemia is present as well, which implies that care plans must be able to handle multiple issues simultaneously. This convergence is a reminder that balancing an outlook on health is of the utmost importance. Educating healthcare professionals about how anemia converges with other chronic disease can guarantee greater compliance with treatment programs—and in most instances, which means better general quality of care (Bolt et al., 2015).

5.1. Types of Anemia

Learning Outcome

- Iron-deficiency anemia;
- Vitamin deficiency anemia;
- Anemia of chronic disease.

Anemia shows itself in so many various forms. Iron-deficiency anemia, for example, happens when your body simply doesn't have enough iron in it to build hemoglobin—the protein employed for carrying oxygen around. Consuming minimal amounts of iron, having trouble absorbing it, or losing it on a regular basis (e.g., from heavy periods or internal bleeding) can do it. Typically, people get tired, look paler than usual, and get breathless quickly. Generally, doctors check serum ferritin and hemoglobin in trying to figure out what's happening proof of why there is so much demand for straightforward, accurate tests (Adibuzzaman et al., 2017). Another kind that likes to receive plenty of attention is anemia of chronic disease (ACD). This happens in patients with chronic inflammation, kidney disease, or even cancer. In general, even if the body's stores look good or even a bit high, inflammation intervenes—disrupting iron recycling and hepcidin signals—ultimately limiting iron to new red cells.

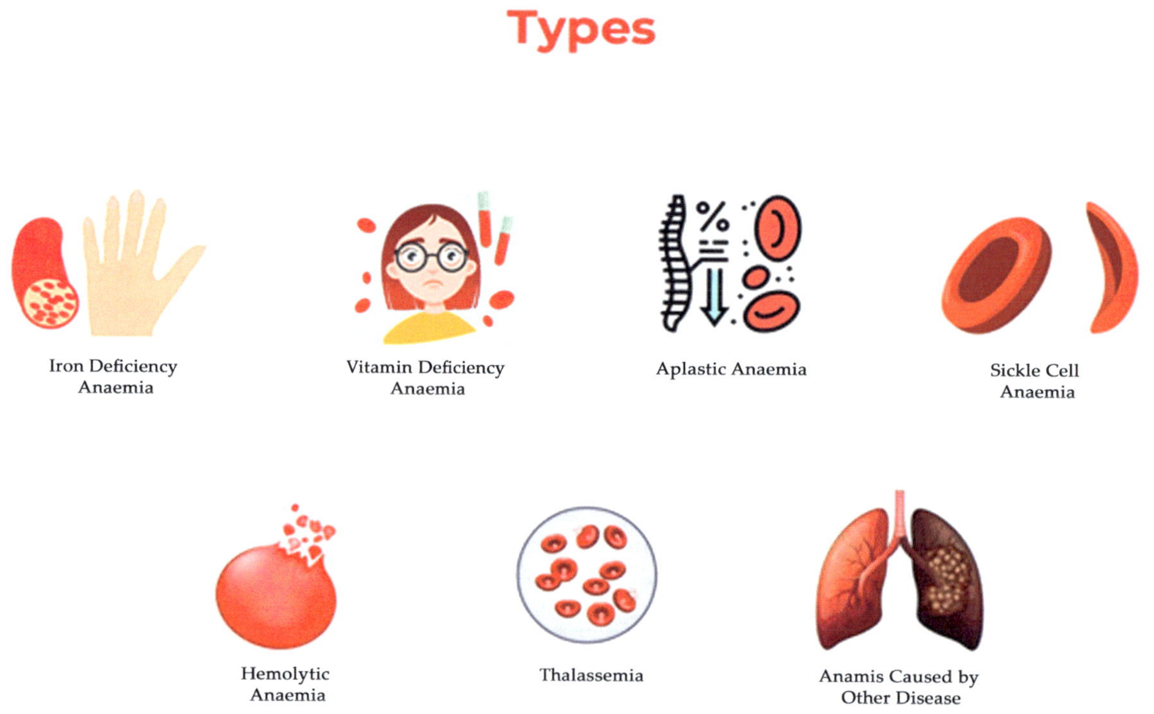

Figure 5.3. Types of anemia.

Source: https://www.lalpathlabs.com/blog/wp-content/uploads/2022/11/Picture23.png.

Symptoms here tend to be less severe, so diagnosis becomes a bit more challenging; doctors have to trust patient history and low-grade inflammatory markers to put the pieces together. In determining ACD separate from iron-deficiency anemia, it is important because the treatment regimens can be quite different (Abdolrahim et al., 2017). Megaloblastic anemia, on the other hand, arises when duplicating DNA is stalled in some way, usually as a result of inadequate levels of vitamin B12 or folate. This results in abnormally large cells and immature red blood cells to be seen in both the marrow and blood. Without those essential vitamins, red cell production doesn't work as it should, which leads to a cascade of blood abnormalities. The patient can have trouble with overall weakness, an oddly painful tongue (glossitis), or even neurological issues—especially when B12 is significantly depleted. In most instances, testing involves vitamin B12 and methylmalonic acid level determinations, which offers proof of the problem. Awareness of these personal attributes enables healthcare professionals to tailor treatment regimes to suit each person, ultimately to improve quality of life (Figure 5.3).

5.1.1. Iron-Deficiency Anemia

Iron deficiency anemia presents as a very common problem, particularly in the run-of-the-mill doctor's office. Approximately half of all cases of anemia are due to low iron, which obviously indicates that a better screening and diagnosis are needed. It may occur due to not consuming enough iron in your diet, added body requirements during pregnancy or other such conditions, or chronic blood loss due to conditions like gastrointestinal bleeding.

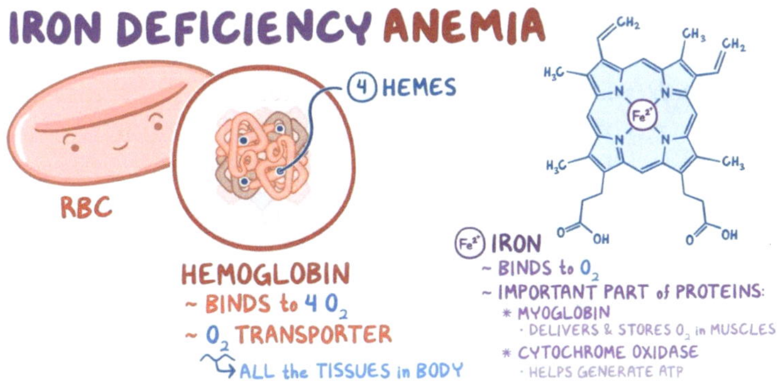

Figure 5.4. Iron deficiency anemia.

Source: https://d16qt3wv6xm098.cloudfront.net/MNI3puZ6RYeK_hB6Wim_RG-6RHSgbyWd/_.jpg.

Resolved to know why the iron is low is significant, since other forms of anemia may occur for quite other reasons. Getting the diagnosis right not only opens the door to specific treatment, but it also plays a role in general health and quality of life—especially among those groups that are more at risk, like children and women of childbearing age (Guzmán et al., 2016). When doctors examine a case of suspected iron deficiency, they take into account a blend of clinical presentations, blood work, and some iron studies. You might be experiencing fatigue, pallor, and generalized weakness, but the real evidence comes in laboratory tests of such as serum ferritin, transferrin saturation and hemoglobin. These numbers are what distinguish iron deficiency from the rest of the anemia; otherwise, good and diligent lab workup is what makes the difference. There is also emerging evidence that if IDA is left untreated, it could lead to worse things—cognitive, developmental, even physical—issues in children, for example. So, a timely and correct diagnosis really makes a huge difference in mitigating those negative effects (Adair et al., 2015). Treatment of this disease is simply a matter of building up the body's iron store through better diet and, if needed, supplementation. Most advice is to stock up on foods rich in iron, including red meat, legumes, and leafy greens, and most mentions vitamin C as a sidekick that helps iron absorption. In advanced cases, doctors even prescribe oral or intravenous iron supplements. However, the underlying cause of iron loss—i.e., digestive diseases or menorrhagia—also needs to be treated so that it doesn't recur. Ultimately, its treatment from a holistic point of view not only eliminates symptoms but also benefits overall health conditions more, potentially lowering the rate at which IDA occurs in the general population (Guzmán et al., 2016) (Figure 5.4).

5.1.2. Vitamin deficiency anemia

Without crucial vitamins, literally, our blood system becomes out of balance. Too little of those nutrients – either from lacking in our diet or from our bodies just not being very good at absorbing them – can result in a form of anemia that really messes things up. One good example is when vitamin B12 is lacking, typically resulting in megaloblastic anemia in which red cells get larger than usual. At times it's because the body is missing a helper protein (an intrinsic factor deficiency, as in pernicious anemia) or because of other digestive absorption issues, and yes, a lack of enough folate can have the same effects on blood.

The ultimate effect is less oxygen delivery, which leaves people feeling drained, weakened, and simply less alive in life. Determining this vitamin-anemia is therefore important if treatment is to take hold. More than an order of one test is required to uncover the source of vitamin deficiency anemia. Physicians will often pair serum nutrient testing with a complete blood count in an effort to untangle the differences – like a higher than usual mean corpuscular volume (MCV) that suggests low levels of either folate or vitamin B12. It's simply a matter of putting the puzzle pieces together: a patient's history, their baseline diet, and any indication that their gut isn't digesting things properly all figure in. With most cases, a careful lab workup and close attention to the patient's lifestyle, as new evidence suggests (Groer et al., 2002), help clinicians develop a diagnosis far removed from guesswork.

Adding supplements and some strategic dietary adjustments usually finish off the whole plan for raising those vitamin levels where they need to be. Treatment strategies have changed along with our understanding of nutrition and patient counseling coming into adulthood. It's not just doctors on the front lines anymore – pharmacists chime in as well by making sure that patients are equipped with the knowledge necessary to make better dietary choices and follow through with their treatment plan.

The call for increased collaboration in healthcare is highlighted by new professional training programs (Kucera et al., 2014). These training programs assist all in achieving a greater understanding of the identification and management of different anemias, especially those linked with vitamin deficiencies. By treating both mitigating symptoms and investigating the cause of why an individual would be deprived of the benefits of vitamins, our healthcare system is slowly improving the recovery of patients and becoming more active in nutritional well-being (Figure 5.5).

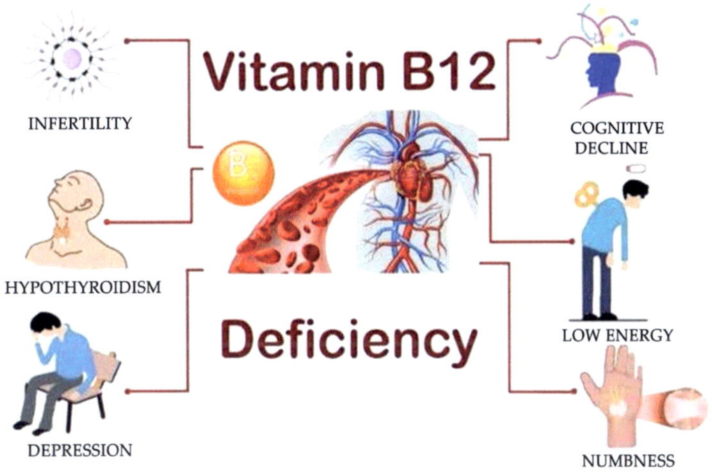

Figure 5.5. Vitamin deficiency anemia.

Source: https://bizimages.withfloats.com/tile/636a1944d09eb5000122bcc5.jpg.

5.1.3. Anemia of Chronic Disease

Chronic disease really does upset a mess in how our blood is made. Sometimes, when a person is combating infections, autoimmune disorders, or even cancer, their body releases inflammatory cytokines which end up disrupting iron regulation and red blood cell production. IL-6, for instance, just pops out of nowhere and increases hepcidin, which in turn kind of slams shut the door on iron acquisition in the gut and pins release from macrophages. So instead of just being short on iron, you've got this complicated battle between long-term inflammation and how the body makes heme—a complicated process that needs high-detail testing to sort out (Conlon et al., 2013). While ACD does occur quite often, it is often ignored or misinterpreted as some other form of anemia. It's usually necessary to distinguish it from iron deficiency anemia simply because the treatment process actually varies very greatly. In ACD, serum ferritin levels usually function at the normal or even higher levels—complete opposite of IDA's low levels. This lack of congruence, one that clinicians actually use when ordering lab work, tells us that even when iron stores look normal or above normal, something is still wrong with red cell production. Basically, pouring more iron in isn't going to cut it, so clinicians are going to have to figure out what is wrong with the patient's chronic issues before proceeding with treatment (Brys et al., 2015). As far as ACD management goes, the most critical thing to do is address the cause of whatever's causing it. In most instances, treating the underlying chronic disorder typically will cure the anemia itself. For example, being able to get control of that chronic inflammation or curing cancer can raise hemoglobin levels without actually doing anything for the anemia per se. In some cases—most notably when the anemia is incredibly severe—doctors will resort to erythropoiesis-stimulating drugs, but they have to balance these benefits against issues like thromboembolic events. This holistic methodology, taking into account the overall health of the patient along with laboratory values, reaffirms that ACD is not merely a lab test. Rather, it is an indicator of systemic inflammation in a broad sense, eventually resulting in better patient outcomes (Conlon et al., 2013) (Figure 5.6).

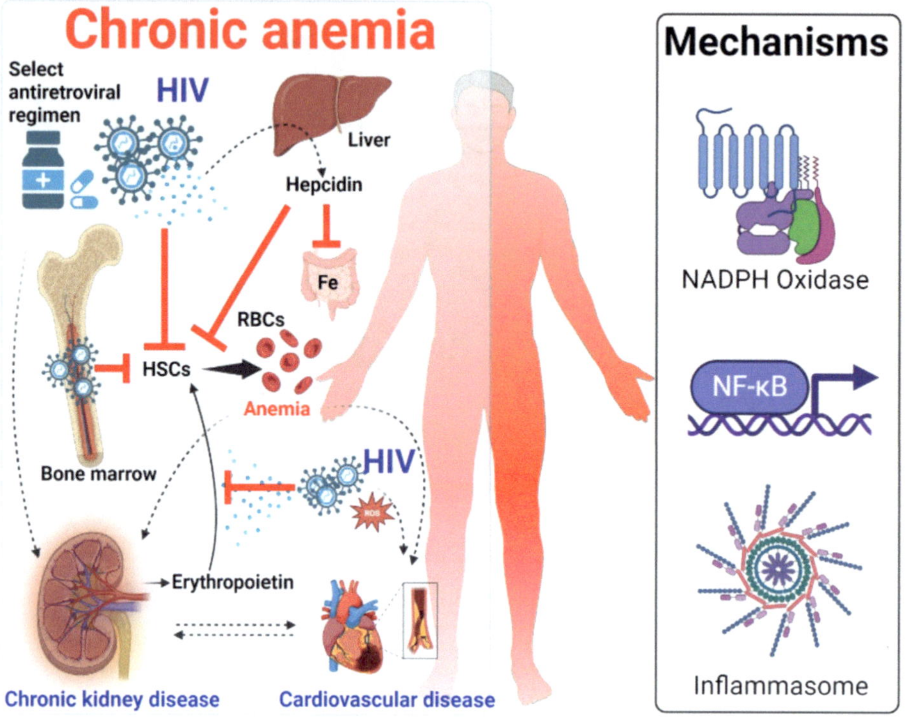

Figure 5.6. Anemia of chronic disease.

Source: https://pub.mdpi-res.com/viruses/viruses-16-00542/article_deploy/html/images/viruses-16-00542-ag.png?1711799140.

Test Your Knowledge

1. What are the major classifications of anemia based on red blood cell size and morphology?
2. How does iron-deficiency anemia differ from megaloblastic anemia?

5.2. Causes of Anemia

Learning Outcome

- Nutritional deficiencies;
- Genetic disorders;
- Chronic diseases.

There are many things that can trigger anemia – for instance, inadequate nutrients are a big part of the problem. The absence of iron is a large culprit, whether this is due to missing out on required foods or absorption issues. Without enough iron, hemoglobin suffers, and your blood isn't able to get oxygen to where it needs to go as effectively. Pregnant women and children are more acutely affected because their systems need to draw more nutrients in at once. Classifying anemia in terms of these nutritional needs can actually help tailor treatments, and addressing these problems early on can actually change the whole course of the disease and even enhance quality of life (Saputra et al., 2024). Chronic illnesses add another tricky layer to anemia's causes. Diseases like rheumatoid arthritis, kidney disease, or even cancer can disrupt your body – sometimes by lowering erythropoietin or by messing with the way iron works. These kinds of chronic illness often produce broad inflammation, which tends to slow the creation of new red blood cells. It is not surprising that anemia in these instances can be rather complicated in diagnosis; doctors would need to reconcile your laboratory results with your clinical background. Integration of information derived from analytical techniques like RBC histograms and indices, as well as traditional blood smears, gives better understanding of what is wrong and allows for better therapeutic choices (Thyagaraju et al., 2024). Genes have their say in anemia too. In thalassemia or sickle cell anemia diseases, hereditary traits can interfere with normal hemoglobin activity, creating red blood cells that just aren't quite right to look at or work. Testing for these genetic defects is especially important in groups where the conditions are more prevalent. New test methods more recently – even using machine learning algorithms in some cases – have shown potential in offering accurate classification. Such developments not only enhance how we diagnose the problem, but they also open the door to more specific treatments that can actually produce a concrete impact in the management of anemia due to genetic reasons (Saputra et al., 2024) (Figure 5.7).

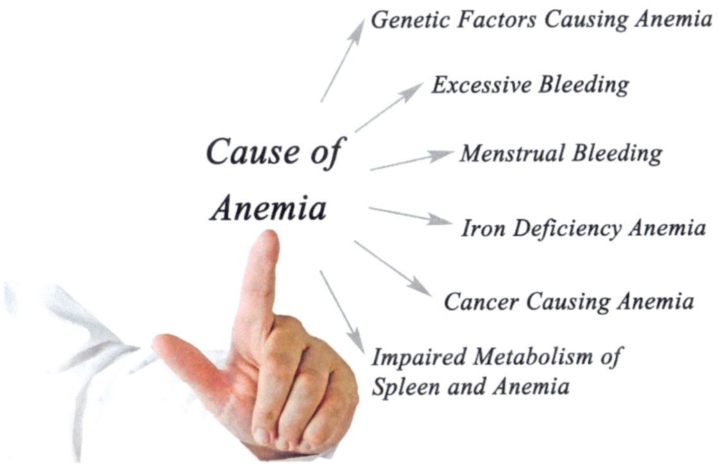

Figure 5.7. Causes of anemia.

Source: https://fytika.com/cdn/shop/articles/anemia.jpg?v=1702919375.

5.2.1. Nutritional deficiencies

Anemia starts with a lack of iron – a nutritional imbalance that seems to occur in some more than others. Children, for example, and those who have chronic kidney disease tend to have trouble with this problem, as insufficient iron causes the usual production of red blood cells to be foiled. In the majority of cases, when young ones fail to get enough iron, it triggers the kind of microcytic, pale anemia that could interrupt their general growth and initiate a multitude of unforeseen issues. In the case of individuals with CKD, it's not only a question of the body being wedded to producing less erythropoietin; nutritional deficiencies seep in, too. In short, being aware of these gaps in nutrients matters if we're ever to prevent and manage the millions of health problems anemia is able to create. Examining anemia through the flawed lens of nutritional lack, the significance of iron—and other basics—becomes apparent. It is as if a deficiency of proper nutrients initiates a chain reaction; studies show that inefficient iron absorption can keep patients in a cyclical process that aggravates the disease, especially in patients with chronic kidney disease and chronic inflammation. Physicians who investigate such nutritional factors are likely to discover more holistic approaches to diagnosis as well as treatment. There are recommendations floating around to help direct diagnosis and prevention, although such guidelines do not always agree, prompting more studies to be conducted in different populations. It is extremely important to modernize clinical practice in the fight against nutritional deficiencies that cause anemia, particularly among children. Experts at a number of Poland's medical societies have recently released an extensive series of recommendations – with some minor discrepancies – to detect and treat iron deficiency in children patients. The recommendations are based on a critical appraisal of the literature with added observational clinical experience, covering issues in children from birth to 18 years of age. Since uncontrolled iron deficiency can potentially speed anemia risk and disrupt developmental milestones, staying on top of screening isn't just recommended—it's imperative. Ultimately, giving healthcare providers a deeper insight into such nutritional impacts means they have improved resources for beating anemia and boosting overall health outcomes.

5.2.2. Genetic Disorders

Understanding how genetic disorders tie into anemia matters a great deal when you're trying to figure out diagnoses and classifications. Genetic quirks often show up in different blood conditions – they can change the way red blood cells are made, how they look, and even how they work. Take thalassemia and sickle cell disease, for example; both are the result of genetic mutations that disrupt hemoglobin synthesis and weaken the durability of red blood cells. In most cases, such genetic defects highlight why pregnant women and newborns need to be screened – early identification of potential issues can mean greater chances for life-saving treatments. As we learn more about genes, it becomes more apparent that targeting those genetic bases with specific diagnostic and treatment methods is key in successful anemia treatment. Genetic disorders such as coeliac disease have also been linked to anemia – one typically founded on autoimmune events that compromise nutrient absorption. The people with coeliac disease could miss out on the most important things like iron simply because the lining of their intestines gets damaged. It has been observed that nearly 26.6% of the coeliac patients end up with at least one other autoimmune disease later, making blood-related problems even more complex. History of autoimmune conditions in the family or long-standing duration of gastrointestinal symptoms can predispose to complications. Thus, screening unexplained anemic patients for coeliac disease is really quite important since early treatment and diagnosis really do make a difference. In so doing, genetics continue to rear their head in discussions of overall health and how we proceed with both diagnosis and treatment. And then there's the case of non-immune fetal hydrops (NIFH), which offers another glimpse into how genetic causes lead to potentially life-threatening anemia. What occurs is that genetic faults, especially such abnormalities as chromosomal aneuploidies, are usually manifested either in the first or second trimester – and then cardiovascular defects take the lead in third-trimester problems. These essentially signify that thorough examination of genetics in prenatal screening is necessary. Including genetic counseling as a routine part of prenatal care will help to offset the risks of perinatal loss and other complications that are associated with NIFH. In general, seeing how these genetic disorders correlate with the various forms of anemia really highlights the need for complete genetic screenings as part of a general health policy (Figure 5.8).

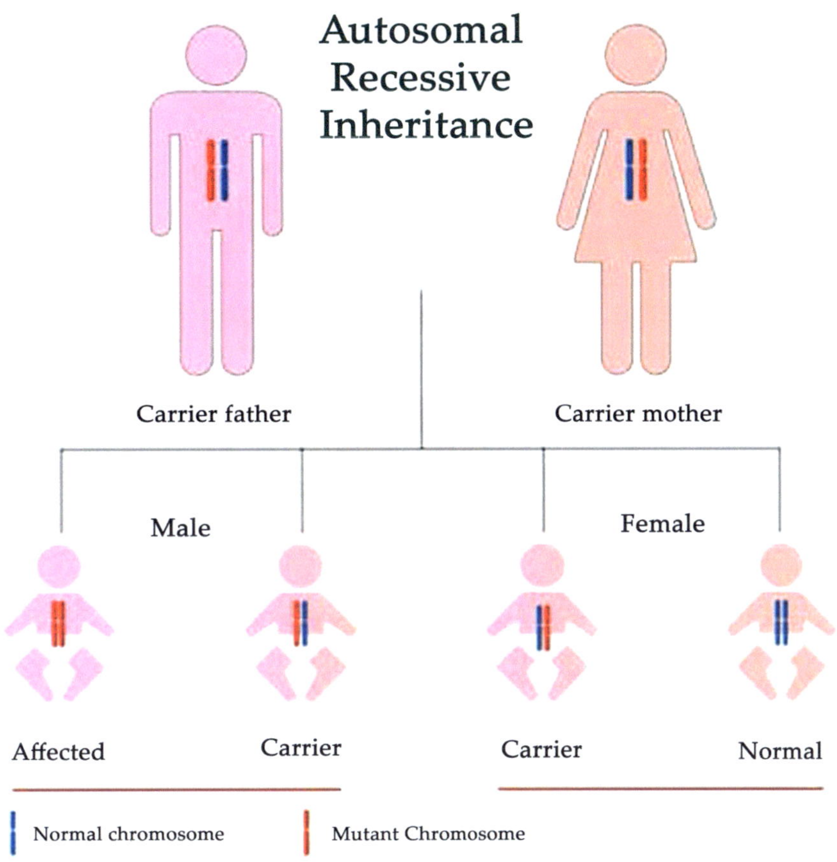

Figure 5.8. Genetic disorders.

Source: https://external-content.duckduckgo.com/iu/?u=https%3A%2F%2Fgeneticeducation.co.in%2Fwp-content%2Fuploads%2F2018%2F08%2FGenetic-inheritance-.002-e1580965491392-449x450.jpeg&f=1&nofb=1&ipt=a34d41596e1d23d34d81ee95e1302b2e740524c8fd4792ba06ede408e55d3553.

5.2.3. Chronic Diseases

Chronic illness actually wreaks havoc with our capacity to recognize and repair such issues as anemia. The combination isn't always straightforward—occasionally autoimmune processes or even tumors produce a complete cascade of blood challenges that further obscure the picture. Think about, for example, hypereosinophilic syndrome (HES), which might occur with autoimmune hemolytic anemia. It's something of a skein of confusion: anemia in a patient may well be a symptom that there is a chronic, underlying condition at work (Brys et al., 2015). Doctors need to dig a little deeper and think again if they are to strike the right note with a diagnosis that is accurate and to establish treatment in the best possible direction. It's not as easy as labeling a hemoglobin decrease as simply anemia; usually, chronic inflammation pushes iron regulation to go out of whack. One of the factors—hepcidin—has been found to spike when inflammation persists, which, in turn, messes up the transport of iron and creates functional iron deficiency, despite normal-appearing iron stores (Conlon et al., 2013). Generally speaking, this nuance speaks to requiring a conservative, sometimes unbalanced approach to operation to determine why one is anemic when it comes to chronic illnesses. Clinicians, by being careful to watch for minor details, can often catch these anomalies before they have become larger problems. It takes more than filling in the boxes on lab work to diagnose anemia in chronically ill patients. The investigation may include all sorts of tests—antibody tests, imaging studies, and even biomarker testing—to enable doctors to get the full picture. When hypereosinophilia or autoantibody-mediated hemolysis is suspected, a complete investigative process becomes really critical. In most cases, these tests start emerging as to how reformation of chronic inflammation and syndromes like HES get entangled in the anemia seen in the majority of patients. All of this points health practitioners in the direction of treatments not only aimed at the low blood count but also at the underlying, chronic conditions that lead to it (Brys et al., 2015).

Test Your Knowledge

1. How do nutritional deficiencies contribute to the development of anemia?
2. What role do chronic diseases and infections play in anemia pathogenesis?

5.3. Symptoms of Anemia

Learning Outcome

- Fatigue and weakness;
- Pale skin and jaundice;
- Shortness of breath.

Anemia comes in so many forms and actually affects one's daily life. The patients would not only come in with fatigue and weakness; this is the case when low hemoglobin causes reduced oxygen to be transported to essential tissues. Shortness of breath on exertion is also something that you would observe since the body is having difficulty compensating for the lack of oxygen. In most instances severity of these symptoms is based on what caused the anemia and how rapidly it occurred. For example, a person with a smoldering, chronic type can gradually acclimate to smaller blood counts, whereas an acute, sudden drop will produce more severe symptoms. These ambivalent signs are what need to be recognized for an instant diagnosis because just going with symptoms may not inform you precisely which form of anemia is involved (Gómez et al., 2025). Consider pernicious anemia, for instance—this form is differentiated by its large red blood cells, typically found due to a vitamin B12 deficiency. Its classic signs normally include weariness fatigue, limb numbness, inexplicable weight loss, and even a sore tongue. In a systematic review, several cases depicted these features, so physicians should be vigilant. Typically, approximately 55% of patients present with tiredness, and approximately one third with nerve symptoms such as decreased sensation. Such a blend of symptoms, in most cases, speaks for itself on why a better understanding of the disease is merited: early diagnosis can do wonders for the prognosis (Seage et al., 2024). Beyond the common body pains, the psychological effects of anemia should not be taken lightly. The majority of patients complain of feeling depressed, anxious, and even having trouble focusing elements that exacerbate the condition overall. It usually becomes a vicious cycle in which the tiredness increases mental pressure, and that stress, once more, also makes things complicated for physical health. A whole assessment that looks into body and mind is generally required in order to fight anemia effectively. Keeping all these varied symptoms in mind makes it simpler for both the patients and healthcare professionals to communicate and collaborate with one another, which can lead to effective diagnosis and improved treatment. Overall, the process of coming to understand this complicated snapshot remains a critical component of establishing what's really going on (Gómez et al., 2025) (Figure 5.9).

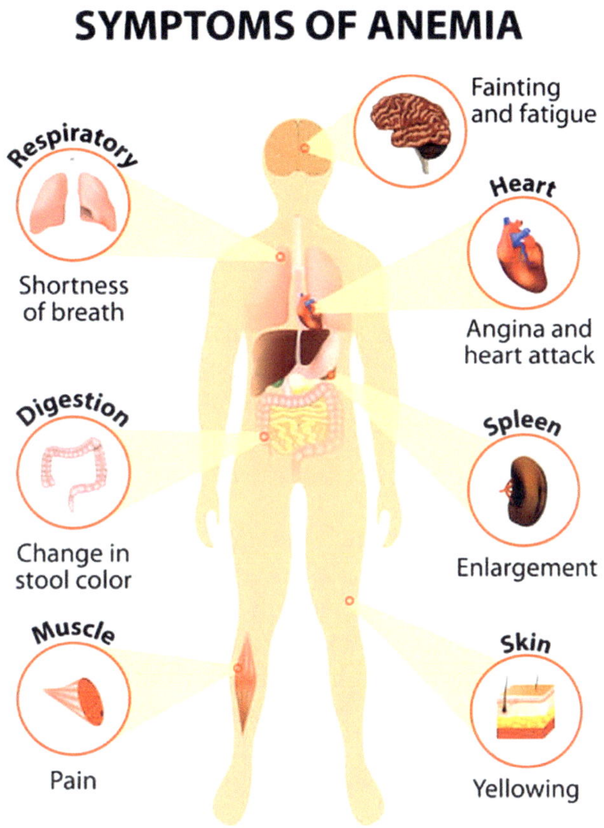

Figure 5.9. Symptoms of anemia.

Source: https://external-content.duckduckgo.com/iu/?u=https%3A%2F%2Fmedlineplus.gov%2Fimages%2FPX000178_PRESENTATION.jpeg&f=1&nofb=1&ipt=de9814053fd5fab24bc94500be0ea3402674ec9e90e4fe7ecf9ae387910a358d.

5.3.1. Fatigue and Weakness

Weakness, fatigue, and anemia all occur together quite often in medicine, and doctors keep a close eye on how they work together. Fatigue is described by most people as feeling simply as plain tiredness—a draining of energy that is not the same for every person with anemia. Weakness more often than not is usually a loss of body strength that disturbs simple daily functions and general quality of life. Low hemoglobin is typically what's behind it since the body is not getting enough oxygen to be able to function. In most cases, being cognizant of the subtle differences in how weakness and fatigue manifest is the key to making the correct decision on diagnosis and treatment (Bejar et al., 2019). As soon as myelodysplastic syndromes or acute myeloid leukemia are introduced into the picture, weakness and fatigue have a tendency to make their ugly appearances as real issues directly reported by patients. Patients detail their daily struggles, and this direct input actually ranks higher in treatment paradigms and quality-of-life assessments. Scientists largely implore equipment that is better suited to detect these sensations—equipment that shows what treatment is actually like for an individual's life. Using well-documented quality-of-life measures enables clinicians to follow these symptoms closely, bridging the chasm between what's picked up on laboratory work and the way patients actually feel. It's a gentle reminder that when patients complain of their weakness and fatigue, it can inform directions of treatment towards reducing their burden (Carlo et al., 2018). In day-to-day clinical work, the detection of fatigue and weakness is not checklist-driven routine—it often spurs investigation for other types of anemia. A thorough examination doesn't only rely on observing the level of hemoglobin; it also keeps a sharp eye on what the patients report to them about weakness and fatigue themselves. Neglecting these symptoms might occasionally lead to misdiagnosis or unsuccessful treatments, further incapacitating a patient's day-to-day performance. Fatigue, compounded with weakness, clearly reveals anemia as not being a condition of a single cause but rather usually comprises several causes. Clinicians would, therefore, be well advised to use a patient-centered approach, one that treats such symptoms as part of a broader story when diagnosing and managing anemia (Bejar et al., 2019).

5.3.2. Pale Skin and Jaundice

Anemia is likely to manifest by way of physical manifestations that signal hidden blood issues—yellowish color and pale skin, for instance. Pale skin commonly presents when hemoglobin or red blood cell count is low, something you can see in iron deficiency anemia and aplastic anemia. It's really just a sign that there isn't enough oxygenated blood making it to the skin. In contrast, jaundice—this yellow pigmentation you might notice on the skin and mucous membranes—is generally caused by an excess of bilirubin in the bloodstream. Most often, elevated red blood cell turnover, as with hemolytic anemias, elevates bilirubin because the liver simply can't process it fast enough. In general, analyzing both of these signs is necessary in order to get the proper diagnosis and set right treatment regimens. Sometimes, the jaundice symptom and pale skin seem to merge in such a way as to make the diagnosis even clearer, for instance, hemolytic anemia caused by glucose-6-phosphate dehydrogenase (G6PD) deficiency. This particular disease, which primarily affects males, typically manifests in infants who have both a yellowish appearance of the skin and a pale face. For example, a clinical case report included a neonate who had shown acute jaundice and 9.8 g/dL pre-transfusion hemoglobin, a clear sign of underlying anemia. Diagnostic tests that recorded elevated indirect bilirubin levels added credibility to the severity of the condition and led doctors to start such interventions as phototherapy. Early treatment of the above symptoms not only prevents immediate risks like acute hyperbilirubinemia encephalopathy but also provides a window for referral for further genetic counseling and regulation of measures to control G6PD deficiency, so that the process of jaundice and anemia is not repeated in the future (Kaddas et al., 2024). It's not a bad plan, also, to step back and consider the cultural and historical dimensions of things, and these can actually add a lot to our understanding of modern medicine. There's a very long history of linking blood to life and health—think about ancient vampire legends—and this has had an impact on how people understand symptoms like pale color and jaundice, tending to link a light color with illness or weakness. Such accounts have a way of conflating the more complex, scientific realities of such afflictions. Overall, the medical community today is seeking to unravel these myths, applying evidence-based practices to the diagnosis and management of anemia, and suggesting that a synthesis of old knowledge with new wisdom might be helpful insofar as it brings us closer to knowledge of these problematic health issues (Schneider et al., 2023) (Figure 5.10).

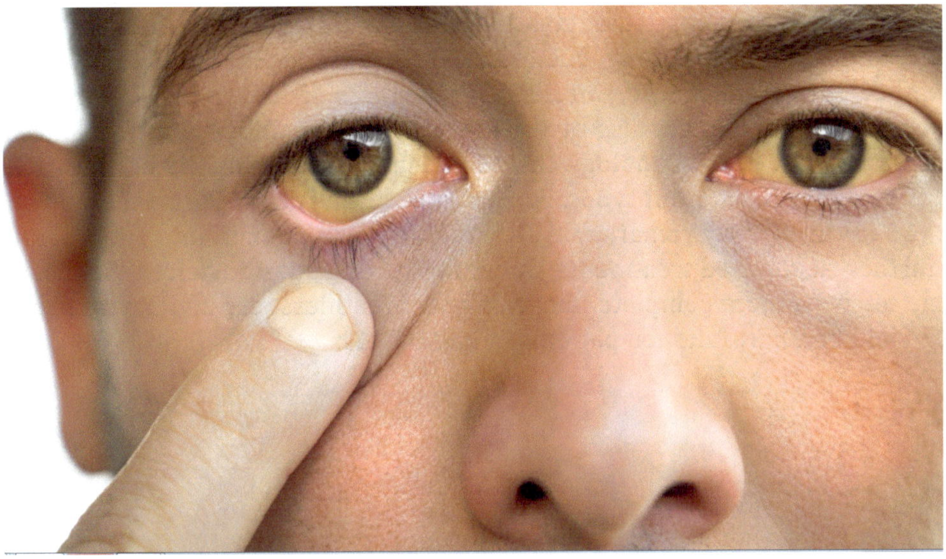

Figure 5.10. Pale skin and jaundice.

Source: https://external-content.duckduckgo.com/iu/?u=https%3A%2F%2Fimages.ctfassets.net%2F4f3rgqwzdznj%2F1gS5nop8hbSeptAlwMgm4u%2F7d9a9288cdb7c71853cf182bf74f4277%2Fcloseup_of_jaundice_eyes-1297312951.jpg&f=1&nofb=1&ipt=17f357966423eb724901c6d3c7464d0e103e05591022e6462c4c58bfe915604c.

5.3.3. Shortness of Breath

Fatigue isn't just a matter of feeling worn out—it often drags along a host of physical cues, with shortness of breath standing out, especially when anemia is in play. Tissues don't get the oxygen they need because of lower hemoglobin levels, and that lack really shows up as breathlessness, particularly when you're moving around. The body tries to make up for the difference, and it is during this time when most individuals become winded suddenly. Generally speaking, research tells us that the connection between hemoglobin content and the efficacy of breathing is very strong in explaining the reason behind the manifestation of the symptom. For example, Gómez et al. (2025) observes that exploring red blood cell details not only helps you concentrate on what is at fault for anemia, but also helps uncover the kind of symptoms like shortness of breath you would expect. How to find and treat this sign, then, can be vital in terms of managing anemia effectively. In everyday clinical practice, not diagnosing anemia is not just a question of the count of blood—it's also a question of balancing how terrible the symptoms are, including breathlessness. The disease tends to show up in a mixed, sometimes patchy way, so doctors will tend to marry the lab results with a careful observation of how the patient feels. They might screen for things like anemia of red blood cells and hemoglobin, and also chart any episodes of hard breathing that sound like heart failure. It's not unusual for that shortness of breath to throw a monkey wrench into the works by occasionally even suggesting a lung issue when it's actually anemia performing its function. Dullah et al. (2025) basically highlights that if the symptom information is accurate, then diagnostic accuracy can be enhanced, particularly in complicated situations. In most cases, ensuring overlapping signs are fully considered can lead to discovering actual causes and confronting them directly. Treating anemia rightfully includes listening to its signals—above all, the shortness of breath one experiences that could indicate underlying illness issues. By tracking both the hemoglobin and patients breathing, doctors can create treatment plans to counteract both the anemia and difficulty breathing. Sure, unrelenting shortness of breath is not only about transient misery—if it continues, but it might also be waving a red flag for underlying problems. Researchers have even been trying out new technology, including machine learning methods, to achieve a more precise picture of anemia's different types. For instance, the Random Forest method showcased by Gómez et al. (2025) was pretty remarkable at breaking down anemia into subtypes, which opens the door for further customized treatments. Generally, getting such advanced diagnostics into daily practice seems to give a more complete image of how breathlessness and anemia are related and, in the end, to yield better results for patients (Figure 5.11).

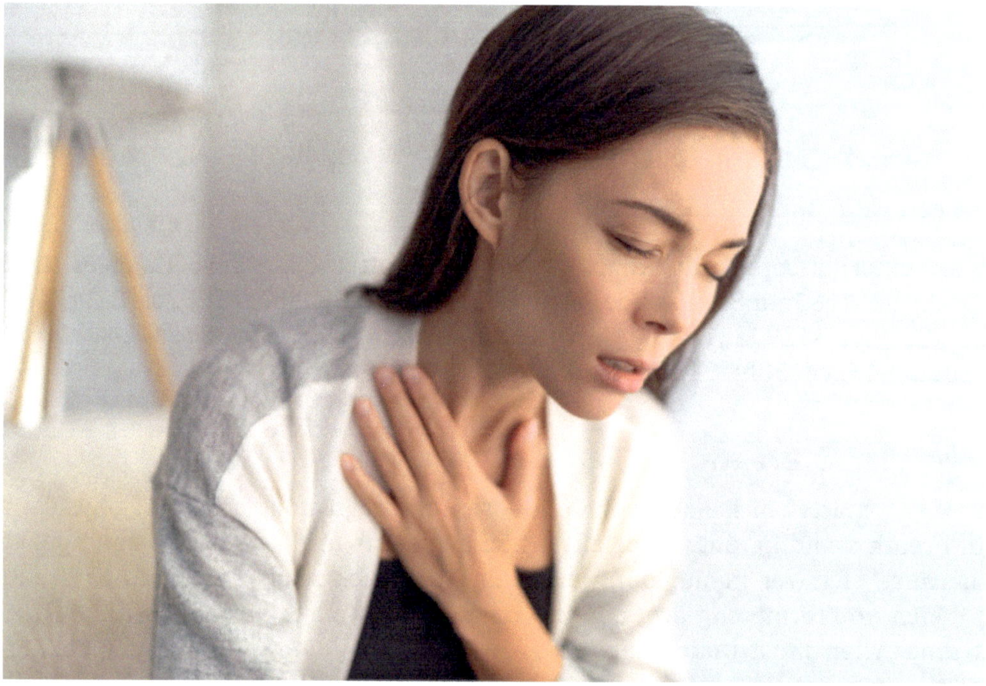

Figure 5.11. Shortness of breath.

Source: https://external-content.duckduckgo.com/iu/?u=http%3A%2F%2Fnurseadvisormagazine.com%2Fwp-content%2Fuploads%2F2020%2F07%2FAdobeStock_339822145-min.jpeg&f=1&nofb=1&ipt=8c91c34c615d31f789bfd77c4abd80e9008998ad01f0554a0489a4399b421d04.

Test Your Knowledge

1. What are the common general symptoms of anemia seen in most patients?
2. How do severe cases of anemia affect the cardiovascular and respiratory systems?

5.4. Diagnostic Methods

Learning Outcome

- Complete blood count (CBC);
- Peripheral blood smear;
- Bone marrow biopsy.

Diagnosis of anemia actually has come a very long way. We used to depend primarily on plain blood tests in the olden days; today, good old methods combined with newer sharper ones take a better picture. A complete blood count (CBC) is still a workhorse tool—giving information like hemoglobin, hematocrit, and red blood cell values—even though it might appear old-fashioned. But adding tests like reticulocyte counts and testing of erythropoietin levels enables doctors to more accurately determine what type of anemia an individual might have. That added knowledge makes a significant difference, especially when making the distinction between iron deficiency and anemia of chronic diseases because each has a different treatment protocol. Glycated hemoglobin, or HbA1c, is no longer diabetes's sole province—it now has a role in diagnosing anemia as well.

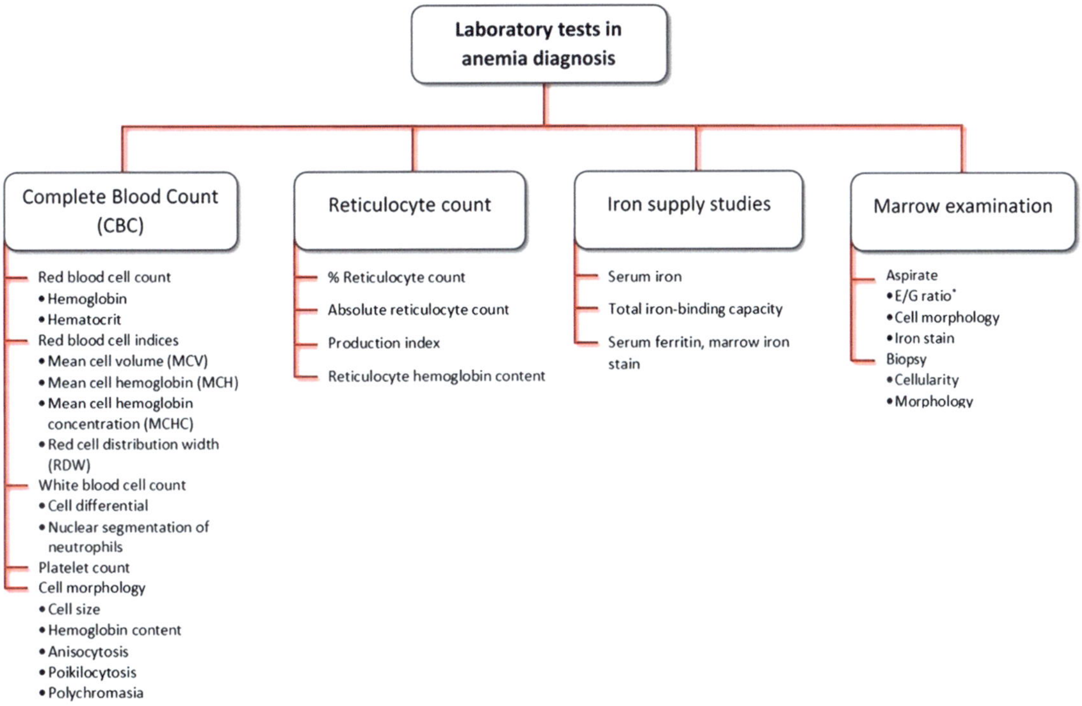

Figure 5.12. Anemia diagnostic methods.

Source: https://cdnintech.com/media/chapter/56750/1512345123/media/F2.png.

The methodologies used in measuring the HbA1c, far back in the late 1970s, were a little archaic; nowadays, the process is much more advanced. As explained by English et al. (2014), making all these processes uniform not only set world standards for the management of blood sugar, but also opened our eyes to its application when the hemoglobin levels are tampered with. By learning how HbA1c actually comes together, doctors can dig deeper into red blood cell development as a whole, filling it out with established and emerging measures to guide treatment. On top of that, new advances like machine learning algorithms, which are transforming medical diagnostics—of anemia along with them. By combining structured data with unstructured data, these algorithms make predictions more accurate; for instance, it is shown in one study on the basis of the MIMIC-III dataset (Band et al., 2019) that they will typically beat standard methods. In the world of anemia, this means diagnoses are finer, interpretations more nuanced, and treatment more personalized. On balance, it's an exciting development that marries good old-fashioned testing to new-fangled technology in a way that appears poised to tailor healthcare to what each patient actually needs (Figure 5.12).

5.4.1. Complete Blood Count (CBC)

One of the first things doctors do is screen for anemia using the CBC. It gives a snapshot impression of a person's blood in a timely manner and usually, a kind of snapshot that indicates what is occurring. You are provided with data like hemoglobin level, red blood cell count, and hematocrit that together help to indicate whether the issue might be iron deficiency or something else related to chronic disease.

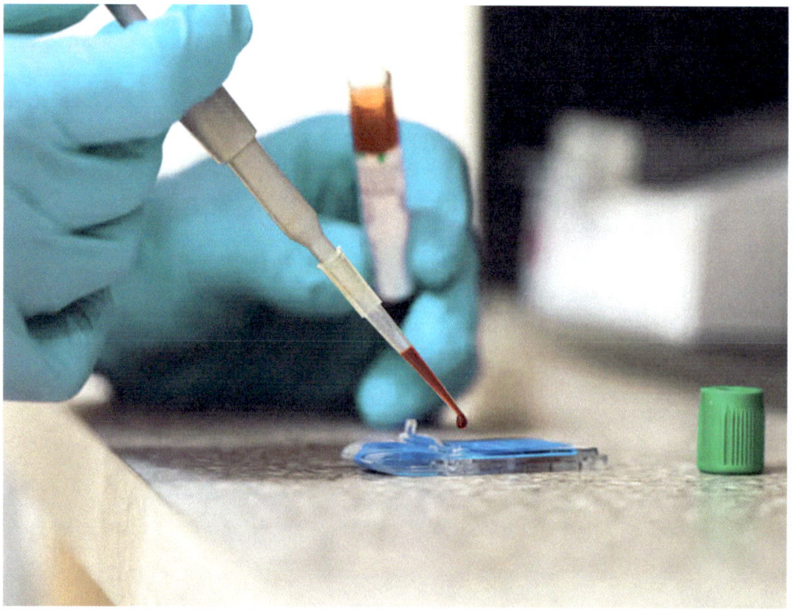

Figure 5.13. Complete blood count (CBC) for anemia.

Source: https://media.post.rvohealth.io/wp-content/uploads/2024/01/testing-blood-in-lab-732-549-feature-thumb.jpg.

Low hemoglobin, for example, will lead towards the diagnosis of iron-deficiency anemia, while abnormal white blood cell counts might signal long-term illness. Further, consideration of the mean corpuscular volume (MCV)—in other words, the average size of red cells—enables clinicians to ascertain the microcytic or macrocytic nature of a case and guide the subsequent treatment (Amalia et al., 2024). Data mining of CBC data has also come a long way in recent years.

In most cases, researchers now sift through huge amounts of blood test results by means of algorithms like the J48 Decision Tree and Random Forest. This not only helps to identify trends but also to correlate blood test data with patient demographics such as age and gender. This therefore places health professionals in a better position to create treatment protocols that really fit an individual's condition. This approach also renders the whole process of diagnosis more scientific and less guesswork, in addition to being a more personalized plan, aimed at facilitating overall efficiency in care provided (Airlangga et al., 2024). Deep learning is also starting to revolutionize the CBC analysis sector. In place of solely relying on traditional metrics, scientists now experiment with models like Convolutional Neural Networks (CNN) and Fully Connected Networks (FCN) in order to enhance detection of various forms of anemia. They employ tricks like data augmentation—and sometimes weighted loss functions—to address issues like class imbalance, which have a tendency of biased results. These technological innovations have the possibility of not just enhancing the precision of diagnosis but also to present the doctors with a virtual second opinion. As the field progresses, combining these new methods with conventional blood testing could be the path to more precise, patient-tailored interventions (Airlangga et al., 2024) (Figure 5.13).

5.4.2. Peripheral Blood Smear

To examine a peripheral blood smear is, for the majority of cases, one of the most significant ways of gaining an idea of what's occurring with the blood in a patient. How red cells look—larger or smaller, darker or lighter—is generally the first to give hints regarding abnormalities like anemia. For example, if most of the red blood cells are microcytic or abnormally pale (hypochromic), iron deficiency is the first thing that is thought; on the other hand, finding predominantly larger, macrocytic cells can be indicative of a folate deficiency or a vitamin B12 deficiency. These observations, simple though they might appear, in fact form the basis for how the condition will be classified and for what follow-up tests will be requested. Interestingly, the blood smear does not just reveal the type of anemia—but also distinguishes between less harmful causes and others that are potentially more worrisome, such as myelodysplastic syndromes or even leukemias. When one presents with myelodysplastic syndromes (MDS), the blood smear is particularly vital. MDS usually occurs with other forms of cytopenias—decreased red cell, white cell, or platelet counts—you can recognize by intensely reviewing blood films. For the most part, the French–American-British (FAB) classification system—the World Health Organization (WHO) later modified it—is based heavily on these morphologic observations because dysplastic findings you find can actually represent more significant underlying pathology. Clinicians are likely to highlight that these microscopic observations not only help in making a diagnosis but also give indications about future development, and hence influence patient-specific treatments (Al-Nehmi et al., 2019). Hypereosinophilic syndrome (HES) adds another layer of complication to the equation. It's marked by an extremely high number of eosinophils, and in some it occurs as an isolated abnormality, while in others it occurs as a bundle with other hematologic diseases. Overall, the peripheral blood smear helps to determine if the eosinophilia is a reactive process—typically secondary to some underlying disorder—or idiopathic and prompts clinicians to consider other possibilities like chronic eosinophilic leukemia or autoimmune anemia. The diversity of the causes of HES underscores the importance of actually taking careful notice of cell forms and counts; indeed, even in those few cases which are linked with autoimmune hemolytic anemia, an understanding of the interplay of eosinophilia with other hematological abnormalities is crucial. Ultimately, the smear not only offers classification but also functions as a guide tool when choosing the best therapeutic option for complex, multi-perspective hematology problems (Brys et al., 2015).

5.4.3. Bone Marrow Biopsy

Bone marrow and anemia go hand in hand. There are also times when routine blood tests just can't give the whole picture, leaving doctors to have to rely on a bone marrow biopsy to really get to the bottom of things. When trying to sort out complications like aplastic anemia or those nasty myelodysplastic syndromes, obtaining a simple sample from the bone marrow can be literally a matter of life and death. In many cases, analyzing a bone marrow aspirate enables physicians to see the cell structure up close and even provides clues as to the underlying process that leads to the anemia. It isn't surprising that the unruly character of anemias often requires more advanced sleight of hand, for instance, getting a bone marrow biopsy to figure out exactly what is happening. Studies seem to suggest that should an aspiration meet with adversity—a dry tap, for example—the biopsy is the second line. This method does not simply count cells; it offers pathologists a chance to test for any underlying malignancies, e.g., acute myeloid leukemia (AML) or other blood cancers, which might be present in conjunction with the anemia. The constant cross-talk between anemia and cancer really emphasizes the importance of getting the proper diagnoses and classifications to allow us to select the right treatments. Drilling down, knowledge of the genetic nuances in blood diseases is critical for good patient care. Where conditions like nonseminomatous germ cell tumors occur with AML, it would follow that inclusion of bone marrow biopsy in the picture is a good idea. The high-powered exome sequencing has even picked up somatic mutations in genes like PTEN and TP53 in such a scenario, suggesting the potential of a common clonal origin obscuring the treatment options. Through these molecular details through marrow analysis, doctors can craft tailored treatments—a strategy that, in most cases, delivers better patient outcomes, as in some recent research (Bhandari et al., 2017; Demeter et al., 2016) (Figure 5.14).

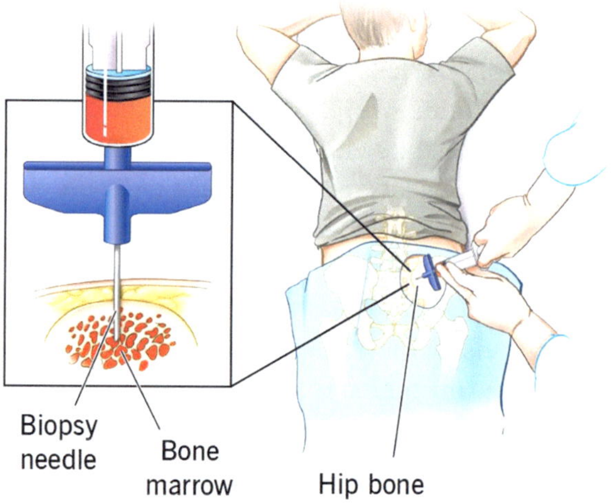

Figure 5.14. Bone marrow biopsy.

Source: https://my.clevelandclinic.org/-/scassets/images/org/health/articles/17735-bone-marrow-biopsy.

Test Your Knowledge

1. How is patient history and physical examination important in diagnosing anemia?
2. What role does the complete blood count (CBC) play in identifying anemia?

5.5. Laboratory Tests

Learning Outcome

- Serum ferritin levels;
- Vitamin B12 and folate levels;
- Reticulocyte count.

Anemia is not necessarily as simple as it sounds to figure out—you actually have to dig through a lot of bloodwork to know the full story. Serum ferritin, for example, is a big part of distinguishing iron deficiency from, say, anemia associated with chronic disease. In one study, which was set up to interrupt the normal diagnostic process, a regression model was built from straightforward demographic and clinical data to predict ferritin levels. The model yielded a moderate r = 0.854, which, all in all, suggests that it might hold its own in the clinic. It even did so well as to be able to sort patients into distinct ferritin categories that doctors might more precisely tailor treatments. All this is to demonstrate how the incorporation of advanced lab tests in with regular diagnostics can actually enhance the precision of how we classify anemia (Varekha et al., 2025). Another way of looking at diagnosing anemia is now through machine learning, which is a new twist on the old lab methods. Researchers accessed a pool of micro-normocytic anemia patients and built a supervised model that scored 99.82% at cutting up anemia types. Especially where low-resource environments don't have the luxury of pricey lab tests. Through the use of models such as Random Forest, doctors aren't restricted to only confirming anemia—but can actually determine whether it's microcytic, normocytic or macrocytic. This extra level of detail not only deepens the understanding of a patient's condition but also helps steer treatment in a more targeted way, blending modern computational methods with tests we've relied on for years (Gómez et al., 2025). Lab tests do more than just diagnose—they're key for keeping tabs on treatment success and patient progress too. Serial monitoring of hemoglobin, reticulocyte count, and iron studies are the pillars of tracking the progression of anemia development, which often provides a clue as to when therapy might need a minor adjustment. As an example, if a patient is receiving iron supplementation, monitoring ferritin allows us to determine whether treatment is effective or whether an adjustment is needed. In addition, a full blood panel may reveal underlying causes like chronic inflammation or nutritional deficiencies. In brief, coordination among these tests helps identify specific categorizations and plays a crucial role in managing anemia overall, and as such, they're really indispensable in modern medicine (Gómez et al., 2025; Varekha et al., 2025).

5.5.1. Serum ferritin levels

Biological variables all together and together tip serum ferritin values, which tell us about the iron contained in a body. Ferritin's not just some random number—it gives a general idea whether or not an individual out of iron or has another form of anemia. Low ferritin in most cases means there's not enough iron, but when there is inflammation in the picture, ferritin will still test high, obscuring the situation slightly. You might say it's not simple to determine what these numbers represent; you have to factor in a recent illness or chronic inflammation before deciding what's really happening with a patient's iron and whether or not treatment is warranted (Zimmermann et al., 2008). The application of ferritin extends beyond diagnosis, influencing actually treatment for victims of anemia. In simple terms, when one is running low on iron, doctors normally advise taking iron supplements and dietary changes to replenish those levels. Tracking ferritin over time enables health professionals to establish whether or not the remedies are effectively working, maintaining iron levels bouncing back as intended. Reliance solely on hemoglobin can lead to an inapt diagnosis as it is non-specific; in addition to that, ferritin and other tests, such as transferrin saturation, offer a more holistic picture (Zimmermann et al., 2008). In day-to-day clinical practice, keeping in mind that values for ferritin are by themselves possessive is essential. These include age, gender, and prior state of health, and they may have an influence on the levels of ferritin and result in improper conclusions on the iron status of the individual. Even if the levels are high, it may not necessarily lead to increased oxygen delivery because more ferritin does not always mean greater oxygen flow. Studies have shown that reduced oxygen levels in iron-deficient individuals may impair their ability to cope with physical exertion, a function for which ferritin needs to be considered in conjunction with other markers of functioning. In general, diagnosing and staging anemia involves a broad perspective—one responsive to what ferritin reveals and where it breaks down (Figure 5.15).

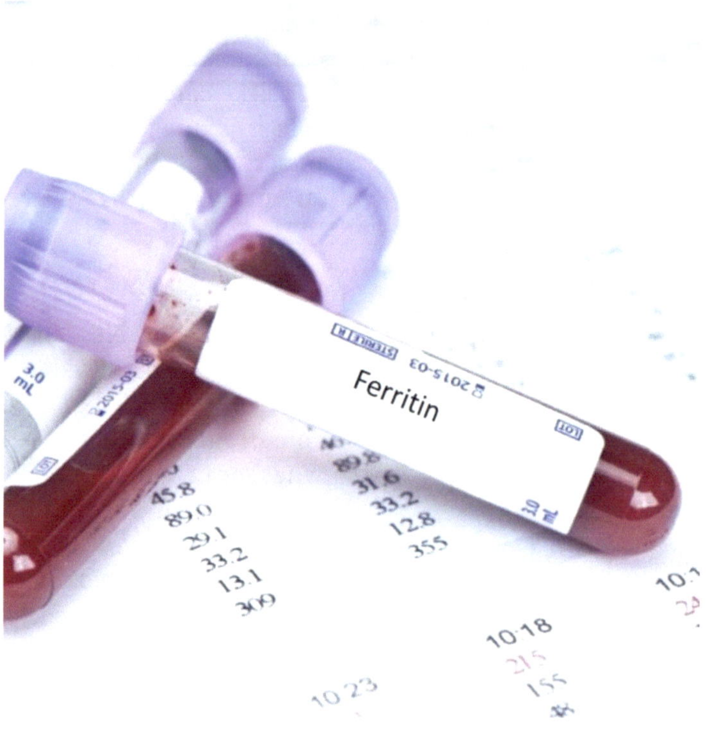

Figure 5.15. Serum ferritin level blood test.

Source: https://www.viplab.in/uploads/blog/1535779819_ferritin%20level.jpg.

5.5.2. Vitamin B12 and folate levels

Vitamin B12 and folate have a rather unexpected function in anemia—watching how they play tricks on the body's functions is the solution. In cases of deficiency, people can become a type of anemia where red blood cells are excessively large and don't function properly. DNA synthesis is impaired in these deficiency states, which impairs the production of new blood cells and decreases oxygen carried around. Sometimes the problem is due to not eating well, and other times it is because the body is unable to absorb these vitamins; either way, the situation gets more complicated. Since anemia can be due to a plethora of issues—nutritional deficiencies merely one of them—it is a good idea to get the laboratory tests for these vitamins, which will assist in identifying the cause and choosing the right treatment option (Tuli et al., 2017). Doctors usually check the levels of vitamin B12 and folate closely, especially in individuals who are at higher risk. Older adults, vegetarians, and those with gastrointestinal disease most often have symptoms of deficiency in vitamin B12. Folate, on the other hand, drops when diets are poor or metabolic demand increases, as it does in pregnancy.

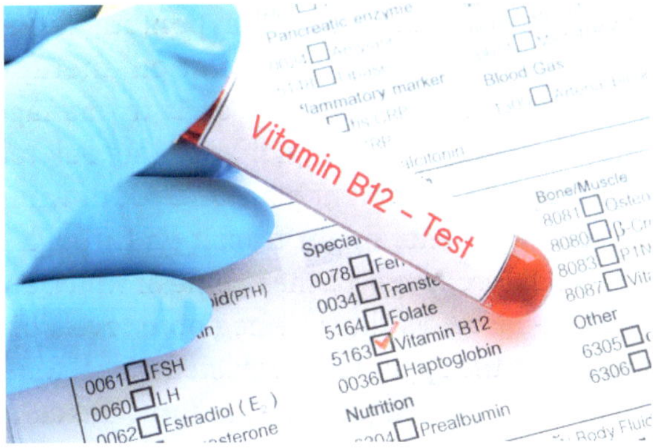

Figure 5.16. Vitamin B12 blood test.

Source: https://millenniumpathologylab.com/wp-content/uploads/2021/11/Vitamin_B12.jpg.

It may not be simply a question of anemia; deficiency also may lead to nerve damage or birth defects in the newborn. That is one of the reasons why targeting the routine screening on these high-risk populations is so important—to catch things early and hopefully prevent more serious complications (Bonham et al., 2023). Overall, B12 and folate testing is a significant part of uncovering anemia. Physicians have to cross-reference the findings from the lab with what they see in the patients, piecing together on an individual's nutritional and blood profile. In the majority of cases, this entails recommending dietary changes or even supplements in order to rectify the imbalance. This form of hands-on, personalized treatment results in improved outcomes and serves as a reminder to every one of just how important prevention is, especially for those at greatest risk. Lastly, the acquisition of control over how the vitamins influence red blood cell production pushes more efficient anemia control and overall patient health (Tuli et al., 2017) (Figure 5.16).

5.5.3. Reticulocyte Count

Bone marrow health is of utmost significance regarding the detection of anemia. The number of reticulocytes serves as a handy gauge of how much at capacity the marrow is producing new red blood cells at – a kind of progress bar of its activity. When those numbers fall, it can mean that the marrow isn't quite operating at maximum potential, like in aplastic anemia or some other marrow disorders. On the other hand, if there is a high count, it typically means the marrow is responding harder to cope with the challenge, which you might notice after a bleed or in hemolytic crises. For the most part, clinicians don't necessarily need to know these numbers—that really provides them with data to modify treatment strategies depending on what's going on behind the scenes. Reticulocyte counts are not only a snapshot diagnosis but also a window to a patient's likely future trajectory. For instance, in a recent non-Hodgkin lymphoma study, a high percentage of patients turned out to be anemic, and those with low reticulocyte counts had much less complete response (Lahkar et al., 2013). Generally speaking, they serve the dual purpose of both informing us about what is happening in the here and now, and implying how well treatment in the future will be likely to work. Clinicians (yes, with the somewhat humorous little spelling error) largely depend on this data to make real-time decisions regarding switching therapy, and add that these numbers are useful for both short-term and long-term care. Technology has actually revolutionized reticulocyte counting. Current hematology analyzers employ sophisticated techniques–such as automated hemocytometry

-to provide such measurements with greater accuracy. Even minute fluctuations in reticulocyte production, indicating one of several flavors of anemia or related issues, become more detectable. With advances in laboratory hematology ongoing, the use of reticulocyte counts grows ever more crucial as a diagnostic and classifying tool for blood diseases. With these advances in technology providing a better picture of what is happening within the bloodstream, patient care and outcomes will surely gain a big boost (d'Onofrio et al., 2021).

Test Your Knowledge

1. How are serum iron studies (iron, ferritin, TIBC) useful in diagnosing iron-deficiency anemia?
2. What laboratory tests are commonly used to detect megaloblastic anemia?

5.6. Treatment Options

Learning Outcome

- Dietary changes and supplements;
- Medications and injections;
- Blood transfusions and other procedures.

Treating anemia usually consists of a mix of approaches that actually depend on what is causing the issue and on what particular patients need. One example of this is in the case of myelodysplastic syndromes (MDS), where the blood is not being produced properly; in such cases, physicians usually start treatment with red blood cell-stimulating drugs, also known as ESAs. Research has shown that, on balance, only a third of patients fare sufficiently well with these medications so that alternative methods are generally required.

One new medication, luspatercept, has more recently been licensed for those lower-risk MDS patients who respond insufficiently to ESAs—its ability to raise hemoglobin levels appears to offer a useful new weapon in our treatment armory (Boccia et al., 2023). Taking a look a little further at the therapy options, it seems that individuals with refractory anemia often do best when a variety of treatments is attempted instead of depending on one. Clinicians at times combine the use of hypomethylating agents, incorporate iron chelation therapy, and incorporate supportive care to manage symptoms and enhance quality of life. Far too frequently, the treatment plan isn't put down in concrete – patients might transition through a string of different approaches, some of which are not ESAs-based, as their hemoglobin levels are tracked and the approach is adjusted in real time; this undoubtedly highlights the importance of being able to change a plan at a moment's notice. Overall, this adaptable method aims to reduce anemia as well as any other problem of MDS (Boccia et al., 2023). For less common issues like the vascular malformations of Blue Rubber Bleb Naevus Syndrome (BRBNS), however, the situation is quite different. This disorder tends to cause severe anemia, mainly because of chronic gastrointestinal bleeding, and thus needs to be managed effectively and promptly. Therapies in such cases might involve surgical removal of the offending vascular lesions, dietary and iron supplementation to fight blood loss, and other supportive care. In such cases, being very familiar with the patient's presentation – and being able to access treatment from several different specialists – is key. By treating the anemia and the resultant vascular problem, doctors are often able to enhance outcomes and minimize the risk of long-term complications.

5.6.1. Dietary Changes and Supplements

When addressing anemia, a shift in diet can be a lifesaver. A diet that increases your consumption of iron, vitamin B12, and folate truly helps spur the creation of red blood cells and keeps your blood factory in full production. Lean flesh foods, liberal quantities of legumes, and leafy greens provide enough iron to keep iron-deficiency disease at bay, whereas eggs and milk—foods high in vitamin B12—are likely to protect against megaloblastic anemia, which may attack in the absence of that vitamin. Ninety percent of the time, eating healthfully gives you the building materials for not just treatment, but also symptom relief from fatigue and weakness that plague so many people (Kucera et al., 2014). As you focus on supplements, it goes without saying that not all nutrients play exactly the same role in every circumstance. Some research in general defines that vitamin B12 will be lower in some groups, especially among patients who have neurodegenerative conditions (Christine et al., 2019). While proper dietary changes are crucial, supplements typically become a significant helper—especially for those who are restrained by restrictive diets or are not able to absorb nutrients. Clinical guidelines sometimes suggest hitting some vitamin and mineral targets to boost the output of red blood cells, implying that supplements can be a convenient sidekick to a good diet. You need to monitor nutrient levels regularly as well. It lets you adjust your plan if needed and tailor it to the type and etiology of anemia you are treating. For instance, while iron supplements can be wonders for someone with iron-deficiency anemia, they might be hazardous to you if you have a condition such as aplastic anemia, where more iron can be more of a threat. That is why doctors usually prescribe regular blood tests—to test and determine whether your food changes and supplements are really doing something. In general, combining smart food choices with targeted supplements tends to form a good strategy for fighting anemia (Kucera et al., 2014) (Figure 5.17).

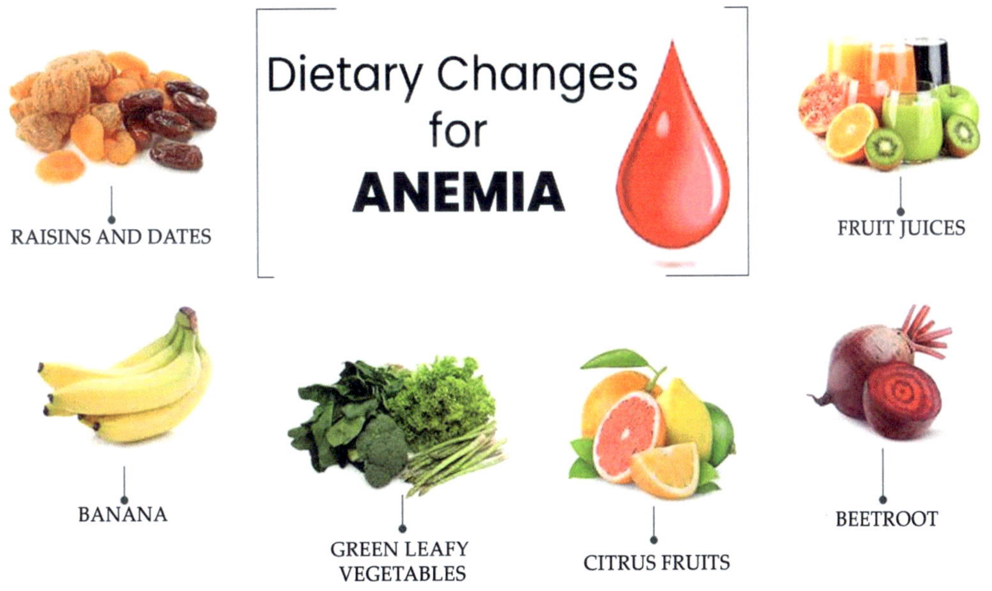

Figure 5.17. Dietary changes and supplements for anemia.

Source: https://cdn.shopify.com/s/files/1/0586/8234/3501/files/dietary-changes-for-anemia.jpg?v=1716285649.

5.6.2. Medications and Injections

The treatment of anemia is usually a process of balancing different meds and injections, usually based on the offender causing the condition. As an example, myelodysplastic syndromes or chronic disease anemia usually results in the use of drugs that promote blood production—more commonly referred to as erythropoiesis-stimulating agents (ESAs). ESAs are basically the ones who prod the bone marrow to increase the level of red blood cells, which consequently removes that uncomfortable fatigue and weakness. The patients can notice the difference in their everyday life with a rise in hemoglobin levels. It is not a matter of a cell increase, though; the doctors also watch out for side effects like elevated blood pressure or occurrence of thromboembolic events, for which they might need to make a change in the dose or even alter the treatment plan. There are a few diseases, including anemia with myelofibrosis, for which drugs like ruxolitinib have certain unique advantages. Ruxolitinib, an inhibitor of JAK, is fairly broad in application, treating such symptoms as an enlarged spleen and others at the same time. It has the potential to lead to shrinkage of the spleen and symptom relief, which can make the patients more adherent to treatment. However, there is concern that the treatment itself could cause anemia in a dose-related fashion. In all but a few cases, which takes careful monitoring, and sometimes doctors even give extra help with drugs like ESAs or danazol. All of these factors contribute to the worth of matching treatment regimens to individual patients' specific needs, such as the extent of the anemia and any accompanying medical issues. Shots and methods of injection also are evolving as an integral part of anemia management. Consider IV iron formulations, for example, which are gaining favor in clinics due to the fact that they address iron deficiency without the stomach issues that routinely accompany pills. Recent investigations have mostly demonstrated that intravenous iron is able to rapidly raise serum ferritin and transferrin saturation, ultimately helping improve hemoglobin levels. And for injectable ESAs, these provide a rapid, effective means for those who can't afford oral meds. Research on the best dosing regimens and means of encouraging patient compliance remains ongoing - all of which attests to how integral these injection-form treatments have become to treating anemia for a broad range of patients in general.

5.6.3. Blood Transfusions and Other Procedures

Blood transfusions are often the first consideration in the management of anemia. In patients severely impacted by conditions like myelodysplastic syndromes (MDS), a transfusion is not just some kind of band-aid—it really does make their day-to-day better, both their energy and how they feel about themselves. MDS patients depend on transfusions to remove the symptoms of low hemoglobin, not just giving some physical relief but seeming to lift their mood. In most cases, that surge of hemoglobin is absolutely beneficial, and if you overlay on top of it the growing cost of ongoing transfusion therapy, the bottom line doesn't remain unseen, as more recently documented (Berger et al., 2008). It isn't merely a case of the blood transfusions, though. A full array of tests, including bone marrow biopsies, nutrition tests, and even genetics, is used in finding the cause of anemia. With these tests, one can map out what is causing the condition, either a deficiency in nutrition, some chronic ailment, or even a genetic cause. For example, using an advanced diagnostic approach is essential while trying to distinguish between iron deficiency anemia and anemia related to chronic disease. That kind of specificity in the diagnosis enables health care providers to improve interventions, keeping up with newer strategies for better patient outcomes (Agabiti et al., 2017). The management of anemia, especially with complicating factors like MDS, actually needs collaboration. Health care professionals need to weigh the near-term advantages of transfusion treatments against consideration of the patient's overall medical situation—other diseases can change hospitalization and even mortality rates. Sometimes poor record-keeping within health systems introduces a secondary level of complexity in keeping track of the patients' course (Agabiti et al., 2017). Lastly, quality improvement of these systems is needed so that such therapies as transfusions are part of an overall, managed method of diagnosing and treating this difficult disease (Figure 5.18).

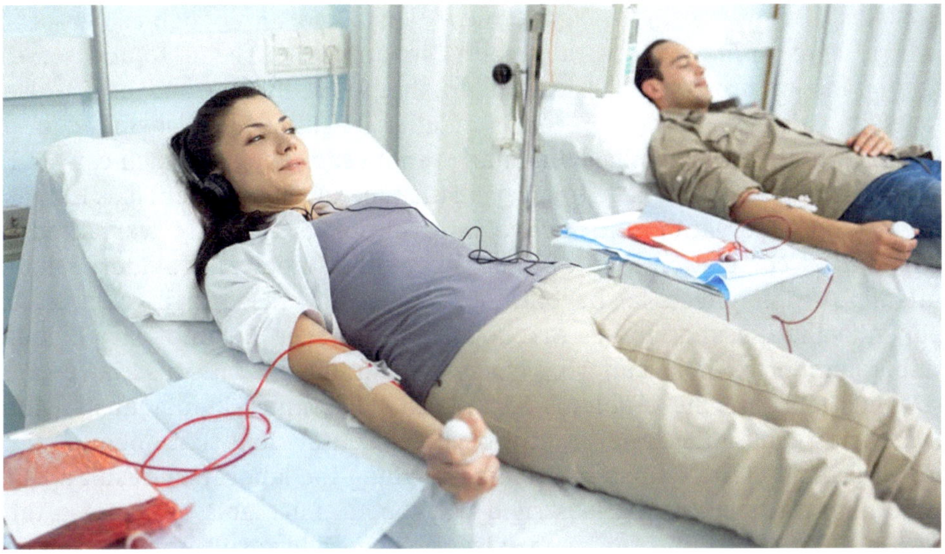

Figure 5.18. Blood transfusions and anemia.

Source: https://i0.wp.com/post.medicalnewstoday.com/wp-content/uploads/sites/3/2020/06/GettyImages-151340032_header-1024x575.jpg?w=1155&h=1528.

Test Your Knowledge

1. What are the common treatment strategies for iron-deficiency anemia?
2. How are vitamin B12 and folate deficiency anemias managed?

Summary

Years of research on anemia have taught us a lot about how it's sorted and spied. It's pretty obvious that identifying the exact cause—whether it is nutritional deficiencies or a chronic illness in progress—is important when it comes to choosing a treatment that really works. Causes are ubiquitous, so instead of the one-size-fits-all approach, patients need a dive in; patients who come in with fatigue, washed-out look, or just plain general weakness usually leave with numerous tests and check-ups. Most of the time, knowledge of these twists and turns enables doctors to match up care better, which tends to improve overall health. New research seems to add some unexpected complexities, too, and to propose a knotted dance between anemia and other diseases in the body. Some reports suggest that certain forms of anemia—like the form found in autoimmune gastritis—may activate threats for other ailments, even diseases like stomach cancer. For example, some studies show that patients with atrophic gastritis will develop higher risks for gastric tumors, so an astute, ongoing observation with active intervention is typically warranted (Annibale et al., 2015). This kind of correlation kind of underscores that medical providers should be on the lookout for anemia's ripple effects far beyond low counts. And there is the complicated interplay between the anemia and digestion issues that adds another layer of complexity. Evidence suggests that a reasonable number of those suffering from autoimmune gastritis also have gastrointestinal issues—those which obscure the problems for treatment as much as diagnosis (Annibale et al., 2017). If you look at it from this angle, what it becomes self-evident that doctors might be forced to take a more all-around view of a patient's state, weighing the laboratory result against intestinal health. By combining these clues in a less rigid way, doctors are able to create a total care plan that treats both the Band-Aids and the deeper issues, generally resulting in better outcomes.

Anemia is not a cookie-cutter condition – it's a set of circumstances that call out for a second look. There are several kinds—iron deficiency, vitamin B12 deficiency, and even aplastic anemia—each pointing to its own set of causes. Iron deficiency, for example, usually comes from nutritional deficiency or chronic blood loss, while aplastic cases may arise due to the bone marrow not working properly or due to exposure to specific chemicals. These minor differences make a world of difference in mapping out a course of treatment that addresses the root problem instead of masking the symptoms. On a general note, newer advancements in medical technology, such as machine learning working through high volumes of patient data, have played a major role in streamlining the manner in which we predict and distinguish between anemia types (Band et al., 2019). Exploring deeper into diagnosis, a general blood test is the cornerstone in figuring out what's happening. The CBC—short for complete blood count—is holding up valuable data like hemoglobin levels and red blood cell measurements indicating both the nature and severity of the anemia. Iron studies, a screening of serum iron, ferritin, and total iron-binding capacity, also uncover the ins and outs of iron metabolism. These overlapping yet distinct tests allow doctors to piece together a plan that may range from changes in diet to supplementing or more complex treatment, depending on the test results. Combinatorial therapy in most cases assures appropriate and timely therapy for patients battling anemia (Berger et al., 2008). Patient-specific factors also come into play; gender, age, and existing conditions can change the presentation of anemia and how it is managed. For instance, older patients are more likely to be susceptible to myelodysplastic syndromes, more likely to need blood transfusions and lifelong treatment—issues that will affect quality of life and healthcare costs. To recall these nuances is to help clinicians decide which tests are most relevant and how rapidly to act. By embracing the heterogeneity of anemia's etiologies, health care providers can better individualize their methods of management and improve outcomes while being more judicious in use of resources (Berger et al., 2008).

KEY TERMS FROM THIS CHAPTER

- Anemia
- Aplastic anemia
- Bone marrow examination
- Folate
- Hematocrit
- Hemoglobin
- Hemolytic anemia
- Iron deficiency anemia
- Macrocytic anemia
- Mean corpuscular volume (MCV)
- Microcytic anemia
- Normocytic anemia
- Pernicious anemia
- Reticulocyte count
- Serum ferritin
- Sickle cell anemia
- Thalassemia
- Vitamin B12

Critical Thinking Questions

1. **Which of the following is a classification of anemia based on red blood cell (RBC) size?**
   a. Hemolytic anemia
   b. Macrocytic anemia
   c. Aplastic anemia
   d. Iron-deficiency anemia
2. **What laboratory test is commonly used first to help diagnose anemia?**
   a. Urinalysis
   b. Complete Blood Count (CBC)
   c. Liver Function Test
   d. Erythrocyte Sedimentation Rate (ESR)
3. **Microcytic hypochromic anemia is most commonly caused by:**
   a. Vitamin B12 deficiency
   b. Folic acid deficiency
   c. Iron deficiency
   d. Aplastic anemia
4. **Which test differentiates between vitamin B12 and folate deficiency in macrocytic anemia?**
   a. Ferritin
   b. Reticulocyte count
   c. Serum B12 and folate levels
   d. ESR
5. **In normocytic normochromic anemia, the mean corpuscular volume (MCV) is typically:**
   a. Less than 80 fL
   b. Greater than 100 fL
   c. Between 80 and 100 fL
   d. Unmeasurable

Answers to Critical Thinking Questions

1. (b); 2. (b); 3. (c); 4. (c); 5. (c)

Short Answer Questions

1. How is anemia defined in clinical practice (based on hemoglobin levels)?
2. What are the three main classifications of anemia based on red blood cell size (MCV)?
3. What are common causes of microcytic anemia?
4. Which laboratory tests are typically ordered to investigate anemia?
5. How can a reticulocyte count help differentiate between types of anemia?

References

1. Abdolrahim, M., Jazayeri, H. E., Rabiee, M., Rajab, et al. (2017). Evaluation of glycated albumin (GA) and GA/HbA1c ratio for diagnosis of diabetes and glycemic control: A comprehensive review. https://core.ac.uk/download/213086982.pdf (accessed on 1st July 2025).
2. Adair, L. S., Attard, S. M., Gordon-Larsen, P., et al. (2015). Implications of iron deficiency/anemia on the classification of diabetes using HbA1c. https://core.ac.uk/download/345220514.pdf (accessed on 1st July 2025).
3. Adibuzzaman, M., Ahamed, S. I., Ahsan, G. M. T., Chu, et al. (2017). A novel real-time non-invasive hemoglobin level detection using video images from smartphone camera. https://core.ac.uk/download/213087142.pdf (accessed on 1st July 2025).
4. Agabiti, N., Aloe Spiriti, M. A., Andriani, A., Breccia, et al. (2017). A population-based study on myelodysplastic syndromes in the Lazio Region (Italy), medical miscoding and 11-year mortality follow-up. The Gruppo Romano-Laziale Mielodisplasie experience of retrospective multicentric registry. https://core.ac.uk/download/127588182.pdf (accessed on 1st July 2025).
5. Airlangga, G. (2024). Comparison of deep learning architectures for anemia classification using complete blood count data. https://core.ac.uk/download/620625385.pdf (accessed on 1st July 2025).
6. Al-Nehmi, A. W., Hamid, G. A., & Shukry, S. (2019). Diagnosis and classification of myelodysplastic syndrome. https://core.ac.uk/download/322440498.pdf (accessed on 1st July 2025).
7. Amalia, D., Prasetiawan, I., & Setiawan, J. (2024). Data mining techniques for predictive classification of anemia disease subtypes. https://core.ac.uk/download/604529764.pdf (accessed on 1st July 2025).
8. Annibale, B., Carabotti, M., Conti, L., et al. (2018). Risk factors associated with the occurrence of autoimmune diseases in adult coeliac patients. https://core.ac.uk/download/188824534.pdf (accessed on 1st July 2025).
9. Annibale, B., Carabotti, M., Esposito, G., et al. (2017). Upper gastrointestinal symptoms in autoimmune gastritis: A cross-sectional study. https://core.ac.uk/download/80312104.pdf (accessed on 1st July 2025).
10. Annibale, B., Corleto, V. D., Di Giulio, E., et al. (2015). Occurrence of gastric cancer and carcinoids in atrophic gastritis during prospective long-term follow-up. https://core.ac.uk/download/54520617.pdf (accessed on 1st July 2025).
11. Badura, K., Janc, J., Wąsik, J., Gnitecki, S., Skwira, S., Młynarska, E., Rysz, J., et al. (2024). Anemia of chronic kidney disease—A narrative review of its pathophysiology, diagnosis, and management. *Biomedicines, 12*. https://www.semanticscholar.org/paper/47c222851a11c0973dca7c2d04170d1ffc5b7833 (accessed on 1st July 2025).
12. Band, C., Gao, X., Lam, M., et al. (2019). Multimodal machine learning for automated ICD coding. https://arxiv.org/abs/1810.13348 (accessed on 1st July 2025).
13. Bejar, R., Bell, J. A., Cano, S., et al. (2019). A pragmatic patient-reported outcome strategy for rare disease clinical trials: Application of the EORTC item library to myelodysplastic syndromes, chronic myelomonocytic leukemia, and acute myeloid leukemia. https://core.ac.uk/download/323066928.pdf (accessed on 1st July 2025).

14. Berger, K., Gattermann, N., Hofmann, W. K., et al. (2008). Myelodysplastic syndromes: Aspects of current medical care and economic considerations in Germany. https://core.ac.uk/download/16432340.pdf (accessed on 1st July 2025).

15. Bero, L., Cooke, G. P. E., Doust, J. A., et al. (2013). Expanding disease definitions in guidelines and expert panel ties to industry: A cross-sectional study of common conditions in the United States. https://core.ac.uk/download/196601152.pdf (accessed on 1st July 2025).

16. Bhandari, A., Maharjan, S., Osti, B. P., et al. (2017). Bone marrow aspiration cytology in the diagnosis of hematologic and non-hematologic diseases in a multi-specialty hospital in Nepal. https://core.ac.uk/download/539912767.pdf (accessed on 1st July 2025).

17. Bhide, A., Khalil, A., Kulkarni, A., Thilaganathan, B., Dempsey, E., Sileo, F. G., Hutchison, A. A., et al. (2020). Non-immune fetal hydrops: Etiology and outcome according to gestational age at diagnosis. https://core.ac.uk/download/322366720.pdf (accessed on 1st July 2025).

18. Boccia, R., Xiao, H., Miteva, D., Che, M., Gu, T., McBride, A., Glassberg, M., et al. (2023). Real-world patient characteristics, treatment patterns, and outcomes in patients with lower-risk myelodysplastic syndromes who have been treated with luspatercept. *Blood*. https://www.semanticscholar.org/paper/320383b2f2f575eaa112ef3f17c85226896c6963 (accessed on 1st July 2025).

19. Bolt, D. M., Fink, J., Greenlee, R. T., et al. (2015). The relationship of individual comorbid chronic conditions to diabetes care quality. https://core.ac.uk/download/323070914.pdf (accessed on 1st July 2025).

20. Bonham, K. S., Bowness, P., Britton, G. J., et al. (2023). Alterations in the gut microbiome implicate key taxa and metabolic pathways across inflammatory arthritis phenotypes. https://core.ac.uk/download/578154334.pdf (accessed on 1st July 2025).

21. Boselli, C., Cavaliere, D., D'Andrea, V., et al. (2018). Surgical treatment of gastrointestinal stromal tumors of the duodenum: A literature review. https://core.ac.uk/download/188824368.pdf (accessed on 1st July 2025).

22. Brys, A. K., Sheth, M. R., Sohn, D. D., et al. (2015). Diagnostic and therapeutic considerations in idiopathic hypereosinophilia with warm autoimmune hemolytic anemia. https://core.ac.uk/download/323075654.pdf (accessed on 1st July 2025).

23. Cardenas, D., Castillo Sequera, J. L., Rivera, J., et al. (2024). Early prediction model for anemia in infants using clinical data from Perú applying supervised machine learning algorithms. https://core.ac.uk/download/641599099.pdf (accessed on 1st July 2025).

24. Chaber, R., Helwich, E., Lauterbach, R., Mastalerz-Migas, A., Matysiak, M., Peregud-Pogorzelski, J., Styczyński, J., et al. (2024). Diagnosis and treatment of iron deficiency and iron deficiency anemia in children and adolescents: Recommendations of the Polish Pediatric Society, the Polish Society of Pediatric Oncology and Hematology, the Polish Society of Neonatology, and the Polish Society of Family Medicine. *Nutrients, 16*. https://www.semanticscholar.org/paper/149ef149322e747ff5fa0f6cce3395f5cecdc293 (accessed on 1st July 2025).

25. Chadwick, C., Dietiker, W., Kim, C., et al. (2019). Characterization of vitamin B12 supplementation and correlation with clinical outcomes in a large longitudinal study of early Parkinson's disease. https://core.ac.uk/download/305124307.pdf (accessed on 1st July 2025).

26. Conlon, C., Goldacre, M. J., Goldacre, R., et al. (2013). Associations between selected

immune-mediated diseases and tuberculosis: Record-linkage studies. https://core.ac.uk/download/30696542.pdf (accessed on 1st July 2025).

27. d'Onofrio, G. (2021). Full-field hemocytometry: Forty years of progress seen through *Clinical and Laboratory Hematology and the International Journal of Laboratory Hematology*. https://core.ac.uk/download/604623263.pdf (accessed on 1st July 2025).

28. Demeter, R. T., Duncavage, E. J., Griffith, M., Griffith, et al. (2016). A common founding clone with TP53 and PTEN mutations gives rise to a concurrent germ cell tumor and acute megakaryoblast leukemia. https://core.ac.uk/download/212861571.pdf (accessed on 1st July 2025).

29. Dullah, A. U., Utami, P., & Unjung, J. (2025). Asthma classification using an adaptive boosting model with SVM-SMOTE sampling. *Journal of Information System Exploration and Research*. https://www.semanticscholar.org/paper/6c3a14091255392b9de0fb29ded59d82591f484e (accessed on 1st July 2025).

30. English, E., Garry, J. W., & Milosevich, E. T. (2014). *In vitro* determination of hemoglobin A1c for diabetes diagnosis and management: Technology update. https://core.ac.uk/download/41992337.pdf (accessed on 1st July 2025).

31. Gómez, J., Parra, U. C., Salas Álvarez, D., Hernández, R. V., & Ramirez-Gonzalez, G. (2025). Anemia classification system using machine learning. *Informatics*. https://www.semanticscholar.org/paper/135f4f046e648306d69794def187091bcde76482 (accessed on 1st July 2025).

32. Groer, M., & Phillips, K. D. (2002). Differentiation and treatment of anemia in HIV disease. https://core.ac.uk/download/268728550.pdf (accessed on 1st July 2025).

33. Guzmán Llanos, M. J., Guzmán Zamudio, J. L., & Llanos de los Reyes-García, M. J. (2016). Significado de la anemia en las diferentes etapas de la vida. https://core.ac.uk/download/352679546.pdf (accessed on 1st July 2025).

34. Kaddas, A. H., Nurkholis, M. I., Ridha, N. R., Syahrurrahman, et al. (2024). Hemolytic anemia due to glucose-6-phosphate dehydrogenase deficiency in neonate. https://core.ac.uk/download/618069877.pdf (accessed on 1st July 2025).

35. Kisiel-Cybula, E., Sionek-Wręga, I., Jakubowska, E., Ślemp, J., Pakuła, A., Kuźma, K., Bierć, K., et al. (2024). Trigeminal neuralgia – Impact on daily activities and sports, treatment options that enable a pain-free life. *Journal of Education, Health and Sport*. https://www.semanticscholar.org/paper/e6ed9147e5b1faa95f90a1b8e76c791118c5ab6d (accessed on 1st July 2025).

36. Kjeldsen, A. D., Evans, A. M., Friedman, A. N., Phillips, B. E., Silva, B. M., O'Driscoll, B. R., Mason, C. G., et al. (2014). Arterial oxygen content is precisely maintained by graded erythrocytosis responses in settings of high/normal serum iron levels, and predicts exercise capacity: An observational study of hypoxaemic patients with pulmonary arteriovenous malformations.

37. Kucera, A., Smith, B., & Tsu, L. V. (2014). Anemia and the role of the pharmacist. https://core.ac.uk/download/215741022.pdf (accessed on 1st July 2025).

38. Lahkar, K. (2013). A prospective single center study of the frequency and patterns of anemia in non-Hodgkin lymphoma, with special reference to its impact on response to treatment and chemotherapy-related toxicity. https://core.ac.uk/download/287236448.pdf (accessed on 1st July 2025).

39. Lenarcik, M., Pachlewski, J., & Mróz, A. (2021). Bean's syndrome (blue rubber bleb nevus

syndrome–BRBNS) as a gastrointestinal bleeding–Case report and review of the literature. *Polish Journal of Pathology, 72*(2), 190–194. https://www.semanticscholar.org/paper/b58e06eee962461be3a3a5e81f9027beedafddb0 (accessed on 1st July 2025).

40. Saputra, D. C. E., Muryadi, E. I., Futri, I., Win, T. A., Sunat, K., & Ratnaningsih, T. (2024). Revolutionizing anemia classification with multilayer extremely randomized tree learning machine for unprecedented accuracy. *International Journal of Robotics and Control Systems.* https://www.semanticscholar.org/paper/5cf56a3439de4001401329002fd78d8fea99df2b (accessed on 1st July 2025).
41. Schneider, K. M. (2023). What's at stake: Is it a vampire or a virus? https://core.ac.uk/download/588591391.pdf (accessed on 1st July 2025).
42. Seage, C. H., Bennett, A., Ward, N., Semedo, L., Plattel, C. H. M., Suijker, K. I. M., Vis, J. Y., et al. (2024). A systematic review of symptoms of pernicious anemia. *Food and Nutrition Bulletin, 45*(1_suppl), S34–S39. https://www.semanticscholar.org/paper/d6d0db7bd0d526372739732f713bf75ef582e521 (accessed on 1st July 2025).
43. Thyagaraju, B., & Doddagowda, S. M. (2024). A comparative study of peripheral smear findings with RBC indices and automated analyzer generated RBC histograms in the diagnosis of anemias. *Journal of Health and Allied Sciences NU.* https://www.semanticscholar.org/paper/826a877f41c3658eabe29a7d895fff919479a40d (accessed on 1st July 2025).
44. Tuli, A., & Yenilmez, E. D. (2017). Laboratory approach to anemia. https://core.ac.uk/download/322432622.pdf (accessed on 1st July 2025).
45. Vachhani, P., Repp, J., Hamer-Maansson, J., Braunstein, E. M., Bhatt, V., & Al-Ali, H. (2024). Clinical outcomes in patients with myelofibrosis treated with ruxolitinib and anemia-supporting medications. *Blood.* https://www.semanticscholar.org/paper/d65af03981708ccc8d8468726166b7429e8766bc (accessed on 1st July 2025).
46. Varekha, N. V., Stuklov, N., Gordienko, K. V., Gimadiev, R., Shchegolev, O. B., Kislaya, S. N., Gubina, E. V., et al. (2025). Development of a method for differential diagnosis of iron deficiency anemia and anemia of chronic disease based on demographic data and routine laboratory tests using machine learning technologies. *Onomatology.* https://www.semanticscholar.org/paper/930c05038b73760229db40ada827a2c95efa0f34 (accessed on 1st July 2025).
47. Zimmermann, M. B. (2008). Methods to assess iron and iodine status. https://core.ac.uk/download/pdf/29257923.pdf (accessed on 1st July 2025).

WHITE BLOOD CELL DISORDERS

6

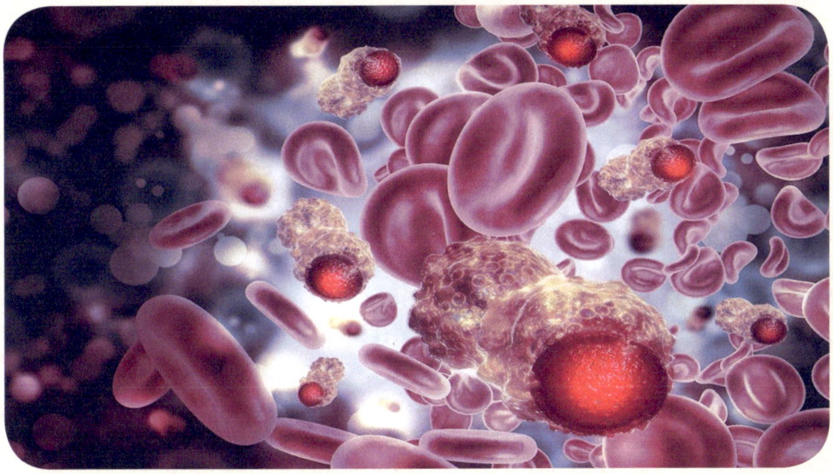

LEARNING OBJECTIVES

After studying this chapter, you will be able to:

1. Explain the types of white blood cells;
2. Discuss about common white blood cell disorders;
3. List the causes of white blood cell disorders;
4. Explore the symptoms and diagnosis white blood cell disorders;
5. Describe the treatment options for white blood cell disorders;
6. Illustration of prognosis and living with white blood cell disorders.

Introduction

White blood cell disorders strike us in a variety of unexpected ways. They appear in the guise of leukemia, lymphoma, and other cytopenias, and when these cells, so necessary for fighting infection, do not act as they should, our bodies can really be in trouble. Sometimes genetic idiosyncrasies, autoimmune reactions or even environmental influences cause this aberration, making both diagnosis and therapy a genuine headache. In most cases, not just the overt symptoms are significant but also the underlying, complex issues underneath that we have to dig through. Being on top of these problems ahead of time and having an interdisciplinary, multi-team approach is the key, which is why staying current on the latest research and best practices is a hard requirement for healthcare providers. Take autoimmune hemolytic anemias, for example, especially warm autoimmune hemolytic anemia (wAIHA). This illness, while rare, can be quite severe—autoantibodies end up killing red blood cells, causing acute anemia, dragging fatigue along, and even leaving the way open to blood clots, as some recent studies have shown. Fatigue is a huge factor in this case, then, so drawing upon measures such as the Functional Assessment of Chronic Illness Therapy-Fatigue (FACIT-Fatigue) scale becomes extremely important. While this scale works for the majority of people, its use in wAIHA remains something that needs further digging into, suggesting that maybe we need more targeted measures in order to truly gain insight into outcomes for patients (Scippa et al., 2023).

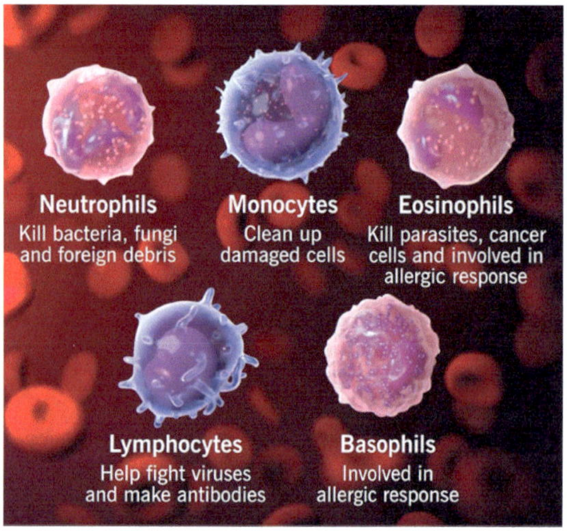

Figure 6.1. White blood cell disorders.

Source: https://my.clevelandclinic.org/-/scassets/images/org/health/articles/21871-white-blood-cells-function.

And then there is antiphospholipid syndrome (APS), which is a disease that is receiving considerable focus of late. This autoimmune disease—manifested by repeated clots and pregnancy complications due to antiphospholipid antibodies—demonstrates how white blood cell failure can impact our integrity of vessels and our overall well-being. Even find cases with neurological disturbances, like mini-strokes or memory faults, which only makes it more confusing by relating immune dysfunction to systemic disturbances. The APS criteria direct us towards utilizing precise laboratory tests and careful risk assessment, along with personalized anticoagulation treatments for each patient (Wong et al., 2021). All these advanced interactions remind us, quite precisely, that continued research is the key to improving care as well as clinical outcomes (Figure 6.1).

Definition of White Blood Cells

White blood cells (WBCs) are right at the center of our immune systems, working round the clock against infections and foreign invaders. They're primarily made in the bone marrow and some lymphatic tissues, and frankly, they exist in a variety of flavors—lymphocytes, monocytes, neutrophils, eosinophils, and basophils—each serving some different purpose. Lymphocytes typically are responsible for sensing and fighting pathogens, and neutrophils fill the role of ground troops when inflammation hits hard. No wonder then that if these cell types run amok in numbers or function, a chain reaction of trouble can follow, underlining just how crucial they are to maintaining us in health and in charge of disease. Abnormal cell morphologies or WBC counts typically reflect earliest-warning signals of other blood disorders. Peripheral blood smears, morphologically examining cells visually, are usually employed by experts to achieve an integrated overall picture even with the availability of automated hematology analyzers. The complexity of such cells means an experiential examination is sometimes necessary, especially in cancer patients where disease or treatment might change the shape of cells (Liu et al., 2024). New techniques in the majority of cases like machine learning and deep learning are transforming the field with models like Capsule Network (CapsNet) being able to outperform conventional methods for accuracy. These new tools not only accelerate cell classification but also suggest broader applications in clinical laboratories, marking a significant improvement in diagnostic hematology. For clinicians treating white blood cell disease, it is essential to have a complete knowledge of what sustains these cells. Leukopenia or leukocytosis, which reflect dramatic cell count changes, can profoundly impact the body's ability to fight off infection. Otherwise, the presence of other abnormal lymphocytes or even myeloblasts is a clear message of likely malignancies such as leukemia or lymphoma. Really, both the shape and the behavior of these cells need to be known. Scientists, for instance, are currently using self-supervised models that learn from the forms of cells to improve classification performance without needing infinite manual confirmation (Gaikwad et al., 2025). With research ongoing and technology advancing, these tactics could be very important not only in the early detection of WBC complications but in generating treatment regimens that are truly meaningful to the patient.

Importance of White Blood Cells in the Immune System

White blood cells have a monumental role in protecting our body--even though the immune system is full of different players, these cells (also known as leukocytes) take center stage. They fend off unwelcome visitors like bacteria, viruses, and fungi. Not only do these cells sense and eliminate intruders, but they also help set the defense strategy in motion as a whole. For example, T cells and B cells—both white blood cells—lie at the heart of a form of "memory" reaction in that when the infection returns, the reaction is both more rapid and more specific. For the most part, activity and activity is what maintains order and keeps disease at bay. It's not just about fighting germs, however; white blood cells are also busy with inflammation and tissue repair. They do occasionally muck it up, though—over- or under-responding—and the lack of symmetry can be problematic. In dire cases, such as sepsis, too much white blood cell activity can even start to kill the body, illustrating how finely tuned their performance is. In most cases, even illnesses like depression seem to share this coexistent relationship with inflammation, with abnormal cell counts indicating underlying biological alterations (Sealock et al., 2021). Examining further into disorders of these defense cells, their importance becomes even clearer. When regulations of normal white blood cell formation or function are not followed, such diseases as leukemia, immunodeficiency, or even autoimmune disease are likely. It's fascinating—at the beginning of sepsis, there may be a sudden spike in these cells, only to have their levels decrease later, which can in turn exacerbate organ issues (Wang et al., 2021). Both protector and potential source of mischief—this dual function truly speaks to how complex their role is. Understanding these irregularities not only helps us understand individual diseases better but also guides concepts for therapies that could help even out the immune system (Figure 6.2).

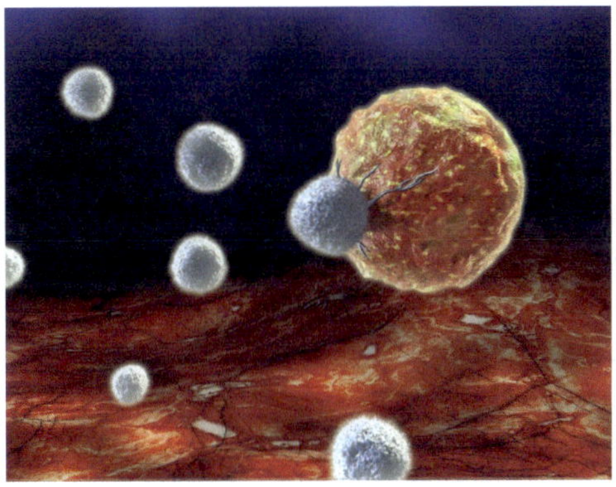

Figure 6.2. Importance of white blood cells in the immune system.

Source: https://cdn.mos.cms.futurecdn.net/jo5gNvX8LVUbdJeeVVC4tU-1200-80.jpg.

Overview of White Blood Cell Disorders

White blood cells are at the forefront of our protection. They have so many things to do, actually, that a problem with their number or ability can cause all sorts of issues. For example, if their number goes down—leukopenia, we refer to it—typically leaves the body open to infection, and if their number goes up—leukocytosis—typically indicates some kind of inflammation. It's clear that having knowledge of such differences is vital for the diagnosis of a condition as well as determining the ideal treatment approach. The way we distinguish these diseases seems complex, but it does matter in the treatment of blood diseases. Just in the past few years, there have been new tricks like state-of-the-art imaging and even machine learning stepping into the mix to help doctors get a better idea of what is going on, which ultimately leads to better patient care and outcomes. Diagnostic tools have had a serious overhaul recently, overall transforming our approach to white blood cell issues. Deep learning has turned the tables on traditional methods that simply could not compete with the subtleties between various cells. Capsule Network studies—normally called CapsNet—have proven to be able to greatly increase accuracy, sometimes even exceeding the more standard Convolutional Neural Networks when defining spatial data in blood smear images. This increased precision paves the way for faster diagnoses and eventually sooner and more successful treatments. The latest computer simulations are now giving clinicians a method of attaining a new degree of diagnostic precision, which in many cases is equivalent to better outcomes and a better understanding of blood diseases (Gaikwad et al., 2025). White blood cell disorders manifest themselves in all possible guises, ranging from relatively innocuous conditions to potentially life-saving cancers like leukemia and lymphoma. In a majority of instances, advanced analysis methods—think Computer-Aided Diagnosis of Hematologic Disorders Detection Based on Spatial Feature Learning Networks with Hybrid Model (CADHDD-SFLNHM), for example—are transforming the manner in which we detect and classify them. This strategy, which pre-processes the images of blood cells before leaving them to the work of convolutional neural networks, has achieved some very high accuracy levels in distinguishing one from the other disorder. Such technical innovations prove why the application of artificial intelligence and machine learning into the everyday practice of medicine is so important. It not only amends the past rules but also establishes new possibilities in healthcare, robustifying and making diagnostic skills stronger and more reliable (Jamal et al., 2025).

6.1. Types of White Blood Cells

Learning Outcome

- Neutrophils and their role in fighting infections;
- Lymphocytes and their function in adaptive immunity;
- Monocytes and their contribution to inflammation.

Our immune system is built up by a mixture of white blood cells that play different roles in keeping us healthy and removing intruders. Lymphocytes, for example, are of two main kinds—T cells and B cells. T cells are the ones which directly attack infected or even cancerous cells, and B cells help by creating antibodies that aid in detoxifying toxins and unwanted pathogens. The thing that each of these cells has a specialty is actually what our immune responses can be so complicated, that both types team up in some sort of spontaneous, yet efficient, agreement. In most cases, understanding the ways these cells work together is the basic not only to understanding normal immune function, but also to understanding disorders that occur when things do go awry. Switching gears slightly, of all the granulocytes, neutrophils are really the stars. They're by far the most common white blood cells and are a first line of defense against infection—especially against bacterial and fungal infections. They can race to an infection site and perform phagocytosis;

that is, they essentially engulf and digest invading microbes in a process that's both miraculous and absolutely necessary. Though eosinophils and basophils are less common, they're just as important. Eosinophils most often deal with parasitic infections and help manage allergic responses, while basophils trigger inflammation by spewing forth histamine and other chemicals. And finally, there are the monocytes, large and important white blood cell players that gear up when they hit the tissues—they're likely to become macrophages or dendritic cells. Macrophages are more like a ramshackle cleanup squad, devouring not just pathogens but also dead or dying cells, while dendritic cells have the role of presenting antigens, really filling the gap between our innate and adaptive immunity. To see monocytes transform into these specialist cells is really revealing just how adaptable our immune defenses are. And if monocytes fail to function properly or are thrown out of balance, then all sorts of disorders can arise—something particularly relevant when addressing health management for diverse groups, such as children who at times experience special blood-related issues (Chalmers et al., 2009) (Figure 6.3).

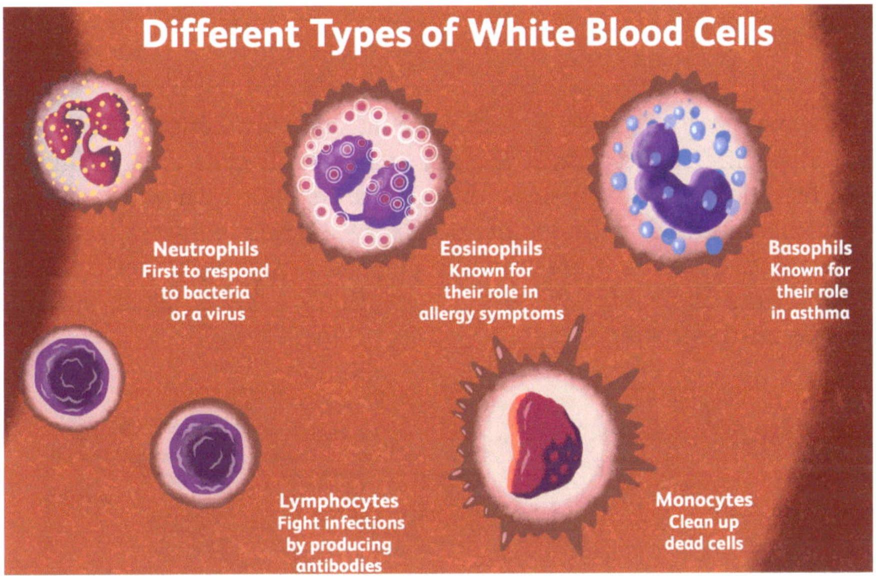

Figure 6.3. Types of white blood cells.

Source: https://www.verywellhealth.com/thmb/rBW3UTFMMboJ-fKGWxQfmPTkjcc=/1500x0/filters:no_upscale():max_bytes(150000):strip_icc()/understanding-white-blood-cells-and-counts-2249217_final-0587074073ce4709b41e42a08db0f596.gif.

6.1.1. Neutrophils and Their Role in Fighting Infections

Neutrophils are one of the stars when our body gets hit with an infection. They show up nearly at once, exiting circulation to flood into areas of trouble. The cells quickly engulf intruders—a process most of us call phagocytosis—although the whole process is far more sophisticated. They use everything from reactive oxygen species to a mixture of enzymes to incapacitate bacteria and fungi. Neutrophil toll-like receptors also seem to over-speed their assault on grievous infection (Chomel et al., 2024). Sometimes, though, this defense of speedy reaction can go into overdrive and create problems of its own. They don't just limit themselves to simply gorging microbes. Neutrophils also emit a range of signals—cytokines, chemokines, and so forth—that summon additional immune cells to the battle. In most cases, such signals not only strengthen the local immunity but also induce a more systemic, body-wide response. Oddly enough, such cells have been observed to release sticky traps, referred to as neutrophil extracellular traps (NETs), that capture wayward pathogens. But when NETs get dysregulated, nearby tissues become the target of collateral damage, a process well-documented in inflammatory diseases (Saini et al., 2023). Things begin to go awry when the balance is disturbed. Diseases that lower the counts of neutrophils or impair their function—like congenital neutropenia or certain dysfunction syndromes—can leave the body vulnerable to recurrent serious infections. Research has more recently also looked into how these cells, quite paradoxically, can also contribute to long-lasting inflammation and even cause autoimmune tissue damage. By examining the way neutrophils get activated and what they communicate via, scientists hope to find targets in order to fine-tune immune responses without leaving us open to infection (Chomel et al., 2024). With the science becoming deeper, neutrophils are still at the center of the controversy as to how to balance the speed of defense and overall health even if sometimes their actions aren't all rainbows and unicorns.

6.1.2. Lymphocytes and Their Function in Adaptive Immunity

Lymphocytes are the mainstay of our body's adaptive immune protection. These major white blood cells launch a quite specific counterattack against intruders. B cells and T cells–maturing in the bone marrow and thymus, respectively–lead this charge in their own ways. When pathogens are present, B cells become plasma cells that manufacture antibodies to neutralize invaders and T cells approach infected targets or assist other immune players. Antigen-presenting cells, by displaying pieces of these pathogens as proof, initiate the activation of this defense, making its specificity and strength close to on-the-fly-like.

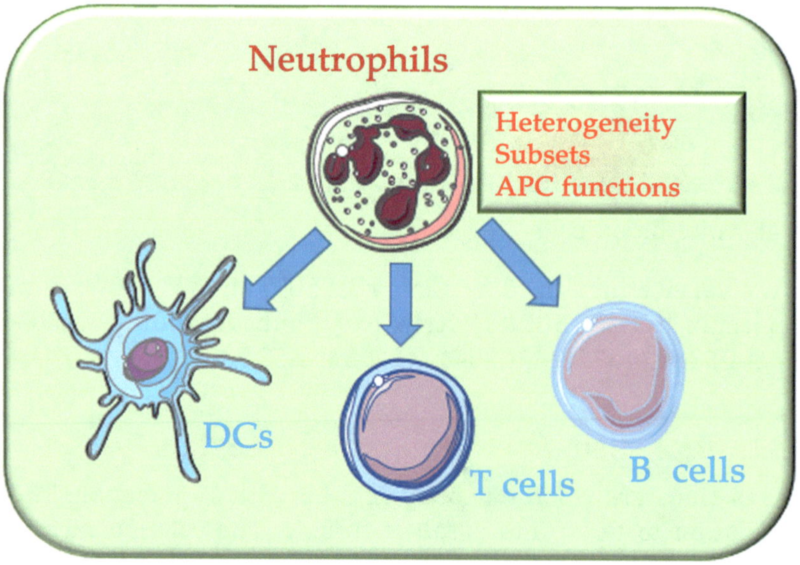

Figure 6.4. The regulatory roles of neutrophils in adaptive immunity.

Source: https://media.springernature.com/lw1200/springer-static/image/art%3A10.1186%2Fs12964-019-0471-y/MediaObjects/12964_2019_471_Figa_HTML.png.

With all these parts working together, the system not only keeps infection at bay but also produces immunological memory so that a repeat performance by the same bug elicits a faster, more intense response. Lymphocytes in fact double as security guards. They're not just busy keeping existing infections at bay but also patrol the body searching for abnormal cell growth, like cancer. Consider cytotoxic T cells, for example—they find and kill renegade cells either by direct contact or through the secretion of toxic granules. Helper T cells come next, which support the actions of B cells and other protectors through the release of cytokines that modify and enhance the total immune response. Together, all these varied functions illustrate just how indispensable lymphocytes are to our body's balance, and they are our keystone species of adaptive immunity. Because they can adapt to ever-changing threats as well as detect cancer growth early on, they are indispensable as a defense against infection and cancer. Of course, sometimes balance is lost. In other cases, excessive active lymphocytes can create autoimmune diseases where the immune system accidentally attacks and inflames healthy tissues. In contrast, when these cells are not properly active, that can result in immunodeficiency, which can make the body vulnerable to opportunistic infections. This back-and-forth is really highlighting the complexity of managing lymphocyte functions—and how terribly wrong things can become. They should be understood in order to develop new therapies, for instance, advanced biotherapies designed to restore normal immune function and reduce disease loads; it's a bridge between basic immunology and applied clinical therapy (Chong et al., 2013; Gallucci et al., 1995) (Figure 6.4).

6.1.3. Monocytes and Their Contribution to Inflammation

Monocytes play an enormous role in our immune defense by becoming structures like macrophages and dendritic cells after they move into tissue. They're huge, living cells that help detect and swallow up invaders, cell waste, and dying cells – an immune injection into the healing process. As soon as the inflammation starts, these cells swarm to infected or injured areas and start secreting an array of pro-inflammatory signals, including TNF-alpha and IL-1β. This wave of signals, in the majority of cases, further intensifies the inflammation by recruiting more white blood cells and enhancing local defenses. In particular, when monocytes are not performing as they should, the consequence is chronic inflammation, a testament to their dual nature and a confirmation of their importance in many white blood cell pathologies. Delving further, research has shed more light on the involvement of monocytes in inflammation by presenting variability in their count in different diseases. For example, research has identified that individuals with methamphetamine or spice cannabis use disorder have much higher levels of monocytes than healthy controls, indicating some form of system-wide inflammation and changed immune function (Sehlikoğlu et al., 2024). This elevation in monocyte numbers may be interpreted as a marker of an increased inflammatory state that may be driving disease advancement. And indeed, the markers associated with monocyte activity tend to correlate with physical health conditions as well as psychological struggle, highlighting the intricate interplay between inflammation, immunity, and general health. For the most part, these discoveries are fairly illuminating, particularly when it comes to how unbalanced monocyte function would be used as some sort of marker for immune disorders in general. Apart from simply causing inflammation, monocytes also seem to influence immune markers related to immediate behavioral status, such as suicidal behavior. Recent evidence (Voros et al., 2024) shows that certain markers, like the monocyte-lymphocyte ratio (MLR), show quite marked fluctuation in individuals with acute psychiatric illnesses, and this may imply that monocytes could influence physical as well as psychological health. Increased MLR has even been associated with enhanced suicide risk, essentially placing these cells on the list of potential markers for psychiatric assessments. This combination of immunology and psychology highlights that monocytes do more than the usual function in inflammation and proposes avenues by which our body's inflammatory reactions can influence mood and behavior. Together, these suggestions ignite interest in exploring the roles of monocytes in physical and mental health, and in particular, white blood cell abnormalities (Figure 6.5).

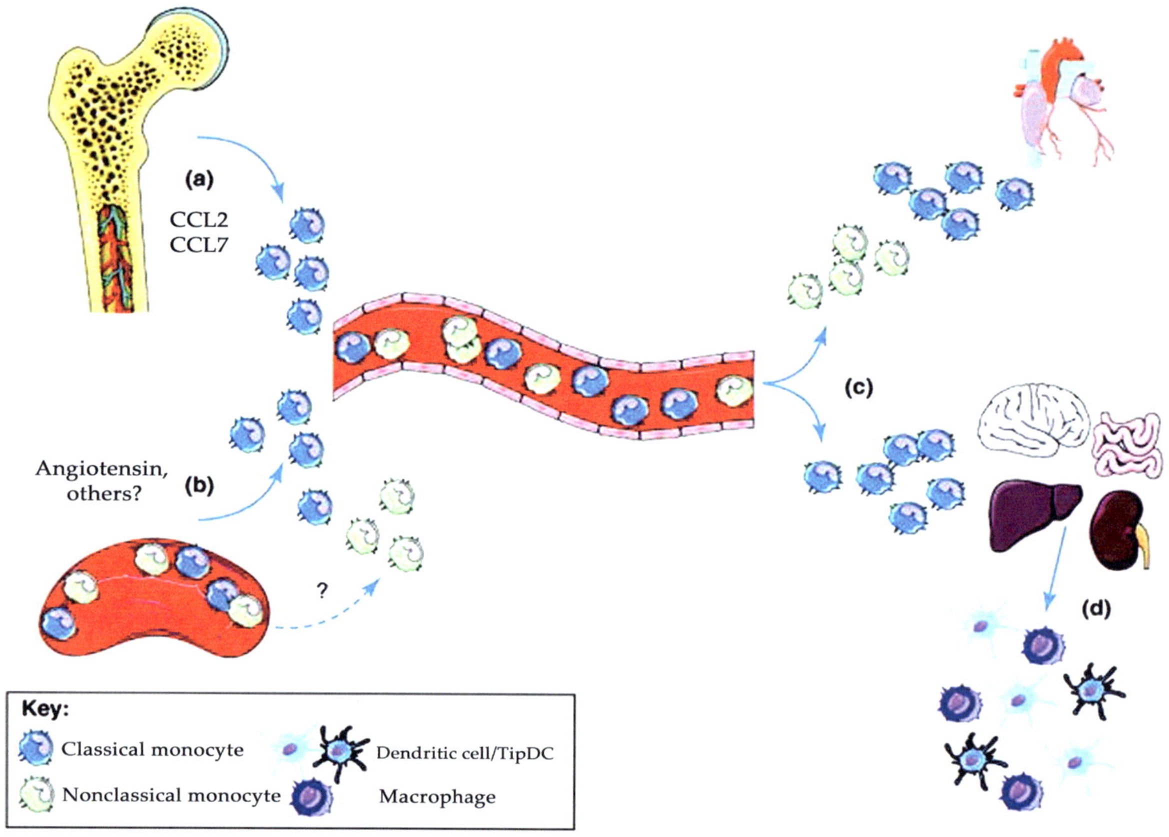

Figure 6.5. Monocyte trafficking in acute and chronic inflammation.

Source: https://ars.els-cdn.com/content/image/1-s2.0-S1471490611000780-gr1.jpg.

Test Your Knowledge

1. What are the five main types of white blood cells, and what are their primary functions?
2. How do granulocytes differ from agranulocytes in structure and role?

6.2. Common White Blood Cell Disorders

Learning Outcome

- Leukemia: types and characteristics;
- Lymphoma: distinction between Hodgkin and non-Hodgkin;
- Myelodysplastic syndromes: causes and symptoms.

White blood cell disorders are extremely diverse and can actually interfere with the way our blood works, usually hitting a person's overall health pretty hard. Leukemias, for example, are cancers where the body ends up making much too many immature or defective white blood cells—cells that just aren't doing their job well. This over-production interferes with the immune system and, quite frankly, leads to all kinds of systemic issues. In a majority of cases, you observe that acute lymphoblastic leukemia (ALL) occurs mostly in children, proving that sometimes the youngest are hit the worst; on the other hand, chronic lymphocytic leukemia (CLL) occurs in the old, proving that age does play a role in how these problems happen and how things turn out. It's not just the cells that turn cancerous—the spin-off effects also affect patients' lifestyles and mental lives, and their families as well. Another huge category to look at is myeloproliferative neoplasms (MPNs). The MPNs are overproduction conditions of one or more of the three primary blood cell types: red cells, white cells, or platelets, and they usually go undetected with overt symptoms at first. Disease conditions such as polycythemia vera, essential thrombocythemia, and myelofibrosis fall under the MPN umbrella, and they usually develop as a result of genetic mutations that interfere with normal hematopoietic stem cell function. All too frequently, these are only found by chance based on routine blood tests, but over time—and as these MPNs progress—patients can develop catastrophic issues like blood clots (thrombosis) or even transformation to acute leukemia. You could say that mutations in the JAK2 gene play a central part in all of this, and in most cases, getting these genetic factors under control is the key to personalized, beneficial treatments. And then there are the lymphoproliferative diseases like the lymphomas that are worth mentioning when white blood cell issues are at hand. Lymphomas start when lymphocytes turn malignant and begin to proliferate wildly, resulting in bungling overgrowths of the lymphatic system. We generally speak of two broad categories: Hodgkin lymphoma and non-Hodgkin lymphoma. Hodgkin lymphoma is defined by those characteristic Reed-Sternberg cells and frequently occurs with symptoms like swollen lymph nodes and noticeable "B" symptoms—like fever and weight loss—that cannot be ignored. On the other hand, non-Hodgkin lymphoma is a mixed bag wherein disease behavior and reactions to treatment can be very unpredictable. New developments in immunotherapy and targeted therapy—like clever use of monoclonal antibodies and even CAR T-cell therapies—have totally flipped the game around, promising much for many who have to fight these powerful diseases.

6.2.1. Leukemia: Types and Characteristics

Leukemia typically manifest as an abnormal expansion of white blood cells that are unresponsive - a condition that complicates both diagnosis and treatment of the condition. Rather than expanding in nice and neat groups, it branches off into two broad categories: acute and chronic. In the majority of cases, acute forms like Acute Lymphoblastic Leukemia (ALL) or Acute Myeloid Leukemia (AML) develop very fast, necessitating immediate, quick interventions. Meanwhile, chronic types - take CLL and CML as examples - progress more slowly along, sometimes giving doctors some latitude to adjust several treatment approaches in the process. For the most part, knowledge of the basics of what causes these diseases and how they manifest in patients is crucial in adjusting treatments and improving outcomes. Getting a timely and correct diagnosis really can make all the difference when it comes to tackling leukemia. Traditional methods – such as blood tests and bone marrow exams – are often resource-intensive and can take longer than we'd like. Lately, though, new approaches have started to appear; recent studies have tossed around ideas like automatic diagnostic prediction systems that lean on advanced image analysis. By combining the use of machine learning algorithms with digital image processing, researchers have now pushed the game to new heights when it comes to identifying and separating abnormal blood cells related to leukemia. Convolutional neural networks (CNNs), for example, have in certain cases reached as high as 99% in correctly identifying acute leukemia, demonstrating the kind of potential these digital technologies bring to speeding up the diagnosis process and making treatment protocols more exacting (Ilyas et al., 2024). Scientists also closely monitor how white blood cell activity is associated with inflammation. For instance, white blood cell count to mean platelet volume ratio, or WMR. It originally gained researchers' interest as a potential marker in metabolic disease research, but now many consider it to be a potential lead in leukemia as well. Some research has shown that increased WMR might be associated with worse prognosis, implying that inflammation may be more significantly implicated than hitherto thought in the etiology and pathogenesis of these conditions. As we continue to learn more about such associations, further research is apparently in the pipeline – we will soon perhaps be able to use such markers not only to forecast the behavior of the disease, but also to tailor individual treatment even more precisely in this very difficult field of blood disorders (Wang et al., 2024) (Figure 6.6).

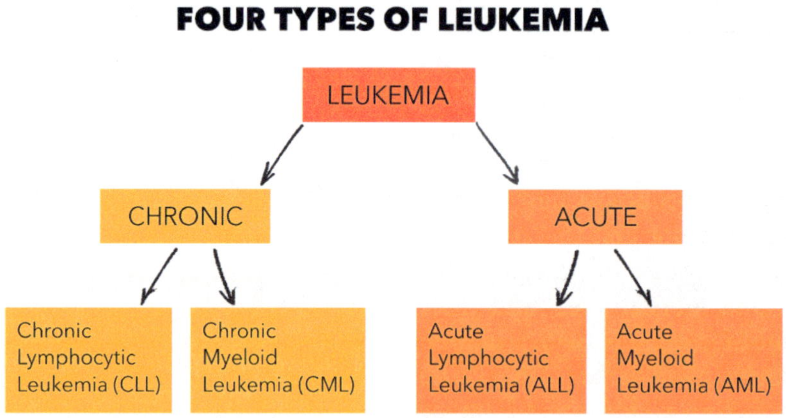

Figure 6.6. Leukemia.

Source: https://www.medstarhealth.org/-/media/project/mho/medstar/services/leukemia/leukemia_diagram_170330.png?h=918&iar=0&w=1622&hash=CDD2E3E08DBEECF85D2D87B8492905A7.

6.2.2. Lymphoma: Distinction Between Hodgkin and Non-Hodgkin

Lymphoma boasts some characteristic cell clues that separate Hodgkin lymphoma (HL) from non-Hodgkin lymphoma (NHL). Reed-Sternberg cells – those large, oddly shaped lymphocytes – are found almost exclusively in HL, while NHL is a toss-up, being mostly of B and T cell descent. Doctors don't just eyeball the cells; they also go on to probe immune markers and even genetic cues. HL tends to respond better to treatment, overall, than most of the types of NHL, so an individualized plan is typically warranted. The different cell behaviors necessitate a string of tests to determine the optimum treatment, so thorough diagnostics are needed. Because each type demands a special approach, specialists need to modify their plans to fit the specific patient. Population studies show that the epidemiology and prognosis of Hodgkin and non-Hodgkin lymphomas can be substantially different, even because of a mixture of such influences as genetic susceptibility and environmental idiosyncrasies.

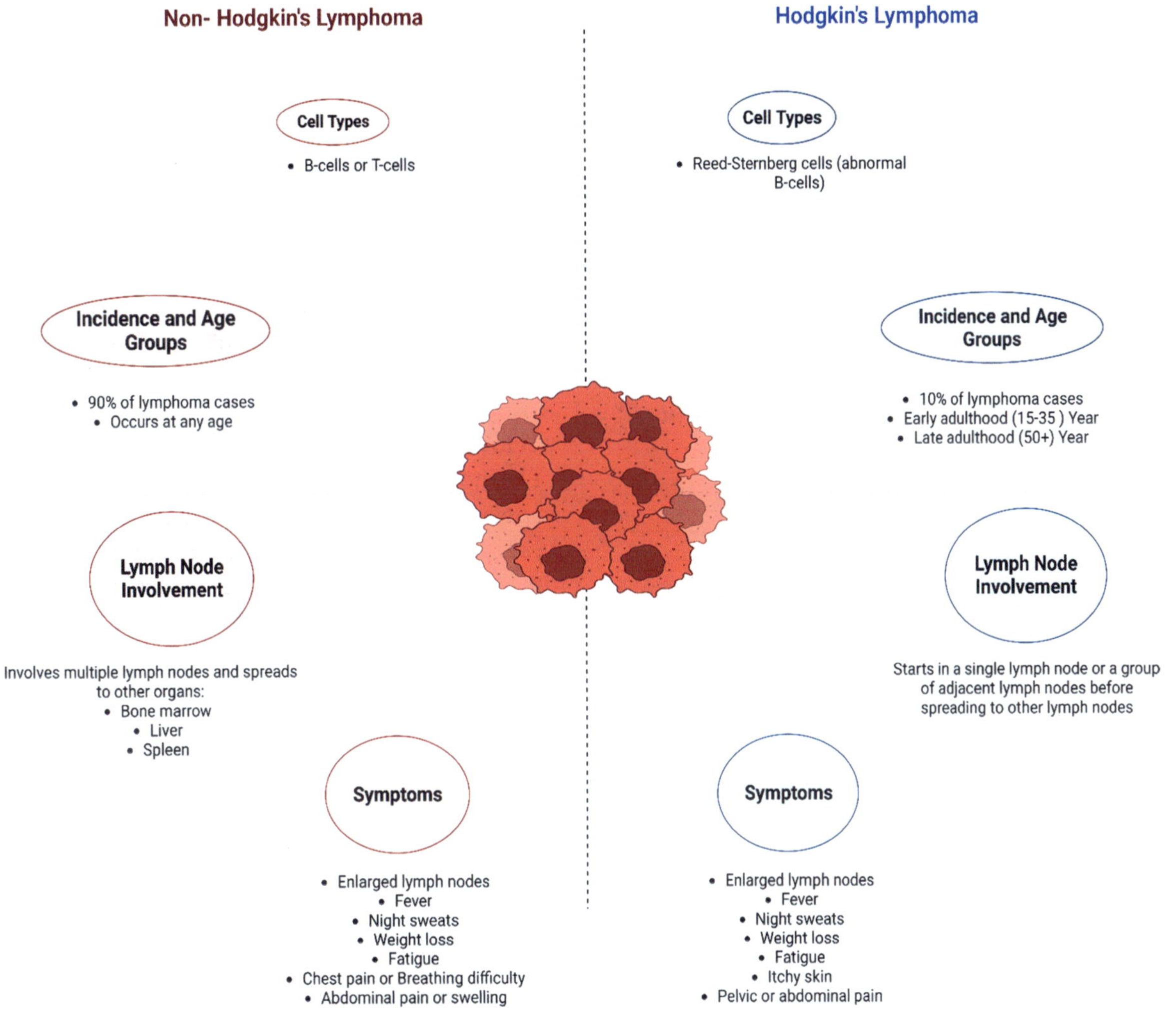

Figure 6.7. Distinction between Hodgkin and non-Hodgkin.

Source: https://www.researchgate.net/publication/379079590/figure/fig1/AS:11431281230343986@1710894752395/Key-differences-between-Hodgkins-lymphoma-and-non-Hodgkins-lymphoma.png.

It's interesting how ethnic background and heredity have been source of controversy around inherited susceptibility, prompting further investigation of lymphoma's etiology. The human leukocyte antigen (HLA) complex, for example, is involved in both diseases. Some HLA variants, in most cases, are linked strongly with Hodgkin lymphoma – making distinctions between Epstein-Barr virus–positive and -negative subtypes – while for NHL, a multifactorial assortment of low-risk genes can add up to rise susceptibility. In most cases, such subtle interactions make each diagnosis unique. These findings underscore the importance of further investigation into the interplay between environmental and hereditary factors in lymphoma, which could provide avenues for earlier diagnosis and more specific treatment approaches. Fluctuations in the immune system definitely play a role in the progression of both HL and NHL. Patients with conditions like common variable immunodeficiency (CVID) characteristically have more non-Hodgkin diagnoses, and it is implied, therefore, that there is some correlation between a weakened immune force and the onset of lymphoma. Statistics also exhibit a significant – sometimes several-fold – rise in NHL in these patients. Therefore, what in our immune responses might promote these cancers is quite important to establish. Granted, the precise interaction between our immune systems and cancer cells remains a mystery to keep scientists busy. Even though the unclean processes behind these events are objectionable, and even though they need more research, there are hints that immune-mediated pathways might alter the immediate surroundings of lymphatic cells and how they grow and live. This information not only tells us about lymphoma but also highlights immune checkpoints' central function in cancer evasion, as explained by Agostini et al. (2018) and Jarrett et al. (2015) (Figure 6.7).

6.2.3. Myelodysplastic Syndromes: Causes and Symptoms

Genetic mistakes paired with external factors seem to trigger myelodysplastic syndromes (MDS)—a combination of blood diseases where cells just plain don't turn out correctly. Stem cells that produce blood cells develop abnormalities that interrupt the process of regular cell production, so blood cells end up weirdly dysplastic. In nearly all studies, researchers have observed that somatic mutations—those that disrupt genes that are part of epigenetic control—seem to be at the center of it. Abnormalities in genes like TET2, ASXL1, and DNMT3A hint at an inborn susceptibility that can be worsened by external exposures, be it chemicals or even radiation. All of this paints a messy picture that really calls for more digging into these underlying issues if we're ever going to develop therapies aimed directly at these genetic glitches (Fan et al., 2021). Patients with MDS will often have a complete set of frightening symptoms that can actually become a burden to daily life. There are usually low cell counts in the blood, so anemia, low white cell count, and fewer platelets. Anemia is usually expressed as the inability to perform something and weakness due to a lack of hemoglobin, while low white cell counts make a person prone to infections. In addition, low platelets also typically result in further bruising and bleeding, making it even more complicated. Regular blood tests will typically pick up these abnormal counts and also abnormally shaped cells within the bone marrow, so a full hematologic workup is required. Most times, these problems end up significantly impacting quality of life, so ongoing monitoring and supportive therapy becomes the norm (Erik et al., 2019). The prognosis for an MDS patient can veer pretty far, depending on a combination of genetic idiosyncrasies and the way symptoms present. Risk assessment is crucial—after all, patients in the high-risk category tend to have a significant possibility of turning into acute myeloid leukemia (AML). Advances in molecular genetics in recent times have brought forth various biomarkers that, more often than not, sharpen our predictive powers and guide treatment decisions. New treatments, such as drugs that regulate methylation pathways and certain immunomodulators, promise to strike against aberrant cell behavior. And, lastly, individually designed treatment courses based on increased insight into the individual's specific genetic makeup are slowly gaining acceptance, with the promise of better outcomes. In general, the incorporation of such genetic data into regular clinical practice remains an important component of improving treatment in those combating MDS (Fan et al., 2021) (Figure 6.8).

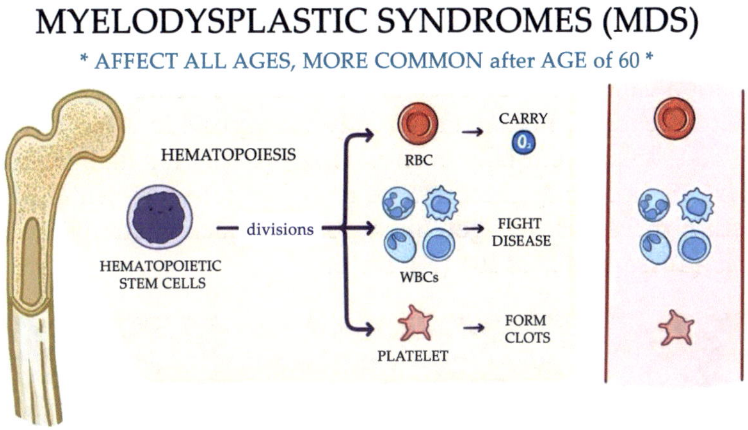

Figure 6.8. Myelodysplastic syndromes.

Source: https://d16qt3wv6xm098.cloudfront.net/eTHlOWMkS1G6Yur70nY-eZa1SSGXg7kL/_.jpg.

Test Your Knowledge

1. What are the key differences between leukocytosis, leukopenia, and leukemia?
2. How does lymphoma differ from leukemia in terms of origin and progression?

6.3. Causes of White Blood Cell Disorders

Learning Outcome

- Genetic factors and hereditary conditions;
- Environmental influences and exposure to toxins;
- Viral infections and their impact on white blood cell production.

Environmental and genetic factors interact with each other in ways that set the stage for white blood cell disorders. Genes that are born with mutations can drive a patient toward leukemias or lymphomas. For instance, kids who have Down syndrome or people who have Fanconi anemia typically seem to be at more risk for blood cancer—cancer where white blood cells start growing in abnormal patterns. It's not entirely in the genes, though; radiation or chemical poisons can, on occasion, trigger or worsen these genetic quirks. Oddly, most people who have a history of blood cancers in their families are, in most instances, much more at risk for these side effects, which reminds us that a combination of genetic and environmental factors is at work here (Tessa et al., 2020). Infection chimes in too. Think about chronic viral infections: Epstein-Barr virus (EBV) in particular has a tendency to interfere with the normal routine of cells, which can in turn lead to a range of lymphoproliferative syndromes, both non-Hodgkin and Hodgkin lymphomas.

The virus disrupts the functioning of the cell in such a way as to cause lymphocytes to overgrow. To make matters worse, long-term bacterial infections might send the immune system into overdrive, at times leading to such conditions as chronic lymphocytic leukemia (CLL). These chronic infections have the potential to slowly manipulate the immune environment, making way for the development of blood malignancies and highlighting why patients who are at risk must be given enough attention (Leonard et al., 2005). Autoimmune diseases are another aspect of this story. Autoimmune diseases such as systemic lupus erythematosus (SLE) or rheumatoid arthritis can cause the body's defense mechanism to fail and turn against its own healthy white blood cells. This disorganization can lead to cytopenias—basically, a deficiency of certain types of white blood cells. The resultant chronic inflammation may even provide a basis that allows pathologic clonal expansions to take hold, eventually even paving the way for malignancies. Clarifying these intricate, mutual interactions among autoimmune complications and white blood cell dysfunction is critical in formulating therapies that genuinely react to such challenges and allow patients to manage their diseases (Tessa et al., 2020) (Figure 6.9).

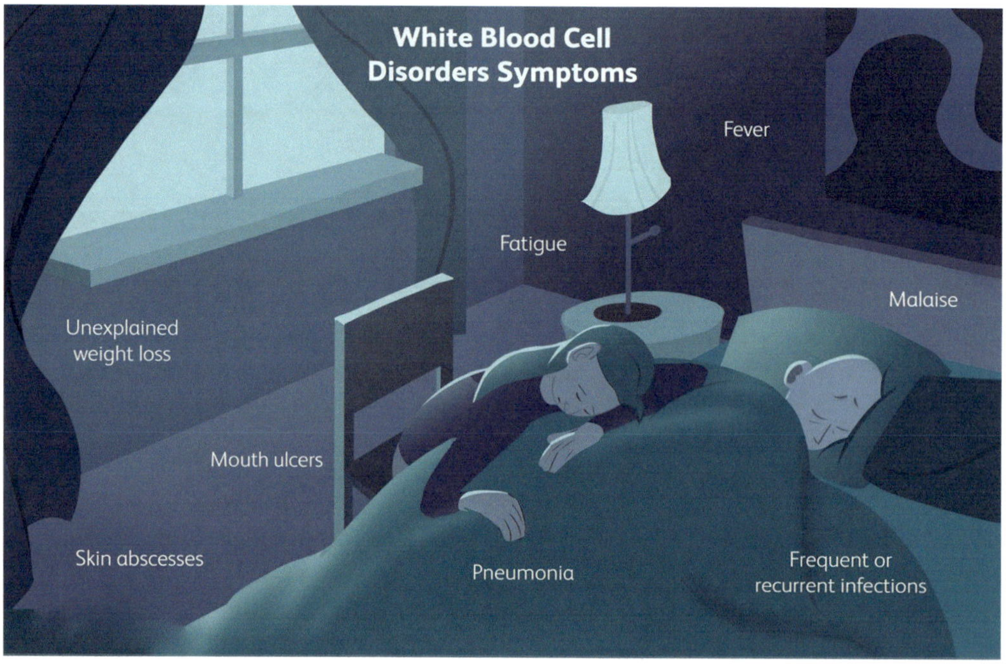

Figure 6.9. Causes of white blood cell disorders.

Source: https://www.verywellhealth.com/thmb/pZ3lGnCeLqWhPlArQdMkuhPxwFU=/1500x0/filters:no_upscale():max_bytes(150000):strip_icc()/white-blood-cell-disorders-overview-4013280_final-ab4ee51345a3425f9b0a2488d2d6af4d.jpg.

6.3.1. Genetic Factors and Hereditary Conditions

Genetic defects may occasionally throw a monkey wrench into the normal functioning of white blood cells. Gene mutations—like those seen in leukemias or lymphomas—may interfere with the normal messages received by cells telling them to proliferate or divide, and in some instances lead to over-multiplication. In fact, such alterations in cellular communication generally have a way of feeding malignant processes in the end. Family history, which in the majority of cases implies concealed blood issues, represents a red flag, directing us to genetic counseling and familial screening as easy tools for prevention at an early stage (Baniamer et al., 2024). In the end, it's a sophisticated dance between our genes and the action of our cells that truly matters. Hereditary blood diseases can offer another interesting twist when considering the ways genetics affect our results of health. Diseases such as inherited thrombotic disease, for example, bring to mind that when genes related to clotting factors get out of whack, the normal hemostatic processes of the body are interrupted. Take hemophilia A and B, for example—these are due to a lack of particular clotting factors and may make things so complicated that white blood cell issues become even harder to handle (Baniamer et al., 2024). Discerning these variations in the genes typically leads to treatments tailored to the individual, usually resulting in more effective and less hazardous care. From this view, investigating the genetic basis for these diseases not only sharpens diagnostic accuracy but also has an impact on tailored care that can significantly make a patient's prognosis better. Sometimes the tale becomes cloudy when we add environmental influences into our genetic blueprint. New science overall shows that people with certain genetic traits may have virtually all different symptoms when the usual environmental cues come into play. Even experiments have hinted that when genetic traits—such as those associated with some red blood cell diseases—are combined, they can subtly alter the expression of a disease, making it a moving target to diagnose and treat. This is why it all seems so important to incorporate both genetic screening and environmental factors into an overall plan. By closely observing the way our genes nudge the behavior of these disorders, healthcare professionals can create more proactive and informed plans—ultimately striving to help those suffering from white blood cell problems and their accompanying hereditary conditions (Figure 6.10).

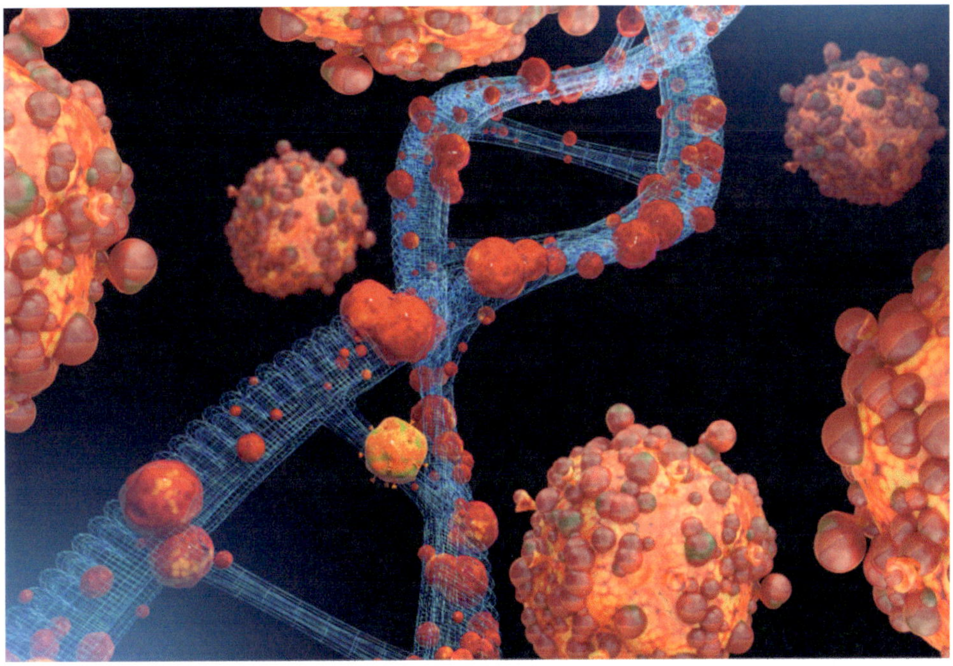

Figure 6.10. Genetic factors and hereditary conditions.

Source: https://www.veritasint.com/blog/wp-content/uploads/2022/11/hereditary-disease.jpg.

6.3.2. Environmental Influences and Exposure to Toxins

Environmental pollutants at critical development stages pose a severe threat to health—especially concerning how our immune system and white blood cells work. Take this: ordinary foods have the potential to be infested with aflatoxins, which in turn may induce harmful effects. Some research indicates that when a pregnant mother becomes exposed, her white blood cells in the baby result in changes in DNA methylation—sort of a gentle, long-term signature on genes that regulate immune function. It's like our environment and genetic design are in a tangled dance that affects long-term health. This confusion truly necessitates us taking greater heed and attempting to stem toxin exposure. If you think about how these toxins act, they have a tendency to induce a kind of chronic, low-grade inflammation—a small spark that can potentially lead to an immune response chain reaction. For example, inflammation might start laying the groundwork for disorders that disrupt white blood cell function. And here's a kicker: white fat, so often pushed to the periphery in these discussions, has a role too by releasing inflammatory cytokines. That long-term inflammation, caused by environmental toxins, somehow raises the risk for autoimmune diseases, in which the body is disoriented and attacks itself. Charting these intricate pathways might eventually yield novel treatments that tackle inflammation and immune disorders simultaneously. And then there's everything else on top of this, day-to-day lifestyle choices—what we load up on with every meal, particularly high-fat foods. These diets have the potential to add to the adverse effect of toxins such as aflatoxin, pushing people toward obesity and metabolic syndrome, diseases with a direct link to immune function changes. Obesity, for instance, is often linked with lower insulin sensitivity, which in its turn seems to feed into the inflammatory process and immune regulation issues. With obesity increasing worldwide, it's absolutely imperative to understand how these environmental factors play off each other with disorders of the white blood cells. As a whole, understanding more about these dynamics has the ability to guide public health strategies that promote healthy immune systems from the very beginning of childhood right through adulthood.

6.3.3. Viral Infections and Their Impact on White Blood Cell Production

Viruses will have a sneaky way of interfering with the production of white blood cells. They use every kind of sneaky trick to avoid our defenses, often attacking the very cells that have a tendency to proliferate in order to protect us—like hematopoietic stem cells and lymphocytes. This disruption generally decreases the number of these critical defenders, making the body more vulnerable and pushing it in the direction of immunosuppression. Take, for example, feline leukemia virus (FeLV): aside from causing lymphocyte cancers, it disrupts bone marrow function, which predisposes to secondary infection. In general, this viral trickery disassembles our natural immunity and sets off a ripple effect on health in general, which in fact merits further research into how viruses disrupt blood cell development (Ackley et al., 2012). In humans, the picture can be even more desperate. HIV, for instance, targets specifically CD4+ T lymphocytes—those forceful leaders of our immune system—and slowly this barrage draws their numbers down to dangerous levels. Losing these cells not only puts our ability to fight infection in jeopardy; it also interrupts the production of other white blood cells, creating further imbalance. When the immune function derails, people become more susceptible to every kind of opportunistic infection and leukemia. Recent studies further indicate, in most cases, a possible relationship between viral infection-induced neuroinflammatory effects and white blood cell dysfunction, which actually makes it much more complex to manage patient care

(Brew et al., 2017). When viruses disrupt white blood cell production, the impact doesn't stop at cells; it destabilizes treatment regimens and patient outcomes in general. To treat these disorders, one has to address both the original damage caused by the virus and the secondary immunosuppression that follows. Therapies like HIV antiretroviral therapy are designed to activate immune response and encourage regrowth of white blood cells, but the virus's insidious capability to escape detection remains an ongoing challenge. In general, knowledge of the many ways viruses disrupt blood cell dynamics is crucial in the creation of therapies that can keep up with constantly shifting virus strategies and the development of new pathogenic diseases (Ackley et al., 2012; Brew et al., 2017) (Figure 6.11).

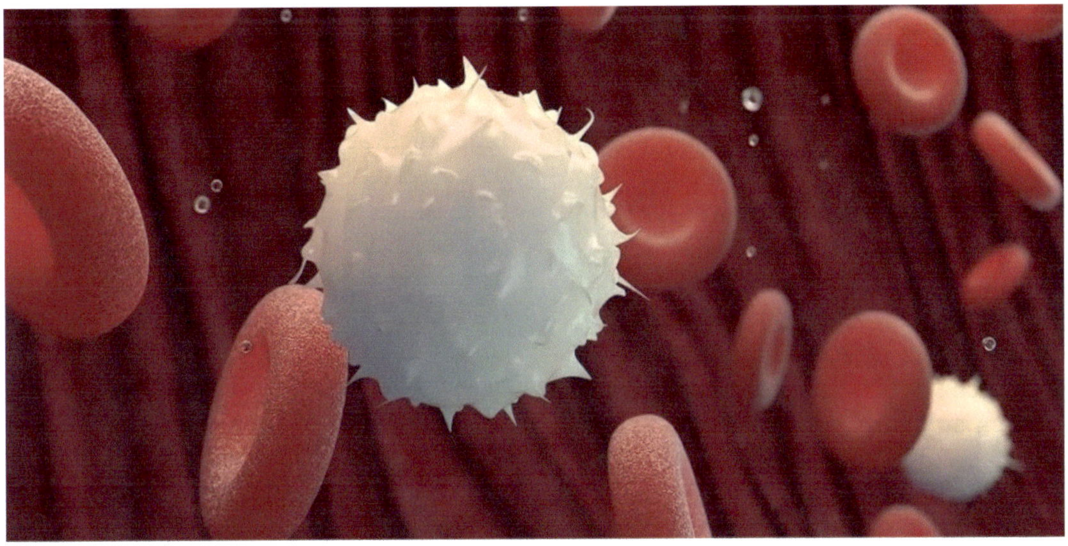

Figure 6.11. Viral infections and their impact on white blood cell production.

Source: https://maxlab.co.in/categoryimage/1667373426.jpg.

Test Your Knowledge

1. How can infections lead to abnormal WBC counts?
2. What role do genetic mutations play in the development of leukemia and other WBC cancers?

6.4. Symptoms and Diagnosis

Learning Outcome

- Common symptoms associated with white blood cell disorders;
- Diagnostic tests: blood tests and bone marrow biopsy;
- Importance of early detection and monitoring.

White blood cell diseases have the propensity to present along with a combination of symptoms that have the capability to utterly perplex the whole process of diagnosis. For instance, in leukemia, you can have an unexpected rise in abnormal white blood cells that disrupts normal blood cell formation. Patients tend to complain of persistent tiredness, becoming ill more frequently than usual, or having bruises and bleeding for which they cannot explain. The reason that such symptoms are so elusive is that they are often so benign in character, so there is a real danger of misdiagnosis or even delay before the real issue is found, which usually requires a blanket examination of the system. With the help of tools like direct imaging and laboratory testing is key to isolating the different types of these disorders, and early identification of such warning signs is crucial—especially in aggressive ones like leukemia, where every moment counts (Ilyas et al., 2024). Diagnosis of such conditions involves a combination of approaches. You begin with a judicious clinical assessment, include several laboratory tests, and tend to toss in some imaging tests as well. For instance, simple blood work up that addresses the leukocyte counts and differentials will suffice to begin with, and then a bone marrow biopsy can follow to further assess the nature and extent of the issue. Generally, when one encounters leukemia, dividing it into subtypes like Acute Lymphoblastic Leukemia (ALL) or Acute Myeloid Leukemia (AML) not only directs how the treatment should be attempted but also provides some indication of what may or may not be in store for the future. Experimental diagnostic methods utilizing machine learning and image processing have been researched recently in order to hasten the process and improve accuracy, taking the workload off that comes as standard from regular, time-absorbing tests (Devi et al., 2024). There is a need to obtain the diagnosis right when it comes to disorders within white blood cells. More advanced methods—like computer-based systems with digital image processing—have started to show effectiveness. Thanks to the application of convolutional neural networks, researchers have been able to achieve very high accuracy, so diseases like leukemia can be detected much earlier in a few cases. These technological innovations not only address the loopholes present in traditional methods but also pave the way for speedier and improved treatment techniques. With advancements continuing to arrive on the scene, incorporation of new technology into standard diagnostic practice will continue to redefine how such disorders are diagnosed, eventually leading to enhanced overall care for the affected (Ilyas et al., 2024).

6.4.1. Common Symptoms Associated with White Blood Cell Disorders

White blood cells really do have an important role to play in our immune system, and when they're out of whack or their numbers or function are off, there is trouble. Fatigue typically presents first—it's not a tired feeling but a sign that the body's ability to fight off infection has been compromised due to abnormal WBC counts. People can be found to be suddenly exhausted and more prone to falling ill, especially in cases like leukemia or lymphoma when the creation of such cells goes awry. Coupled with that, unintentional weight loss is likely to tag along as well, along with both the physical and emotional problems people have to deal with. Recurrent infections, almost like unwanted guests, also tend to appear when these cells do not function properly. Since white blood cells are meant to seek out and kill intruders, anything going wrong on their part can lead to repeated or even complete cycles of illness—and with regimens that simply fail to work. Neutropenia, a reduction in the count of neutrophils, often plays a huge role in such issues. Kanaya et al. (2024) also mentions that patients that have chronic episodes of low neutrophils will be at higher risk for complications if they are subjected to more aggressive therapies and that early recognition of these signs is crucial in the treatment of the disorder. Unexpected bruising or bleeding also can happen, implying that the body's clotting support is off balance—usually because of low platelet counts compromising effective bone marrow function, such as with aplastic anemia or acute myeloid leukemia. These symptoms often are disconcerting, sometimes causing a great deal of anxiety and offering one additional level of difficulty for patient management. And then splenomegaly; if the spleen is enlarged—usually with conditions such as lymphomas—it can cause pain or a chronic feeling of fullness in the stomach that progressively erodes on overall quality of life. Bodnar et al. (2024) supports the argument that it is absolutely critical to truly understand these signs because addressing these related challenges is critical to providing holistic and thoughtful patient care (Figure 6.12).

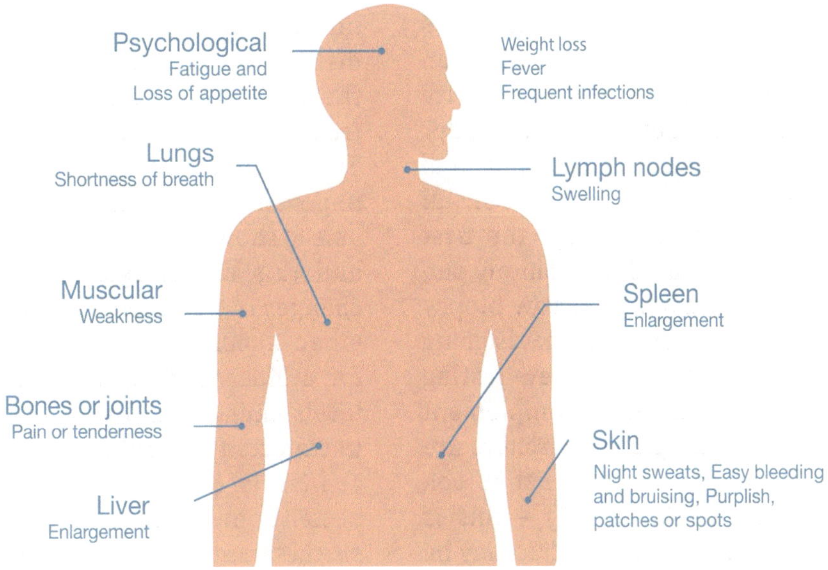

Figure 6.12. Common symptoms associated with white blood cell disorders.

Source: https://images.everydayhealth.com/images/cancer/leukemia/what-are-common-symptoms-of-leukemia-1440x810.jpg.

6.4.2. Diagnostic Tests: Blood Tests and Bone Marrow Biopsy

White blood cell disorders are sly, but usually the first sign emerges in a routine blood test. Doctors usually start there because these tests give us an immediate sense of how our immune system is doing – in essence, they track things like the total number of total white blood cells and how those cells are apportioned among the different types. In the majority of cases, the CBC is adequate to raise an eyebrow about something like leukemia, lymphoma, or even multiple myeloma. In some cases, when other proteins or markers turn up on serological tests, it indicates something such as MGUS (Monoclonal Gammopathy of Undetermined Significance), which is usually monitored closely to avoid any fall into something bad like multiple myeloma (Huang et al., 2024). So, in a general sense, blood work is pulling double duty with the goal of establishing an initial diagnosis and tracking the disease's progression in time. There are moments when a blood test simply doesn't paint the whole picture, and that's when a bone marrow biopsy usually comes into play. This method – admittedly somewhat invasive – involves the removal of a minute amount of bone marrow, most commonly from the hip bone, and then further analysis of the hematopoietic (blood-forming) cells. The test allows experts to examine such things as cell form, cell division rate, and the presence of any unremarkable or abnormal cells. This kind of information is important in confirming suspicion for diseases like leukemia, various lymphomas, or even myelodysplastic syndromes. In the majority of cases, the ability to detect the disorder stage (sometimes demonstrating chromosomal abnormalities in diseases like essential thrombocythemia) helps in deciding the best course of treatment (Oh et al., 2024). Simply put, putting the blood test and bone marrow biopsy together provides a clearer view of what is going on. Medicine is ever-evolving, and new testing methods are being developed to complement these older tests. For example, researchers are investigating liquid biopsy techniques that look for circulating tumor DNA (ctDNA) – this is generally a non-invasive procedure that may be able to replace bone marrow biopsies one day. Not only is this method less risky and painful for patients, but it also holds promise when it comes to diagnosing disorders like monoclonal plasma cell diseases. By incorporating targeted methylation sequencing by doctors, they can gain more information regarding genetic changes and disease progression pathways in the case of MGUS as well as multiple myeloma (Huang et al., 2024). Generally speaking, with increasing research yielding exciting new technologies, clinicians should soon be capable of more precise detection and monitoring of white blood cell disorders, all of which would eventually translate into earlier interventions and more specific therapy.

6.4.3. Importance of Early Detection and Monitoring

Detecting white blood cell issues in their earliest stages is really important—it can literally mean the difference for how well a patient does. Leukemia or lymphoma tends to sneak up quietly with barely noticeable warning signs. Routine blood work now and then picks up on small changes in cell numbers or abnormal cell shape changes, alerting doctors in advance. New diagnostic tests, including micro-fluidic systems, are making it easier to catch even subtle signs of infection or cancer. These technologies improve disease management more effectively and lower the massive emotional and economic cost of treating advanced diseases (Azad et al., 2016). Tracking these markers over a period is just as important. Follow-up tests on a regular basis are able to show changes in the amount of leukocytes, and this encourages the clinicians to make changes in treatments accordingly. For instance, when a person is undergoing chemotherapy for a blood cancer, monitoring how white cell levels change can avoid complications such as unexpected infections or bleeding due to low cell levels. Regular monitoring also provides a better opportunity to detect a relapse early on, so the treatment can be resumed early. Good knowledge of these blood details leads to more individualized management of the patient—something particularly important in children, who may react differently from grown-ups (Chalmers et al., 2009). Last but not least, early diagnosis and monitoring are the foundation stones of effective management of white blood cell disorders. Advanced devices such as lab-on-chip technologies drive these processes forward by producing complex profiles of the blood at speeds faster than ever and at lower cost. This new method not only improves consistency and accuracy but expands the roster of conditions that can be monitored, from various types of cancers to others. As medicine continues to move toward personalized medicine, building a solid foundation in early detection and follow-up will be critical to making new therapies more effective, hopefully resulting in better survival and quality of life for patients with these complex diseases (Azad et al., 2016; Chalmers et al., 2009) (Figure 6.13).

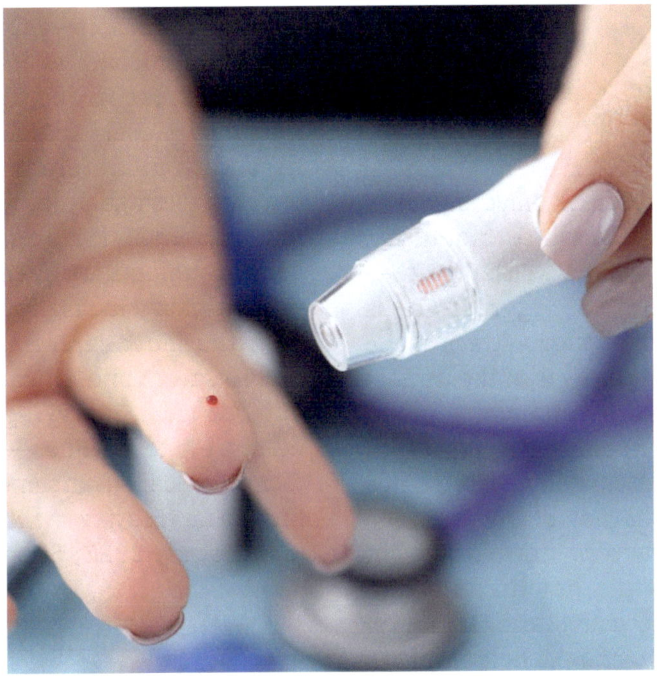

Figure 6.13. White blood cell count test.

Source: https://external-content.duckduckgo.com/iu/?u=https%3A%2F%2Ffirebasestorage.googleapis.com%2Fv0%2Fb%2Fglycan-age.appspot.com%2Fo%2Fmagazine-articles-white-blood-cell-count-test-4-white%2520blood%2520cell%2520test%2520%2520-%2520pic2.jpg%3Falt%3Dmedia%26token%3D173d82db-557f-4a63-acaf-65828b5ecb79&f=1&nofb=1&ipt=cd4c1ab0ad85769fe6950735b1996fc7f16ea4cea710b37b0104d3a12fec1b4f.

Test Your Knowledge

1. What are the most common clinical symptoms of WBC disorders such as leukemia?
2. How does a complete blood count (CBC) assist in diagnosing WBC abnormalities?

6.5. Treatment Options

Learning Outcome

- Chemotherapy and its role in managing disorders;
- Radiation therapy and its applications;
- Stem cell transplantation as a potential cure.

Medical tech and new research have basically transformed how we treat white blood cell disorders. Chemotherapy is still the go-to—especially for something as aggressive as leukemia, where specialized meds attack those cancer cells. Accurate diagnosis is of the utmost importance here, with different white blood cell problems being in need of varying types of treatment. It's a delicate balancing act, since white blood cells—the heroes of our immune systems—mean that doctors have to target the bad cells exactly while not harming the good ones. AI tools, like convolutional neural networks, are also now starting to help improve diagnostic accuracy and open the way for more precise and improved treatments. Taken as a whole, such innovations are reflective of a turn towards not only the treatment of the symptoms but also the underlying causes that result in the disorders (Saini et al., 2023). Immunotherapy has also been producing some creative ideas. New drugs like monoclonal antibodies and CAR T-cell therapy are gaining popularity, particularly for conditions such as lymphoma and some leukemias. Using the use of genetically altered immune cells, these methods aim to possess a high specificity against infected cells but leave most healthy tissues intact. Current studies still study the potential use of integrating traditional methods with such novel immune mechanisms to increase overall effect. Also, there's a buzz building up on using AI to enable faster diagnosis—scrutinizing patient information with static classification models can often pave the way for swift, more effective reactions (Sharma et al., 2023). Personalized medicine is maturing, pushing treatment strategies toward a progressively personalized path. Genetic testing and biomarker analysis are also increasingly important for determining the optimal treatment strategy based on the patient's specific condition—yes, one and all. This shift enables clinicians to individualize treatments, from chemotherapy to immunotherapy, so that they closely match the disorder at hand. In addition, developments in gene editing technologies like CRISPR are opening up exciting new avenues for repairing the underlying genetic defects of such diseases. Even these revolutionary ideas, however, need to be tested with the most careful, high-stringency testing before safety and efficacy can be assured. Last but not least, marrying proven methods with these new techniques—brought on by ongoing technological advancements—is the wave of the future in treating white blood cell disorders (Saini et al., 2023; Sharma et al., 2023).

6.5.1. Chemotherapy and Its role in managing disorders

White blood cells link to our immune system in ways that make their disorders cure unexpectedly tricky. When they overgrow uncontrollably in diseases like leukemia and lymphoma, chemo is the go-to choice. Chemo strikes those dividing cells directly, slowing disease progression and allowing the body to overcome infection once more. Studies, for example, show that having adequate views of the amount and shape of these cells is crucial to determining a diagnosis and deciding upon what type of chemo course of treatment would be best for a specific patient's unique case (Saini et al., 2023). Even treating these diseases, however, relies on having a solid grasp of the underlying principles of chemo. Take combination therapies: treating together to assault numerous pathways has shown, in most cases, that you not only maximize the effect but minimize the chance of resistance—a problem with conventional methods. Beyond that, the treatment landscape is evolving; medical image analysis is now gaining much attention for tracking patient response. Techniques like deep learning help classify and segment white blood cells with a level of detail that really offers fresh insights into both a patient's overall health and how effective their treatment might be (Vivek et al., 2023). As our understanding of white blood cell disorders deepens, the role of chemotherapy keeps changing with new findings emerging all the time. Active research is typically investigating the balance between how well treatments work and how safe they are, especially since patients can be made more vulnerable to infection after chemo. For this reason, other treatments—supportive care or even new immunotherapies—are being investigated to try and improve outcomes while closely watching general health. In this more sophisticated approach, the merging of new diagnostic methods with new treatment therapies promises a future where survival and quality of life can be truly improved. It seems that, through their implementation, chemo may be maximized as an even better, more tailored treatment regimen for each specific disorder (Saini et al., 2023) (Figure 6.14).

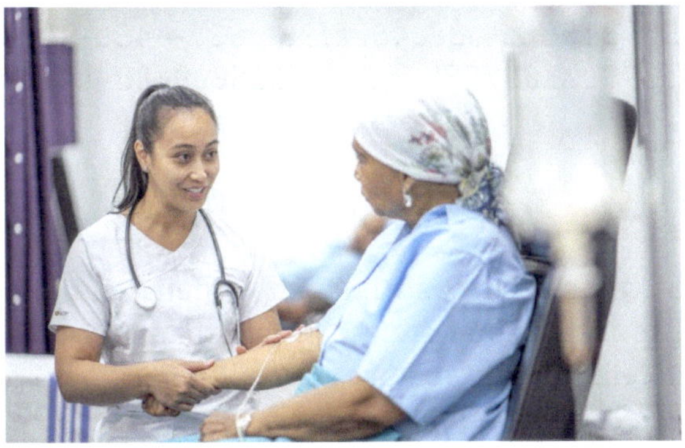

Figure 6.14. Chemotherapy.

Source: https://external-content.duckduckgo.com/iu/?u=https%3A%2F%2Fwww.fmchealth.org%2Fapp%2Fuploads%2F2019%2F10%2Foncology-960x600.jpg&f=1&nofb=1&ipt=27ec09fcf92cfe4d7ff4e98ec8d74290fe00f11d35055ca4370d9b34de04b394.

6.5.2. Radiation therapy and Its applications

Knowing the way our immune system operates is crucial when battling cancer, particularly diseases associated with white blood cells. Radiation isn't a sledgehammer that kills tumors indiscriminately – it may also amplify the efforts of immune cells such as lymphocytes. Quite frequently, an abnormally active JAK/STAT pathway ultimately aids cancer cells in evading our defenses. Generally speaking, when radiation is applied, it can destroy this unwanted signal, making tumors more susceptible to assault (Hu et al., 2021). Doctors most often use this tactic in combination with immuno-therapeutic agents on the hope that the therapy will destroy cancer cells and rally the body's own fight against disease. Inflammation and cancer quite nicely combine in bizarre manners. Chronic inflammation – usually a sign that the immune system is slightly awry – can potentially offer a fertile environment upon which tumors might flourish. In these situations, radiation sometimes causes an acute episode of localized inflammation that aids in maturation of dendritic cells and facilitates antigen presentation, effectively revivifying the anti-tumor response. In most cases, such as MAPK and TLR, these pathways ultimately became involved in this radiation-induced flare, paving the way for targeted therapy. Combining radiation with cytokine therapy or other novel agents might then ensure a more balanced approach to resolving the inflammatory context in white blood cell malignancies, enhancing patient survival and overall quality of life (Zhao et al., 2021). Radiation therapy is reaching out beyond traditional treatment of cancer, too. For blood cancer, leukemias, and lymphomas, directed radiation sometimes zaps the rogue cells without killing the normal production of blood cells—if used judiciously. This delicate dance can be a double-edged sword indeed; it promises hope and threat at the same time, so that doctors must beware of allowing unwelcome side effects to best them. Technological advancements in radiography have, in a majority of cases, increased precision in the delivery of radiation, thereby reducing damage to the adjacent healthy tissue. Treatment timing during the immune body cycle can also be crucial; knowing JAK/STAT and other pro-inflammatory signals might allow for a solution that is better able to leverage the immune response. Research, gradually but irresistibly, are unraveling the complex interweave of the relationships between radiation, inflammation, and dysfunction of white blood cells—toward more promising frontiers of future therapy (Hu et al., 2021; Zhao et al., 2021) (Figure 6.15).

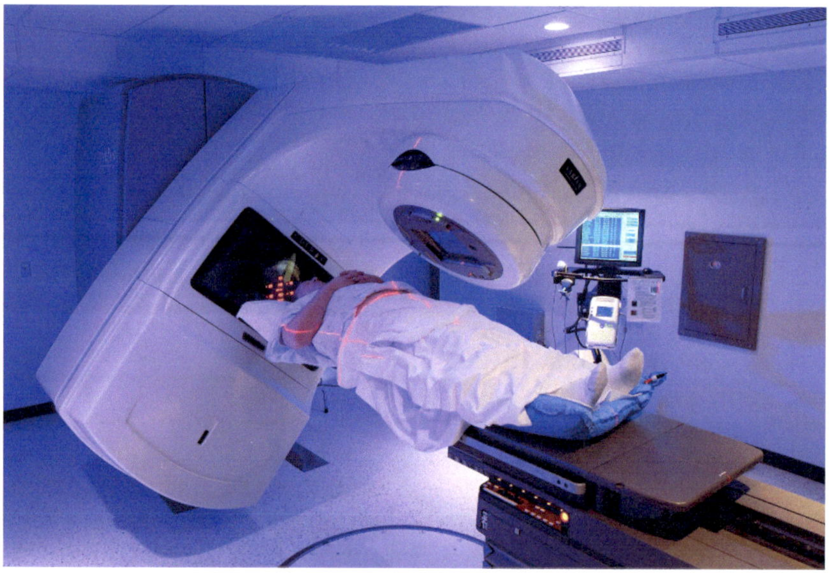

Figure 6.15. Radiation therapy.

Source: https://external-content.duckduckgo.com/iu/?u=http%3A%2F%2Fuserscontent2.emaze.com%2Fimages%2F0492d6fd-9f0c-4859-99d2-b9855931588a%2Fe46bef78-e827-445d-920d-3fdd2e8bf3f0.jpg&f=1&nofb=1&ipt=1de33314aa85fca3990ba0877882bc773da268e96884a4eeea831991c7235487.

6.5.3. Stem Cell Transplantation as a Potential Cure

White blood cell disorders have taken a giant leap in the recent past. Instead of being satisfied with mere drugs, therapies now take a sensational leap in terms of stem cell transplants. During this procedure, doctors introduce hematopoietic stem cells to help restart normal blood flow and immune function in patients suffering from diseases like severe combined immunodeficiency (SCID) or certain leukemias. It's not just a matter of giving an opportunity for a cure; it also relieves complications related to faulty or non-existent white blood cells. It basically replaces the bone marrow with healthy cells to create a brand new, working immune system that treats the core of most blood problems. It's also remarkable that these transplants are working in white blood cell-related disorders involving brain conditions like Krabbe disease or X-linked adrenoleukodystrophy. In all these conditions, there is a lack of the vital enzymes that leads to the things going awry at the cellular level, gradually eroding the nervous system. There are many studies that show infusions of hematopoietic stem cells can reverse some of those long-term effects—lessening inflammation and even reversing small blood vessel alteration in the brain. In Krabbe disease, for example, the treatment has been found to improve symptoms and keep the brain's functions in place (Cappello et al., 2016). There is more to this picture. Stem cell transplants are not just about masking blood counts; they imply a whole new way of thinking concerning white blood cell diseases. Instead of just treating the symptoms, this strategy targets the underlying causes, which typically results in better patient recovery and overall well-being. A more detailed investigation of the way genetic idiosyncrasies disrupt white matter and nerve well-being has even led to transplant procedures that are more or less tailored to each individual. Research, for instance, has cited improvement in microvascular function post-procedure, suggesting that hematopoietic stem cells can assist in modulating not only blood components but also brain microenvironment—specifically in conditions like X-linked adrenoleukodystrophy (Lauer et al., 2017) (Figure 6.16).

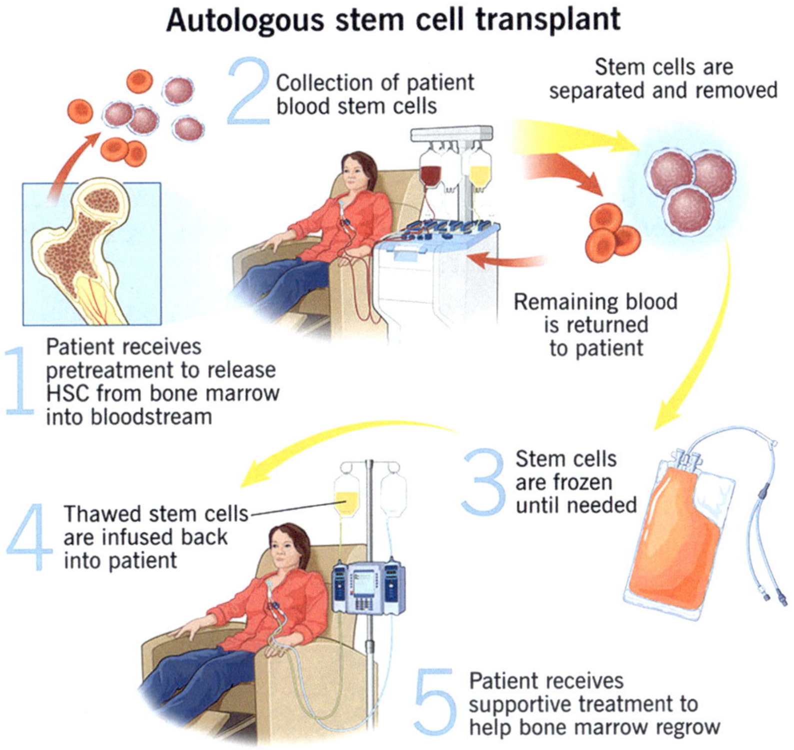

Figure 6.16. Stem cell (bone marrow) transplant.

Source: https://my.clevelandclinic.org/-/scassets/images/org/health/articles/autologous-stem-cell-transplant.

Test Your Knowledge

1. How are bacterial or viral infection–related WBC disorders typically managed?
2. What are the main treatment approaches for leukemia and lymphoma?

6.6. Prognosis and Living with White Blood Cell Disorders

Learning Outcome

- Factors influencing prognosis and survival rates;
- Psychological impact on patients and families;
- Support systems and resources available.

It takes living with a disorder of white blood cells – especially leukemia – to its logical conclusion, issues that extend far beyond that original diagnosis or first treatment. Kids with acute lymphoblastic leukemia (ALL) in general do extremely well – 90% event-free survival if they're under the age of ten, usually – and that's partly due to the developments in using more than one chemotherapy drug and finding levels of risk to treat each patient based on that. Yet the threat of relapse never truly vanishes; it involves follow-ups for years to come. Survivors are likely to end up needing close observation since the intensive treatments can then cause difficulties like memory bumps, musculoskeletal problems, or a second malignancy. All these factors imply that treatment can't solely focus on one aspect—there needs to be an action that takes care of both body and psyche as patients struggle to rebuild their lives after intervention (Joel, 2019). Care for a white blood cell disorder rearranges daily life not just for the patients themselves but also for their families. Long-term health issues quite frequently need constant management and readjustment.

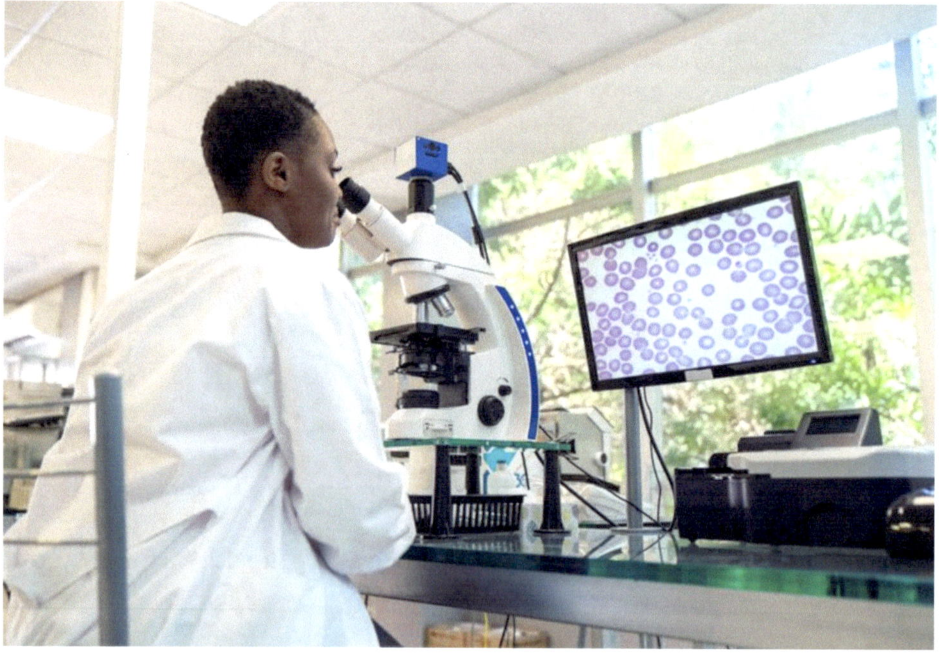

Figure 6.17. Prognosis and living with white blood cell disorders.

Source: https://external-content.duckduckgo.com/iu/?u=https%3A%2F%2Fwww.verywellhealth.com%2Fthmb%2FdMXyppAQlim8TZjoRuT6jQWmn7Q%3D%2F750x0%2Ffilters%3Ano_upscale()%3Amax_bytes(150000)%3Astrip_icc()%2FGettyImages-1371706582-bc5587bb36984911ac604d1f399969b0.jpg&f=1&nofb=1&ipt=1df0f3c1ed3d72f809c97c306c03760067b6b3fd14110035105ad5a9781cb1ad.

For example, children treated for leukemia commonly experience such problems as ongoing fatigue and heightened susceptibility to becoming infected, problems which are physically draining and emotionally distressing. Sometimes this even interrupts the routine habits – like adapting to school or sports – with physical limitations or even illness fear holding them back. And don't count out the psychological toll; most survivors have incidents of depression or anxiety that complicate things further. In such cases, having good support – either familial or societal – is absolutely essential in helping them gradually return to a normal life (Villanueva, 2019). As medication advances further and further, the entire game of coping with such white blood cell disorders is altering too. New treatment options – including targeted immunotherapies and precision medicine approaches – now provide better results and fewer side effects. This change to more personalized care is particularly encouraging for patients with chronic myelogenous leukemia (CML) and acute myeloid leukemia (AML). The way that newer drugs, such as tyrosine kinase inhibitors, have redefined the disease's treatment is nothing less than revolutionary; it's led to tighter disease control and a markedly improved quality of life. All the same, the long-term implications of these new treatments are still being worked out, so there needs to be continuing follow-up to identify any late-onset complications. In short, in treating white blood cell disease patients nowadays, the strategy has to deal with both the medical side and a broader, more extensive support network for mental health alongside overall quality of life (Joel, 2019) (Figure 6.17).

6.6.1. Factors Influencing Prognosis and Survival Rates

White blood cell disorder results are all wrapped up in a mix of variables that don't quite fit into one neat equation. Age, gender, and other illness come into the picture – and, given an equal shuffle of the deck, younger people generally do better because their systems are healthier and there is less excess baggage to carry. No wonder that other problems like heart complications throw a monkey wrench into the works; these secondary illnesses can cloud the immune system and make treatment less effective. Ironically, even a higher white blood cell count, which would otherwise appear desirable, can in fact be an indicator of a worse prognosis. Take a step back and view the general picture, and clinical data like how far along the disease is and what kind of treatment they've had are relevant. As a rule, where in the disorder the disorder is diagnosed determines what comes next. The sooner it's diagnosed, the more hopeful the treatment options – sometimes even curative – and the worse, the less hopeful. Chemotherapy, stem cell transplantation, and other therapies are not equally suitable for everyone but vary depending on the type of disorder, and delayed or inappropriate treatment generally results in decreased survival. This close relationship between clinical manifestations and treatment essentially requires careful, individualized attention. Some recent research has thrown a more discerning eye on laboratory tests as pointers to what lies ahead. Moderate alterations in white blood cell numbers, platelet numbers, and even fibrinogen levels can indicate the direction the disease will take. Elevated white blood cell levels were correlated with lower chances of survival and even determined risk-scoring models for patients presenting with chronic illness in one study (Yamanaka et al., 2025). Similarly, tumor features and in-hospital data such as hematocrit and platelets are also linked with global survival in esophageal cancers, affirming the importance of thorough, comprehensive blood tests (Rui et al., 2024). Lastly, these blood markers are not only static snapshots of current health but are useful aids to doctors when making decisions on treatments for each patient (Figure 6.18).

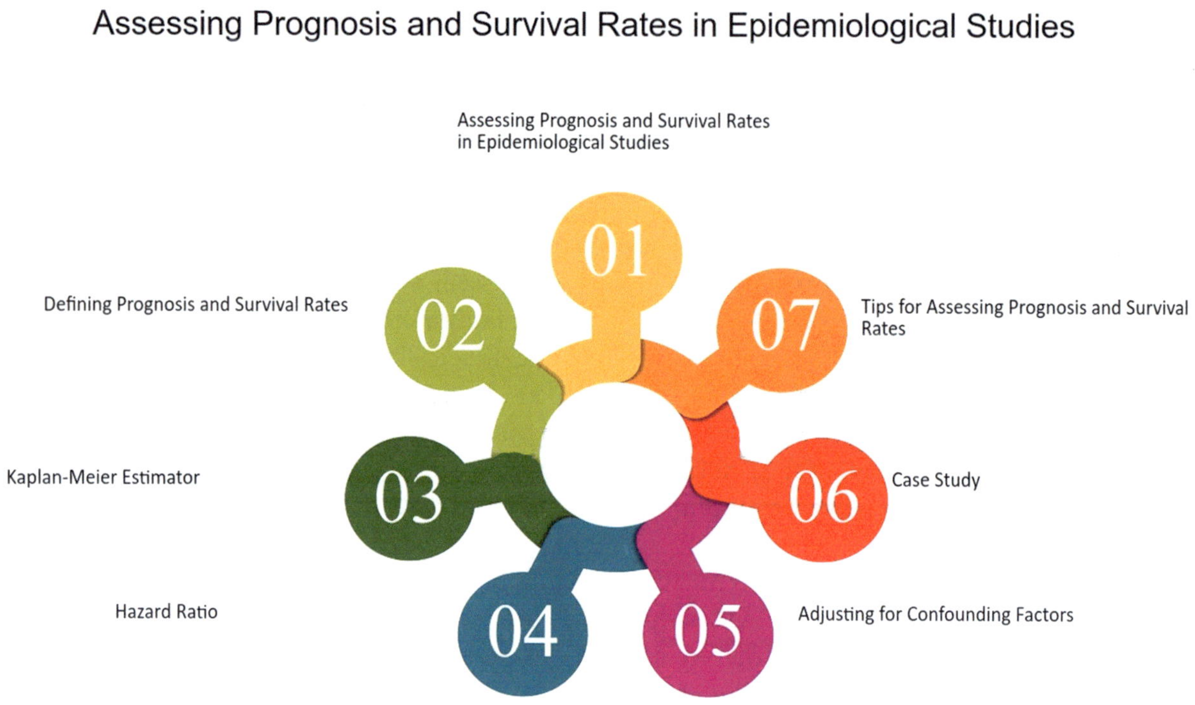

Figure 6.18. Prognosis and survival rates.

Source: https://fastercapital.co/i/Survival-analysis-in-epidemiology--Unraveling-Disease-Dynamics--Assessing-Prognosis-and-Survival-Rates-in-Epidemiological-Studies.webp.

6.6.2. Psychological Impact on Patients and Families

White blood cell diseases attack not just the body— they really shake someone up in the head. When a patient is diagnosed with leukemia or lymphoma, there tends to be a flurry of feelings—fear, worry, even bouts of depression that just won't subside. Most patients are left wondering what the next step is, caught in a never-ending cycle of fear. The whole process can be made even more daunting by navigating through a medical system riddled with confusing terminology and rigid protocols, and before long, isolation creeps in—especially when exhaustion or prolonged hospitalization diminishes usual socializing. More often than not, being able to get a handle on these emotional battles becomes part of the overall treatment plan, because being able to keep the mind in hand actually makes a big difference when being able to stay on the course of care. A diagnosis doesn't just end with the ill individual—it radiates out and often finds family members having to bear a significant emotional burden as well. Occasionally the everyday family routine gets totally out of whack, with loved ones ending up being forced to play the roles of full-time caregivers and being drained emotionally as a result. It's not even the disruption in daily routine; anxiety about money and how things will even run day-to-day only add to the stress. Parents, especially parents with young kids, can become stressed and frustrated, constantly fretting about long-term health and all-around well-being. In the majority of cases, this kind of pressure can even start to creep into everyday conversation in the home. A bit of counseling—a session or a local support group—can sometimes mitigate that stress to some degree, where family members can heal and get on with their lives together. These problems all reflect the reason why it is so important for treatment plans to go beyond merely physical in nature and include healthy mental care. In most cases, care teams that include psychological support in addition to medicine have a profound effect on both patients and families. These strategies are not just about the relief of distress but also help individuals in adopting better ways to cope with stress. Having mental health professionals present in consultations enables patients to express concerns and fears—happens where the medical facts are sorted out as well. Also, when loved ones participate in supportive therapies, it creates a sort of safety net around the patient, something many believe is necessary to recovering from tough times. Nowadays, experts affirm that taking care of someone's mood is as crucial as curing the physical illness, making a strong case for care that integrates concepts from every type of discipline.

6.6.3. Support Systems and Resources Available

Most people with white blood cell disorders are encircled by a chaotic array of support systems that can really make a difference in overall care. Medical professionals intervene early—guiding treatment protocols and even guiding people to specialists like hematologists who interpret the particulars of the disease. Support groups for patients, surprisingly enough, become mini-communities where individuals become attached to each other through shared ups and downs, occasionally speaking in ways that soothe that inner loneliness and anxiety. Access to the proper information is, for most, a large piece of the patient and caregiver puzzle. Simple leaflets, hands-on workshops, and even webinars on the internet can clarify what those symptoms and treatment schedules actually mean—but, frankly, the technical jargon still gets all mixed up at times. Groups committed to blood disorders even add in the latest research results and clinical trial data, keeping families up to date on new approaches to treating the condition. This blend of factual directness and ongoing reports works to enable patients to be masters of their own treatment plan. Financial realities can't be ignored either. Often, the cost factor in attending to white blood cell disorders presents as severely as do the medical issues, so a number of organizations offer support in the way of grants, scholarships, or patient advocacy programs designed specifically to lighten that load. Insurance policies baffling at best sometimes have patients in a situation whereby they have to rely on the use of counseling services to understand what their coverage is. More often than not, putting together emotional, educational, and financial support—grudgingly somewhat of a patchwork—does indeed make individuals more resilient and overall better quality of life through these horribly difficult times (N/A, 2023; Visseren et al., 2021).

Test Your Knowledge

1. How does early detection influence the prognosis of WBC cancers like leukemia?
2. What lifestyle modifications can support patients living with chronic WBC disorders?

Summary

White blood cell disorders are messy and complicated; they demand a mix of approaches if we're to really get a grip on what's going on. There's a crazy amount of variety in these cells—and each one does its part in our immune system—so even a small glitch can turn into a big health issue. There appears to be evidence from research linking oxidative and nitrosative stress—more or less those toxic peaks of reactive substances—to being central to such conditions, something that shows up in a broad variety of disease settings. For example, some patient cases show increased blood levels of reactive oxygen species and nitric oxide, which imply the mechanisms involved in terms of cell malfunction and even cell death. All of this speaks, in most cases, to the potential of targeting these pathways in creating treatment modalities for white blood cell disorders (Arese et al., 2015). New discoveries in genomic and epigenetic science are uncovering new potential for new therapies. When genes regulating the white blood cells fall into disarray, any number of disorders are possible, making it necessary to know the general genetic and epigenetic landscape. Investigating how metabolic hiccup is connected to immune function, it's clear that such diseases as obesity tend to amplify white blood cell issues even more. Advances in DNA methylation—one of those interesting niches of genetics—give us important information about how our environment drives gene expression in blood-forming cells, opening the door to more targeted treatments (Kang et al., 2019). In summary, the complexity of white blood cell disorders calls for the excavating deep into their molecular, genetic, and even environmental interrelationships. Clinicians and scientists really need to work together with one another, bridging the chasm between basic research and routine clinical practice, and taking advantage of new technologies to improve both diagnosis and treatment. With the advance of technology, the merger of knowledge of oxidative stress and epigenetics appears to hold the key to progressing personalized medicine. Looking at the whole picture, medicine as an enterprise has a greater chance of helping patients and developing resistance to immune system breakdowns. Our future therapies depend ultimately on coping with such complexities—unstable and messy as they are—with solutions based firmly on hard scientific research.

White blood cell diseases really rock the boat inside the body. These illnesses derange the immune system in a manner that disrupts its normal rhythm. Most times, illnesses like leukemias, lymphomas, and myelodysplastic syndromes come as a surprise – one moment it's an onset of immature white cells that keeps normal blood components from maturing properly, and the very next moment it's all about cancerous tumors forming in lymph tissue. It's hard not to appreciate that managing these diseases needs a full armory of different tools, from high-tech imaging and even molecular definition, each one individually tailored to the specific personality of the individual patient. The influence of these diseases isn't just felt by one person, either; they have a ripple effect out into our broader healthcare system and even into society's view of disease management. With greater demand for novel treatments, science is generally constricting its attention to the small molecular mechanisms driving these conditions. More recently, the breakthroughs in cell-based medicines and immunotherapies have opened up new realms, and even sometimes you hear the discussion regarding the possibility of the gut-brain axis being combined with immunity and more systemic issues. A bird's-eye view—while there are some small contradictions here and there—is relevant, as lifestyle choices, preventive medicine, and even schooling will all reduce the risk in the future. In the future, most are focusing on improving diagnostics and outcome for white blood cell disorders. Further research on genetic clues and environmental influences is, on the whole, significant for recognizing those who could be at greater risk. At the same time, novel biotechnological approaches may well reveal the hidden dynamics of cells, aiding in further fine-tuning therapies. Synergistic interactions between fields like microbiology and immunology–as noted by current studies–apparently are paving the way for interventions that not only move medicine forward but also offer enhanced, wholistic care for patients (John et al., 2019; Percie et al., 2020).

KEY TERMS FROM THIS CHAPTER

- Acute lymphoblastic leukemia (ALL)
- Basophilia
- Bone marrow biopsy
- Chronic myeloid leukemia (CML)
- Hodgkin's lymphoma
- Leukocytosis
- Lymphocytosis
- Lymphopenia
- Myelodysplastic syndromes (MDS)
- Acute myeloid leukemia (AML)
- Blast cells
- Chronic lymphocytic leukemia (CLL)
- Eosinophilia
- Leukemia
- Leukopenia
- Lymphoma
- Monocytosis
- Neutropenia

Critical Thinking Questions

1. **Which of the following conditions is characterized by an abnormally low white blood cell count?**
   a. Leukocytosis
   b. Leukopenia
   c. Polycythemia
   d. Thrombocytosis
2. **What is the primary function of white blood cells?**
   a. Carry oxygen
   b. Form blood clots
   c. Fight infections
   d. Transport nutrients
3. **Which WBC disorder involves uncontrolled production of abnormal white blood cells in the bone marrow?**
   a. Leukemia
   b. Lymphoma
   c. Anemia
   d. Hemophilia
4. **Eosinophilia is an increase in eosinophils and is commonly associated with:**
   a. Viral infections
   b. Bacterial infections
   c. Parasitic infections and allergies
   d. Bleeding disorders
5. **A differential white blood cell count is used to:**
   a. Measure hemoglobin
   b. Determine platelet count
   c. Identify proportions of different types of WBCs
   d. Measure blood glucose

Answers to Critical Thinking Questions

1. (b); 2. (c); 3. (a); 4. (c); 5. (c)

Short Answer Questions

1. What is the normal range of WBC count in adults?
2. Define leukocytosis and name two common causes.
3. What is leukopenia, and what conditions can lead to it?
4. What are the characteristic features of acute lymphoblastic leukemia (ALL)?
5. How does chronic myeloid leukemia (CML) differ in presentation and lab findings from acute leukemias?

References

1. 2023 Alzheimer's disease facts and figures. (2023). *Alzheimer's & Dementia, 19*, 1598–1695. https://doi.org/10.1002/alz.13016 (accessed on 1st July 2025).
2. Aas, M., Blokland, G. A. M., Chawner, S. J. R. A., Choi, K., et al. (2016). Summaries of plenary, symposia, and oral sessions at the XXII World Congress of Psychiatric Genetics, Copenhagen, Denmark, 12–16 October 2014. https://core.ac.uk/download/227054289.pdf (accessed on 1st July 2025).
3. Abd Wahab, M. B. A., Mahmood, S., Mohamad Rus, M. A., Mustar, M., et al. (2020). Quality control improvement at Jana DCS Sdn. Bhd. https://core.ac.uk/download/12007130.pdf (accessed on 1st July 2025).
4. Ackley, R., Anderson, L., Barlough, J., Barnett, S., Barr, M., Beatty, J., Beatty, K., et al. (2012). Clinical aspects of feline retroviruses: A review. https://core.ac.uk/download/16431899.pdf (accessed on 1st July 2025).
5. Agostini, C., Cinetto, F., Crescenzi, L., Milito, C., et al. (2018). Gastric cancer is the leading cause of death in Italian adult patients with common variable immunodeficiency. https://core.ac.uk/download/168406648.pdf (accessed on 1st July 2025).
6. Alsamri, J. M., Alqahtani, H., Al-Sharafi, A. M., Darem, A. A., Nazim, K., Sattar, A., Alshammeri, M., et al. (2025). Computer-aided diagnosis of hematologic disorders detection based on spatial feature learning networks using blood cell images. *Scientific Reports, 15*. https://www.semanticscholar.org/paper/85efd72bd4ae0dd88ba4299e1e9c2c31d0e7d04c (accessed on 1st July 2025).
7. Arese, M., Buscarinu, M. C., Chessa, L., Coarelli, G., et al. (2015). Evidence for detrimental cross interactions between reactive oxygen and nitrogen species in Leber's hereditary optic neuropathy cells. https://core.ac.uk/download/54529895.pdf (accessed on 1st July 2025).
8. Azad, M., Goudarzi, M., Mobarra, N., Sahmani, M., et al. (2016). Microchips and their significance in isolation of circulating tumor cells and monitoring of cancers. https://core.ac.uk/download/52205560.pdf (accessed on 1st July 2025).
9. Baniamer, A., Hamdan, A. M., AlGhzawi, M. R., Alfaqeh, M. T., Yaseen, S. Y., Alshtawi, S. M., Alomush, H. Y., et al. (2024). Understanding inherited bleeding disorders: Genetic mutations in blood coagulation factors and regulatory proteins. *Journal of Hematology and Oncology Research*. https://www.semanticscholar.org/paper/a14d6683f9c539cf6126def22b96ffb4a4bee2ac (accessed on 1st July 2025).
10. Bao, E. L., Cheng, A., & Sankaran, V. G. (2019). The genetics of human hematopoiesis and its disruption in disease. *EMBO Molecular Medicine, 11*. https://doi.org/10.15252/emmm.201910316 (accessed on 1st July 2025).
11. Barrett, T. J., Lee, A. H., Xia, Y., Lin, L. H., Black, M. A., Cotzia, P., Hochman, J. S., et al. (2020). Platelet and vascular biomarkers associate with thrombosis and death in coronavirus disease. *Circulation Research, 127*, 945–947. https://doi.org/10.1161/circresaha.120.317803 (accessed on 1st July 2025).
12. Bodnar, S., Brander, T., Avigan, Z. M., Genthe, W., Melnekoff, D., Laganà, A., Houldsworth, J., et al. (2024). Enhanced detection of pathogenic germline variants in plasma cell disorders: Impact of a targeted genetic counseling referral pathway. *Blood*. https://www.semanticscholar.

org/paper/054e7ae5c6a0ca54900f5e88690b58be88bd1c52 (accessed on 1st July 2025).

13. Borgen, A. (2020). Health related effects of wheat varieties. https://core.ac.uk/download/323144679.pdf (accessed on 1st July 2025).
14. Brew, B., Ellero, J., & Lubomski, M. (2017). Interventions for neurocognitive dysfunction. https://core.ac.uk/download/84111210.pdf (accessed on 1st July 2025).
15. Cappello, V., Marchetti, L., Parlanti, P., Landi, S., Tonazzini, I., Cecchini, M., Piazza, V., et al. (2016). Ultrastructural characterization of the lower motor system in a mouse model of Krabbe disease. *Scientific Reports, 6*. https://doi.org/10.1038/s41598-016-0001-8 (accessed on 1st July 2025).
16. Chalmers, E. A., & Halsey, C. (2009). Hematological investigations in children. https://core.ac.uk/download/110273.pdf (accessed on 1st July 2025).
17. Chomel, L., Vogt, M., Demiselle, J., Le Borgne, P., Tschirhart, M., Morandeau, V., Merdji, H., et al. (2024). TLRs1-10 protein expression in circulating human white blood cells during bacterial and COVID-19 infections. *Journal of Innate Immunity, 16*, 216–225. https://www.semanticscholar.org/paper/2375e6de96c5c630d3604885d4e4e0bf5f7201a3 (accessed on 1st July 2025).
18. Chong, S. Y. C., Fu, Y. H., Kurien, P. A., Ptáček, L. J., et al. (2013). Sick and tired: How molecular regulators of human sleep schedules and duration impact immune function. https://core.ac.uk/download/322310899.pdf (accessed on 1st July 2025).
19. Cryan, J. F., O'Riordan, K. J., Cowan, C. S. M., Sandhu, K. V., Bastiaanssen, T. F. S., Boehme, M., Codagnone, M. G., et al. (2019). The microbiota-gut-brain axis. *Physiological Reviews, 99*, 1877–2013. https://doi.org/10.1152/physrev.00018.2018 (accessed on 1st July 2025).
20. Devi, J. R., Kadiyala, P. S., Lavu, S., Kasturi, N., & Kosuri, L. (2024). Enhancing acute lymphoblastic leukemia classification with a rapid and effective CNN model. *2024 Third International Conference on Distributed Computing and Electrical Circuits and Electronics (ICDCECE)*. https://www.semanticscholar.org/paper/4d2b0cc30325041b4751f63ca970e0a99796f96d (accessed on 1st July 2025).
21. Fan, B. E., Cao, L., Gallardo, C. A., Lee, S. S. M., Koh, L. W., Goh, L. L., Ong, K. H., et al. (2021). Myeloid and lymphoid vacuolation in *VEXAS* syndrome. *American Journal of Hematology, 96*, 1056–1057. https://doi.org/10.1002/ajh.26098 (accessed on 1st July 2025).
22. Gaikwad, P. S., Zope, M., Mahale, P. P., & Deshmukh, R. K. (2025). Developing next-generation CapsNet models for enhanced white blood cell classification in medical diagnostics. *Journal of Information Systems Engineering and Management*. https://www.semanticscholar.org/paper/20cb2f06f9c40f99d99755c3d5409d6dfe2af881 (accessed on 1st July 2025).
23. Gallucci, B., Bierut, M., & McCarthy, D. O. (1995). The immune system. https://core.ac.uk/download/213081395.pdf (accessed on 1st July 2025).
24. Hernández-Vargas, H., Castelino, J. M., Silver, M., Dominguez-Salas, P., Cros, M., Durand, G., Le Calvez-Kelm, F., et al. (2015). Exposure to aflatoxin B1 in utero is associated with DNA methylation in white blood cells of infants in The Gambia. *International Journal of Epidemiology, 44*(4), 1238–1248. https://www.semanticscholar.org/paper/14d77485fb13eebcdf07cdf6dfa6520aa2a63078 (accessed on 1st July 2025).

25. Hu, X., Li, J., Fu, M., Zhao, X., & Wang, W. (2021). The JAK/STAT signaling pathway: From bench to clinic. *Signal Transduction and Targeted Therapy, 6*. https://doi.org/10.1038/s41392-021-00791-1 (accessed on 1st July 2025).
26. Huang, Y., Thakkar, R. D., Kappes, K., Steffen, K., Venn, O., Shaknovich, R., Liu, Q., et al. (2024). Novel liquid biopsy approach for detection and characterization of disease progression of plasma cell disorders. *Blood*. https://www.semanticscholar.org/paper/02861c341a63bf06251260e6d5209407c7057b29 (accessed on 1st July 2025).
27. Ilyas, M., Bilal, M., Malik, N., Khan, H. U., Ramzan, M., & Naz, A. (2024). Using deep learning techniques to enhance blood cell detection in patients with leukemia. *Information*. https://www.semanticscholar.org/paper/42b1ec5e8ed9a684e5f566049c4f1b332747678b (accessed on 1st July 2025).
28. Jarrett, R. F., & McAulay, K. A. (2015). Human leukocyte antigens and genetic susceptibility to lymphoma. https://core.ac.uk/download/46558899.pdf (accessed on 1st July 2025).
29. Joshi, V. C., & Mehta, M. (2023). White blood cell segmentation using DeepLabv3+ for improved hematological disease detection. *2023 IEEE Region 10 Symposium (TENSYMP)*. https://www.semanticscholar.org/paper/25a6dcde3e4d37e609b148f2c077de6b8b4a99e5 (accessed on 1st July 2025).
30. Kanaya, M., Mukai, Y., Kobayashi, M., Kajikawa, S., Suzuki, T., Yokoyama, E., Izumiyama, K., et al. (2024). Combination of low white blood cell count and impaired renal function is a risk factor for higher concentrations of venetoclax and prolonged neutropenia in AML patients with venetoclax combined regimen: Real world experience in the Japanese cohort. *Blood*. https://www.semanticscholar.org/paper/1aa5d9d9f2d1f6ba677144325bab5f6e8805cec0 (accessed on 1st July 2025).
31. Kang, S., & Ma, X. (2019). Functional implications of DNA methylation in adipose biology. https://core.ac.uk/download/323080862.pdf (accessed on 1st July 2025).
32. Kaplan, J. A. (2019). Leukemia in children. *Pediatrics in Review, 40*, 319–331. https://doi.org/10.1542/pir.2018-0192 (accessed on 1st July 2025).
33. Lauer, A., Da, X., Hansen, M. B., Boulouis, G., Ou, Y., Cai, X., Pedrotti, A. L. C., et al. (2017). ABCD1 dysfunction alters white matter microvascular perfusion. *Brain, 140*, 3139–3152. https://doi.org/10.1093/brain/awx262 (accessed on 1st July 2025).
34. Liu, Z., Castillo, S., Han, X., Sun, X., Hu, Z., & Yuan, Y. (2024). Adaptive self-supervised learning of morphological landscape for leukocytes classification in peripheral blood smears. *2024 IEEE EMBS International Conference on Biomedical and Health Informatics (BHI)*. https://www.semanticscholar.org/paper/a7aa7e0bfd260ed0158f202d992a878ad932622a (accessed on 1st July 2025).
35. Oh, Y. B., Lee, Y. E., Lim, H., Kwon, Y. J., Choi, Y. J., Park, J., Choi, H. J., et al. (2024). White blood cell count, neutrophil to lymphocyte ratio and serum lactate dehydrogenase level associated with thrombosis risk prediction in essential thrombocytosis. *Blood*. https://www.semanticscholar.org/paper/8fd3e3920e12bbe9285af2db7e826bbaee83cde1 (accessed on 1st July 2025).
36. Palić, I., & Palić, D. (2025). An overview of neuroprotective strategies in preterm neonates. *Preventive Pediatrics*. https://www.semanticscholar.org/paper/922cac43a6faa5b0667e07fe798bb040fef42df6 (accessed on 1st July 2025).

37. Percie du Sert, N., Ahluwalia, A., Alam, S., Avey, M. T., Baker, M., Browne, W. J., Clark, A., et al. (2020). Reporting animal research: Explanation and elaboration for the ARRIVE guidelines 2.0. *PLoS Biology, 18*, e3000411. https://doi.org/10.1371/journal.pbio.3000411 (accessed on 1st July 2025).

38. Priya, V. (2020). White adipose tissue. *Definitions*. https://www.semanticscholar.org/paper/74368315352db12a7ec6233234f885ba1d92052f (accessed on 1st July 2025).

39. Russo, F., Iscaro, A., Marra, R., Nostroso, A., Rosato, B. E., Dionisi, M., Esposito, F. M., et al. (2024). Evaluating the clinical impact of hemoglobinopathy and hereditary red blood cell disorder co-inheritance in a cohort of 315 patients. *Blood*. https://www.semanticscholar.org/paper/1ec36503dc548f0134adf5e2825641fbb8b0286a (accessed on 1st July 2025).

40. Saini, A., Guleria, K., & Sharma, S. (2023). A deep learning-based convolutional neural networks model for white blood cell classification. *2023 4th International Conference for Emerging Technology (INCET)*. https://www.semanticscholar.org/paper/fee279ce86627438ee0983f979fcd099079eff73 (accessed on 1st July 2025).

41. Scippa, K., Mangrum, R., Martin, S., Cueto, D., Bryant, A., Schantz, K., & Pease, S. (2023). Establishing content validity of the FACIT-fatigue scale in patients living with warm autoimmune hemolytic anemia: Results from qualitative interview studies. *Blood*. https://www.semanticscholar.org/paper/8939ebab3b461971b85d60190689a7a9868f04a4 (accessed on 1st July 2025).

42. Sealock, J., Lee, Y. A., Moscati, A., Venkatesh, S., Voloudakis, G., Straub, P., Singh, K., et al. (2021). Use of the PsycheMERGE network to investigate the association between depression polygenic scores and white blood cell count. *JAMA Psychiatry, 78*, 1365–1365. https://doi.org/10.1001/jamapsychiatry.2021.2959 (accessed on 1st July 2025).

43. Sehlikoğlu, Ş., Yıldız, S., Kazğan Kılıçaslan, A., Kurt, O., Göçüm, E., & Han Almiş, B. (2024). Evaluation of complete blood cell count parameters and their role in inflammation in patients with methamphetamine and synthetic cannabis use disorder. *Psychiatry and Clinical Psychopharmacology, 34*, 134–143. https://www.semanticscholar.org/paper/c68d65665bac4e2a954a8f06291ec25be479db9d (accessed on 1st July 2025).

44. Sharma, G., Anand, V., Chauhan, R., Garg, N., & Gupta, S. (2023). Deep learning-based blood cell disease classification: A CNN-enhanced approach for accurate hematological diagnosis and treatment. *2023 2nd International Conference on Futuristic Technologies (INCOFT)*. https://www.semanticscholar.org/paper/9bef4167ccbdb2a7614fea745021adc6584458b6 (accessed on 1st July 2025).

45. Shultz, L. D., Lyons, B., Burzenski, L., Gott, B., Chen, X., Chaleff, S., Kotb, M., et al. (2005). Human lymphoid and myeloid cell development in NOD/LtSz-*scid IL2Rγnull* mice engrafted with mobilized human hemopoietic stem cells. *The Journal of Immunology, 174*, 6477–6489. https://doi.org/10.4049/jimmunol.174.10.6477 (accessed on 1st July 2025).

46. Villanueva, A. (2019). Hepatocellular carcinoma. *New England Journal of Medicine, 380*, 1450–1462. https://doi.org/10.1056/nejmra1713263 (accessed on 1st July 2025).

47. Visseren, F. L. J., Mach, F., Smulders, Y. M., Carballo, D., Koskinas, K. C., Bäck, M., Bénétos, A., et al. (2021). 2021 ESC guidelines on cardiovascular disease prevention in clinical practice. *European Heart Journal, 42*, 3227–3337. https://doi.org/10.1093/eurheartj/ehab484 (accessed on 1st July 2025).

48. Voros, V., Saghy, E., Molnar, C., Kovacs, M., Peto, B., Kovacs, S., Zemplényi, A., et al. (2024). Certain immune parameters may have a significant impact on suicidal behavior–A naturalistic study among psychiatric in-patients. *European Psychiatry, 67*, S349–S350. https://www.semanticscholar.org/paper/10a7e88db8da3fd61138ddbca17b688c022a73b2 (accessed on 1st July 2025).

49. Wang, R., Li, C., Da, Q., Yue, Y., Jing, L., Guo, R., Cui, Y., et al. (2024). Analysis of the influencing factors in the long-term survival of esophageal cancer. *Frontiers in Oncology, 13*. https://www.semanticscholar.org/paper/86247680b1eb875218ab510b72e296fe0dada96a (accessed on 1st July 2025).

50. Wang, Y., Miao, Y., & Wan, Q. (2024). Association of white blood cell count to mean platelet volume ratio with type 2 diabetic peripheral neuropathy in a Chinese population: A cross-sectional study. *BMC Endocrine Disorders, 24*. https://www.semanticscholar.org/paper/a79483ad974bd4ad52b793d67c27db1834670831 (accessed on 1st July 2025).

51. Wang, Y., Xu, M., Peng, Y., Zhang, D., Tong, J., & Li, Y. (2021). Novel insights into the potential mechanisms of N6-methyladenosine RNA modification on sepsis-induced cardiovascular dysfunction: An update summary on direct and indirect evidences. *Frontiers in Cell and Developmental Biology, 9*. https://doi.org/10.3389/fcell.2021.772921 (accessed on 1st July 2025).

52. Wong, P., Rhys, T., Mangat, P., Beynon, H., & Stratton, R. (2021). P02 Doctor, I just don't feel alright. *Rheumatology Advances in Practice, 5*. https://www.semanticscholar.org/paper/7fc745179d2ba916740738ecf83edcc5a16fbf94 (accessed on 1st July 2025).

53. Yamanaka, T., Higashitani, M., Matsui, A., Jujo, K., Murata, N., Kodama, T., Mizuno, A., et al. (2025). Investigation of factors for a poor prognosis in Rutherford 4 patients who undergo endovascular treatment. *International Heart Journal*. https://www.semanticscholar.org/paper/33757253848cc9b201246fb7bfbb5524abe709df (accessed on 1st July 2025).

54. Zhao, H., Wu, L., Yan, G., Chen, Y., Zhou, M., Wu, Y., & Li, Y. (2021). Inflammation and tumor progression: Signaling pathways and targeted intervention. *Signal Transduction and Targeted Therapy, 6*. https://doi.org/10.1038/s41392-021-00658-5 (accessed on 1st July 2025).

HEMOSTASIS AND COAGULATION

7

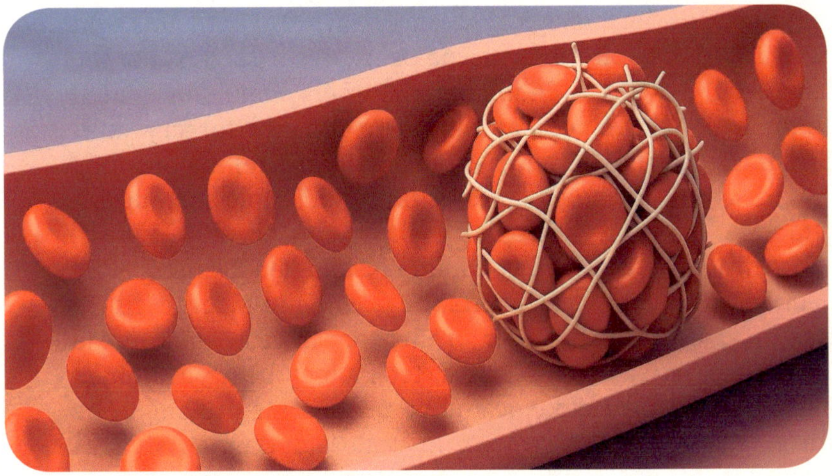

Introduction

Blood clotting plays a vital role in keeping our bodies balanced—our vessels stay strong and tissues remain healthy. These processes, quite simply, not only stop us from bleeding too much when injuries occur, but they also help avoid clots that might clog our systems, sometimes causing thrombosis. In many cases, both clot-promoting and clot-inhibiting factors are jostling together in our bloodstream, each doing its bit. Our bodies build a solid fibrin framework by an active mixture of cells, chemical messengers, and a number of pathways. Studying these interactions gives us insight into various health problems and—if you think about it—accounts for why we really must pay closer attention to how they're handled when disease occurs. Research continues to develop, and the role of blood clotting markers in the clinical setting becomes more and more obvious, particularly in the management of long-term sickness and infection-related issues. Example: CAP serves as a reminder that an ongoing tendency to clot can

LEARNING OBJECTIVES

After studying this chapter, you will be able to:

1. Discuss about the hemostasis process;
2. Define coagulation cascade;
3. List the factors influencing coagulation;
4. Explore the disorders of hemostasis;
5. Illustrate the laboratory assessment of coagulation;
6. Identify the treatment and management of coagulation disorders.

still be present even once recovery seems to be complete. Increased levels of these markers, like D-Dimer and thrombin-antithrombin complexes, have been found to tend to correspond with more cardiovascular fatalities, sometimes long subsequent to the initial symptoms. That such a frequent correlation exists indicates that closer monitoring of these hemostatic markers may be the solution to better long-term patient care, as indicated by studies on acute infection and cardiac disease (Kaynar et al., 2011). And then there's the intriguing twist of alternative therapies—like phytomelatonin from green algae, for instance, which gives blood clotting research a new twist. Preliminary evidence shows that consumption of a regular ethanol extract of green algae might boost blood parameters, including clotting factors, at least in animals. The preliminary evidence indicates that natural compounds can enhance our adaptation mechanisms for coagulation. The positive effects seen on different markers of blood open new doors for traditional medicines to supplement present therapies. With every advance in understanding these complex interplays, integration with some novel natural substances can very well pave the way for more personalized measures in treating clotting disorders (Devi et al., 2016).

Definition of Hemostasis

Bleeding control is a survival issue. When an artery is injured, the body instantly constricts it—prompted by discharged chemical signals—to slow blood flow. Platelets then rush to the area and stick to the damaged surface, forming a plug that's temporary. This union of cell response and biochemical signals starts what we call primary hemostasis, setting the stage for what follows in stopping bleeding. Following the initial patch, secondary hemostasis proceeds with a protein cascade. The clotting factors within the plasma are triggered by the provisional plug, and ultimately fibrinogen is transformed into fibrin, building a stable mesh across the plug. Not only does this barrier stabilize the patch but it also seals off the breach effectively. By and large, it is essential to know these facts when working with bleeding disorders or with atypical clotting conditions. RS models are now providing new insights—demonstrating that tiny variations in natural inhibitors can at times cause conditions such as thrombophilia or thromboembolism (Bendjeddou et al., 2024). Technological advances have also shed new light upon these mechanisms. Technologies like the Virtual Endoluminal Surgery Simulator (VESS) have been developed to enhance surgery skills and training, especially in controlling bleeding during procedures like endoscopic submucosal dissection (ESD) (Bayrak et al., 2019). Such technologies combine hands-on training with computer simulation, enabling surgeons to evaluate their proficiency in real time. In the majority of cases, technology being combined with biological understanding is proving to be a breakthrough in understanding as well as regulating the complexities of blood clotting (Figure 7.1).

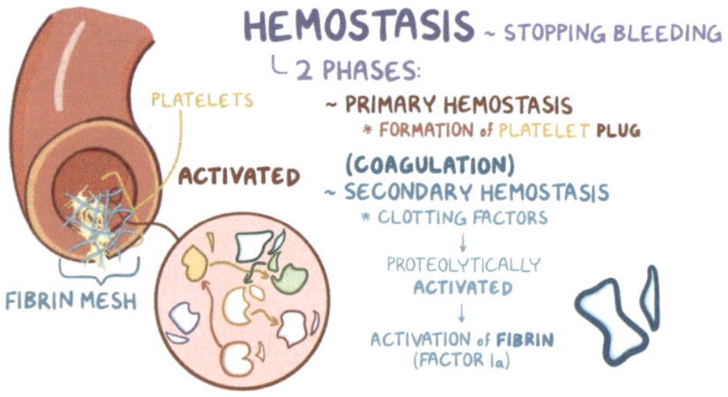

Figure 7.1. Hemostasis.

Source: https://external-content.duckduckgo.com/iu/?u=https%3A%2F%2Fd16qt3wv6xm098.cloudfront.net%2FrDwE2voSQ3a27ZmkkxauhcpZQDeXynqg%2F_.jpg&f=1&nofb=1&ipt=bb335d7a021f5b12fb3fb3f50df9ca19e393fb889c81e5aecc6bb36ce3972201.

Importance of Coagulation in the Human Body

Coagulation serves to keep our blood vessels healthy—it's kind of our body's first line of defense against dangerous bleeding. When one of those vessels gets injured, platelets and the other clotting factors rush in, setting off a cascade that eventually leads to a tight clot. Not only does this seal up the bleeding in an instant, but it also acts to start tissue repair and rebuilding. Periodically, when that concerted effort goes awry—e.g., in circumstances that predispose to red cell destruction (hemolysis) or careless clotting—it can result in uncontrolled bleeding or even acute clotting, which typically only serves to demonstrate how crucial a smooth-operating clotting apparatus is to our well-being. As a case in point, ailments that promote these issues can completely undermine healing and recuperation following surgery, underscoring the significance of a general well-tuned system of coagulation. Recent research has begun examining the mechanisms of clotting in various medical contexts. Experiments suggest that plasma levels of fibrinogen, which some would like to be manipulated, can have an influence over the risk of bleeding in surgery. Keeping this process precariously balanced in most situations during surgery is most important. Interestingly, toxin preconditioning like that with *Crotalus atrox* venom has been shown to augment the production of fibrinogen, thereby increasing the ability of the blood to clot in compromised conditions. Such observations point out that clotting is not an easy body process—it's a big issue in the context of targeted therapy too. Modulation of fibrinogen by new mechanisms can reduce surgical risk and improve recovery of patients, practically minimizing complications secondary to uncontrolled hemorrhage (Applegate et al., 2017). Beyond the operating room, researchers are exploring if naturally occurring compounds might affect coagulation, an area that's attracting some attention in mainstream medicine. Green algae studies, for instance, indicate that certain phytochemicals can modulate blood parameters positively, thus giving hemostatic activity a supportive boost. These findings point to a bigger picture in which old school and new school can work together in preventing clotting. Putting together the knowledge of hematology with the knowledge of hemostasis provides a scope for practitioners to create more integrated ways of diagnosing and treating bleeding disorders. Ultimately, the main purpose that clotting helps to ensure our vessels remain intact makes it a significant topic—not just in studying everyday body functions but also when developing therapeutic methods and continuing ongoing medical discourse (Devi et al., 2016).

7.1. The Hemostasis Process

Learning Outcome

- Stages of hemostasis;
- Role of blood vessels in hemostasis;
- Importance of platelets in the hemostatic process.

After an injury, a messy cascade is triggered. Endothelial cells are disrupted—they expose underlying collagen and start releasing a whole bunch of signals that activate platelets, so they clump together and form an initial plug. Nicotine, surprisingly, has a quite large role here; through activation of the PAR4 receptor, it enhances platelet clumping and granule release. In the majority of cases this receptor's activity elevates intracellular calcium—a critical signal for normal platelet function—suggesting that nicotine may push the clotting process along in ways that will surprise us (Wu et al., 2025). It's also necessary to consider clotting as part of an overall context. In thinking about diseases such as COVID-19, patients exhibit a bifurcation in their clotting activity. Generally speaking, patients with mild ones manage an overactive state of clotting, whereas those with severe ones tend to have reduced, hypocoagulable, reactions. These variations, in all honesty, present a difficult challenge for doctors since critical cases are at risk for bleeding complications. Techniques like turbidimetry and thromboelastography help doctors assess plasma hemostasis, although admittedly these tests are not perfect (Elena et al., 2024). Summing it all up, the clot-dissolving mechanism is as important as the clot-forming one.

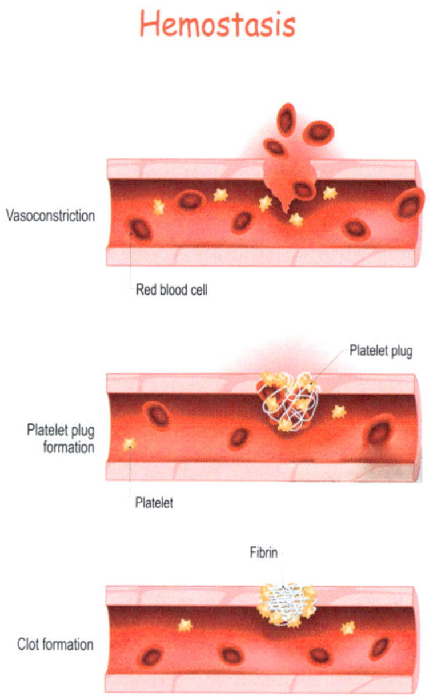

Figure 7.2. Hemostasis process.

Source: https://study.com/cimages/multimages/16/plateletplug.jpg.

The switch between clot formation and dissolution depends on a delicate equilibrium between clot-promoting and anti-clotting factors. Platelets, for instance, aren't only busy forming clots; they assist in repairing and re-establishing blood flow after injury. In this regard, signals from such agents as nicotine might direct the system toward an equalized hemostasis or, in the event of a mistake, trigger excessive clotting. Such a closer investigation of how multiple mediators modulate platelet activity, then, might reveal new avenues for treating both bleeding and thrombotic disease. More studies have continued to shed some light—though quite an erratic one—at the various twists of clotting processes in varied states of health (Wu et al., 2025) (Figure 7.2).

7.1.1. Stages of Hemostasis

When a blood vessel ruptures, the body quickly activates an emergency process to close the wound. In no time, the vessel narrows—a kind of sudden pinch that slows down blood flow to the injured part. Later, inner substance like collagen and other adhesive substances come to the surface, inviting platelets to stay. These platelets then pile up into quite a disorganized fashion, forming what seems to be a weak white plug that lays the groundwork for a later stronger clot. The interaction between these piling-up cells and the inner vessel lining is highly important; even minor mistakes in this process will at times lead to issues like untimely clots or too much blood loss. For the most part, being aware of these early nuances is important to looking at the bigger picture of how our body responds to damage. When that initial patch forms, a secondary chain reaction begins—the coagulation cascade. Most often, this starts with the conversion of prothrombin to thrombin, an enzyme that behaves almost like a master switch. Thrombin then gets the task of converting fibrinogen, a soluble plasma protein, into fibrin, spinning a more resistant network in conjunction with the adhesive platelets. Strange as it may seem, thrombin also amplifies the entire process by switching on additional platelets and clotting factors. Its function can be adjusted by factors such as the amount of natural blood thinners circulating in the bloodstream, so this aspect is a sensitive balancing act. In the final phase of this process, the clot becomes mature and subsequently slowly degrades through fibrinolysis so that normal blood flow is not obstructed once healing is well established. The clot is remodeled here—a process that may be interrupted in liver disease or following procedures like an orthotopic liver transplant. On rare occasions, elevated concentrations of tissue-type plasminogen activator (t-PA) break down clots too quickly and cause what we call hyperfibrinolysis—a situation that can greatly complicate hemostatic management. Such technologies as thromboelastography (TEG) and rotational thromboelastometry (ROTEM) appear to be valuable tools for monitoring clot activity in real time—an especially important capability in neonatal practice, where clotting behavior tends to differ from that observed in adults. All in all, watching this dynamic process shows us a lot about the way our bodies react to bleeding, and it teaches better treatment methods in the clinic (Argentiero et al., 2021; Bontempo et al., 1989) (Figure 7.3).

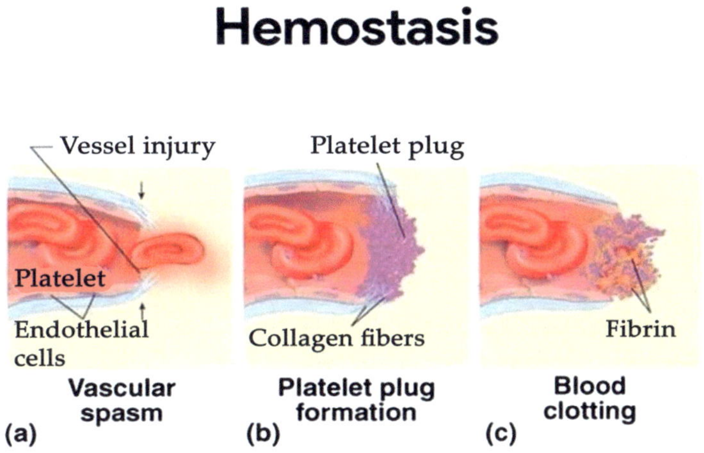

Figure 7.3. Stages of hemostasis.

Source: https://external-content.duckduckgo.com/iu/?u=https%3A%2F%2Fcdn.medizzy.com%2FAISyngodzqt24mRd2n5s5xMlrxQ%3D%2F680x508%2Fimg%2Fposts%2F44c9af0e-020e-4731-89af-0e020e4731e5&f=1&nofb=1&ipt=b491e5fc676addb98246dbfed9bc33-38d87c04be62179d746b9b92853aeeac01.

7.1.2. Role of blood vessels in hemostasis

Blood vessels and the surrounding cells set the hemostatic process in motion in a relatively active way. When a vessel is struck by trauma, its internal membrane—nearly the endothelium—instantly wakes up and sends out a flurry of chemical messages to direct the reaction. The vessel-lining cells produce chemicals that activate platelets to clump together and also uncover sticky molecules that beckon the platelets. This transition is critical: platelets progress from a resting state to one in which they tenaciously adhere to injured tissues, rapidly forming a temporary plug. In the vast majority of cases, this initial burst of activity not only halts blood loss but serves as the foundation for later stages of coagulation. Clearly, that inner lining isn't lingering for the sake of entertainment; it triggers the whole process by providing the correct signals. Blood vessels aren't just giving a platelet surface to stick to—they're actually controlling the blood pressure and flow past the injury, too. Most of the time, the smooth muscle of the vessel wall will immediately contract, restricting blood to the injured area—a process we call vasoconstriction. This is quite an important response since it reduces blood loss as the more involved cellular processes get started. Damaged endothelial cells also release substances like endothelin, which actually narrows the vessels further, showing that blood vessels are not just passive responders in the case of clotting regulation but are actually active contributors. Basically, they regulate the overall clotting dynamics and do not just wait passively for things to happen. Blood vessels again have an integral role to play as the body shifts attention from clumping the platelets to healing the tissue. The mechanism changes over to simple clumping to spinning a fibrin mesh that consolidates the plug. Both activated platelets' and damaged vessel lining's enzymes—utilize tissue factor, for example—help to bring about the transition in the clotting cascade. Interestingly, the way in which blood vessels interact with these coagulation factors relates to the vessel as a whole being healthy; the slightest dysfunction in the endothelial function will lead to serious complications when there is trauma. For instance, when the vessel lining does not work properly it can cause excessive fibrinolysis, something that has been seen, for instance, in cases like orthotopic liver transplantation (Bontempo et al., 1989). Broadly speaking, it is essential that such interaction is comprehended if we want to develop therapy for bleeding disorders and achieve efficient coagulation (Carestia et al., 2016).

7.1.3. Importance of platelets in the hemostatic process

Platelets and blood vessel walls ally together in a surprisingly important partnership to prevent bleeding. During a wound, the cells that make up our blood vessel walls spring into action and lay open collagen along with other fragments of the extracellular matrix that attract platelets—this initial stickiness is what sets the whole process in motion. Within seconds, platelets flow to the wound and start to change their shape and release signals to bring in even more platelets. The mad activity, combined with clotting factors, finally constricts into a firm plug that seals tiny breaches and keeps the blood from being lost. Apart from some special circumstances, this rapid platelet response is vital so that there can be a satisfactory barrier formed to shelter the critical blood supply whilst healing takes place (Neubauer et al., 2021). Platelets do not just clump at a wound. They also direct the whole clotting process. The moment they're activated, these tiny cells release granules full of clotting material that triggers both thrombin generation and fibrin synthesis—two key ingredients of a tight clot. While they do that, they also keep pro-clotting and anti-clotting signals in balance, typically nudging the lining of a blood vessel with gentle encouragement.

Overall, this balance is particularly important in disease states like COVID-19, where it's all too easy for everything to tip into over-clotting or unexpected bleeding. This equilibrium, though delicate, is the cornerstone of understanding platelet regulation of hemostasis and how their dysregulated function can be behind significant bleeding or clotting disorders (Colling et al., 2020). Closer examination of platelet function offers an insight into not only normal physiological function but also the manner in which things are disrupted during disease. If platelets do not behave as expected, the outcomes may vary from a trivial issue with bleeding to life-threatening thrombosis. In systemic disease such as COVID-19, research has noted that platelets sometimes become overactive—essentially, they go into overdrive and aggravate the clotting issue, in some cases resulting in complications such as venous thromboembolism. It would appear that these observations underscore the need for more research into how platelets get activated and affect the rest of the clotting machinery. By demystifying platelet complexity, researchers and clinicians can better comprehend how to act when balance is disrupted, ultimately maximizing treatment for victims (Neubauer et al., 2021) (Figure 7.4).

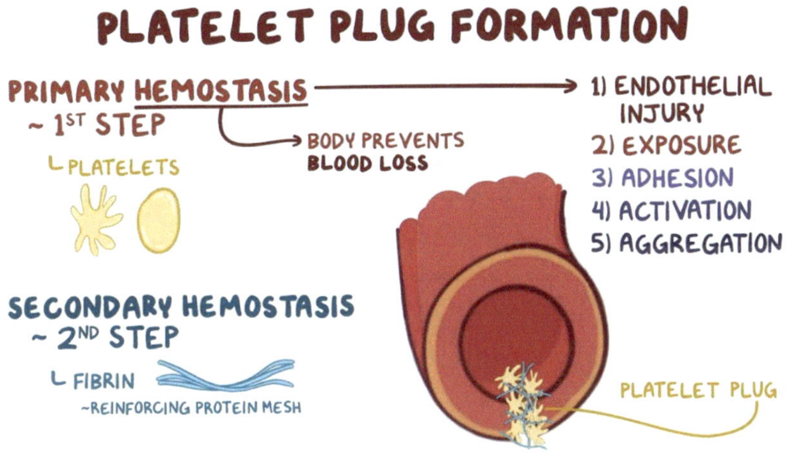

Figure 7.4. Platelets in the hemostatic process.

Source: https://d16qt3wv6xm098.cloudfront.net/GnStjWilTkmG4GkMjcsBhr45QuumZBYj/_.jpg.

Test Your Knowledge

1. What are the three main stages of the hemostatic process, and how do they interact?
2. How does vascular spasm contribute to the prevention of blood loss?

7.2. Coagulation Cascade

Learning Outcome

- Intrinsic pathway of coagulation;
- Extrinsic pathway of coagulation;
- Common pathway and fibrin formation.

The process of blood clotting is not just a simple reaction—it's a series of complex enzyme-catalyzed steps that builds an insoluble barrier when there is injury. It all starts when damage signals invite the platelets to aggregate, and subsequently, the internal and external pathways, in a parallel manner. They eventually merge. In most cases, this merging causes fibrinogen to change into fibrin, forming a kind of net that holds everything in place. Slight glitches in this delicate chain can lead to issues like thrombosis or too much bleeding. Researchers, in most cases, now point out that conditions such as multiple sclerosis (Fornasiero et al., 2019) may be affected by these clotting factors in ways we're only beginning to understand. The link between this clotting cascade and the immune system came back into focus in the past decades. People have learned that mediators like thrombin and factor X aren't just busy with hemostasis—these seem to trigger inflammatory responses, too. Most of the time, seeing these clot signs in other diseases implies a subtle exchange between clotting and immune responses. For example, in multiple sclerosis, immune and clotting processes have been found to be affecting each other much more than ever thought (Fornasiero et al., 2019). This means that in order to really comprehend blood clots, you need to consider the interaction between a wide range of functions in the body and not compartmentalize clotting as an isolated event. Computational techniques, especially reaction systems (RSs), have, in most cases, revolutionized the manner in which scientists investigate the dynamics of blood clotting. Instead of relying solely on conventional mechanisms, scientists can now use software like BioReSolve to model the behavior of different clotting factors and inhibitors in order to investigate complicated interactions. This exercise, though a bit unconventional at times, has yielded new insights regarding diseases such as thrombophilia and thromboembolism. Briefly, it seems that, in general, computational biology not only deconstructs these intricate processes but also helps design particular treatments—a consideration which may actually come into play when dealing with coagulation disorders (Figure 7.5).

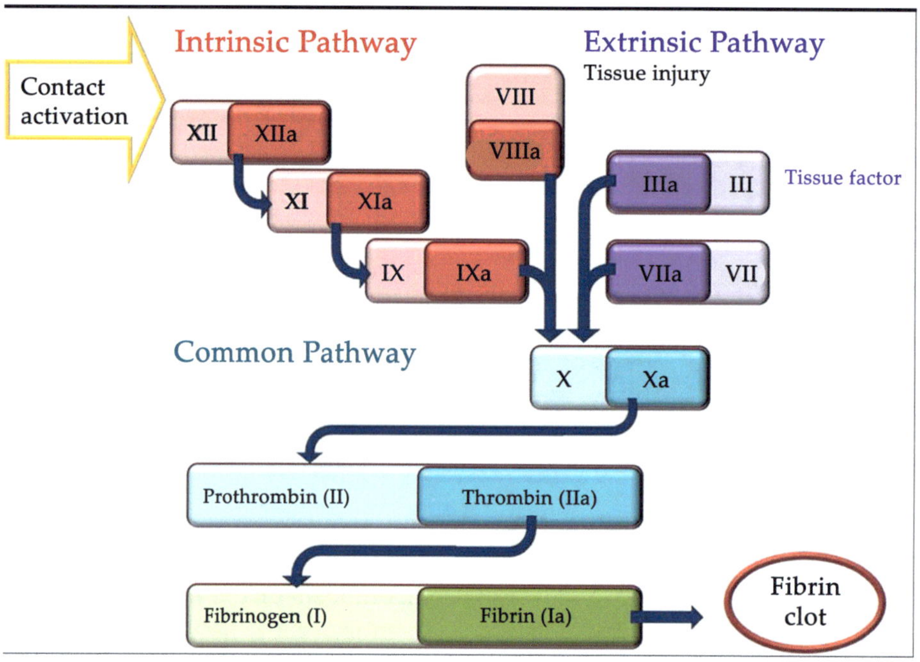

Figure 7.5. Coagulation cascade.

Source: https://www.researchgate.net/publication/381361545/figure/fig1/AS:11431281251517672@1718244830856/A-schematic-overview-of-the-coagulation-cascade-The-coagulation-process-can-be-triggered.ppm.

7.2.1. Intrinsic pathway of coagulation

Coagulation through the intrinsic pathway is triggered when a blood vessel is damaged—it's among the body's quick reactions to blood loss. When blood touches negatively charged surfaces, a chain reaction is triggered. Factor XII is triggered first, which sets off a chain of activation that then engages factor XI, and then factors IX and X join the fray. At the end of this cascade, thrombin emerges; it is responsible for turning fibrinogen into fibrin to create a stable clot, and even gives a kick to trigger the extrinsic pathway. For the most part, this double function is geared to maintain bleeding in check and help with healing, showing that this pathway is very important to our overall blood balance. The path is not only about inhibiting bleeding—it also intersects with other health issues, especially when inflammation or immune response come into the equation. Recent studies in general have shed light on the fact that coagulation factors tend to get mingled with inflammatory mediators, so some of the intrinsic pathway may affect the way our immune system will respond. For example, research in multiple sclerosis shows that elements like thrombin and factor XII can interfere with our natural immunity, a possibility that could initiate neuroinflammation into overdrive.

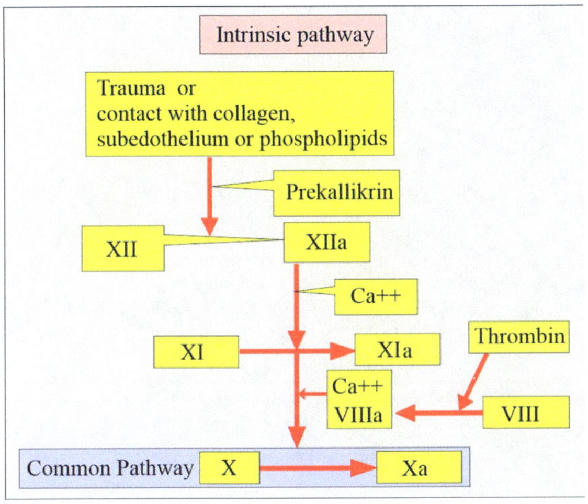

Figure 7.6. Intrinsic pathway of coagulation.

Source: https://labpedia.net/wp-content/uploads/2020/01/Intrinsic-pathway-cycle-1.jpg.

This shows that while the main role of the intrinsic pathway is the control of hemostasis, its influence on immune regulation too leaves us with a glimpse that more is required in the way of illumination of such interactions and their clinic implications (Fornasiero et al., 2019). Though critical to its purpose, trying to use the intrinsic pathway to effect therapy isn't without intrigue. Emerging advances—like those with hemoglobin-based oxygen carriers—have questioned how coagulation balance is achieved, especially in coagulopathy and some platelet disorders. These considerations remind us that monkeying around with coagulation needs to be done cautiously or else balance will be achieved in the direction of too much clotting. Furthermore, the art of understanding the subtlety of how this pathway is entwined with the general systemic responses—i.e., when working with resuscitation in regions with limited medical interventions—is crucial in producing better patient outcomes. Future research, in most cases, has no option but to face such complexities to formulate treatments that take advantage of the inherent pathway without causing unexpected risks (Holtby et al., 2014) (Figure 7.6).

7.2.2. Extrinsic pathway of coagulation

When a blood vessel is wounded, the body jumps into action to prevent bleeding in the first instance. The extrinsic coagulation pathway is triggered immediately—largely—to deal with tissue damage. TF, or tissue factor, is released by the injured cells and comes into contact with factor VII in the bloodstream; they form a TF-VIIa complex that speeds up events. This cascade activates factor X to function, which in turn feeds into thrombin generation and mobilizes fibrinogen into conversion to fibrin. Basically, this rapid chain forms a rapid plug that keeps blood loss under control from the onset, and this is a critical component of overall hemostatic control. How this pathway fits into the entire clotting process is intriguing. Unlike the intrinsic, slower pathway, the extrinsic path responds essentially at once—it fills the virtually instantaneous space between damage and clotting. Upon activation of factor X, both initiators of the extrinsic and intrinsic pathways lead into so-called the common pathway. In most cases, it is necessary for the coordinated action, which allows the body to react in due time to limit blood loss in trauma without a loss of control. Platelets get their turn here, as well, by responding instantly by adhering to naked collagen when a blood vessel is severed.

They form a transient plug—a type of speed bump, physical barrier—that is soon stabilized by a fibrin network formed in the course of the coagulation cascade. The interaction of platelets, tissue factor, and sequence of clotting factors uncovers how complex and dynamic hemostasis is. This multifunctional response not only is responsible for rapid cessation of bleeding but also prevents clotting from becoming uncontrolled, pointing to the delicate balance that needs to be struck in order to maintain vascular integrity (Bronowski et al., 2020; Oliveira et al., 2018) (Figure 7.7).

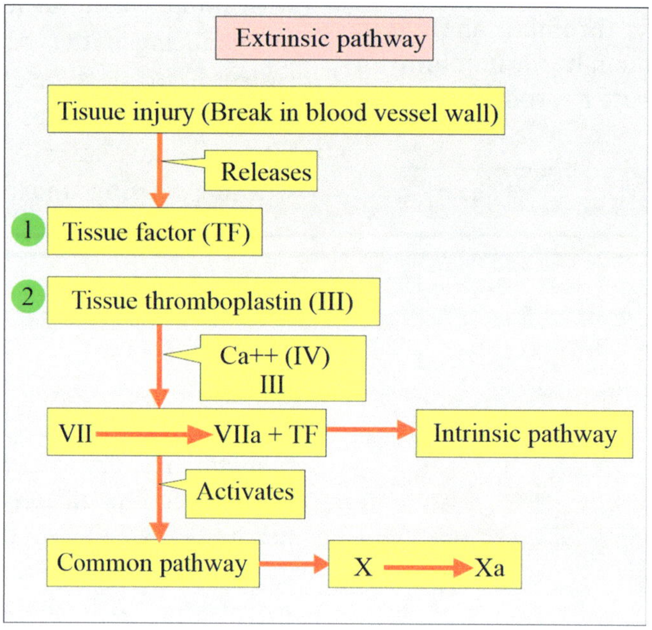

Figure 7.7. Extrinsic pathway of coagulation.

Source: https://labpedia.net/wp-content/uploads/2020/01/Extrinsic-pathway-cycle-1.jpg.

7.2.3. Common pathway and fibrin formation

Blood coagulation is a fascinating mix of biology that goes on just under our skin. Our vessels stay intact thanks to a cascade of events in which cells and molecules get along and have things happen that just work. The process isn't cut into neat steps – it's more of a mix of the intrinsic and extrinsic pathways that come together in what's known as the common pathway. Factor Xa then takes over at a certain point and catalyzes prothrombin to thrombin, which catalyzes fibrinogen into strands of fibrin. This from liquid to a type of gel process works really effectively in solidifying your initial platelet plug better, on the whole, and keeping you from losing too much blood when you are cut. All is not quite so straightforward, though. Fibrin does not happen by chance; it is part of an actively maintained dance, emphasizing how much attention the body gives to balancing things. Thrombin, seemingly paradoxically, is both an enabler for clotting and a self-regulator to prevent too much buildup in the first place. In most cases, a little give-and-take like that prevents clots from forming where they shouldn't. You'll even notice things like tissue factor playing a role in this cascade, initiating clotting only when absolutely necessary (Bronowski et al., 2020). This careful, sometimes redundant game of cat and mouse shows you just how much we need our clotting processes to be so finely tuned to maintain cardiovascular health. Step back and take a look at the bigger picture, and you'll also be impressed with some evolutionary flair. Certain animals – take mammals that hibernate as an example – have evolved unique adaptations such that their blood still clots properly even as their metabolism slows nearly to a stop and their body temperatures fall. Research finds that even with all the variations, the basic components of the clotting mechanism itself differ little from one species to the next (Cullinan et al., 2015). Most commonly, awareness of such natural mechanisms not only informs us about the complex processes by which our bodies respond to injury but also stimulates us to novel ways of regulation of clotting in the clinical setting.

Test Your Knowledge

1. What are the differences between the intrinsic, extrinsic, and common pathways of the coagulation cascade?
2. How does thrombin function as a central enzyme in the coagulation process?

7.3. Factors Influencing Coagulation

Learning Outcome

- Genetic factors affecting coagulation;
- Environmental factors and their impact;
- Medications that influence coagulation.

Blood clotting isn't so simple as many would believe—it's a dance of a number of factors from within and without your body. The health of your blood vessels is one of the key players here. When the inner lining, the endothelial cells, is healthy, it releases signals such as nitric oxide and prostacyclin that keep platelets in check and provide blood vessels with a little leeway. If something causes damage to the tissue, the underlying collagen is exposed, which stimulates platelets to stay and trigger the clotting cascade. Meanwhile, the balance of chemicals in your blood that either prevent or favor clots creates the whole process tending one way or another. Overall, the awareness of this dynamic is essential for coming up with treatments—especially for patients who have stents, where the risk of clots is enormous (Kalaskar et al., 2023). Your genes add another piece to this complex picture. Usually, how your body stops bleeding depends very much on what you are born with. Small differences in clotting factor genes allow for creating diseases such as hemophilia, where the body is defective in creating clots. And there are gene variations that regulate platelet response to stress, so responses to clotting vary slightly in each individual. Apart from genetics, diet, exercise, and even medication you're taking can regulate expression of clotting genes. Vitamins K and D, through their natural function in the assembly of clotting factors, can also control tendencies to bleed. Taking these genetic and lifestyle variables together not only makes sense of individual health risk but also directs more specific medical decisions (Oliveira et al., 2018). Last but not least is the role of bioactive agents, which is particularly tantalizing in the field of medical devices. Take stents, for instance—newer stents have traditionally been coated with bioactive coatings that more closely match up with blood. The coatings can contain clot-fighting drugs and be surface-modified so that they moderate reactions that could form clots. Innovations like nano-coatings have only started to appear, with much potential in changing the way that these devices interact with blood. The surface properties, including how charged or hydrophilic they are, play a critical role in the manner in which platelets respond once they have been in contact. Ongoing research on these interactions not only further refines device design but can also be shown to enhance safety and duration during procedures, especially in interventional cardiology (Kalaskar et al., 2023).

7.3.1. Genetic factors affecting coagulation

Coagulation genetics matters because it teaches us about how our bodies keep flowing blood in balance. Tiny molecules called microRNAs—small fragments of non-coding RNA—are in the spotlight right now because they quietly regulate our genes. They've even been linked to venous thrombosis and could potentially be markers for clotting disorders. One study from the Genetic Analysis of Idiopathic Thrombophilia (GAIT-2) Project, for example, identified microRNAs (miRNAs) such as hsa-miR-885-5p and hsa-miR-192-5p and their role in blood clotting. The discovery of 1,323 genetic variations that change the levels of such miRNAs gives us a better understanding of how our genes interfere with hemostasis and points to—quite temptingly—routes that could raise an individual's susceptibility to clot formation (Rodríguez et al., 2020). Genetic oddities also jumble up how our clotting mechanism functions, particularly when considering the intrinsic and extrinsic limbs of the cascade. For the most part, studies indicate that normal gene variations can alter how factors like Factor IX and von Willebrand Factor function—both quite important in clotting. When these factors malfunction, they sometimes cause prothrombotic characteristics. It's a complex waltz, really; knowing the genetics of these factors may allow us to understand conditions such as acute ischemic stroke, in which coagulation is a significant player. As our understanding continues to improve, the addition of genetic hints will also hopefully be instrumental in refining antithrombotic therapy while balancing bleeding risks (Ceulemans et al., 2024). Consider inherited diseases such as hemophilia, for example—they elegantly demonstrate how significantly genes can influence blood clotting. Genetic mutations in the clotting factor genes can result in excess bleeding or incorrect clotting, pointing to just how sensitive this balance really is. New genetics tests not only raise our diagnostic capabilities but also introduce a gateway to tailored treatments engineered just for you; occasionally the same gene mutations even emerge during risk analysis. Overall, all these findings highlight, in a very human way, that genetics plays a vital role in hemostasis and also in coagulation, directing future research towards tackling bleeding and clotting hazards more effectively (Rodríguez et al., 2020) (Figure 7.8).

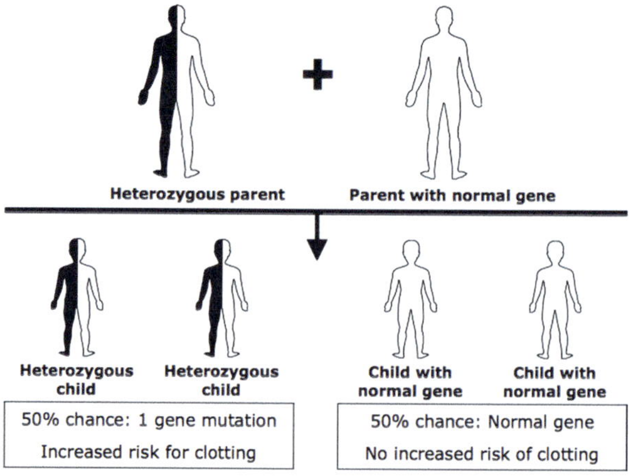

Figure 7.8. Genetic factors affecting coagulation.

Source: https://www.stoptheclot.org/wp-content/uploads/2013/11/Screen-Shot-2013-11-21-at-3.21.35-PM-300x221.png.

7.3.2. Environmental factors and their impact

Hemostasis and coagulation don't just work on the body's internal systems; they're also very sensitive to what's occurring in our environment. Temperature, humidity, and even toxin exposure – all of which can nudge the chemistry of clotting and dissolution in some fairly unexpected ways. Take a warmer day as an example; that extra heat has the potential to make some of the enzymes more active, maybe tipping the balance towards a thicker blood in some people. This is especially important when conditions are not being consistent—think of outdoor athletes or workers who work in uncooperative weather. Toxins like heavy metals and industrial chemicals may interfere with the normal role of platelets and make the lining of blood vessels irregular, disrupting the balance. In most cases, understanding how the environment affects clotting is crucial in designing treatments that are able to effectively manage coagulation disorders. It's not just what we have in the air surrounding us—what we eat plays a major role here as well. Nutritional inadequacies can lead to the inability of the body to produce the clotting factors it needs. Vitamins, including vitamin K, and minerals such as calcium are very core in keeping these functions in balance. Research generally shows that communities without access to a well-balanced diet experience more with bleeding or clotting problems. Addressing these gaps, then, isn't just about nutrition—it's a step toward tuning up the whole coagulation system to stave off heart issues. The way our eating habits and our environment weave together really drives home how health solutions need to consider both what's inside us and what we're exposed to. New evidence also hints at a cold prospect: changing the immediate environment of an injury may help in healing and smooth out clotting issues. A few of the new treatments now consist of scaffolds loaded with growth factors that seem to get the job done where it must occur. These scaffolds change the immediate setting of the wound, improving healing and minimizing the difficulties that come as a result of faulty hemostasis. This kind of strategy is true innovation, especially in clinics that are managing chronic, recalcitrant wounds. Through a synergistic combination of biomaterials and active biological substances in therapy protocols, we might really be tackling both problems of optimizing coagulation as well as healing acceleration. Further research in the majority of cases suggests that a shift in comprehending the interaction between the environment and our body might actually revolutionize the way we treat blood diseases and wound healing (N/A, 2021; Tottoli et al., 2020).

7.3.3. Medications That Influence Coagulation

It is a delicate dance to regulate blood clotting, with numerous drugs available to either start the clotting process or prevent it. Warfarin, for instance, an old friend vitamin K antagonist, is widely used in the upkeep of thromboembolic issues in the long term. Still, overall, its narrow margin of safety and the constant balancing act between certain foods and other drugs in use make the administration of it a fine art. When doctors need to reverse its anticoagulant properties on an emergency basis, they can fall back on options like fresh-frozen plasma or prothrombin complex concentrates, although these also carry their own complications—sometimes in the form of uncoordinated infusion issues or delayed onset. In more recent times, there has been a growing call to examine newer agents that would reverse these effects more rapidly, indicating that studies in this area of patient care are not only warranted but already under way. In over-anticoagulation—particularly when warfarin is a bit too zealous—giving recombinant factor VIIa (rFVIIa) has been a promising intervention. Several studies indicate rFVIIa lowers the international normalized ratio (INR) quickly, with no serious side effects normally associated with more traditional therapy in the form of fresh-frozen plasma. Because it can resupply procoagulant factors into the bloodstream with measurable speed, rFVIIa seems to be an extremely attractive option in acute clinical settings where immediate hemostasis is a necessity. All the same, however, supporting evidence for rFVIIa remains in its infancy, and prudence is certainly to be recommended before sweeping changes to usual protocols are introduced. Clinicians, most often, must balance potential instant gains with potentially unforeseen dangers—highlighting the need for further controlled trials to establish firmly its role within practice (Deveras et al., 2002). It also helps to have a sound grasp of the finer points of blood clotting, specifically in the setting of postpartum hemorrhage (PPH). Pregnant patients, as might be anticipated, have higher concentrations of clotting factors, which creates a characteristic clotting profile that could make bleeding harder to control than in the nonpregnant patient. Routine investigations, though commonly used, may not always represent the true state of coagulation in such cases due to the peculiar physiological alterations occurring in pregnancy. Therefore, some parameters such as fibrinogen are also points of focus while predicting possible hemorrhagic complications (Solomon et al., 2014). Researchers are also more actively pursuing the optimization of testing methods—like point-of-care devices like thromboelastography—that give more active feedback regarding a patient's coagulability, and might inform more specific and efficacious interventions in emergency crises within PPH and other kinds of surgical disasters (Figure 7.9).

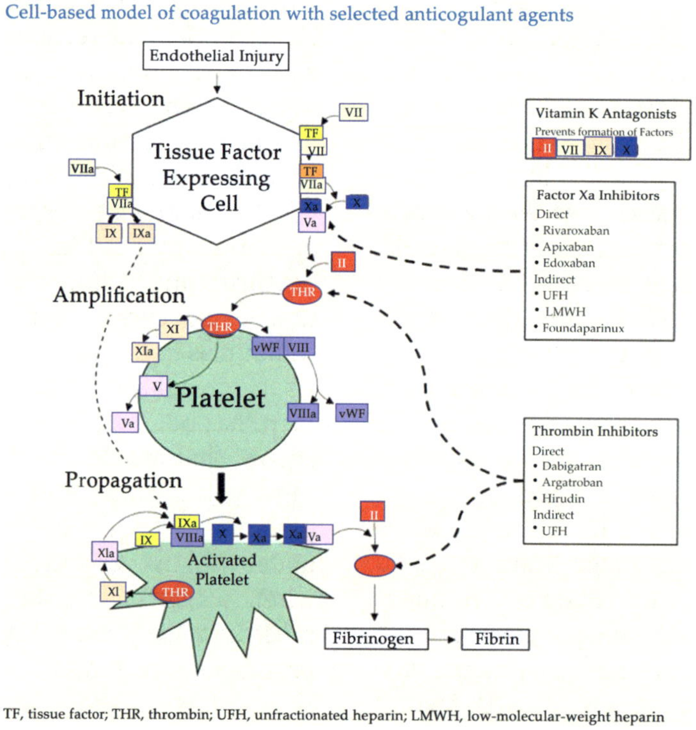

Figure 7.9. Drugs affecting coagulation.

Source: https://ars.els-cdn.com/content/image/1-s2.0-S147202992100196X-gr1.jpg.

Test Your Knowledge

1. How do vitamin K and calcium ions contribute to the coagulation process?
2. In what way do anticoagulant proteins (such as protein C and antithrombin) regulate clot formation?

7.4. Disorders of Hemostasis

Learning Outcome

- Hemophilia and its types;
- Thrombosis and its implications;
- Other bleeding disorders.

The body's clotting system works like a delicate dance—different processes mesh to keep blood vessels sturdy and stop heavy bleeding. Sometimes, though, this balance goes off, and the body either clots too readily or doesn't clot enough. It usually boils down to a mix of factors we're born with, conditions that crop up later, or even things in our surroundings. For instance, people with congenital clotting disorders (say, hemophilia) show that even a small genetic flaw can lead to huge bleeding issues. In the meantime, chronic conditions—chronic is perhaps too strong a term, but diseases like diabetes—can disrupt platelet binding to vessel walls, further adding to the whole clotting process. In most cases, they all work together, and it becomes relatively clear that being aware of these problems is going to be beneficial to knowing about overall health. Small vessel flow and how platelets respond is relevant when something happens wrong with clotting. An example of diabetic foot syndrome is a good one: this will mess up small-sized vascular tubes and upset the clotting ratio. It is not uncommon that patients show some form of overzealous platelet response, which ends up causing unwanted clots.

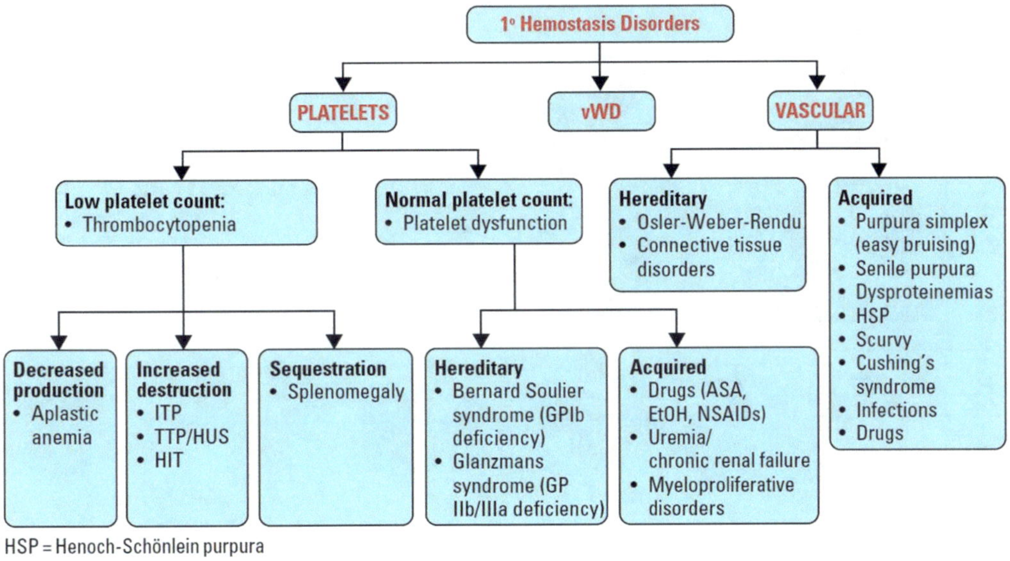

Figure 7.10. Disorders of hemostasis.

Source: https://encrypted-tbn0.gstatic.com/images?q=tbn:ANd9GcR_Gam67cTRLlZkUvbKVUFGaRpBKjjz48nTuA&s.

Their causes are an interwoven mix of dysregulation of clotting and metabolic dysbalances. A study revealed that approximately 65–80% of patients with diabetes also experience cardiovascular complications—a statistic that underscores both the extent and frequency of these issues. Understand these facts can become tricky at times, but it plays a role in organizing better ways of preventing and treating the disorders. With treatment, the approach is two-fold: you must stop the clots from forming as a problem, but not inhibit the body from closing an injury when necessary. Healthcare workers often opt for drugs like anticoagulants, antiplatelet medications, and even clotting factor replacements depending on the situation, so each is individually tailored to the patient's idiosyncrasies. Patients with an underlying condition may hide or even exacerbate the clotting problem, so each strategy is individually designed. New research even factors in gene therapies and other emerging medicines that try to counteract the system into balance. Overall, this continually shifting context—yes, it can get a little out of control—highlights the importance of continuous education and vigilant surveillance in healthcare to ensure improved outcomes (Figure 7.10).

7.4.1. Hemophilia and Its Types

The clotting process has much underlying complexity to explain why people bleed excessively—hemophilia being a good example. It isn't neatly categorized, but hemophilia does predominantly occur in two forms: one where factor VIII is missing (hemophilia A) and another involving a lack of factor IX, commonly called Christmas disease.

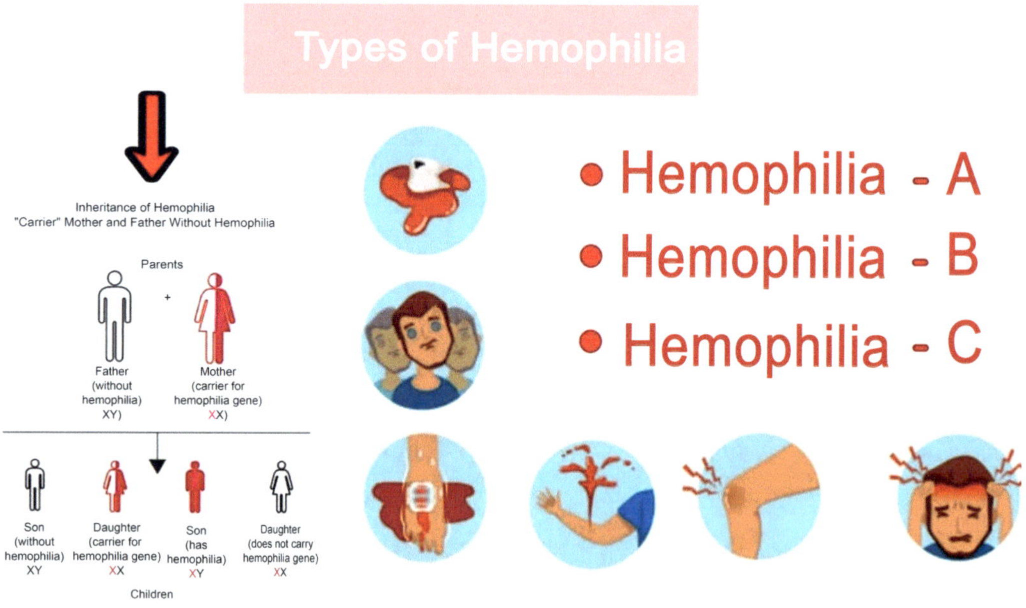

Figure 7.11. Hemophilia and its types.

Source: https://medsurgeindia.com/wp-content/uploads/2023/06/Types-of-Hemophilia.webp.

When these key components are not present in sufficient amounts, even a minor wound or a routine operation can lead to uncontrolled bleeding. In short, by understanding how the body typically manages a bleed, surgeons can better engineer treatments to improve the quality of life and prevent life-threatening complications. Treatment, in most cases, is a matter of replacement therapy. Doctors use factor concentrates as a replacement for what the body cannot naturally supply, usually to gain control over bleeding episodes. There's just one catch—in certain patients, the immune system may start rejecting these transfusions by developing so-called inhibitory alloantibodies. This immunological complication, for the most part, complicates treatment, raises the risk of secondary complications, and even raises management costs. Recent research has highlighted the importance of further investigating these inhibitors, especially since other inherited bleeding disorders have not been so precisely documented (Franchini et al., 2017). Uncovering why patients develop these antibodies might just lead to more targeted treatment options. Other than the treatments themselves, the whole scenario calls for proper patient examination and sane prevention measures, particularly in environments where bleeding is more likely, like when conducting surgery or dental work. Numerous studies emphasized the importance of having a proper natural clotting mechanism in upholding patient safety during invasive procedures. A detailed history, if at times laborious, may be the key to preventing future complications—emphasizing the value of both keen diagnostics and comprehensive treatment protocols. When you join the dots of the big picture of inherited clotting disorders—not just hemophilia A and B, but disorders such as Von Willebrand disease—you're basically looking at a collaborative effort to maximize both safety and treatment efficacy (Lozano et al., 2011) (Figure 7.11).

7.4.2. Thrombosis and Its implications

Thrombosis is a sloppy subject that plays an enormous part in how our bodies stop bleeding, especially if you include heart health. It likes to get started when clotting is caused in all the wrong directions, and then that can lead to some not-so-good things like heart attacks and strokes. There's a feeling growing now that inflammation—yes, the same inflammation that causes atherosclerosis—is closely linked with clotting. On other occasions, that inflammation not only stores plaques but also makes more likely that acute, destructive clot events will arise when plaques burst. In the patient and laboratory studies, in the majority of cases, however, are showing that inflammation is prompting platelet adhesiveness and actually causing the development of clots by way of tissue factors, thereby determining overall thrombotic outcomes. In short, a greater grasp of this connection can offer new possibilities to target clot-related issues with atherosclerosis and other inflammatory disorders (D'Ugo et al., 2016). The action of thrombosis is not limited to acute cardiac emergencies; its role percolates through chronic diseases like liver disease, where the fine balance of clotting can really go haywire. For example, in severe chronic liver disease the liver's management of clotting factors becomes all muddled—think proteins like von Willebrand factor (VWF), the enabler of platelets to coalesce into clots. Elevated levels of VWF, in the majority of cases, act as a kind of red flag for portal hypertension and signify heightened risk for thrombotic events. Of especial interest is the interaction between ADAMTS13 and VWF, an enzyme that degrades VWF into fragments; when ADAMTS13 activity is absent, patients seem to suffer more clot risk, thus worsen liver-related complications. Therefore, management of thrombosis not only requires immediate medical intervention but also a deeper understanding of its biochemical pathogenesis (Karsdal et al., 2023). Aside from addressing outright clot danger, there's a new notion that anti-inflammatory therapies may be particularly key to alleviating thrombosis. Typically, studies indicate that by suppressing the inflammatory reaction of the body, one can decrease both the frequency and intensity of clotting events—particularly in individuals who already have ongoing inflammation. This form of therapy can even calm down those unstable atherosclerotic plaques, preventing them from rupturing and activating a potentially life-threatening chain reaction. And these types of treatments can even normalize the way the body forms and then breaks down clots (the thrombotic and fibrinolytic systems), something that would be particularly helpful for patients with conditions like obesity where traditional risk factors aren't always apparent. More generally, building on our current understanding of thrombosis and its-reaching consequences seems essential to the creation of new therapies aimed at reducing both harm and loss of life from these complications (D'Ugo et al., 2016) (Figure 7.12).

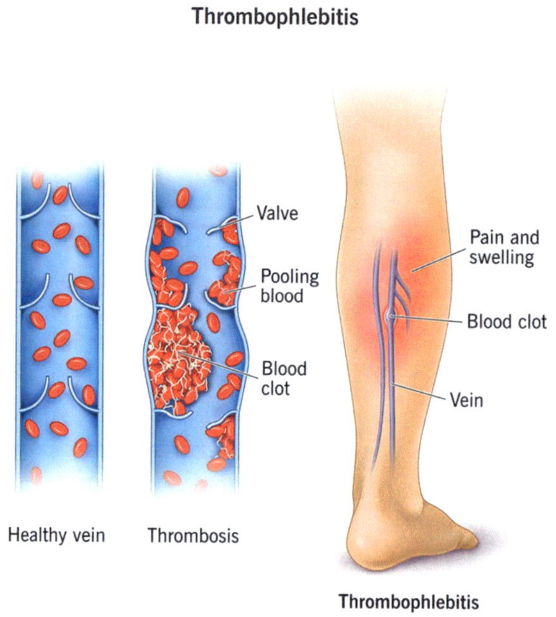

Figure 7.12. Thrombosis and its implications.

Source: https://my.clevelandclinic.org/-/scassets/images/org/health/articles/23311-thrombophlebitis.

7.4.3. Other Bleeding Disorders

Hemostasis isn't limited to hemophilia A or B—there's an entire cohort of less frequent inherited bleeding disorders that throw additional complications into the mix. These disorders sometimes produce undesirable surprises, like the development of inhibitors (basically, alloantibodies to clotting factors rather than the usual ones). Hemophilia inhibitors have been researched extensively, yet we still don't fully comprehend how these inhibitors are formed in patients with factor V, VII, XI, and XIII deficiencies. Because these conditions are so rare, overall, the picture of these conditions is still unclear and life is made harder for doctors and researchers. Overall, these knowledge gaps are worth filling because inhibitors can be a genuine monkey wrench in terms of treatment—raising bleeding risks and, by default, healthcare costs (Franchini et al., 2017). Liver disease adds its own twist. With cirrhosis, the liver's production of critical clotting factors crashes, putting patients in the tricky position of being able to bleed easily but also have clotting problems—a paradox. Surgery for such conditions isn't straightforward either; doctors have to work around the complex interwoven complications of the underlying blood diseases, which means taking extra precautions.

Most of the time, understanding how liver deterioration affects the body's coagulation system is a crucial part of the equation because omitting this could lead to serious events like bleeding in the digestive tract or even hepatic encephalopathy, illnesses which have some major risks for illness and death (Bacalbaşa et al., 2019). It's not all about physiology, though—the psychological and social ramifications weigh heavily too. People who have these rare conditions often fight with uncertainty and fear, especially the constant specter of a severe bleeding attack looming over their heads. This emotional weight is sometimes further added to by the shame of visible symptoms or the need for constant medical care. And, quite frankly, the struggle to obtain specialized treatment because the condition is so rare can make people feel very isolated. The more we are aware and know about these problems of bleeding, the more it seems that health systems really do need to consider not just the physical but also the emotional and social side of care—helping patients to cope with their own problems in a more holistic, supportive way.

Test Your Knowledge

1. What are the key differences between bleeding disorders (e.g., hemophilia) and thrombotic disorders (e.g., DVT)?
2. How does von Willebrand disease affect platelet function and clotting?

7.5. Laboratory Assessment of Coagulation

Learning Outcome

- Common tests for coagulation;
- Interpretation of coagulation test results;
- Role of laboratory professionals in coagulation assessment.

Blood clotting isn't as simple as it may sound. Tests in the lab that simply test how well our body is doing with hemostasis and coagulation can teach us a great deal about an individual's clotting health. You perform tests like prothrombin time (PT) and activated partial thromboplastin time (aPTT) – they essentially test the extrinsic and intrinsic pathways, respectively – and have them done routinely to detect any abnormalities, which can be indicative of such conditions as hemophilia or thromboembolic issues. Dependence on these tests is largely on the manner in which they're conducted, the nature of the reagents used, and even sample handling, without mentioning patient-specific idiosyncrasies. Technology has become a lot better in the past several years to the extent that it's much simpler to delve into the nitty-gritty of coagulation factors. In general, the Clauss method is still utilized to quantify fibrinogen levels by essentially seeing how fibrinogen reacts with thrombin to form a fibrin clot. There are, however, hindrances—different reagents and equipment have a tendency to create inconsistency in the results. Some studies (Gaffney et al., 2002) indicate greater values seen in clinical situations such as DIC or while undergoing thrombolysis, which, honestly, makes things more difficult for experts to interpret the results. In most cases, keeping these differences in mind not only enhances the trust in laboratory findings but also helps clinicians make better-informed choices while dealing with clotting diseases. There's also been the shift towards molecular and antigen-based tests that add more layers to the way we assess coagulation. Enzyme-linked immunosorbent assays (ELISAs) and immunonephelometric assays have come onto the scene as new-generation options that can measure specific clotting factors more accurately. While these more recent assays do appear to hold their own against older methods, they have their own set of bugs as well, including antigen level fluctuations—at times even affected by small fibrinogen breakdown. Interaction among these different assays is rather complex at times, with occasional inconsistencies in readings (Gaffney et al., 2002) that may leave clinicians scratching their heads. Finally, selecting the best testing strategy becomes necessary in order to treat patients effectively and maximize treatments with the understanding that no method is perfect (Figure 7.13).

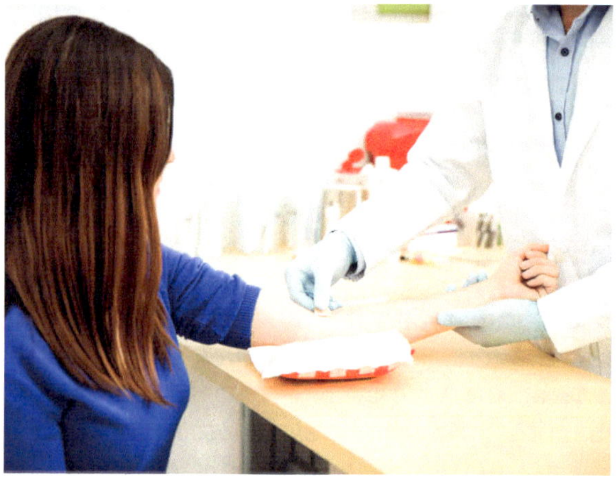

Figure 7.13. Laboratory assessment of coagulation.

Source: https://media.post.rvohealth.io/wp-content/uploads/2020/08/coagulation-tests_thumb.jpg.

7.5.1. Common tests for coagulation

Understanding blood clotting isn't just about memorizing lab tests—it's a bit more involved than that. You've got tests like Prothrombin Time (PT), Activated Partial Thromboplastin Time (aPTT) and even the Platelet Count (PC) all playing a part. Generally speaking, PT is aimed at the extrinsic route, basically keeping an eye on factor VII, whereas aPTT dives into the intrinsic side by checking factors like VIII and IX. These tests are not only used to detect problems; they also help monitor blood-thinning drugs during surgeries, manage bleeding disorders, and sometimes warn that something is amiss and requires a closer look and an altered care plan. In everyday practice—especially in obstetrics—use of these tests turns out to be a real lifesaver.

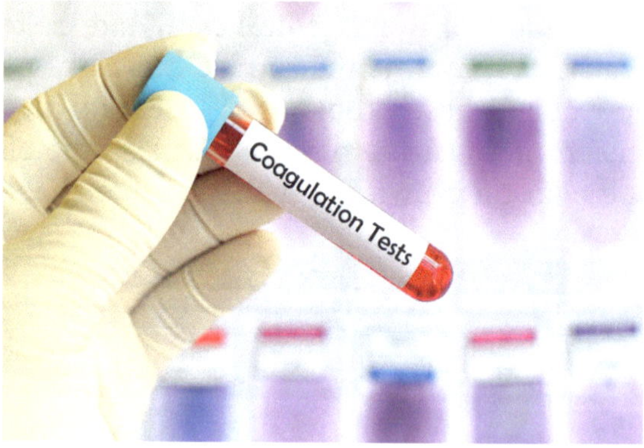

Figure 7.14. Common tests for coagulation.

Source: https://boraxediagnostics.com/wp-content/uploads/2023/10/clotting-profile.jpeg.

Take the case of screening platelet count before conducting neuraxial block in preeclampsia patients among females; in one study, it was shown that almost all patients were screened before they got epidural or spinal anesthesia (Butwick et al., 2013). Such routine screening points towards the need for more open yet standardized testing protocols that push clinicians toward better decisions. Of course, testing will vary slightly from one practitioner to another, so creating guidelines that we can all concur on seems really important if we're going to deal with each patient's risk factors properly. Coagulation becomes hugely complex with all the different pathways and random surprise — inhibitors. In severe hemophilia A and B, for instance, patients can develop alloantibodies against the clotting factors they are given, a surprise that can significantly threaten success with treatment and also general safety (Franchini et al., 2017). Not only do these inhibitors complicate bleeding management but also increase complications and healthcare costs. Detection of such setbacks early by way of regular testing enables alteration of treatment plans in real-time. With advancing familiarity with inhibitors in inherited bleeding disorders, it is increasingly clear that full batteries of clotting tests should guide therapies individually tailored to each patient's specific requirements (Figure 7.14).

7.5.2. Interpretation of coagulation test results

Coagulation test results aren't as straightforward as they seem. Patients arrive with a mix of attributes—age, medication, and overall health—which all can modify the numbers. Blood thinner drugs, for example, can bias results if not accounted for, and different laboratories may perform tests slightly differently. This is to note that procedures like activated partial thromboplastin time (aPTT) and prothrombin time (PT) are especially worthy of mention; really, though, clinicians should remember how these components occlude. Overall, recalling these things can assist in making what the tests say really concur with what's really going on with the patient—even though there is some redundancy here in the ideas. New technology, including high-throughput sequencing (HTS), has pretty much turned the whole process around; they've increased detection of rare bleeding and clotting disorders significantly. For one study that involved 2,396 patients, a significantly high percentage rate of molecular diagnosis was reported, which measures the great impact of new technology. Normally, this is not dealt with by an individual—teams across numerous disciplines sit to discuss the patient's clinical presentation along with genetic data together. Variants become ascribed the classification Pathogenic or sometimes merely indefinite, much like a sign that general tests might miss. In most cases, modern genetic testing is a starting point for identifying inherited bleeding or clotting disorders (Downes et al., 2019). Even with all of those bright ideas, there is room for mistake, especially if you consider what happens before and after the actual analysis. Pre-analytical mistakes, like the manner samples are collected or preserved, can bias the entire test, sometimes misleading clinical judgment. And then, unless the review process afterwards is perfect, the final report might not even represent a patients clinical status. These types of errors can lead to interventions that are not exactly correct and even potentially harm. And so it is that conscientious quality control in laboratories is so imperative—just doing enough to address those loose ends. Recognizing and resolving such difficulty goes a long way to understanding a patient's coagulation profile and guiding better treatment options (Favaloro et al., 2012).

7.5.3. Role of laboratory professionals in coagulation assessment

Laboratory professionals have a key role to play when it comes to figuring out the complex web of blood clotting and stopping bleeding. They spring into action by examining plasma samples for missing factors or unexpected inhibitors that might indicate conditions like thrombosis or hemophilia. In most cases, these professionals do not only conduct tests for detecting bleeding disorders but follow up on treatments as well—like anticoagulant use. Their work, accurate and reliable as it is, actually makes critical decisions regarding patient care, directly affecting individuals. And then there are numerous of these professionals integrating newer technologies into their routine practice. Point-of-care devices have appeared, facilitating quick measurement of blood's ability to clot—a true life-saver in situations of high-pressure stress like cardiopulmonary bypass surgeries (Paniccia et al., 2003). Occasionally, the result of a rapid test can spur the care team into averting uncontrolled blood loss. The union of new technology and traditional lab processes not only boosts productivity at the workflow level but also ties in with improved patient safety, enabling health teams to strike at complications before they get away. Their impact extends far beyond any single diagnosis. By examining clotting profiles for various populations, clinical laboratory scientists help identify trends that would indicate rising risk for thrombotic events or other clotting issues. For example, data collected after events such as community-acquired pneumonia—where markers like D-dimer and thrombin-antithrombin complexes can foretell long-term mortality risk (Kaynar et al., 2011)—all play a part in a broader picture of our hemostatic systems. In all, these results not only guide care today, but also inform research and therapy to come, continually nudging public health in the correct direction (Figure 7.15).

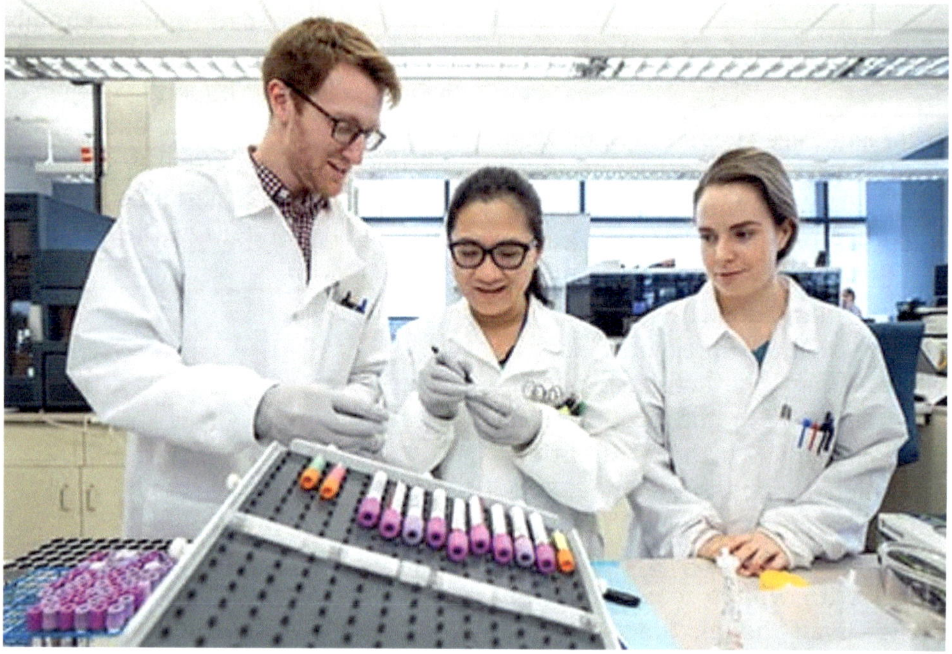

Figure 7.15. Laboratory professionals' collaboration supports accurate and timely patient testing.

Source: https://myadlm.org/~/media/project/myadlm/myadlm/images/publications/cln/articles/2024/janfeb/yale_20200311_2563115_alteredmd_500.jpg?h=333&w=500&hash=0B3EC875E6EA216037814210F3424B0A.

Test Your Knowledge

1. How do PT (Prothrombin Time) and INR help assess the extrinsic pathway of coagulation?
2. What does an aPTT (Activated Partial Thromboplastin Time) test indicate about the intrinsic pathway?

7.6. Treatment and Management of Coagulation Disorders

Learning Outcome

- Pharmacological treatments;
- Non-pharmacological interventions;
- Importance of patient education and management.

Coagulation disorders are complex and generally necessitate that treatment should be specific to the unique situation of each patient. How bad the issue is, what kind of clotting factor is missing, and even overall well-being are all considerations for how it is treated. Hemophilia A and B, for example—since they exclude factor VIII or IX—often involve giving patients concentrates of them. More recent ideas, including taking the clotting factors instead of by IV injection, are being considered to make blood-clotting more effective without the usual needle procedure; this may even help individuals more easily stick to their treatment plan. Most currently, studies have shown that drugs given orally can engender a form of tolerance (Alpan et al., 2007) to enable hemophilia treatment less invasively. In total, this shift points to just how much more we have to try novel ways of treating these disorders. Cooperation certainly enters into play in treating coagulation issues. Frequently, an array of medical professionals—hematologists, internists, and so on—take over and determine what's actually happening before developing a plan that is tailor-made for the patient. Their professionalism is especially crucial when complications develop from other co-related health issues, and these are bound to disrupt normal treatments. Take dental treatment adjustments in patients with bleeding disorders; it's a clear indication that teamwork is a key factor. When specialists speak freely—even if their vocabulary isn't always textbook—patients experience care that weighs medical risks against everyday life (Blanco et al., 2014).

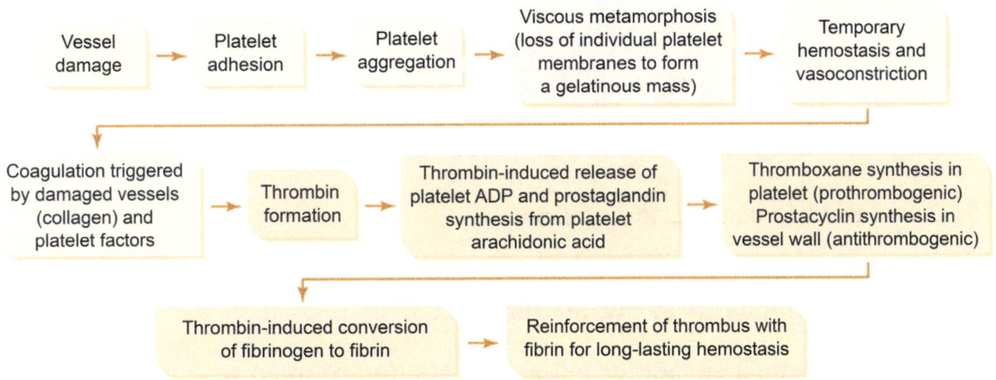

Figure 7.16. Treatment of coagulation disorders.

Source: https://basicmedicalkey.com/wp-content/uploads/2017/04/B978032306812300016X_gr1.jpg.

Generally speaking, this kind of cross-specialty teamwork is critical to better outcomes and to riding out the emotional roller coaster of chronic disease. Medical care isn't the whole story, however; patient education and patient and family support count, as well. If people get the full picture about what their illness is all about, they're more likely to be constructively involved in managing it. Plain instructions including potential difficulties, pre-treatment precautions, and reasons for staying with the treatment can really boost a patient's confidence. And sometimes going to a support group to share experiences and coping tips can lighten the emotional load of enduring long-standing bleeding issues. Together, merging sound medical management with authentic education not only increases quality of life but recognizes that treating coagulation challenges is at least as much of a journey for the patient as it is a clinical challenge (Figure 7.16).

7.6.1. Pharmacological Treatments

The body reconciles clotting and regulation daily, and it is especially important when medication gets involved. Medications avoid unnecessary bleeding or promote clotting where needed; in some cases, the necessity to apply clot-busting medication and specific methods arises in conditions like acute ischemic stroke—interventions that in most cases occur in conjunction with other steps to reduce bleeding risk (Ceulemans et al., 2024).

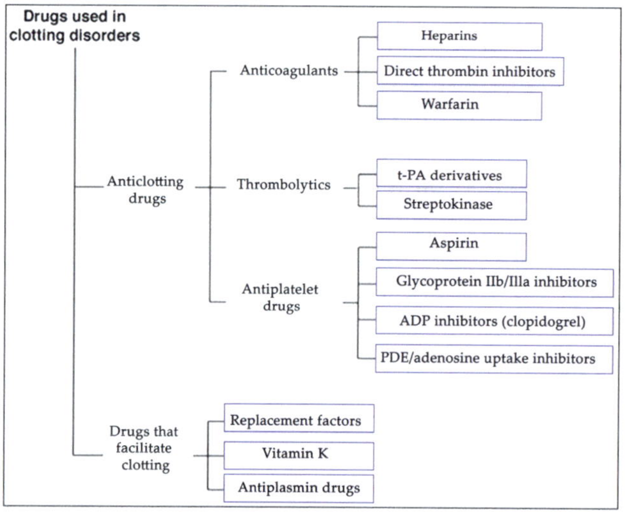

Figure 7.17. Drugs used in coagulation disorders.

Source: https://doctorlib.org/pharmacology/pharmacology-examination-board-review/pharmacology-examination-board-review.files/image169.jpg.

More often than not, you'll encounter initial intervention coupled with later, expertly balanced treatments that emphasize the two-sided nature of managing hemostasis. Traumatic trauma, for instance, may disrupt the normal rhythm of clotting—a situation known as trauma-induced coagulopathy (TIC). With severe trauma, the body's response may get out of balance and increase the risk of life-threatening, frequently preventable, bleeding. It is here that doctors need to be cautious, mixing anticoagulants with anti-platelet medication in such a way as to allow clotting while not enhancing further bleeding. More recent strategies such as state-of-the-art transfusion methods and novel medications are being tried in order to improve the prognosis of these patients; generally, the procedures involve searching for the ideal balance (Brännström et al., 2021). Outside the classic blood thinners, the world of pharmacological interventions still expands. There are new agents being created to not just prevent clots, but also to cause clots safely—a determinant factor in complex cases such as acute ischemic stroke, where the dynamic relationship of blood vessels and platelets is anything but straightforward. Coupled with standard therapy, these developments grant clinicians more instruments to tailor treatments to individual needs. Oftentimes, understanding of the interaction between various drugs helps in the overall idea of managing short-term crises as well as the longer-term states. With all these advancements, there is genuine hope for better results and ultimate revision of clinical guidelines (Ceulemans et al., 2024) (Figure 7.17).

7.6.2. Non-Pharmacological Interventions

Hemostasis management is not just grabbing a bottle of drugs. Sometimes non-drug approaches—like tracking blood loss—actually come into practice, especially when the stakes are high. Childbirth, for example, is generally a good thing to track for blood loss with measured collectors that follow guidelines intended to prevent postpartum hemorrhage (PPH). Such active observation opens up possibilities of rapid intervention by nurses and doctors to stem the harm caused by over-bleeding. Practices such as a successful uterine massage or a gentle tug on the umbilical cord at the very end of labor are also suggested, intermixing hands-on therapy with traditional procedures (Vladimír et al., 2025). Another approach these days is based on assembling an interdisciplinary team of care providers. Much of the time, physicians will start making customized plans well ahead of a difficult delivery, so they can intervene early and avert problems. This shared strategy doesn't just help during labor, but also treats conditions like anemia, which can have the potential to increase the risk for PPH, in most cases. The need to treat anemia antepartally with iron therapy serves as a reminder that effective control of the blood is best achieved by addressing underlying health issues. In short, care that involves finding solutions beyond simple immediate intervention can truly be life-changing for maternal outcomes in such cases (Vladimír et al., 2025). A newer approach seems to emerge in cardiac care, where access site control is changing the game. Hospitals are shifting towards performing catheterizations using the wrist (transradial access) instead of the traditional femoral route, a modality that is endorsed by cardiovascular specialists that is usually associated with fewer vascular complications and better patient safety. There are even recent advances in pressure application—like using air-bladder bracelets to achieve radial hemostasis—highlighting non-drug modalities rapidly evolving. Blending these new habits into everyday life is essential in controlling blood clots at the same level and preventing risks in a range of different medical settings.

7.6.3. Importance of Patient Education and Management

Blood coagulation and having blood available at hand is the most critical for high-quality patient care, even if it seems to be chaotic. Patients receiving clear, straightforward information about their coagulopathy disorders are likely to be compliant. Take Factor XIII (FXIII), a plasma enzyme that functions to promote wound healing. When individuals are made aware of this and other such issues, they will be more inclined to be attentive to something being wrong and worry less about unexplained bleeding. In most cases, this type of practical, everyday education empowers patients to take back control of their care and build self-care abilities. Overall, when patients are well-educated, bleeding risk management and postoperative recovery are a lot easier (Žunić et al., 2024). Too often, the whole topic of coagulation disorders appears muddled and convoluted, so care plans must also be adaptable and ongoing. Frequent checks and minor treatment adjustments are frequently necessary, especially for those patients at most risk who can't fully grasp their condition. With treatments that break down such complexities—offering personalized resources and concrete explanations—patients can fill in gaps that keep them from fully obeying advice. Overall, this individualization bridges the divide between medical terminology and everyday understanding that leads to better blood management and a better quality of life for those enduring clotting complications (Abdullah et al., 2024). Putting patients at the center of their own education is game-changing. As patients become familiar with their illness and the treatments offered, they necessarily become more proactive in managing themselves. Discussion of lifestyle changes on a daily basis, common complications, and simple monitoring of their recovery de-mystifies the clinical condition. This active, at times unorthodox approach enables physicians to note areas of concern earlier, advancing compliance as well as overall patient satisfaction. At large, where there is comprehensive patient education, it not only empowers individuals—it ultimately makes the entire healthcare system healthier (Žunić et al., 2024).

Test Your Knowledge

1. What role do anticoagulant drugs (e.g., heparin, warfarin) play in managing clotting disorders?
2. How are replacement therapies used in the treatment of hemophilia?

Summary

Hemostasis and coagulation keep our blood vessels intact and serve to stop bleeding, and honestly, it's a pretty grimy affair when you think about it. Platelets, our lining of the blood vessels, and all of these clotting factors all sort of dance in a tango, if you will—when one misses a step, the whole process can become upset, leading, in most situations, to such issues as clots that aren't expected or excessive blood loss. Studies have even gone so far as to indicate that if these systems don't work exactly as they ought, they might contribute to problems ranging from thrombotic episodes to bleeding disorders. Methods such as low-frequency vibration piezoelectric hemocoagulography—when combined with standard tests—occasionally reveal surprising information about patients with specific diseases, underscoring the value of having diagnostic methods tailored to each case (Amosova et al., 2013). Take more specifically diseases like diabetes mellitus, and one can see that there is a whole new level of complexity within the involvement of hemostasis. Various studies, e.g., Korobko et al. (2016) highlight that patients with diabetes overall have an increased risk of cardiovascular complications because their clotting processes simply aren't as uniform as they should be. It may be difficult to believe at first, but these disturbances can increase the likelihood of heart issues arising, prompting healthcare workers to monitor coagulation status carefully. By addressing the underlying reason behind these coagulopathies, doctors can better manage the risk factors related to diabetes without losing track of other subtle potential warning signs in the process. Overall, delving into how our body prevents bleeding not only sheds more light on simple physiological processes but also advances medical practice across a multitude of fronts. New diagnostic methods coupled with a balanced understanding of the pathology itself truly open the door to treatment protocols that are more responsive to the needs of each individual patient. The growing body of knowledge from both hemostatic tests and ongoing research adds to our overall body of knowledge that informs decisions made by clinicians on a daily basis. With new information still emerging, it seems more and more necessary to keep examining these dynamics, even if this involves accommodating a few oddities along the way.

Blood clotting is a delicate, sometimes sloppy mechanism. Platelets, clotting proteins, and even the blood vessel walls co-operate—sometimes in a disorganized manner—to close off an injury and prevent our circulatory liquid from escaping. Any defect in one of the components, like a missing or misplaced protein, could lead to conditions like hemophilia or deadly clotting elsewhere (thrombosis). For the most part, having an idea of how these elements interact enables us to design improved treatments; indeed, when doctors are able to view these interactions, they can make interventions that address the very specific level of balance. It is really more of a broad strategy that prevents overclotting and bleeding from happening. Keeping track of markers like fibrinogen is another important element in preventing bleeding risk. Studies have shown that fibrinogen levels, too low or too high, are often correlated with the degree of bleeding that happens and even with how many transfusions might ultimately be needed, especially in orthopedic procedures. For example, one study discovered that lower fibrinogen prior to surgery was correlated with later increased bleeding, which would serve as a handy planning tool for transfusion plans and other intervention measures. In most cases, this form of monitoring does indeed make a concrete contribution to patient outcomes for risky procedures, and that is why prudent evaluation is so important (Carling et al., 2011). Another crucial component to the formula is ensuring that health disparities are being addressed—a requirement when it comes to effective clotting care, especially when confronted with large-scale public health issues. The Finnish reaction to the COVID-19 pandemic is a good illustration: by segregating health information into more limited, focused bits, they were able to target and help those most in need, like people with lower incomes or certain racial groups. For the majority of cases, the blending of social comprehension and health surveillance enables carers to predict more effectively what is required from populations, thus ensuring public health interventions are more effective in crises. Overall, this people-centered but data-driven strategy not only demonstrates that planning can make a difference, but also stresses that justice cannot be displaced as the epicenter of governing matters of blood clotting.

KEY TERMS FROM THIS CHAPTER

- Anticoagulants
- Bleeding time
- Clot retraction
- Clotting factors
- Coagulation
- Fibrin
- Fibrinogen
- Hemophilia
- Hemostasis
- International normalized ratio (INR)
- Platelet aggregation
- Platelets (Thrombocytes)
- Prothrombin
- Prothrombin time (PT)
- Thrombin
- Thrombosis
- Vitamin K
- Von Willebrand factor (vWF)

Critical Thinking Questions

1. **What is the first step in the process of hemostasis?**
   a. Platelet aggregation
   b. Coagulation cascade
   c. Vascular spasm
   d. Fibrin clot formation
2. **Which of the following is responsible for forming the initial plug at the site of a blood vessel injury?**
   a. Red blood cells
   b. White blood cells
   c. Platelets
   d. Plasma
3. **The coagulation cascade is divided into which two main pathways?**
   a. Intrinsic and extrinsic
   b. Internal and external
   c. Primary and secondary
   d. Active and passive
4. **Which vitamin is essential for the synthesis of clotting factors II, VII, IX, and X?**
   a. Vitamin A
   b. Vitamin B12
   c. Vitamin D
   d. Vitamin K
5. **Hemophilia is a disorder primarily associated with deficiency in:**
   a. Platelets
   b. Fibrinogen
   c. Clotting factor VIII or IX
   d. Red blood cells

Answers to Critical Thinking Questions

1. (c); 2. (c); 3. (a); 4. (d); 5. (c)

Short Answer Questions

1. What are the three major steps of hemostasis?
2. What role do platelets play in the hemostatic process?
3. Name two important coagulation factors involved in the intrinsic pathway.
4. What laboratory tests are used to assess coagulation status, and what do they measure?
5. What does an elevated prothrombin time (PT) indicate?

References

1. Abdullah, N., & Mohamed Ludin, S. (2024). Structured module development for self-instillation eye drop technique: Enhancing patient education and adherence in glaucoma care. *International Journal of Education, Psychology and Counseling*. https://www.semanticscholar.org/paper/ecd7d6b5725f34388cfe5b9eed807336e2ad5a84 (accessed on 1st July 2025).
2. Alpan, O., Kamala, T., Matzinger, P., Velander, T., et al. (2007). Oral treatment of hemophilia. https://core.ac.uk/download/286364420.pdf (accessed on 1st July 2025).
3. Amosova, A. V., Bazhora, Y. I., Chesnokova, M. M., Tarabrin, V. E., et al. (2013). Features of the hemostasis system state in patients with pulmonary tuberculosis detected by the method of low-frequency vibration piezoelectric hemocoagulography. https://core.ac.uk/download/237163513.pdf (accessed on 1st July 2025).
4. Applegate, R., Bull, B. S., Gren, E. C. K., Hay, D. L., et al. (2017). *Crotalus atrox* venom preconditioning increases plasma fibrinogen and reduces perioperative hemorrhage in a rat model of surgical brain injury. https://core.ac.uk/download/323070684.pdf (accessed on 1st July 2025).
5. Argentiero, A., Caminiti, C., Cannata, G., Esposito, S., Perrone, S., & Zani, E. M. (2021). *TEG*® and *ROTEM*® traces: Clinical applications of viscoelastic coagulation monitoring in neonatal intensive care unit. https://core.ac.uk/download/534986439.pdf (accessed on 1st July 2025).
6. Arrieta Blanco, J. J., Cabrerizo Merino, M. del C., Martínez López, F., Oñate Cabrerizo, A., et al. (2014). Inherited, congenital and acquired disorders by hemostasis (vascular, platelet & plasmatic phases) with repercussions. https://core.ac.uk/download/71027397.pdf (accessed on 1st July 2025).
7. Bacalbașa, N., Banu, P., Bălălău, C., Ghinghină, I., et al. (2019). The risk of bleeding and encephalopathy in surgical patients with liver cirrhosis. https://core.ac.uk/download/216811033.pdf (accessed on 1st July 2025).
8. Bayrak, C., Cetinsaya, B., Cohen, J., De, L. T., et al. (2019). A task and performance analysis of endoscopic submucosal dissection (ESD) surgery. https://core.ac.uk/download/288845951.pdf (accessed on 1st July 2025).
9. Becker, R. C., Blanco, A. N., Blomback, M., Cambas, B., Chantarangkul, V., Chitolie, A., et al. (2003). Guidelines on fibrinogen assays. https://core.ac.uk/download/9349786.pdf (accessed on 1st July 2025).
10. Bendjeddou, A., Brodo, L., Falaschi, M., & Tiezzi, E. B. P. (2024). A computational model of the secondary hemostasis pathway in reaction systems. https://core.ac.uk/download/618720731.pdf (accessed on 1st July 2025).
11. Bontempo, F. A., Kang, Y. G., Knot, E. A. R., Lewis, J. H., et al. (1989). Systemic effects of tissue plasminogen activator-associated fibrinolysis and its relation to thrombin generation in orthotopic liver transplantation. https://core.ac.uk/download/12204422.pdf (accessed on 1st July 2025).
12. Brännström, A. (2021). Translational studies on mechanical hemostasis and coagulopathy in trauma. https://core.ac.uk/download/427718044.pdf (accessed on 1st July 2025).
13. Bronowski, A., Kosmalska, M., & Znajewska-Szulc, K. (2020). Hemostasis–Compendium for students. https://core.ac.uk/download/587244800.pdf (accessed on 1st July 2025).

14. Butwick, A., & Sultan, P. (2013). Platelet counts and coagulation tests prior to neuraxial anesthesia in patients with preeclampsia: A retrospective analysis. https://core.ac.uk/download/29416263.pdf (accessed on 1st July 2025).

15. Carestia, A., Kaufman, T., & Schattner, M. A. (2016). Platelets: New bricks in the building of neutrophil extracellular traps. https://core.ac.uk/download/161267511.pdf (accessed on 1st July 2025).

16. Carling, M., Jeppsson, A., Wessberg, P., Henriksson, A., Baghaei, F., & Brisby, H. (2011). Preoperative fibrinogen plasma concentration is associated with perioperative bleeding and transfusion requirements in scoliosis surgery. *Spine, 36*, 549–555. https://www.semanticscholar.org/paper/efe7852b5ac62cebd8c497ba4d655eb0f0a836ea (accessed on 1st July 2025).

17. Černý, V., Pařízek, A., Bláha, J., Blatný, J., Ďulíček, P., Gumulec, J., Janků, P., et al. (2025). Diagnosis and treatment of peripartum haemorrhage, consensus of the interdisciplinary working group by the modified ACCORD method. *Ceska Gynekologie, 90*(1), 72–89. https://www.semanticscholar.org/paper/2e1ffe2ad8b76323a024b32b7a044cc91612e920 (accessed on 1st July 2025).

18. Ceulemans, A., Nagy, M., Spronk, H. M. H., Ten Cate, H., et al. (2024). Current and potentially novel antithrombotic treatment in acute ischemic stroke. https://core.ac.uk/download/620780628.pdf (accessed on 1st July 2025).

19. Claramunt Lozano, A., Gavaldá Esteve, C., & Sarrión Pérez, M. G. (2011). Dental management in patients with hemostasis alteration. https://core.ac.uk/download/71058980.pdf (accessed on 1st July 2025).

20. Cluj-Napoca, S. F., Robert, E. B. V., Keskimäki, L. K., Tynkkynen, L. K., et al. (2023). Power and politics of health system data: How data shape responses and equity during pandemics. *The European Journal of Public Health, 33*. https://www.semanticscholar.org/paper/d6dd3f2ceeb49d92b596991dd84ceac0398d38d9 (accessed on 1st July 2025).

21. Colling, M., & Kanthi, Y. (2020). COVID–19-associated coagulopathy: An exploration of mechanisms. *Vascular Medicine, 25*, 471–478. https://doi.org/10.1177/1358863x20932640 (accessed on 1st July 2025).

22. Cullinan, K. (2015). The effects of hibernation on the hemostatic properties of the American bullfrog, *Rana catesbeiana*. https://core.ac.uk/download/222987869.pdf (accessed on 1st July 2025).

23. Deveras, R., & Kessler, C. (2002). Reversal of warfarin-induced excessive anticoagulation with recombinant human factor VIIa concentrate. *Annals of Internal Medicine, 137*, 884–888. https://www.semanticscholar.org/paper/9153e9e4387acc63295c6771d32734aaf4c8847c (accessed on 1st July 2025).

24. Devi, A., Putri, Z. A., Salamah, N., & Sejati, D. (2016). Sub chronic toxicity of green algae (*Spyrogyra* sp.) ethanolic extract on hematologic parameters. https://media.neliti.com/media/publications/300556-subchronic-toxicity-of-green-algae-spyro-313aa6ab.pdf (accessed on 1st July 2025).

25. Downes, K., Megy, K., Duarte, D., Vries, M. J. A., Gebhart, J., Hofer, S., Shamardina, O., et al. (2019). Diagnostic high-throughput sequencing of 2,396 patients with bleeding, thrombotic and platelet disorders. *Blood*. https://www.semanticscholar.org/paper/fca7ecf802c7f64eaf3cb94a7a54c4ad7a048bf2 (accessed on 1st July 2025).

26. D'Ugo, E., De Caterina, R., & Libby, P. (2016). Inflammation and thrombosis–Testing the hypothesis with anti-inflammatory drug trials. https://core.ac.uk/download/154875897.pdf (accessed on 1st July 2025).

27. Estes, J. W. (1962). Modern concepts of the platelet in health and disease. https://open.bu.edu/bitstream/2144/26002/1/Estes_J.%20Worth_1962_web.pdf (accessed on 1st July 2025).

28. Favaloro, E., Funk, D., & Lippi, G. (2012). Pre-analytical variables in coagulation testing associated with diagnostic errors in hemostasis. *Lab Medicine, 43*, 1–10. https://www.semanticscholar.org/paper/1f1f0633a4c441d96d77c39c5011499c81833b85 (accessed on 1st July 2025).

29. Fornasiero, A., Ristori, G., Salvetti, M., Buscarinu, M. C., Ferraldeschi, M., Umeton, R., et al. (2019). Genome-wide multiple sclerosis association data and coagulation. https://core.ac.uk/download/195777097.pdf (accessed on 1st July 2025).

30. Franchini, M., Liumbruno, G. M., Marano, G., Mengoli, G., et al. (2017). Inhibitors in patients with congenital bleeding disorders other than hemophilia. https://core.ac.uk/download/153367572.pdf (accessed on 1st July 2025).

31. Gaffney, P. J., Howarth, D., Kitchen, S., Lawrie, A., et al. (2002). A performance evaluation of commercial fibrinogen reference preparations and assays for Clauss and PT-derived fibrinogen. https://core.ac.uk/download/9349559.pdf (accessed on 1st July 2025).

32. Gracheva, E. S., Abdullina, R. R., Mustafin, I. G., & Abdulganieva, D. (2024). Analysis of plasma hemostasis and the role of micro vesicles in the coagulation process in patients with COVID-19. *Kazan Medical Journal*. https://www.semanticscholar.org/paper/e3b549a84441b9097367003fa5a7f5a1fb1464fe (accessed on 1st July 2025).

33. Holtby, R. J., Jahr, J. S., & Roghani, K. (2014). Effects of hemoglobin-based oxygen carriers on blood coagulation. https://core.ac.uk/download/323078517.pdf (accessed on 1st July 2025).

34. Kalaskar, D. (2023). Surface engineering of bioactive coatings for improved stent hemocompatibility: A comprehensive review. https://core.ac.uk/download/590344682.pdf (accessed on 1st July 2025).

35. Karsdal, M., Leeming, D. J., Lisman, T., Mandorfer, M., et al. (2023). Von Willebrand factor processing in patients with advanced chronic liver disease and its relation to portal hypertension and clinical outcome. https://core.ac.uk/download/597521727.pdf (accessed on 1st July 2025).

36. Kaynar, A. M., Toschke, A. M., Serhan, C. N., Meier, C. R., Cowper, D. C., Angus, D. C., Halm, E. A., et al. (2011). Elevated hemostasis markers after pneumonia increases one-year risk of all-cause and cardiovascular deaths. https://core.ac.uk/download/12212391.pdf (accessed on 1st July 2025).

37. Korobko, E. (2016). Hemorheological failure in the pathology of cardiovascular complications in patients with diabetic foot syndrome. https://core.ac.uk/download/322516355.pdf (accessed on 1st July 2025).

38. Neubauer, K., & Zieger, B. (2021). Endothelial cells and coagulation. *Cell and Tissue Research, 387*, 391–398. https://doi.org/10.1007/s00441-021-03471-2 (accessed on 1st July 2025).

39. Oliveira, S. R., & Tavares-Dias, M. (2018). A review of the blood coagulation system of fish. https://core.ac.uk/download/45520875.pdf (accessed on 1st July 2025).

40. Paniccia, R., & Prisco, D. (2003). Point-of-care testing of hemostasis in cardiac surgery. https://core.ac.uk/download/pdf/3254920.pdf (accessed on 1st July 2025).

41. Rodríguez Rius, A. (2020). Study of the regulatory mechanisms of gene expression in venous thromboembolic disease: microRNAs. https://core.ac.uk/download/429683606.pdf (accessed on 1st July 2025).

42. Seto, A., & Kern, M. (2018). Radial hemostasis: Harder, better, faster, stronger? *Catheterization and Cardiovascular Interventions, 92*, 325–326. https://www.semanticscholar.org/paper/c819a8204713c4555ee6facb34c76e3d64cbd2ab (accessed on 1st July 2025).

43. Solomon, C., Collis, R., & Collins, P. (2014). Hemostatic monitoring during postpartum hemorrhage and implications for management. *Obstetric Anesthesia Digest, 34*, 32. https://www.semanticscholar.org/paper/1e204d3995d777486df2ec2091bdd53f8f40d289 (accessed on 1st July 2025).

44. Tottoli, E. M., Dorati, R., Genta, I., Chiesa, E., Pisani, S., & Conti, B. (2020). Skin wound healing process and new emerging technologies for skin wound care and regeneration. *Pharmaceutics, 12*, 735–735. https://doi.org/10.3390/pharmaceutics12080735 (accessed on 1st July 2025).

45. Wu, X., Liu, Y., Zou, C., He, F., Guo, F., Liu, S., Fan, Y., et al. (2025). Nicotine's impact on platelet function: Insights into hemostasis mechanisms. *Frontiers in Pharmacology, 15*. https://www.semanticscholar.org/paper/6d19039cf41893ea123d6b1f8b7ccb5e800f7bab (accessed on 1st July 2025).

46. Žunić, M., Vreča, N., & Bevc, S. (2024). The role of factor XIII in patient blood management. *Blood Coagulation & Fibrinolysis, 35*, 325–333. https://www.semanticscholar.org/paper/019992fc9118f8a0f731b4ae1d7549a04dacf007 (accessed on 1st July 2025).

RENAL FUNCTION TESTS

8

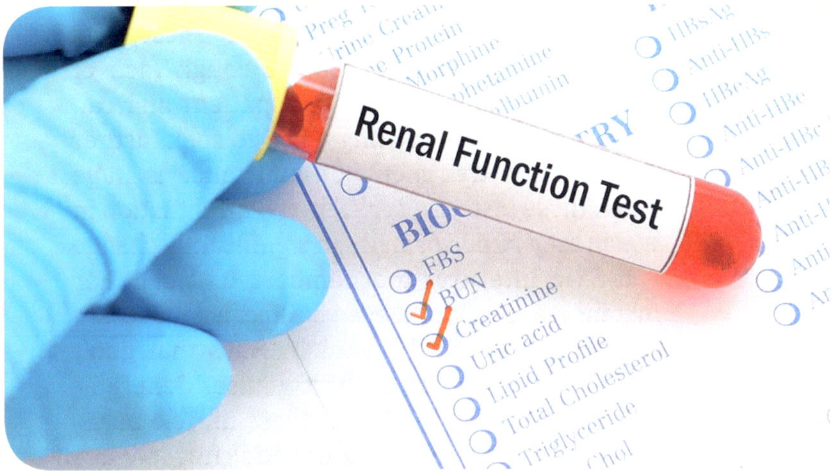

LEARNING OBJECTIVES

After studying this chapter, you will be able to:

1. Illustrate the anatomy and physiology of the kidneys;
2. Explain the types of renal function tests;
3. Identify the Interpretation of test results;
4. Discuss the common renal diseases and conditions;
5. Focus on the advances in renal function testing;
6. Explore clinical applications of renal function tests.

Introduction

Our body's balancing act is not just a matter of keeping things neat—it's also a matter of balancing fluid levels, electrolytes, and acid–base balance, all of which put emphasis on the importance of kidney tests. Kidneys are more than blood filters or producers of urine—they also control blood pressure and even help produce red blood cells by releasing hormones. Most of the time, it is this hectic work that makes tests to determine how well kidneys function become our initial warning system to detect issues before they get serious. It really shows that it is critical to understand exactly how our kidneys function for good overall health. When doctors treat the problem that accompanies kidney problems, they rely heavily on these tests. GFR and serum creatinine levels are very commonly the basis of keeping track of kidney function, and other markers sometimes double up as well to ensure greater confidence in results. For instance, consider the natriuretic peptide (NP) system, which has been the subject of extensive research into its role in heart and kidney arrangements, and how it serves to remind us of that knowledge regarding the functioning of the kidneys is constantly evolving. Newer research on interactions between cardiac hormones and kidney function stresses the need to stay open to adapting test methods so that they always stay in tune with the latest developments in medical science (Volpe et al., 2022). Clinical guidelines also urge clinicians to include kidney function tests as a routine part of patient management.

Overall, recommendations from ESC and similar authoritative bodies emphasize evidence-based intervention in preventing and treating kidney issues (Konstantinides et al., 2014). Guidelines are more than a recipe book; they are practical assistants that can assist patients by alerting them to possible problems early on. With the advancing science, ongoing education—and yes, occasionally even the odd bit of minor idiosyncrasy in style—will help practitioners navigate the bewildering aspects of kidney pathophysiology and ultimately support enhanced kidney function as well as enhanced systemic health (Figure 8.1).

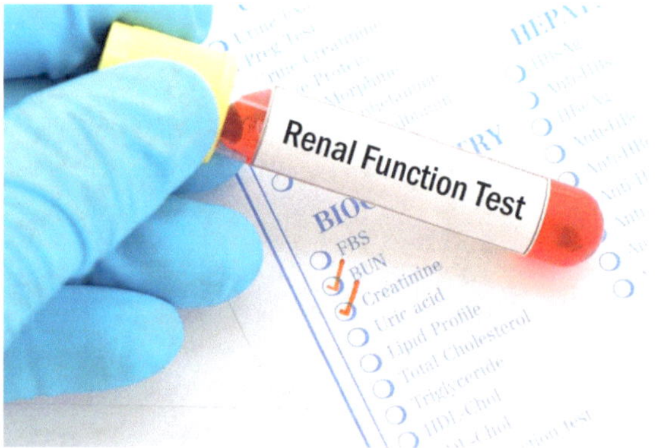

Figure 8.1. Renal function test.

Source: https://blog-revamp.s3.ap-south-1.amazonaws.com/wp-content/uploads/2023/08/13005555/image2-22-1024x683-1-1.jpg.

Definition of Renal Function Tests

Kidney function assessment is a major part of determining and managing an array of medical conditions. It is really just a set of checks to see how the kidneys are performing, giving signs of underlying conditions. More frequently, doctors analyze such markers as blood urea nitrogen (BUN) and serum creatinine in order to develop an understanding of how well the kidneys are filtering, and the eGFR is a leading figure that shows with accuracy how well waste is being eliminated from the blood. These tests collectively provide us with a rough idea of the overall kidney status of a patient and can guide decisions regarding when to seek further diagnosis or treatment. Circumstance is huge when these tests are performed—the situation in which they're performed can significantly change what we interpret the numbers to mean. For instance, age, sex, and even build can shift serum creatinine and BUN values in ways that don't necessarily leap out at first glance. Generally, older individuals might have less muscle mass, so lower creatinine values do not always correlate with actual kidney function. Diabetes and hypertension, among other conditions, are likely to place increased stress on the kidneys, hence routine kidney checks are common in such cases. It's a two-way system: these tests not only show current kidney function but also help track small, incremental variations that allow doctors to make adjustments in treatment regimens as required for best results. There are many ways of testing for kidney disease, and it isn't just a question of doing routine blood work. Urinalysis, to name a few, appears as a convenient tool to observe the efficiency of the kidney in concentrating urine and eliminating excess material. The presence of proteins or even minute amounts of blood in the urine may suggest glomerular injury or other unsuspected complications. And then there are certain tests like the creatinine clearance test, which provides another angle by observing the efficiency of creatinine removal from the blood. In the majority of clinical situations—especially with patients having long-standing disease—this dual approach detects key changes with time. For instance, a patient who has a history of renal cell carcinoma might demonstrate changing markers that merit further observation on treatment (Floris et al., 2024; Rosemar et al., 2020).

Importance of Renal Function in Overall Health

Kidneys are not garbage dumpers—actually, they function to maintain the body in equilibrium. Kidneys control water levels and mix electrolytes so that cells keep humming along and metabolism is normal. When kidney function does start to falter, you might see imbalances like excess potassium (hyperkalemia) or a lack of sodium (hyponatremia), which puts added stress on the heart and nerves. Generally, a decrease in the glomerular filtration rate (GFR) or the efficiency with which the kidneys filter blood can pave the way for chronic kidney disease (Ahmed et al., 2024). Regular checks, most often than not, enable doctors to act in time before the situation spirals out of control. Besides filtering, kidneys become functional during the hormone game. They secrete substances such as erythropoietin, which basically gooses the bone marrow into making red blood cells so that tissues can get the oxygen they need. As kidney function begins to deteriorate, erythropoietin levels fall, and anemia, exhaustion, and a general sense of waning energy follow. Simultaneously, kidneys control blood pressure by the renin-angiotensin-aldosterone system, and when that balance is disrupted, high blood pressure raises its nasty head—telling one of greater cardiovascular risk. That's why routine kidney checkups are such an insightful look at cardiovascular health, especially among those who are already at risk (Ahmed et al., 2024). In old individuals the interplay between the function of kidneys and overall health really comes into sharp perspective. With age, the kidneys' flexibility sometimes declines, which frequently comes with greater frailty, such as weaker muscle strength and decreased mobility. A few research papers—such as the FRASNET study—indicate that a lower estimated GFR is highly related to frailty in individuals aged over 75 (Lanzani et al., 2024). Overall, these findings push us toward a more holistic whole-person model for healthcare that incorporates kidney function into the larger picture of aging and frailty. Being serious about kidney health can make preventive care sharper and, ultimately, improve the quality of life in the long run.

8.1. Anatomy and Physiology of the Kidneys

Learning Outcome

- Structure of the kidneys;
- Functions of the kidneys;
- Role of the kidneys in homeostasis.

Kidney structure is actually quite fascinating – it basically acts as your body's primary cleaner of the blood. In each of the two kidneys, there are roughly 1 million tiny filters called nephrons that make the blood into urine; these small soldiers have a foamy network in which the glomerulus does the major work first by sieving through blood plasma based on size and charge, letting water, ions, and tiny molecules but not big proteins and cells. Following are the tubular segments that aid in recycling what the body actually needs and discarding the rest. The whole process, which is required for fluid, blood pressure, and electrolyte balance, is precisely why it is so crucial to understand how kidneys are built prior to attempting to interpret the results of renal function tests. Kidneys don't just dispose of trash – they also have a significant role in keeping blood pressure at a constant level and even secreting hormones. Where the tubule and glomerulus meet is the juxtaglomerular apparatus, a sensor that perceives an alteration in blood pressure and then releases renin, an enzyme that triggers the renin-angiotensin-aldosterone system (RAAS).

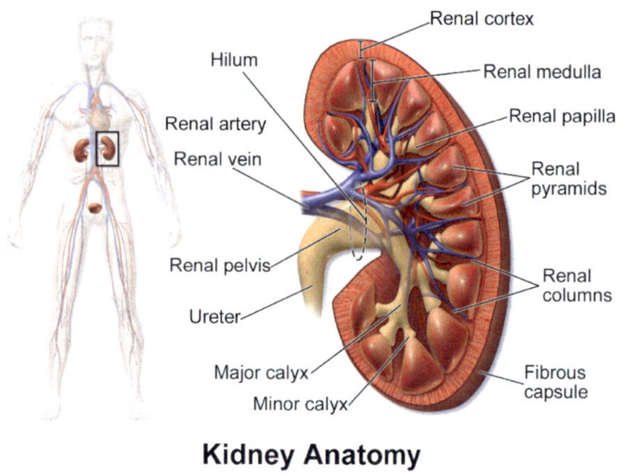

Figure 8.2. Anatomy and physiology of the kidneys.

Source: https://upload.wikimedia.org/wikipedia/commons/d/d6/Blausen_0592_KidneyAnatomy_01.png.

In most cases, this cascade raises blood volume and pressure. Also, they manufacture erythropoietin—a hormone that encourages the bone marrow to produce more red blood cells when oxygen levels fall, thereby directly impacting how well oxygen circulates. All these functions highlight just how much kidneys do to keep our body in balance, which is why checking their function is important so much. The interaction of kidney anatomy, their functionality, and the evaluations that challenge them has been of interest within clinical and research circles. Research such as the ASSESS-AKI study has investigated what happens when an acute kidney injury occurs and how it may influence long-term kidney function (Go et al., 2010). Gain a greater understanding of kidney form and function that helps doctors decode markers like serum creatinine and estimated glomerular filtration rates (eGFR); these are vital to diagnosing issues like chronic kidney disease or acute kidney failure. Contrary to expectations, meta-analyses conducted in recent times have shown that daily routines—such as intake of coffee—fail to produce meaningful impacts upon outcomes of kidney tests, such that lifestyle factors can be distinctly separated from actual pathologies (Mazidi et al., 2021). Overall, comprehension of how each of these factors falls into place is critical for both the assessment of kidney function and patient treatment strategies (Figure 8.2).

8.1.1. Structure of the kidneys

Keeping in mind kidney tests, it's clear that knowing how these organs are built really matters. Each kidney—typically a bean-shaped gem—is home to roughly a million tiny processing machines known as nephrons. These tiny workhorses of our own body contain structures like the renal corpuscle, which simply wraps around a lattice known as the glomerulus within Bowman's capsule. The glomerulus begins blood purification, initiating urine production. This setup, which is complicated, permits the kidney to select what to reabsorb and what to release in order to maintain harmony in the body. Nephrons group mainly in the outer portion, or cortex, and the various roles they play are why these tests are able to spot problems if there is a problem. Kidneys segment into two broad regions—the outer cortex and the inner medulla—each with its own distinct functions. In the cortex, there are most of the renal corpuscles and the corkscrew-shaped proximal convoluted tubules where most filtering and reclaiming is done. The medulla houses structures such as the loop of Henle and collecting ducts that are involved in thickening and concentrating the urine. With such rough-and-ready organization, kidneys govern everything from electrolytes and fluid balance to levels of acid and blood pressure through the renin-angiotensin-aldosterone system. Even minimal change in these regions can disturb how the kidney operates—nephron injury may lead to elevations in levels of creatinine and blood urea, which indicates chronic disease as with increased blood urea nitrogen and creatinine levels (Hadeel et al., 2024). In conditions such as diabetic nephropathy, the architecture of the kidney can actually become flawed. You may notice alterations in the medulla, such as tubular atrophy or interstitial fibrosis, which have drastically impaired filtration efficiency. When nephrons go on the fritz, the body will sometimes make up for it by raising glomerular pressure and volume—though that only succeeds in causing more damage in the end. Doctors will typically turn to imaging or even microscopic inspection to have a closer look at such structural flaws. Research primarily suggests that patients with diabetic nephropathy will record higher levels of cystatin C, which is a marker of ongoing kidney injury and loss of function (Navirius et al., 2023). Understanding these structural components not only allows for unscrambling test results but also for quicker diagnosis and treatment, as a reminder of how learning kidney anatomy remains so worthwhile.

8.1.2. Functions of the kidneys

Kidneys are not garbage disposals but do so much more by keeping our inner balance in harmony. They deal with water and salts like sodium and potassium quietly by-passing blood through millions of tiny filters called nephrons. Sometimes, hormones such as antidiuretic hormone (ADH) and aldosterone come into play, controlling the ratio depending on whether we're hydrated or need salt.

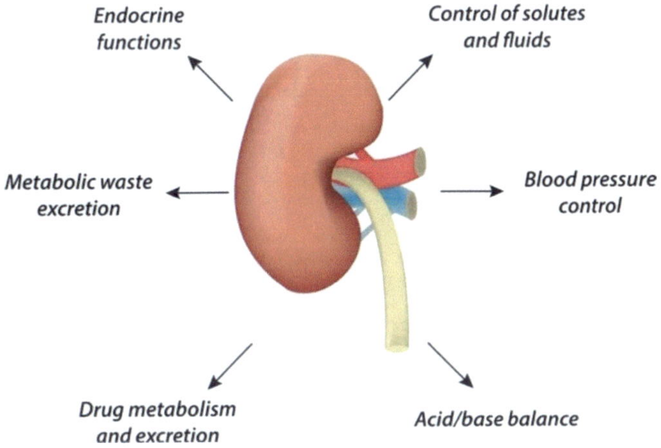

Figure 8.3. Functions of the kidneys.

Source: https://d2jx2rerrg6sh3.cloudfront.net/image-handler/picture/2016/6/The_Kidney_shutterstock_228646804.jpg.

When even a small mistake is made here, it can snowball and affect blood pressure and overall health, showing just how much these organs tip on a daily basis. Simultaneously, kidneys play a crucial role in keeping the body's pH at exactly the right spot. Overall, they handle acidity by removing hydrogen ions and storing bicarbonate—a task that keeps our chemistry in check. It is in these conditions like metabolic acidosis or alkalosis that often occur in combination with kidney problems that this balancing effect is even more significant. For instance, in chronic kidney disease, an impaired capacity to exclude hydrogen ions can tip the system in the direction of acidosis, thereby impairing normal cell functioning and metabolism. It is why the measurement of acid–base status is generally a good reflection of overall renal status. The kidneys play their part on the hormonal side of things, too. They release erythropoietin, a hormone that encourages the bone marrow to produce more red blood cells when oxygen levels aren't exactly where they should be. They even assist with vitamin D metabolism by activating it into its active state, calcitriol, which is vital for calcium control and strong bones. This combination of functions illustrates how a small dysfunction in the kidneys can affect several systems at once. Kidney tests conducted regularly, therefore, are not merely about detecting issues with waste removal—wholly, they are a window into the entire body's balance and health (Figure 8.3).

8.1.3. Role of the Kidneys in Homeostasis

Kidneys are the genuine article—they shore up our insides by regulating a whole lot more than trash. Small workhorses known as nephrons, constantly scanning our blood, take what they need and dump what they don't. Clever sorting dictates electrolyte status, water composition, and even pH levels just so. Like, when sodium and water are reabsorbed, blood pressure adjusts accordingly—and that's a big part of heart health.

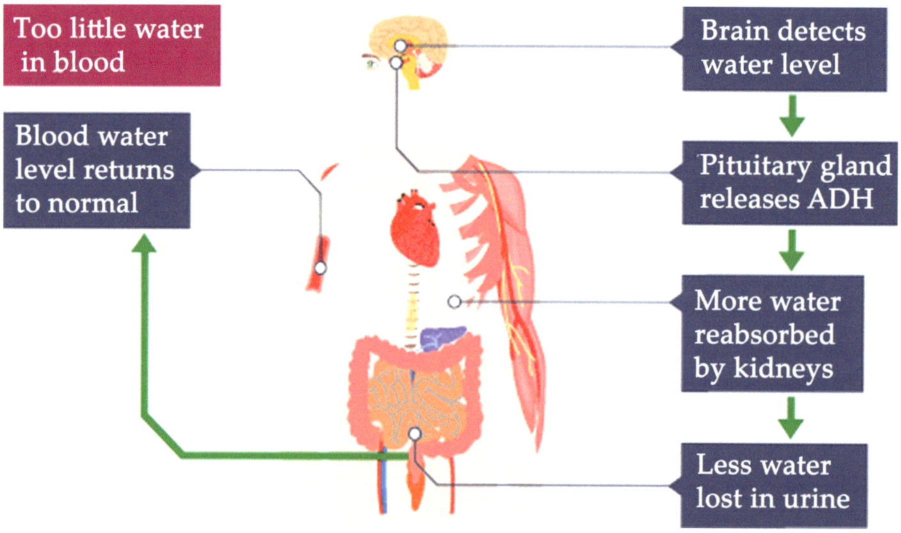

Figure 8.4. The role of the kidneys in homeostasis.

Source: https://bam.files.bbci.co.uk/bam/live/content/z2tmng8/medium.

They handle acid by expelling hydrogen ions or recovering bicarbonate, adjusting our pH level. Kidneys are typically more impressive in their flexibility to our shifting demands in most conditions. How they readjust fluids through internal feedback loops is even more captivating. When blood pressure drops—even slightly—the renin-angiotensin-aldosterone ploy is used, which stimulates kidneys to hold onto more sodium and therefore more water. That extra fluid boosts blood volume and relieves pressure through a signal-based feedback mechanism. And let's not forget, kidneys also urinate out erythropoietin, a hormone that employs ironmongery as a euphemism when oxygen is low: "time to make more red blood cells." Overall, their function is so much more than just throwing out trash; they're busy maintaining all from fluid levels to blood health in equilibrium. There is another twist in the kidney drama that science still discovers—its role in immune reactions. For instance, Tamm-Horsfall protein (THP), mostly for its role in the make-up of urine, also acts to regulate local immune responses. THP can modulate the action of immune cells in the kidney known as renal macrophages, sometimes enhancing their ability to clean up debris, and this adjustment appears to help the kidney in responding to trivial damage. Fortunately, keeping kidneys in prime working order isn't just a filtration or fluid homeostasis affair—it's also crucial for enhancing local immune defenses (Figure 8.4).

Test Your Knowledge

1. What are the main structural components of the nephron and their respective functions?
2. How do the kidneys regulate fluid, electrolyte, and acid-base balance in the body?

8.2. Types of Renal Function Tests

Learning Outcome

- Blood tests (e.g., serum creatinine, BUN);
- Urine tests (e.g., urinalysis, 24-hour urine collection);
- Imaging tests (e.g., ultrasound, CT scans).

Understand how efficiently kidneys filter waste and keep us in equilibrium needs a series of tests that are not arranged in an orderly checklist. Clinicians, for instance, most often start by taking a measurement of serum creatinine—a marker that, when increases, generally means the glomerular filtration rate (GFR) is lower than usual. For the most part, this elevation signals that the filtering equipment of the kidney is compromised. At times, doctors also use equations like the MDRD (Modification of Diet in Renal Disease) to estimate GFR; these kinds of techniques provide a more nuanced picture of kidney effectiveness. Together, these tests provide a first, if sometimes inexact, glimpse at a patient's kidney status and help to guide further studies or interventions, most significantly in patients with risk for diabetic kidney disease and metabolic illness (Urbanovych et al., 2024). Urinary tests, too, are brought into the mix—often in seemingly less systematic but no less valuable manners. Take the albumin-to-creatinine ratio (ACR), for example. In diabetic patients, finding more albumin in the urine may be an early, occasionally lifesaving warning sign for diabetic nephropathy; early intervention may even arrest or delay the progression to end-stage renal disease. Measuring protein levels using ACR gives a non-invasive way of following kidney status over time and is thus routine in routine check-ups for high-risk groups. Other urine markers—electrolytes, urea—also play their part by giving information on tubular function or indicating some abnormalities affecting the operation of the kidneys, finally guiding individualized treatment approaches to maximize overall patient outcomes (Phan et al., 2024).

More recently, several sophisticated studies that integrate novel biomarkers such as proadrenomedullin (Pro-ADM) have added greater depth to traditional assessments. Studies overwhelmingly suggest that Pro-ADM levels correlate positively with various clinical markers, introducing a novel observation regarding kidney deterioration, especially among diabetics who are fighting type 2 diabetes and diabetic kidney disease. Pro-ADM monitoring will enhance our insight into renal dysfunction and, in a large majority of clinical situations, become a useful prognostic marker in addition to more conventional markers. By combining the new tests with the old methods, clinicians now have available a richer, more complex diagnostic paradigm, one that points out the ever-changing nature of renal function assessment (Urbanovych et al., 2024).

8.2.1. Blood Tests (e.g., Serum Creatinine, BUN)

When it comes to testing how efficient our kidneys are, it's essential in clinics as well as research facilities – a true linchpin in identifying and managing kidney complications. Blood tests for serum creatinine and blood urea nitrogen (BUN) are among the numerous choices, mainly due to the fact that they allow us to have an idea of how these organs remove waste products. High levels of creatinine, say, generally mean that the filtering system isn't quite up to scratch; doctors will then investigate further into conditions like kidney disease or even an acute kidney injury. A series of experiments has confirmed the relationship between high levels of creatinine and a number of kidney diseases (Mahmoud et al., 2025). Which is why these tests have become a part of the daily practice of monitoring, keeping clinicians ahead in kidney treatment. BUN has a leading role, too, giving insight not only into kidney function but into overall metabolic activity. In most situations, when BUN elevates, it may indicate failing kidneys or enhanced breakdown of protein – conditions at times driven by dehydration, high-protein intake, or other body-wide problems. Sometimes, you'll even see both creatinine and BUN jumping together; for instance, in cases of Proliferative Glomerulonephritis with Monoclonal Immunoglobulin Deposits, where both markers are noticeably high, signaling serious kidney issues (Gokhale et al., 2024).

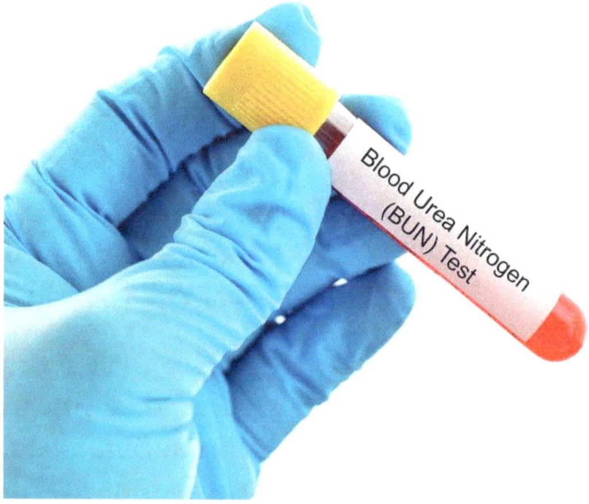

Figure 8.5. A healthcare professional holds a blood sample labeled for a blood urea nitrogen (BUN) test, commonly used to assess kidney function.

Source: https://labs.selfdecode.com/app/uploads/2019/10/bigstock-142429214-min.jpg.

Breaking down how these numbers interact, even if it sometimes feels a bit redundant, really assists healthcare providers in fine-tuning their interventions and treatment plans. Of course, no test is perfect. Creatinine and BUN both can be affected by things outside of the kidneys. For example, creatinine can be lower in people who have less muscle, possibly giving a false impression—meanwhile, BUN can fluctuate wildly depending on what you've eaten or how much you've had to drink, so is somewhat untrustworthy on its own. Physicians prefer to assess these tests in conjunction with imaging tests and urinalysis, hence creating an integrated picture of renal status. Such an integrated, mixed approach enables them to make wise treatment choices and, ultimately, enhance patient outcomes (Figure 8.5).

8.2.2. Urine Tests (e.g., Urinalysis, 24-Hour Urine Collection)

Kidney activity is tested with all sorts of tests, but urine tests truly excel. A simple urinalysis gets the ball rolling by revealing what's in the urine – its composition and characteristics, such as proteins, glucose, and even minute blood residues. It can indicate problems such as kidney disease or diabetes, and most often, it also places the red flag on urinary tract infections while keeping an eye out to see whether treatment is working or not. In the real world, this test generally causes doctors to go after more invasive tests—even when the process does feel a little disorganized at first. Aside from the routine urinalysis, a test that takes a sample of urine over a full 24 hours gives a better picture of kidney function. This method tallies the chemicals your body expels in a day and gives clues not only about how well your kidneys are working but also about your metabolism. Overall, the recommendations of organizations like the European Association of Urology (EAU) and the American Urological Association (AUA) include calcium and oxalate levels tests in case of kidney stones (urolithiasis). For accuracy in pinpointing, patients should be advised to continue a normal meal and drink routine when getting samples (Kushnirenko et al., 2025). The data that is gathered not only helps identify unusual signs but also assists in creating preventive steps as early as possible for future health conditions. The 24-hour test goes one step ahead by measuring important minerals—like phosphorus and calcium—which play crucial roles in deciding disorders such as hyperparathyroidism or renal tubular acidosis. Research mostly shows that stable analytical performance must be maintained; slight variations in pH (if samples are not acidified except under absolute necessity) will impact the results (Canali et al., 2023). Therefore, understanding these slight differences enhances diagnostic precision and even impacts patient care management. With a full battery of urine tests, doctors can prescribe treatment plans that not only treat the active symptoms but penetrate further into the real causes of kidney problems (Figure 8.6).

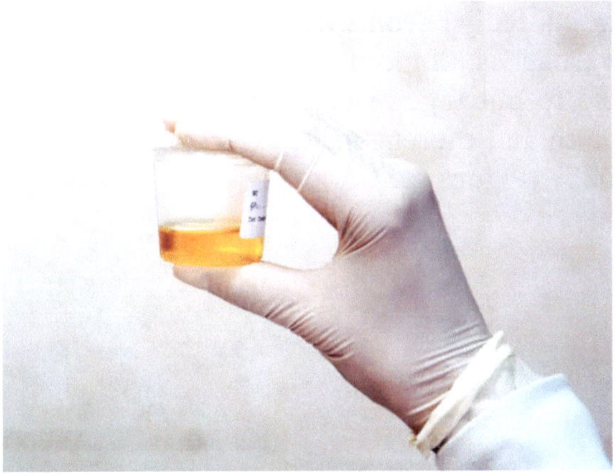

Figure 8.6. A gloved healthcare worker holds a urine sample container, typically used for creatinine clearance or other urinalysis tests to assess kidney function.

Source: https://media.post.rvohealth.io/wp-content/uploads/2020/09/creatinine-clearance_thumb-1-732x549.jpg.

8.2.3. Imaging Tests (e.g., Ultrasound, CT Scans)

Imaging examinations have really transformed the way kidney function is followed. Instead of waiting for and depending on blood work alone, doctors now prefer to observe structures inside the kidneys directly to see if something aberrant comes along. Ultrasound, for instance, is a simple, non-painful examination that offers an on-the-spot view inside the body; it can identify such items as stones, blockages, or even cysts. It's typically easy to access and doesn't incur the risk of ionizing radiation—a huge benefit for pregnant women and children, like. Here and there, scans even direct such interventions as renal biopsies, so it's a routine but necessary part of kidney tests (Kapatia, 2023). CT scans do tend to provide a far more extensive view of kidney anatomy, though. Not only do they help detect tumors or vascular malformations, but also detect abnormal anatomical curvature that can affect kidney function. In crises, this extra information can be invaluable to making a timely decision regarding treatment. With the additional dimension of contrast agents that outline the blood vessels and provide information on blood flow, CT imaging gives physicians another glimpse of kidney function. It's, overall, a valuable addition to regular checkups and illustrates how far imaging tests have come in detecting kidney problems (N/A, 2023). Together, as a combination of lab work and imaging, it gives physicians a better idea of kidney function. Blood tests and urine analysis show how well kidneys handle waste and filter out important substances, and imaging shows structural data and abnormalities. With advancing knowledge regarding kidney disease, the application of these two methods in combination will undoubtedly become widespread—allowing diagnosis and treatment earlier on, with more specific approaches. Clinically, on a day-to-day basis, application of both methods is such that doctors are able to put together a more comprehensive, though sometimes partially messy, vision of kidney health and thereby make informed, better decisions about patient treatment (Kapatia, 2023; N/A, 2023) (Figure 8.7).

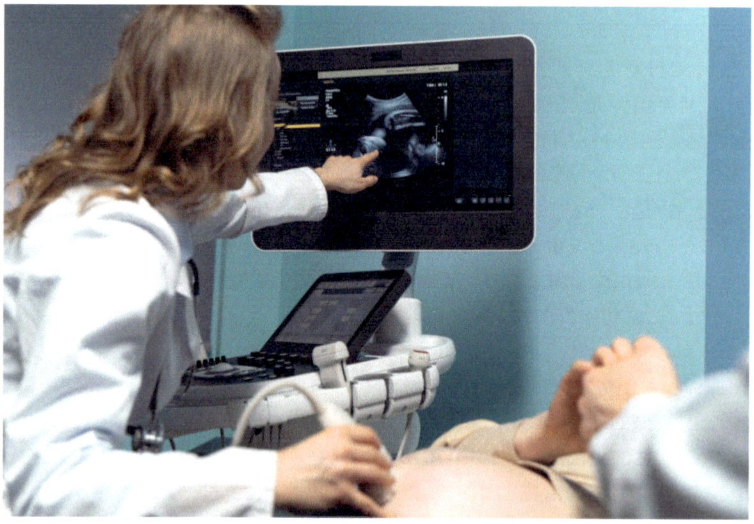

Figure 8.7. A medical professional conducts an ultrasound examination, pointing to the fetal image on the monitor during a routine prenatal checkup.

Source: https://www.mdrcindia.com/uploads/blog/062024//671717737772.jpg.

Test Your Knowledge

1. What is the difference between clearance tests (e.g., creatinine clearance) and blood tests (e.g., serum creatinine, BUN)?
2. How do urine analysis and microscopic examination help assess kidney function?

8.3. Interpretation of Test Results

Learning Outcome

- Normal ranges for renal function tests;
- Factors affecting test results;
- Clinical significance of abnormal results.

Interpretation of the lab tests is absolutely crucial when measuring kidney health—it not only tells us how well the kidneys are working, but it also provides us with an idea as to the equilibrium of the body. Clinicians usually utilize parameters such as serum creatinine, blood urea nitrogen (BUN), and the glomerular filtration rate (GFR) because each has something unique to tell us about kidney function. For instance, a rise in serum creatinine will typically be an early sign of worsening renal function, but one must keep in mind that factors like muscle mass or even diet can drive these values, sometimes making matters more complicated. Kidney function is typically taken into consideration alongside a patient's overall bigger picture situation, such as other ailments they are experiencing. Overall, correlating lab findings with what is observed at the bedside helps to lead clinicians in the direction of optimal management. If the patient has a disorder such as diabetes or COPD, then the number of factors to consider doubles, and laboratory results may suddenly become harder to understand. In a patient study of COPD, mean platelet volume (MPV) even correlated with the severity of an acute exacerbation (Sharma et al., 2021)—a reminder that the whole clinical picture is worth more than a few figures. Nowadays, flash new-fangled technologies like clinical decision support systems (CDSS) are closing the gaps to make the picture less fuzzy. By neatly encapsulating lab results in an integrated presentation, these systems help doctors with a real glimpse of what's happening—down to spotting trends using color warnings and interactive graphs. As an example, in a diabetes-focused dashboard research, renal function data were presented alongside glycemic and lipid profiles, providing a full picture that revealed abnormalities (Sim et al., 2017). In the majority of instances, such technology greatly enhances our capacity to deal with chronic disease complexities and tailor treatment plans over time.

8.3.1. Normal ranges for renal function tests

Knowing what counts as a normal kidney test result matters a lot when checking someone's kidney health or trying to figure out if something's off. Kidney tests usually look at markers like serum creatinine, BUN (blood urea nitrogen), and what's called the eGFR. For most adults, you're looking at creatinine numbers somewhere between 0.6 and 1.2 mg/dL, while BUN tends to be around 7 to 20 mg/dL. eGFR, simply put, is a gauge of how well kidneys are filtering—hopefully, the value should be more than 90 mL/min/1.73 m^2. If the values stray beyond these boundaries, they might suggest declining kidney function or existing disease, which usually prompts doctors to take a closer examination. Variables such as age, gender, and body weight can change these reference values, highlighting that each patient essentially does need an individual check-up. Different normal ranges really do have a profound effect on the way physicians make treatment decisions and take care of patients on a daily basis. For instance, if creatinine decreases below that of normal, the possibility that it might warrant examination of one's food intake, fluid status, or even diseases like diabetes or hypertension is there. Sometimes, chronic kidney disease has a minimal change in eGFR that may not be recognized and differences in muscle mass or dehydration even generate false positives, so the whole situation is a bit messy to untangle. Clinicians, in general, need to take these idiosyncrasies into account to arrive at the proper diagnosis and come up with an appropriate plan for treatment. It all makes sense better when test results are put together with a larger image of the patient's general well-being. Kidney tests also play a significant role when dealing with the dispensation of treatment for kidney issues. Follow-up testing of renal function is most critical in patients with established renal disease or on drugs with the capability to cause stress to the kidneys because even small changes can predict that things are worsening or complications are developing. The American Urological Association, for example, generally recommends checking these markers at intervals to inform treatment and change medicines where needed. Tracking how these values alter over time can be utilized to identify an acute kidney injury or the insidious creep of chronic disease. These so-called normal values, thus, aren't constant numbers for diagnosis—they're part of the day-to-day decisions in nephrology, capturing the ever-changing picture of kidney illness and health (Stephen et al., 2017; Steven et al., 2017) (Figure 8.8).

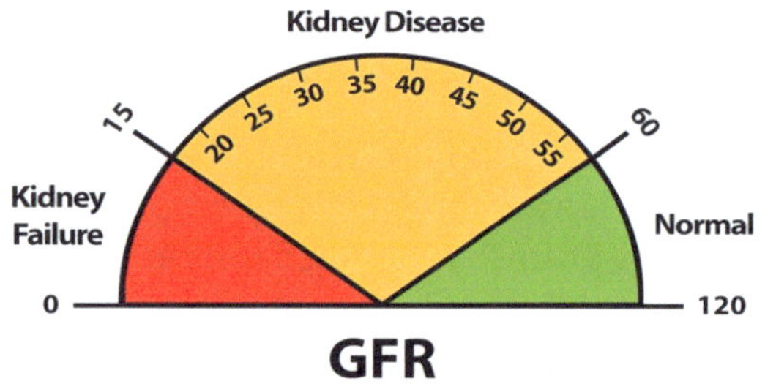

Figure 8.8. Normal ranges for renal function tests.

Source: https://external-content.duckduckgo.com/iu/?u=https%3A%2F%2Fhealthjade.com%2Fwp-content%2Fuploads%2F2018%2F07%2Fkidney-function-test-results.jpg&f=1&nofb=1&ipt=976a0946653179a019bba4fab1bd550d8cf262885adb9cb65dbde7580bc6f4a0.

8.3.2. Factors affecting test results

Kidney tests provide insight into how well the kidneys function, but there are countless variables that can end up skewing the results in bizarre ways. Whoever is getting tested matters—a factor such as their health, for example. Older individuals have some degree of kidney decline, something that can influence the numbers in weird ways. I recall a study with heart failure patients; it so happened that the left ventricular assist device patients were older and had lower preoperative estimated glomerular filtration rates than their heart transplant waiting list counterparts. This sort of difference really demonstrates that you can't consider test numbers in isolation—they need to be considered in the context of what the patient is, as documented by Wen et al. (2025). The method to the test is the other significant factor here. In the majority of cases, how much the lab uses semi-automated or automated techniques will result in insignificant differences in the results. For instance, in one study, analyzers were compared and noticed that while the mean creatinine and urea values appeared to be very similar, some of the measurements had a high bias. Clearly, even when on the surface the two procedures produce apparently similar results, the devil is in the details and it compels the labs to standardize their procedures to produce more reproducible results, as found by Goyal et al. (2024). And then there are extrinsic factors that no one wants to overlook—such as when the sample was obtained or whether the patient is well hydrated. Timing is everything; obtaining a sample after eating or close to the time of medication can easily alter the levels of those important biochemical markers. And if someone is not staying well-hydrated, their urea and creatinine will look higher when they shouldn't be, and a brief misdiagnosis for an acute kidney problem could result. Overall, these other details need to be taken into account. They make the test results actually reflective of the person's health status and not a false positive because of something as ordinary as going without one glass of water.

8.3.3. Clinical significance of abnormal results

Changed renal test results can imply more than just kidney function – occasionally, they can imply more widespread systemic pathology that can need urgent treatment. Abnormal results on tests like serum creatinine, blood urea nitrogen (BUN) and the eGFR can be of extremely practical clinical importance. For example, an increase in creatinine generally points towards an acute kidney injury or chronic kidney condition; doctors can then probe further with imaging tests or even a renal biopsy to ascertain both the cause and the severity of the insult. These test idiosyncrasies may also guide treatment decisions – maybe a referral to an expert working on kidneys or the introduction of kidney-protective measures – all to give the patient a better prognosis (Luck et al., 2017).

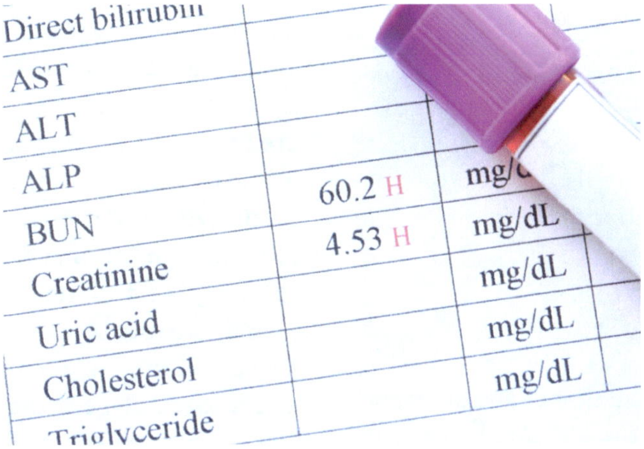

Figure 8.9. Abnormal high renal function test results.

Source: https://external-content.duckduckgo.com/iu/?u=https%3A%2F%2Fwww.infectiousdiseaseadvisor.com%2Fwp-content%2Fuploads%2Fsites%2F16%2F2019%2F01%2Frenalfunctiong9573902201_1448787.jpg&f=1&nofb=1&ipt=5c6ae3e04818f477a5a71be86a316275dd73ffb0bdd1444bc2518619b1103cf9.

Detection of these changes is always important in acting fast and containing the situation properly. Reviewing abnormal kidney test results shouldn't be done in isolation; they must be viewed in the context of the complete clinical picture. A patient's medical history, current medications (because some can drive creatinine up without actual damage) and any existing co-morbid conditions all enter into it. What this does is cause the clinicians to look beyond numbers themselves and relate them to what they are discovering on the physical exam and even what the patients are reporting about the symptoms. This broader lens can help determine if something is an acute hiccup or if it is symptomatic of an underlying long-term issue, and if the issue can be corrected or must be treated immediately (Steven et al., 2017). In most cases, such a mixed view enables healthcare providers to move in the direction of pinning down what is actually causing the abnormal results. Tracking kidney function over time is also required since trends typically tell of slow going downhill or sudden stress-related blips. Every now and then, a rogue abnormal result can be nothing more than a fleeting glitch related to an acute stressor, rather than an ongoing worsening of kidney status.

Close follow-up with targeted testing - and, where needed, focused interventions - can prevent the long-term effects of chronic kidney disease. For example, if a patient is showing persistent deterioration in eGFR, adjustment of medication or modification of lifestyle habits may be needed to further protect the kidneys. By observing these changes regularly - and occasionally accepting some natural fluctuation - doctors are able to institute preventions that prevent kidney disease from progressing too far, ultimately enhancing long-term outcomes (Luck et al., 2017) (Figure 8.9).

Test Your Knowledge

1. How is glomerular filtration rate (GFR) estimated, and what do abnormal values indicate?
2. What does an elevated blood urea nitrogen (BUN) or serum creatinine level suggest about renal function?

8.4. Common Renal Diseases and Conditions

Learning Outcome

- Chronic kidney disease (CKD);
- Acute kidney injury (AKI);
- Glomerulonephritis.

Kidney problems come in all shapes and sizes and at different rates. Often, the delicate balance of the body is thrown off due to complications with the kidneys, and most frequently, chronic kidney disease (CKD) develops slowly. Nephrons—your kidneys' little horses—are gradually damaged, so filtration is out of balance, and creatinine and urea build up in the blood. Diabetes, high blood pressure, and the like frequently spark such problems.

Early kidney function tests are literally a lifesaver by detecting the deterioration before it gets worse, then allowing interventions aimed at saving what is left of the kidney's natural function. In most cases, surveillance has a central role in the treatment of CKD, which has created it a priority in studying and treating renal disease. All kidney issues do not always develop gradually. Acute Kidney Injury (AKI) typically affects hard and fast—typically from dehydration, infection, or even trauma—and, in some lucky cases, can be reversed if caught early. When AKI strikes, waste metabolites start to pile up fast, and laboratory parameters like serum creatinine levels become critical to diagnose the etiology almost instantly. As AKI often happens along with other problems, a team of various medical practitioners is most commonly used to bring the situation under control, balancing kidney assessment with overall patient management. For most cases, which concerted effort is what gets the job done, even though the procedure does feel a little chaotic at times. And then there's glomerulonephritis, a group of diseases affecting the kidney's filtering device—the glomeruli.

This is not isolated; it can follow infections, autoimmune exacerbations, or other systemic illnesses, leading to inflammation that eventually disrupts the functioning of the kidney. Signs and symptoms like hematuria, protein loss, and hypertension are usually present, prompting doctors toward a more detailed workup with renal function studies. Current research, as well as ongoing testing, always points to early identification of glomerulonephritis—and understanding its complex nature—as the key factor for choosing proper treatment options. Together, tracking renal status remains paramount to improving outcomes for patients fighting kidney abnormalities (Figure 8.10).

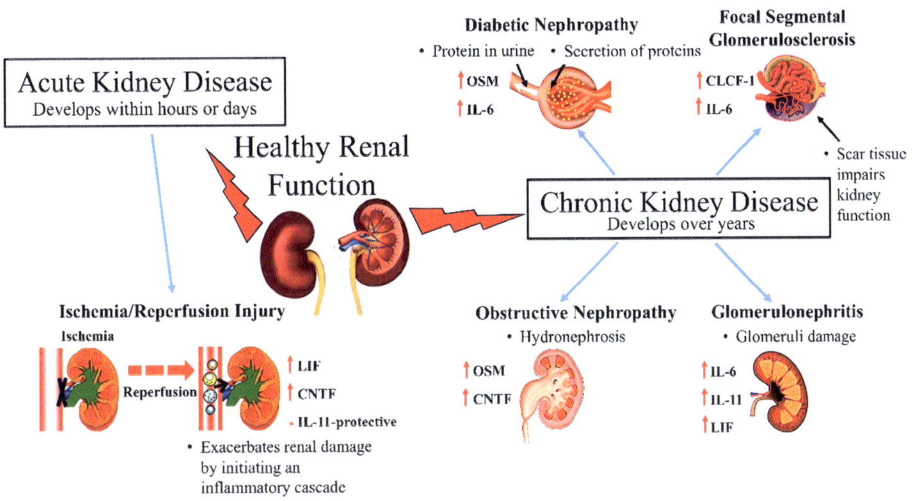

Figure 8.10. Common renal diseases and conditions.

Source: https://external-content.duckduckgo.com/iu/?u=https%3A%2F%2Fwww.mdpi.com%2Fbiomedicines%2Fbiomedicines-07-00019%2Farticle_deploy%2Fhtml%2Fimages%2Fbiomedicines-07-00019-g002.png&f=1&nofb=1&ipt=5cb9236cd547e866dbb316680f09e0d82ac416113d24b662d1aa68558b875a14.

8.4.1. Chronic Kidney Disease (CKD)

Kidney disease is an emerging public health issue—it's a chronic illness bogged down in a lot of etiology. Diabetes, high blood pressure, and even glomerulonephritis all factor into propelling chronic kidney disease forward. Addressing these issues early on really makes a difference; routine kidney exams don't just tell us how much damage has been done, but often determine treatment plans and daily life accommodations. Determining the earlier stages means it's possible to slow the problem and ensure patient well-being, making regular, if sometimes spontaneous, screening for at-risk individuals a requirement. Technology is driving new ideas on how to treat kidney disease you wouldn't have considered. Online support groups and mobile health apps have become new instruments—providing immediate information on health and even motivating patients to stick to their treatment plans. Some studies point out that these web-based resources, apart from making people more compliant with living regimens ordered by physicians, also provide simple communication with physicians and the adoption of simple-to-follow lifestyle recommendations to maintain the kidneys in equilibrium. Most of these techniques are a boon for long-term diseases such as CKD, when being aware of everything all the time and sharing tips is actually essential. With technology on the upswing, incorporating these web-based solutions could become the new standard, revolutionizing traditional approaches to kidney care. Knowing how kidney tests work is a necessity when it comes to monitoring and managing CKD—in most cases, it's simply a matter of reading the correct numbers. Screenings like serum creatinine, the eGFR (which is like a scorecard of kidney function), and urinalyses for protein give an indication of how well the kidneys are coping. eGFR, for instance, actually aids in determining the severity of the issue and directing treatment accordingly. Breaking CKD down into several stages allows doctors to adapt interventions to each patient's unique condition. And watching these numbers change over time gives important feedback on whether or not treatments are succeeding or need a rapid adjustment. Finally, making care based on good test data means it is not guesswork but an ongoing, individualized process—albeit sometimes a little rough around the edges (Figure 8.11).

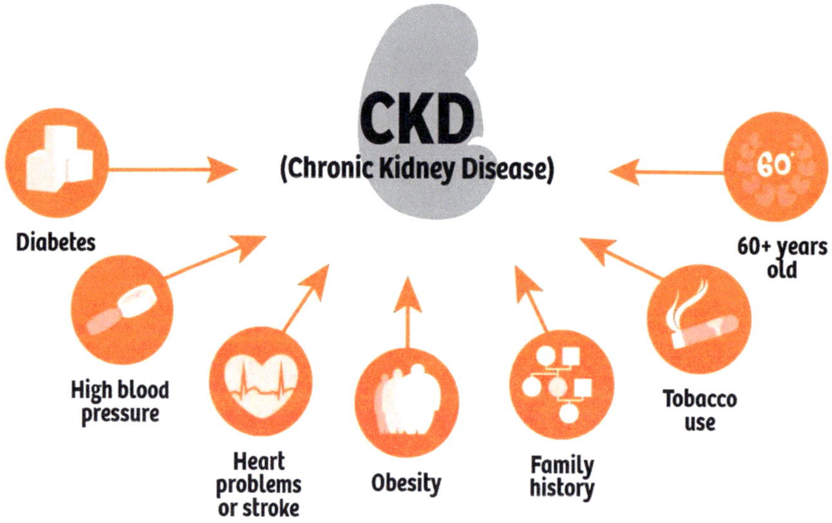

Figure 8.11. Chronic kidney disease (CKD).

Source: https://external-content.duckduckgo.com/iu/?u=https%3A%2F%2Fwww.thevirtualnephrologist.com%2Fwp-content%2Fuploads%2F2023%2F04%2FChronic-Kidney-disease-CKD-risk-factors.jpg&f=1&nofb=1&ipt=c802ce304a3b68167d503340eadefee1c02c0ec1fad5908db938be1a06345640.

8.4.2. Acute Kidney Injury (AKI)

Acute kidney injury (AKI) literally compromises kidney function and raises an eyebrow in clinics and research institutes both. A decrease in the kidneys' functionality suddenly—usually precipitated by states such as dehydration, heart disease, or even toxic exposure—can result in complications such as uncontrolled electrolyte levels and fluid overload. Early identification of the problem is, by and large, the best approach. Simple tests—measuring serum creatinine and observing urine output—give doctors an immediate measure of how well things are going in the kidneys, and this is what determines the action to take to restore normalcy while hopefully not causing long-term damage. Knowing the many facets of AKI essentially becomes crucial; these tests are literally a lifeline when dealing with patients (Black et al., 2016). There are all sorts of reasons that AKI might seem. Let's consider prerenal causes, for instance: when the kidneys are getting too little blood—usually related to dehydration or cardiac disease. Intrinsic AKI is when the kidney tissue gets compromised, possibly after acute tubular necrosis due to a lack of blood flow or toxic substances. And don't forget postrenal AKI, which shows up when something blocks the passage of urine—like a kidney stone or some other kind of obstruction. Appreciating these differences is important because it guides doctors not only in making the diagnosis but also in tailoring the treatment to fit the exact cause, thereby leading to better outcomes (Black et al., 2016). Later research seems to be drawing a linkage between AKI and CKD and reporting some kind of continuum in kidney impairment.

Clinical practice guidelines seem to describe AKI as an acute reduction in kidney function during about a week, and CKD persists for longer than three months. It is this connection that makes a single episode of AKI possibly predispose one to subsequent CKD and thus early intervention is very essential. New terminology such as acute kidney disease (AKD) also emerges to shed some more light on the way kidney disease evolves despite the fact that definitions and guidelines for AKD are still somewhat in limbo. In the vast majority of instances, the same renal tests that are useful in managing AKI also inform a wider understanding of underlying kidney disease processes (Dewitte et al., 2017) (Figure 8.12).

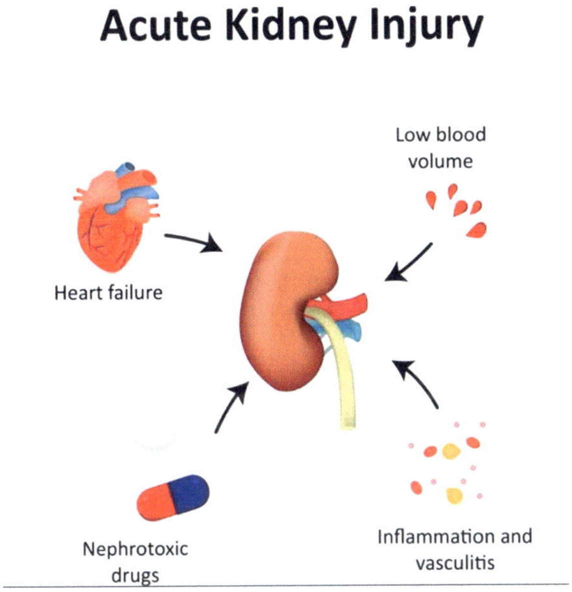

Figure 8.12. Acute kidney injury (AKI).

Source: https://external-content.duckduckgo.com/iu/?u=https%3A%2F%2Fkidneycareep.com%2Fimages%2Fpage%2Faki-acute-kidney-injury-elpaso.jpg&f=1&nofb=1&ipt=ef049f44ffcbdff900387cb8d1d13d424f79da0a5bb1e9ddfdca973729af97e9.

8.4.3. Glomerulonephritis

Glomerulonephritis does disturb kidney function, though—its inflammation gets to play with those filtering structures, the glomeruli, and typically leads to diminished overall kidney function. On most occasions, serum creatinine, blood urea nitrogen, and estimation of the glomerular filtration rate (GFR) become the key parameters to ascertain the severity of the disorder. On some occasions, when things get worse, there is a noticeable protein increase in the urine and even traces of blood. The changes help in the treatment and reveal hints about what is occurring within, just like recent research aimed to accomplish (Ali et al., 2025). The immune component of this condition adds another twist to things. A mix of circulating antibodies and immune complexes usually confirms that the condition is active, sometimes forcing clinicians into specific therapy like immunosuppressive drugs.

In a given study, for example, the use of immunotherapy led to a clear reduction in proteinuria as kidney function also improved—something reflected in better eGFR values (Ali et al., 2025). Apparently, combining data from immune markers and regular kidney tests can indeed be paving the way for more individualized treatment, albeit with the details looking a bit irregularly at first. Rapidly progressive glomerulonephritis is a league of its own—one that needs emergency care. This more severe form is described as a precipitous decline in kidney function, accompanied by symptoms such as huge protein loss and gross hematuria. It is especially difficult when there is an accompanying disease such as systemic lupus erythematosus (SLE) – overlapping complicates the diagnosis. Quick, precise tests are crucial in this case because they are direct immediate treatment regimens that integrate conventional renal assessment with immune studies. This imperfect interdisciplinary methodology can ultimately be a superior hope to avoidable injury and realize improved outcomes in those most immediately at risk (Figure 8.13).

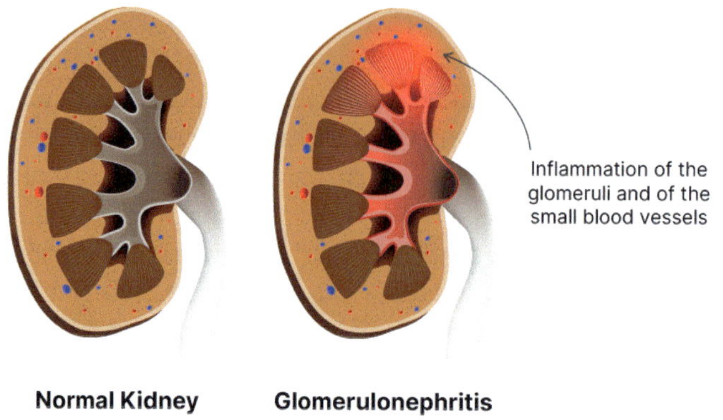

Figure 8.13. Glomerulonephritis.

Source: https://ausmed-images.s3.ap-southeast-2.amazonaws.com/ausmed.com/ausmed-articles/20220509_body_1.png.

Test Your Knowledge

1. What are the differences between acute kidney injury (AKI) and chronic kidney disease (CKD)?
2. How does diabetic nephropathy affect kidney structure and function?

8.5. Advances in Renal Function Testing

Learning Outcome

- New biomarkers for kidney function;
- Technological advancements in testing;
- Future directions in renal diagnostics.

Kidney function testing has had a major makeover in recent years, with new techniques on the horizon that change how physicians interact with patient care. Established markers such as serum creatinine and eGFR remain relevant, but there's growing buzz about newer, more sensitive markers of kidney disease. Urinary biomarkers and new imaging modalities are now in the mix, providing us with a better insight into kidney health. To illustrate, biopsies of kidney mass have started gaining acceptance—an effort endorsed by the recently published American Urological Association guidelines, which overall promote active surveillance founded on each tumor's own characteristics and thus eliminating unnecessary procedures (Steven et al., 2021). All of this indicates a growing tendency toward assessments that fit the individual. There's also been a shift towards non-surgical approaches that tag glomerular filtration rates with more precision. New studies are pointing towards techniques like inulin clearance and novel biomarkers that are more effective at detecting early kidney problems than older tests. Imaging technology—like MRI and newer ultrasound machines—also carries this capacity, enabling doctors to designate kidney issues without the need for surgery. In most cases, early detection of these conditions means quicker intervention and, in the end, better outcomes for patients. The Kidney Disease: Improving Global Outcomes movement even calls for updating our criteria for diagnosis using these new resources so clinicians can do a better job of staying current with the latest developments (Jürgen et al., 2019). With this, our expanding knowledge of the dynamic character of kidney function has seen a fresh re-examination of clinical guidelines. Shifts to the National Kidney Foundation's KDOQI, for example, reflect a demand for more flexible dosing and treatment regimens that actually respond to the individual case of the patient. This is particularly relevant when dealing with conditions like hypertension and diabetes, which have very considerable effects upon kidney function. Overall, these changes—taking genetic predispositions as well as other co-morbidities into account—warped the tradition of care towards a holistic, patient-specific model. Cumulatively, these developments not only enhance the specificity of kidney diagnostics but also lead to a more holistic attitude towards the management of renal wellness in diverse populations (Steven et al., 2021).

8.5.1. New Biomarkers for Kidney Function

Kidney health is growing more and more complex nowadays, and because of that, professionals are now looking for new biomarkers to better enlighten us about the condition of kidneys. Doctors have hitherto depended on markers like creatinine and urea—measures that, while useful over generations, have a tendency to overlook signs of imminent problems. Recently, however, some studies have been pointing to cystatin C; this marker appears to capture the kidney's filtration capability without being affected by changes in muscle mass. In most cases, this allows us to accurately test kidney function in patients whose muscle composition isn't normal. Scientists are also churning around for other biomarkers that can provide an indication of kidney issues even before the old timers start acting up (Luft et al., 2021). There's also vast churning being generated by the domain of electronic records and big data. Thousands of medical records are sorted through nowadays, sometimes barely even more like detective work than traditional research. With the ability to explore these enormous data sets, researchers are discovering patterns that indicate which patients will go on to suffer an acute kidney injury, even potentially preventing serious complications from establishing themselves. It's a blend of technical know-how and a bit of sleuthing that's opening up new pathways to faster diagnosis and, eventually, more accurate treatments (Luft et al., 2020). In spite of all these enticing prospects, a great deal more needs to be done before these new biomarkers can become a daily feature of clinical screening. Yes, there have been many promising candidates, but the practical testing and showing them to work are the hard yards of the endeavor. Scientists are committed—even though sometimes it does feel like a rough ride—to ensuring that these markers actually measure up to their promise in actual application. This is not scholarly jargon; it is a significant shift that could deeply influence kidney issues care, ultimately delivering better care to vulnerable patients (Luft et al., 2021) (Figure 8.14).

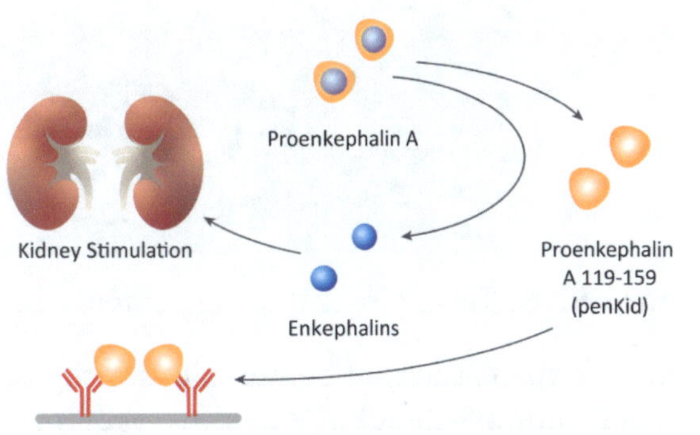

Figure 8.14. Kidney function biomarker.

Source: https://external-content.duckduckgo.com/iu/?u=https%3A%2F%2Fsphingotec.com%2Ffileadmin%2F_processed_%2F5%2F3%2Fcsm_penKid-measurement_healthy_bc36cbd253.png&f=1&nofb=1&ipt=5514e4b9dc60f79ea8b91d4e172803e918c83c51b22c2021ae4f7bc275ec24d6.

8.5.2. Technological Advancements in Testing

Technology's role in medical testing has really shaken the manner in which we test kidney function. The traditional methods, as good as they still are, fall short of capturing those small, subtle changes in how kidneys work. Nowadays, computer systems—ah, those clever new systems—step in to offer more interactive and knowledge-based diagnostic aids that seem to be tailor-made for nephrology. Studies are likely to show that these innovations not only speed up the duration to obtain results but also enhance patient engagement via real-time feedback; hence, patients and doctors can gain so much better overall understanding of kidney health (Bateh et al., 2025). The transition from paper to digital isn't just a baby step—it's a leap of giant proportions making it easy to store and analyze great quantities of data, opening up new avenues to more personalized and responsive care. And it's not always all about digital systems; imaging technology has been improved in real ways too. Take a look at the way grayscale and Doppler sonography have evolved over time. For instance, advanced Doppler imaging now provides us with vital information regarding blood flow in the kidneys—information which is key when considering conditions like chronic kidney disease or even acute kidney injury. In most instances, those Doppler resistive index (RI) values end up being intimately related to a variety of kidney problems, allowing physicians to identify and track minute changes in perfusion and structure (Polaka et al., 2024).

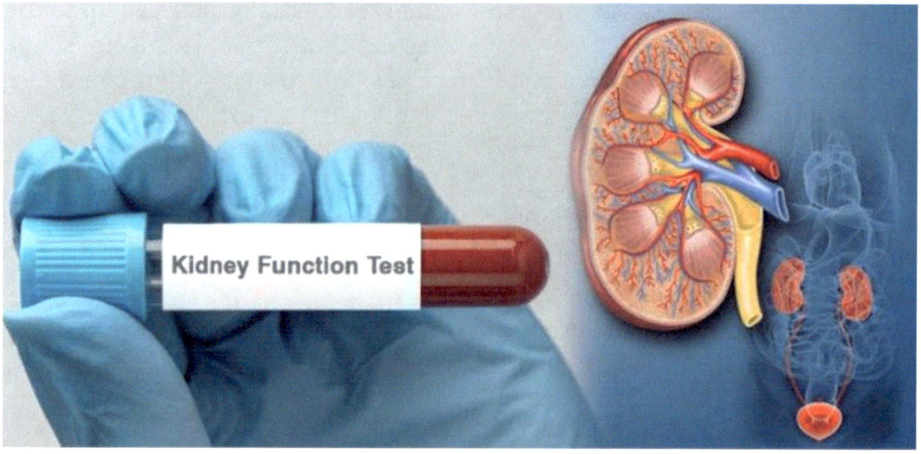

Figure 8.15. Technological advancements in testing for kidney function.

Source: https://external-content.duckduckgo.com/iu/?u=https%3A%2F%2Fwww.ganeshdiagnostic.com%2Fadmin%2Fpublic%2Fassets%2Fimages%2Fblog%2Fbanner%2Fmobile%2F1685609958-Kidney%2520Function%2520Test.webp&f=1&nofb=1&ipt=6cc5e0e7af82203a71f09d8d376ad5057abd8f3ccc3d4540d2b5769f561fa410.

Now, while it does sound a little bit techie, these imaging technologies really do serve a long way toward painting a more precise picture, enabling disease advancement and treatment assessment to be traced more readily over time. Then, of course, there is the trend toward automating lab tests, which has ushered in a new, more precise era of monitoring kidney function. Automated analyzers spit out results faster with fewer human errors, which leaves the clinicians free to do what's most important—result interpretation rather than wowing away sample analysis. Because of such developments in technology, telemedicine and remote monitoring are becoming increasingly viable;

patients can now receive their kidney function analyzed outside a traditional clinic. This shift is especially promising for those that do not have direct access to the healthcare centers, making kidney issues addressed earlier along the process and not later. In general, as our health care system evolves, these technological shifts more often than not point to not just more accurate diagnoses but better patient outcomes in the future (Polaka et al., 2024) (Figure 8.15).

8.5.3. Future Directions in Renal Diagnostics

Kidney screening today has actually taken off in ways nobody could have predicted. Rather than relying primarily on the traditional methods, new methods are revolutionizing the debate over how to monitor kidney health. The older tests are still worth their weight, but sometimes they don't catch the fine-line disturbances—particularly when patients have co-morbid conditions or nearly imperceptible problems. New biomarkers like neutrophil gelatinase-associated lipocalin (NGAL) and cystatin C are showing themselves to be useful by indicating problems before a rise in serum creatinine could, which warns doctors to a useful warning. Apart from that, imaging technology like high-resolution MRI and ultrasound now give us a clearer, if not shiny polished, image of renal architecture and function (Xia et al., 2023). AI is also truly entering kidney care—a new chapter that's as exciting as it is intimidating. Machine learning algorithms sift through huge amounts of data from electronic records and radiological images to make connections that can easily go unnoticed by a human. Overall, these models allow for the prediction of disease patterns, with more individualized treatment plans. They even reduce errors by computing test results without the usual human slips. Of course, bringing AI into a medical setup isn't entirely smooth sailing; thorough validation, data privacy issues, and ethical issues still need some judicious handling (Theilen et al., 2022). In the majority of cases, as these technologies continue to develop, we can expect an underlying shift in how kidney diagnostics are managed. And then there's the fanfare about point-of-care testing (POCT) for kidney function—having test results in hand when every second counts. Quick assessment is especially critical in emergency situations, and portable machines that can monitor kidney markers non-invasively are making that a reality even in remote or underdeveloped areas. By sometimes combining these diagnostics with wearable tech, patients and care teams are made aware of feedback on an ongoing basis, keeping chronic kidney conditions on a tighter leash. Not only does this method allow doctors to more easily keep abreast of problems down the line, but it also gives patients a more hands-on interest in their own treatment. Clearly, the future of kidney diagnosis is set to be based on technological advancements and move towards an integrated, patient-centered approach (Xia et al., 2023).

Test Your Knowledge

1. How are biomarkers such as cystatin C improving the accuracy of kidney function assessment?
2. What role does molecular and genetic testing play in modern nephrology?

8.6. Clinical Applications of Renal Function Tests

Learning Outcome

- Monitoring kidney health in patients;
- Assessing the impact of medications on renal function;
- Guiding treatment decisions in renal disease.

Kidney well-being is monitored by observing many indicators of how well the organ's functioning. Doctors depend significantly on routine kidney tests—also known as RFTs—as a snapshot picture of how well the kidneys are doing, whether an individual is having sudden or long-term issues. They measure markers like blood creatinine and the eGFR, which in most cases actually determines medicine dosing and overall care. It is found that age, gender, and even muscle mass can affect such measurements, so calculating a modified eGFR in some groups often results in values that feel a little truer, which is maybe preferable to informing treatment. Once chronic disease is on the horizon, like diabetes or high blood pressure, regular kidney checks become even more significant. For instance, diabetics are likely to find smaller-sized blood vessel complications that may potentially cause diabetic kidney disease in the future. Regular RFTs thus serve as an early warning system—alerting professionals to those tiny changes before they balloon into major problems. Sometimes, these tests raise a red flag on atypical cases such as non-albuminuric diabetic kidney disease, reminding doctors to think about a patient's overall picture rather than solely hoping on a single result. In the majority of situations, relating these lab results to a physical examination provides a better and more realistic picture of a person's kidney condition, which can affect the planning of care significantly. New research even indicates that kidney tests are shifting upward over and above the usual numbers. Experiments show that kidney function can fluctuate a bit in individuals juggling other health issues, which is why it is important to add those extra facts. Some new biomarkers like neutrophil gelatinase-associated lipocalin (NGAL) or cystatin C are being incorporated recently. Including these additional markers can, in most cases, bring greater accuracy to the sensitivity and specificity of standard tests, enabling doctors to detect early warning signs of complications sooner. All of this new evidence means that refining our approach to kidney exams isn't really about landing a diagnosis—as much as it is about being smart about how we individualize treatment plans, even when minor lapses or slight inconsistencies inevitably creep in between.

8.6.1. Monitoring Kidney Health in Patients

Kidney function is receiving a lot of attention these days, especially because chronic kidney disease cases keep on increasing everywhere in the world. Ultrasound examinations which examine the thickness of kidney tissue are a very effective means of determining how well the kidneys are functioning. In many situations, comparing these thickness measurements between patients with CKD and healthy individuals offers significant information regarding overall kidney function. One study, for instance, found that CKD patients overall had substantially thinner kidney tissues than normal—closely associated with dysfunction in terms of measures like serum creatinine and estimated glomerular filtration rate (Ahmad et al., 2025). Tracking these levels helps doctors detect early alterations so that they can act before the condition worsens. Along with these more traditional tests, newer, minimally invasive methods are beginning to transform the way we track kidney health. Thanks to breakthroughs like near-infrared (NIR) spectroscopy and artificial intelligence (AI)-

driven optical sensing technology, physicians can now acquire quick, real-time images of kidney tissues. In a study involving patients with varying levels of kidney issues, the AI method was extremely precise, sensitive, and specific in detecting severe dysfunction (Divya et al., 2024). These new methods, by rescuing patients from the exposure to painful blood draws or biopsies, not only enhance patient comfort but also push clinical outcomes in the right direction—no matter how futuristic the method might seem at first glance. The blending of both old tests and these new, technology-driven methods really finishes our strategy for kidney care. Regular checks—whether using age-old markers like serum creatinine or diving into modern AI-enhanced imaging—give a fuller picture that helps guide treatment decisions. Timely monitoring catches even subtle shifts in kidney status, which is critical for preventing major complications from CKD. As research and development continue to pave the way for better diagnostics, we're witnessing a gradual shift from invasive procedures to techniques that're more patient-friendly. Finally, the transformation guarantees a future where care is accessible and more effective (Ahmad et al., 2025; Divya et al., 2024) (Figure 8.16).

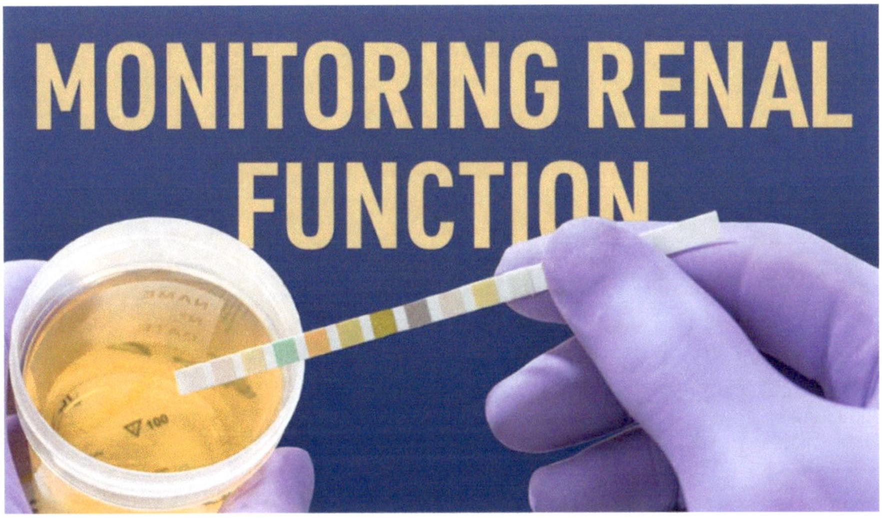

Figure 8.16. Monitoring renal function.

Source: https://external-content.duckduckgo.com/iu/?u=https%3A%2F%2Fausmed-images.s3.ap-southeast-2.amazonaws.com%2Fausmed.com%2Fausmed-articles%2F20181008_cover_V2.jpg&f=1&nofb=1&ipt=3dc3a63f98506f58f3b4dccc785bcfc33beb0c3cdd37ee7e6f96c2509cabb42c.

8.6.2. Assessing the Impact of Medications on Renal Function

Doctors have been curious for a long time about what effect different drugs would have on the functioning of the kidneys. You know, different drugs—NSAIDs, certain antibiotics, etc.—have a tendency to come under a microscope because they act on renal function. Often, the simple tests done regularly for the kidneys (checking serum creatinine and electrolytes, e.g.) will actually yield evidence of stress, and such can literally signal the presence of drug-induced kidney issues. Studies often suggest that long-term NSAID use may on occasion cause acute kidney injury, and it is even more important, accordingly, that such patients on these drugs are monitored closely, although the warning signs may come stealthily. The controversy over creatine supplementing the picture further, especially among athletes. It is a common misconception that creatine is almost risk-free, but there are still risks involved with its effect on kidneys. Interestingly, studies—including employing methods like Mendelian randomization—tend to have little association between kidney injury and creatine levels, with p values above 0.05 (Zhou et al., 2024). This form of evidence propels us toward evidence-based practice and also challenges some unsupported concerns about the safety of creatine, in general. Assessing patients on therapies like hemodialysis, a volume status check reveals yet another layer of kidney care complication. Equipment like bioelectrical impedance analysis (BIA) has been reasonably effective in quantifying body fluid content and even show correlations with measures of heart function (Wang et al., 2024). Astonishingly enough, metrics like Extracellular Water (ECW) do seem to emerge as independent risk factors—meaning that having excess fluid can overload kidney function even more. This interaction, nevertheless, justifies the need for integrating extensive and occasionally mildly differentiated measurement tools into practice as a matter of course in order to be able to identify and manage drug kidney effects and fluid overload and eventually direct towards better patient outcomes (Figure 8.17).

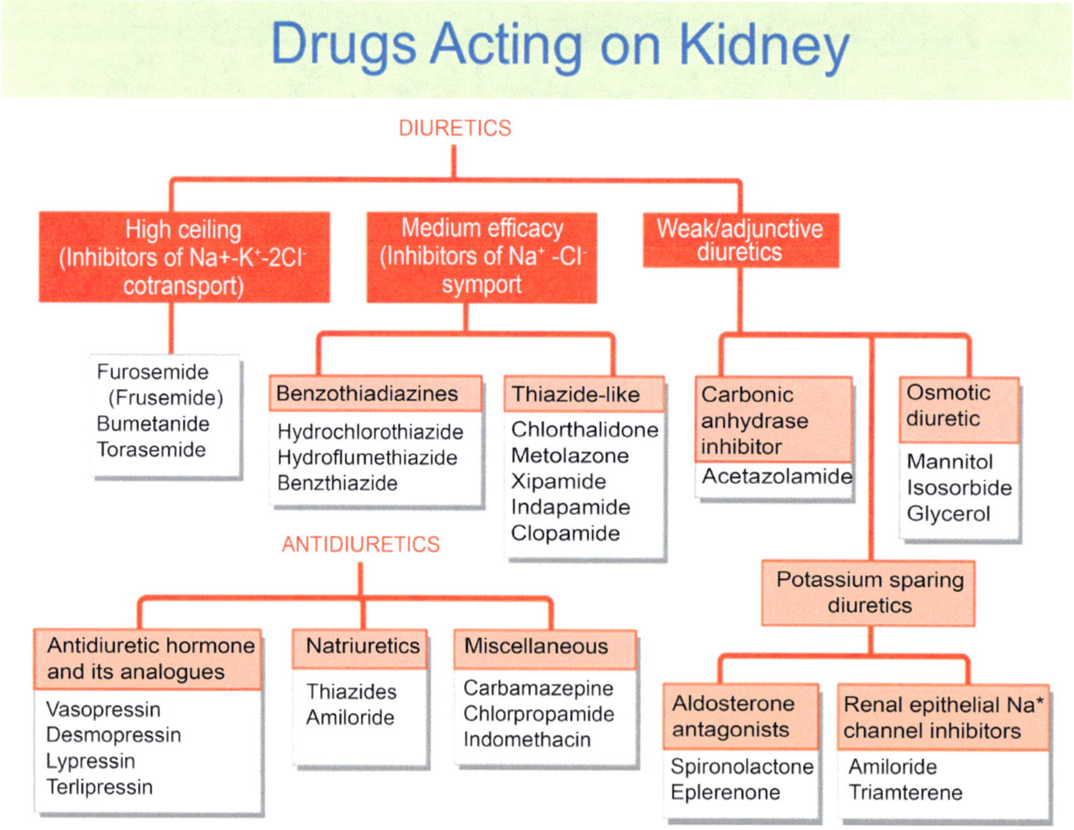

Figure 8.17. The impact of medications on renal function.

Source: https://external-content.duckduckgo.com/iu/?u=https%3A%2F%2Fi1.rgstatic.net%2Fpublication%2F352293557_kidney_drug%2Flinks%2F60c244e54585157774c7b22e%2Flargepreview.png&f=1&nofb=1&ipt=f3aa00b7e3b793528542fa956af5f76e2f1481d8dbc9061305e989935978aa5c.

8.6.3. Guiding Treatment Decisions in Renal Disease

Evaluation of kidney health is paramount when treating kidney disease. Clinicians rely on lab tests because they give an immediate indication of the functioning of the kidneys – a factor that directly influences short-term as well as long-term therapeutic plans. Generally, studies show that kidney function is closely linked with the overall prognosis of patients, especially in serious conditions such as infective endocarditis (IE). For example, when patients present with high creatinine levels alongside low glomerular filtration rates, they often face greater mortality risks—and that really highlights the urgency to act quickly and modify treatment strategies accordingly. Having an idea of what these numbers are, even in simple terms, is helpful for healthcare workers to make the best decisions, such as potential surgeries, when trying to manage the risks of declining kidney function (Balc et al., 2024). It can get more complicated when you include the degree to which patients do know their own conditions, especially in cases with end-stage renal disease (ESRD). In a majority of cases, limited health literacy can keep patients from being assertive in their care and compliant with the treatments they are undergoing.

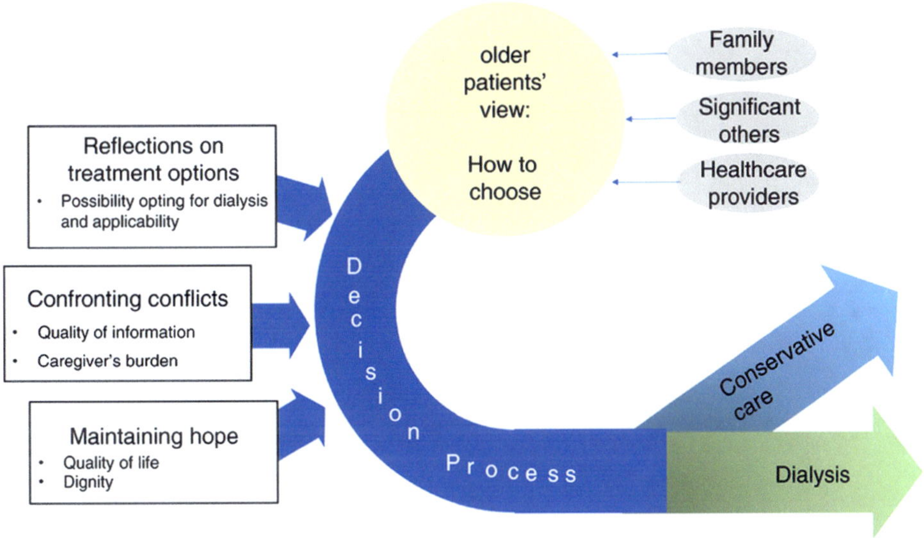

Figure 8.18. Guiding treatment decisions in renal disease.

Source: https://external-content.duckduckgo.com/iu/?u=https%3A%2F%2Fwww.researchgate.net%2Fpublication%2F353018663%2Ffigure%2Ffig2%2FAS%3A1101631286444038%401639660774115%2FTreatment-decision-making-process-in-older-adults-with-end-stage-renal-failure.png&f=1&nofb=1&ipt=6d421734190192701ceae3367fb699d8236c6e679bcae8d3ed0b38476a385976.

Based on recent research, most patients on hemodialysis cannot effectively receive and respond to important health information—information that's important in making well-informed decisions about their treatment. Patients typically appear to have trouble completely comprehending what their illness is all about, what they can do to prevent further deterioration, or how they can get better overall. This means that doctors are not only responsible for monitoring kidney function, but also for improving the way they communicate critical health data so patients are more involved in care decisions (Zahraa et al., 2023). Beyond simply reading test results, a team process is truly essential to treatment planning. When nephrologists, primary care doctors, nurses, and patient educators work together, all aspects of a patient's well-being get some attention – not just the bodily aspect, but also psychological care and lifestyle guidance. In most cases, this teamwork becomes necessary when lab reports indicate that a patient's condition is worsening very rapidly and immediate action is needed. Aligning treatment approaches with integrated patient support enables health care providers to navigate the multifaceted issues of managing renal disease. By so doing, they ensure that the care is integrated, suited to the individual needs of each patient, and maximizes outcomes and quality of life (Balc et al., 2024; Zahraa et al., 2023) (Figure 8.18).

Test Your Knowledge

1. How are renal function tests used in monitoring patients with hypertension and diabetes?
2. In what ways do renal tests guide drug dosing and pharmacotherapy adjustments?

Summary

Kidney tests do a whole lot more than just make sure your kidneys are fine; they literally have a hand in diagnosing issues and deciding treatments for all kinds of issues. They give us clues not only on how mighty the kidneys are, but even on how other diseases could be interfering with them. Take, for example, sickle cell disease individuals—it is not surprising that there is going to be a trace of renal issue in such cases, and thus doctors take quite a generalized approach to treatment to steer clear of the risks posed by renal illness (Qadah et al., 2025). When specialists have a good understanding of these test results, they are able to refine treatments, adjust medications, and even offer some helpful lifestyle tips, all of which help to improve overall health. There's also the situation with chronic disease like diabetes, where tracking kidney function is kind of a big deal when it comes to avoiding complications like diabetic foot ulcers. In the majority of instances, the research has noted that patients with diabetic foot ulcers are most likely to exhibit noticeable differences in their kidney laboratory tests, which will slightly make it harder to manage their care (Sridhar et al., 2025). This overlap truly underscores the reason that it's needed—in most cases—to do routine kidney function tests in people who are already at risk because catching problems early can truly lower the chances of more complications down the line. All things considered, kidney tests have become an important part of modern medicine. They are critical parts of the treatment plan and diagnosis, guiding decisions that generally result in better patient outcomes. Having these tests run regularly and considered with other measures of health raises the chances of finding kidney problems early on, which results in higher preventative care. Because medicine continues to progress, incorporating extensive kidney testing into daily patient care is still of the highest priority for meeting the many challenges associated with chronic diseases.

Kidney tests provide us with an honest idea of how well our kidneys are filtering out our blood. Doctors like to review the glomerular filtration rate (or GFR, as they refer to it) to see if the kidneys are keeping up, but also review such variables as serum creatinine, blood urea nitrogen (BUN), and even do urine tests. Each test throws a bit of light on many areas of kidney function—even an asymptomatic rise in creatinine can point to something being amiss, so more tests are done. Urine tests in some instances provide a hint of dehydration or some other issue, so clinicians order more (Vahanian et al., 2021). These tests are not just to make a diagnosis, though. In summary, they're a valuable instrument for tracking chronic kidney disease (CKD) over time. Regular follow-ups enable doctors to identify minor adjustments that necessitate alterations in treatment protocols. Staging CKD using GFR estimates helps determine the speed with which a treatment would be needed, and with official guidelines, most of the time, it guarantees risks—such as those posed by certain drugs—don't slip through the gap (Jean-Ricco et al., 2017). It is a bit like keeping a well-used engine in tune closely, making sure all of its components are working right. What is most important is that with these tests, kidney problems can be detected early. With diabetes and high blood pressure often hiding behind kidney problems, constant monitoring isn't so unclear. For those who have risk factors, follow-up kidney function testing can lead to individually tailored treatment plans that might even postpone the onset of end-stage kidney disease. More sophisticated testing techniques, such as some new biomarkers, are raising the stakes on accuracy as well. In the end, simply understanding these tests gives clinicians the information they need to make better decisions, which in turn helps everyone (Vahanian et al., 2021).

KEY TERMS FROM THIS CHAPTER

- Blood urea nitrogen (BUN)
- Chronic kidney disease (CKD)
- Creatinine clearance
- Cystatin C
- Fractional excretion of sodium (FENa)
- Glomerular filtration rate (GFR)
- Hematuria
- Microalbuminuria
- Nephrotic syndrome
- Proteinuria
- Renal biopsy
- Renal ultrasound
- Serum creatinine
- Specific gravity
- Urinalysis
- Urine osmolality
- Urine pH
- Urine potassium

Critical Thinking Questions

1. **Which of the following is commonly used to assess kidney function?**
   a. Bilirubin
   b. Creatinine
   c. Amylase
   d. Hemoglobin
2. **What is the primary purpose of the Glomerular Filtration Rate (GFR)?**
   a. To measure liver function
   b. To assess blood pressure
   c. To evaluate how well the kidneys filter blood
   d. To determine oxygen saturation
3. **Which test is most useful for detecting early kidney damage in diabetic patients?**
   a. Serum calcium
   b. Microalbuminuria
   c. Uric acid level
   d. BUN
4. **Blood Urea Nitrogen (BUN) levels are influenced by all the following EXCEPT:**
   a. Protein intake
   b. Dehydration
   c. Liver function
   d. Lung function
5. **Elevated serum creatinine usually indicates:**
   a. Good kidney function
   b. Decreased muscle activity
   c. Impaired renal function
   d. Increased liver detoxification

Answers to Critical Thinking Questions

1. (b); 2. (c); 3. (b); 4. (d); 5. (c)

Short answer Questions

1. What is the primary purpose of renal function tests?
2. What does the glomerular filtration rate (GFR) measure, and how is it typically estimated?
3. What is creatinine clearance, and how does it relate to kidney function?
4. What is the difference between prerenal, renal, and postrenal causes of elevated BUN?
5. What does a urinalysis assess in terms of kidney function?
6. What does the presence of protein or albumin in urine indicate in kidney disease?

References

1. Ahmad, W., Mobeen, H., Ahmad Shah, A. W., Mobeen, N., Rehman, A. U., & Bibi, A. (2025). Comparative ultrasound assessment of renal parenchymal thickness and renal function tests in chronic kidney disease. *Kashf Journal of Multidisciplinary Research*. https://www.semanticscholar.org/paper/924d4f8dc1574c82704467eced465bd4fffec21f (accessed on 1st July 2025).

2. Ahmed, A. R. H., Abdullah, R. A., Wasmi, M. S., Alush, R. A. A., & Mehsun, A. A. (2024). Study of the long-term effects of diabetes on the overall health and quality of life in thalassemia patients. *European Journal of Medical Genetics and Clinical Biology*. https://www.semanticscholar.org/paper/874b6d022374c2130e87ce3ebe86d4f7b7c7413d (accessed on 1st July 2025).

3. AlAni, H. T., & Al-Lami, M. Q. (2024). Evaluation of some biochemical and hematological parameters in patients with chronic kidney disease. *Journal of the Faculty of Medicine Baghdad*. https://www.semanticscholar.org/paper/ac7a7e85761265c34a7db2cd11620bbb95437970 (accessed on 1st July 2025).

4. Ali, L., Shahzad, M., Hayat, F., & Hayat, S. (2025). Immunological aspects of glomerulonephritis advances in diagnosis and treatment: A prospective study. *Journal of Nowshera Medical College*. https://www.semanticscholar.org/paper/b25b340156214671870bee07915d61c4ef52bd3e (accessed on 1st July 2025).

5. Balcı, A. B., Kolay, G., & Yazici, S. (2024). [MSB-09] The impact of renal functions on mortality in patients undergoing surgery for infective endocarditis. *Cardiovascular Surgery and Interventions*. https://www.semanticscholar.org/paper/dbdefd478841669877d4d1dbe407914b6e7cf34c (accessed on 1st July 2025).

6. Bateh, K., Saurman, J., Bartsch, B., Xu, Y., Aboul-Nour, H., Hanson, A., Guan, E., et al. (2025). Abstract TP45: Advancements in digital cognitive assessments for post-stroke patients: A scoping review. *Stroke*. https://www.semanticscholar.org/paper/b6580552b8f35cad104092b93db52d6525207b5f (accessed on 1st July 2025).

7. Biggins, S. W., Angeli, P., García-Tsao, G., Ginès, P., Ling, S. C., Nadim, M. K., Wong, F., et al. (2021). Diagnosis, evaluation, and management of ascites, spontaneous bacterial peritonitis and hepatorenal syndrome: 2021 practice guidance by the American Association for the Study of Liver Diseases. *Hepatology, 74*, 1014–1048. https://doi.org/10.1002/hep.31884 (accessed on 1st July 2025).

8. Black, C., Marks, A., & Sawhney, S. (2016). Discharge after acute kidney injury: Recognizing and managing risk. https://core.ac.uk/download/42130561.pdf (accessed on 1st July 2025).

9. Campbell, K. L., Campbell, Z. C., Chow, C. K., Lee, V. W., et al. (2016). eHealth interventions for people with chronic kidney disease. https://core.ac.uk/download/196601644.pdf (accessed on 1st July 2025).

10. Campbell, S. C., Uzzo, R. G., Allaf, M. E., Bass, E. B., Cadeddu, J. A., Chang, A., Clark, P. E., et al. (2017). Renal mass and localized renal cancer: AUA guideline. *The Journal of Urology, 198*, 520–529. https://doi.org/10.1016/j.juro.2017.04.100 (accessed on 1st July 2025).

11. Campbell, S. C., Uzzo, R. G., Karam, J. A., Chang, S. S., Clark, P. E., & Souter, L. (2021). Renal mass and localized renal cancer: Evaluation, management, and follow-up: AUA guideline: Part II. *The Journal of Urology, 206*, 209–218. https://doi.org/10.1097/ju.0000000000001912 (accessed on 1st July 2025).

12. Canali, D., Zampieri, G., Motta, C. M., Oliveira, D. C., Rosin, C., Argolo, S. V., & Satsuma, W. (2023). B-035 Maintaining the analytical performance of calcium and phosphorus in 24-hour urine without addition of 6n HCl in the pre-analytical process. *Clinical Chemistry*. https://www.semanticscholar.org/paper/b0bc022d4a7882b4b226004d127d555a89437e79 (accessed on 1st July 2025).

13. Coulthard, E., & Hosseini, A. A. (2023). Blood biomarkers: Ready for clinical practice? *Journal of Neurology, Neurosurgery, and Psychiatry, 94*, 409–410. https://www.semanticscholar.org/paper/690f31c61712304d835869d31b80588c8204d2f6 (accessed on 1st July 2025).

14. Crabb, D. W., Im, G. Y., Szabó, G., Mellinger, J. L., & Lucey, M. R. (2019). Diagnosis and treatment of alcohol-associated liver diseases: 2019 practice guidance from the American Association for the Study of Liver Diseases. *Hepatology, 71*, 306–333. https://doi.org/10.1002/hep.30866 (accessed on 1st July 2025).

15. Dagher, P. C., El-Achkar, T. M., Ghosh, J., Hato, T., et al. (2017). Tamm-Horsfall protein regulates mononuclear phagocytes in the kidney. https://core.ac.uk/download/228066343.pdf (accessed on 1st July 2025).

16. Das, U. K., & Chowdhury, E. H. (2024). Male systemic lupus erythematosus, rapidly progressive glomerulonephritis, and iatrogenic acute bone marrow failure: A case report. *International Journal of Scientific Reports*. https://www.semanticscholar.org/paper/36729c8952d2fa848f1a39b31f5b51ce6cb916a1 (accessed on 1st July 2025).

17. Dewitte, A., Ishani, A., Morden, A., Pai, A. B., Schneider, A. G., Lewington, A. J., et al. (2017). Acute kidney disease and renal recovery: Consensus report of the Acute Disease Quality Initiative (ADQI) 16 Workgroup. https://core.ac.uk/download/84041861.pdf (accessed on 1st July 2025).

18. Divya, G., & Vasuki, R. (2024). AI-driven optical sensing techniques for non-invasive kidney function evaluation. *2024 International Conference on Power, Energy, Control and Transmission Systems (ICPECTS)*. https://www.semanticscholar.org/paper/5b72fbac2f6219faeb9b4eb99a4efc087d54f12b (accessed on 1st July 2025).

19. Fernando, J., & Zhou, S. (2015). The role of zinc in renal pathological changes in diabetic status. https://core.ac.uk/download/130975189.pdf (accessed on 1st July 2025).

20. Floege, J., Barbour, S., Cattran, D., Hogan, J. J., Nachman, P. H., Tang, S. C. W., Wetzels, J. F. M., et al. (2019). Management and treatment of glomerular diseases (part 1): Conclusions from a kidney disease: Improving Global Outcomes (KDIGO) controversies conference. *Kidney International, 95*, 268–280. https://doi.org/10.1016/j.kint.2018.10.018 (accessed on 1st July 2025).

21. Floris, R., Demontis, M., Carboni, G., Palmas, S., Boi, A., & Delogu, G. (2024). A case report of an asymptomatic patient with type 2 Wellens' syndrome and renal carcinoma. *European Heart Journal Supplements*. https://www.semanticscholar.org/paper/29cf0134a191b8fbf10068537a184d590b2b9706 (accessed on 1st July 2025).

22. Freitas, R. de A., Santos Filho, M. dos, De Campos, S. N., Correa, L., De Carvalho, W. T. S., De Moraes, M. A., Gomes, V. H., et al. (2020). Malignant tumor of the peripheral nerve sheath in a left Whippet canine kidney. *Acta Scientiae Veterinarian*. https://www.semanticscholar.org/paper/120f12ca4f0af29df528d5baaf0d0c925b6e98fa (accessed on 1st July 2025).

23. Go, A., Parikh, C., Ikizler, T., Coca, S., Siew, E., Chinchilli, V., Hsu, C. Y., et al. (2010). The

assessment, serial evaluation, and subsequent sequelae of acute kidney injury (ASSESS-AKI) study: Design and methods. *BMC Nephrology, 11*, 22. https://www.semanticscholar.org/paper/a2fafd9ced880273320c2d1428de4c257a2f4b8b (accessed on 1st July 2025).

24. Gokhale, V., Mishra, M. P., Yadav, P., & Giduturi, V. N. (2024). Proliferative glomerulonephritis with section monoclonal immunoglobulin deposits: A case report. *Journal of Clinical and Diagnostic Research*. https://www.semanticscholar.org/paper/0c4a7ace8970d0ce8e8cbe002dac449ea143dbc1 (accessed on 1st July 2025).
25. Goyal, A., Singh, K., Shrivastava, R., & Gupta, A. (2024). Comparative analysis of renal parameters test results: Fully automated vs semi-automated biochemical analyzer. *Global Journal for Research Analysis*. https://www.semanticscholar.org/paper/6c477e5fc34250070c84cd8808e02fd4c60aa916 (accessed on 1st July 2025).
26. Jassem, Z. A., & Ashour, I. (2023). Determination of health literacy among end stage renal disease patients. *Pakistan Journal of Medical and Health Sciences*. https://www.semanticscholar.org/paper/9cd0e6d43af214fdbec2d1a8d0d6bcbc73cf80ac (accessed on 1st July 2025).
27. Kapatia, G. (2023). Role of peripheral blood film in renal diseases. *Journal of Human Anatomy*. https://www.semanticscholar.org/paper/c4b4c38207636e857b37d684fcb6cf0ee97d6dde (accessed on 1st July 2025).
28. Konstantinides, S., Torbicki, A., Agnelli, G., Danchin, N., Fitzmaurice, D., Galiè, N., Gibbs, J. S. R., et al. (2014). 2014 ESC guidelines on the diagnosis and management of acute pulmonary embolism. *European Heart Journal, 35*, 3033–3080. https://doi.org/10.1093/eurheartj/ehu283 (accessed on 1st July 2025).
29. Kushnirenko, S., Savytska, L., Rotova, S., Bevzenko, T., & Lysianska, O. (2025). 24-hour urine metabolic profile: Collection technique and procedure, reference values. *Health of Man*. https://www.semanticscholar.org/paper/cd036e1ddf331018614fc738bb5d978f3d8947ae (accessed on 1st July 2025).
30. Lanzani, C., Simonini, M., Citterio, L., Zagato, L., Brioni, E., Damanti, S., Messaggio, E., et al. (2024). #2123 Ageing, renal function and frailty: Analysis of the FRASNET study. *Nephrology Dialysis Transplantation*. https://www.semanticscholar.org/paper/2094e3bae366fe5bb91d67289a1478a08e1ed74e (accessed on 1st July 2025).
31. Luck, S., Wieringa, J. W., Blázquez-Gamero, D., Henneke, P., Schuster, K., Butler, K., Capretti, M. G., et al. (2017). Congenital cytomegalovirus. *The Pediatric Infectious Disease Journal, 36*, 1205–1213. https://doi.org/10.1097/inf.0000000000001763 (accessed on 1st July 2025).
32. Luft, F. C. (2020). Biomarkers and predicting acute kidney injury. https://core.ac.uk/download/516406061.pdf (accessed on 1st July 2025).
33. Luft, F. C. (2021). Biomarkers and predicting acute kidney injury. https://core.ac.uk/download/326810584.pdf (accessed on 1st July 2025).
34. Mahmoud, E., Abdullaziz, I., & Metwally, A. (2025). Comparative evaluation of clinical, ultrasonographic and specific serum biomarkers of traumatic reticuloperitonitis and traumatic pericarditis in cattle. *Alexandria Journal of Veterinary Sciences*. https://www.semanticscholar.org/paper/2fea3c66a08ef08b967d5d33e3be387bd7ac480a (accessed on 1st July 2025).
35. Mazidi, M., Dehghan, A., Mikhailidis, D., Jozwiak, J., Covic, A., Sattar, N., Banach, M., et al. (2021). The association between coffee and caffeine consumption and renal function: Insight

from individual-level data, Mendelian randomization, and meta-analysis. *Archives of Medical Science: AMS, 18*, 900–911. https://www.semanticscholar.org/paper/8e477e6b4f2a5c204b6fa3e010c91058720dc448 (accessed on 1st July 2025).

36. McAdoo, S. P., Tanna, A., Hrušková, Z., Holm, L., Weiner, M., Arulkumaran, N., Kang, A., et al. (2017). Patients double-seropositive for ANCA and anti-GBM antibodies have varied renal survival, frequency of relapse, and outcomes compared to single-seropositive patients. *Kidney International, 92*, 693–702. https://doi.org/10.1016/j.kint.2017.03.014 (accessed on 1st July 2025).

37. Mickhael, H., Mohamed, A., Roushdy, A., & Labib, A. (2020). Ultrasound versus fluoroscopic guided sacroiliac joint injection in patient with chronic sacroiliac joint pain. *Minia Journal of Medical Research*. https://www.semanticscholar.org/paper/7b20aeea15ecc5b09624c8dd76c6333c99cce17c (accessed on 1st July 2025).

38. Navirius, F. J., Pamudji, G., & Herowati, R. (2023). Effect of red betel leaf extract (*Piper crocatum*) on blood glucose levels and kidney histopathology in streptozotocin-nicotinamide induced rats. *Journal La Medihealtico*. https://www.semanticscholar.org/paper/1712512b31cbe0ad78b690445e7f55c7917d24d8 (accessed on 1st July 2025).

39. Phan, K., Chang, K. Y., Haun, T., Gil, A., Pham, J., Truong, P., & Liao, Y. (2024). Effects of heavy alcohol use on fasting glucose and insulin resistance in mid-life adults. *Physiology*. https://www.semanticscholar.org/paper/ac08d8861e5e7bae8f5b61a88bf54144df7f6525 (accessed on 1st July 2025).

40. Polaka, Y., Christina, E. P., Ramakrishnan, K., Mohanakrishnan, A., & Natarajan, P. (2024). A study assessing the role of renal grayscale ultrasonography and flowmetry in correlation with renal function tests across various renal diseases. *Cureus, 16*. https://www.semanticscholar.org/paper/cfc1fb7bd571f8139db7420aa989fd819501cc4b (accessed on 1st July 2025).

41. Qadah, T., & Refaei, A. (2025). Evaluation of the renal function among sickle cell patients: A cross-sectional study. *Italian Journal of Medicine*. https://www.semanticscholar.org/paper/c021cd58daf00e2fac3b31acdc4d64986df0f488 (accessed on 1st July 2025).

42. Ricco, J. B., Bartelink, M. L., Björck, M., Brodmann, M., Cohnert, T., Czerny, M., De Carlo, M., et al. (2017). 2017 ESC guidelines on the diagnosis and treatment of peripheral arterial diseases, in collaboration with the European Society for Vascular Surgery (ESVS). *European Heart Journal, 39*, 763–816. https://doi.org/10.1093/eurheartj/ehx095 (accessed on 1st July 2025).

43. Sharma, K. K., Kumhar, M. R., Shrivastav, M., & Tak, H. (2021). Relationship of mean platelet volume with chronic obstructive pulmonary disease and its severity–An observational study. *International Journal of Advanced Research*. https://www.semanticscholar.org/paper/b4561b864f5b469574a51df7ea085972504d1f26 (accessed on 1st July 2025).

44. Sim, L. L. W., Ban, K., Tan, T., Sethi, S., & Loh, T. P. (2017). Development of a clinical decision support system for diabetes care: A pilot study. *PLoS ONE, 12*. https://www.semanticscholar.org/paper/2f4cdeca04b0ffaf9442045c454d8c2333bc7161 (accessed on 1st July 2025).

45. Sridhar, J., Pratheeba, P., Subburaaj, A. P., Balaji, A., & Deepak, D. (2025). Prevalence, interpretation and management of diabetic lower limb amputation in a tertiary care center. *Journal of Neonatal Surgery*. https://www.semanticscholar.org/paper/762ba823965ee6384045fd965fb43b91833bc67f (accessed on 1st July 2025).

46. Su, H., Yang, M., Wan, C., Yi, L. X., Tang, F., Zhu, H. Y., Yi, F., et al. (2020). Renal histopathological analysis of 26 postmortem findings of patients with COVID-19 in China. *Kidney International, 98*, 219–227. https://doi.org/10.1016/j.kint.2020.04.003 (accessed on 1st July 2025).

47. Theilen, T., Braun, Y., Bochennek, K., Rolle, U., Fiegel, H., & Friedmacher, F. (2022). Multidisciplinary treatment strategies for Wilms tumor: Recent advances, technical innovations and future directions. *Frontiers in Pediatrics, 10*. https://www.semanticscholar.org/paper/003f47e259ecd423fed002874503851f83620428 (accessed on 1st July 2025).

48. Urbanovych, A., & Vereshchynska, A. (2024). Role of proadrenomedullin in the progression of diabetic kidney disease in patients with type 2 diabetes mellitus. *International Journal of Endocrinology (Ukraine)*. https://www.semanticscholar.org/paper/ac05cd9dd08c753a88d1750317588cf386a46233 (accessed on 1st July 2025).

49. Vahanian, A., Beyersdorf, F., Praz, F., Milojevic, M., Baldus, S., Bauersachs, J., Capodanno, D., et al. (2021). 2021 ESC/EACTS guidelines for the management of valvular heart disease. *European Heart Journal, 43*, 561–632. https://doi.org/10.1093/eurheartj/ehab395 (accessed on 1st July 2025).

50. Volpe, M., Gallo, G., & Rubattu, S. (2022). Endocrine functions of the heart: From bench to bedside. *European Heart Journal, 44*, 643–655. https://doi.org/10.1093/eurheartj/ehac759 (accessed on 1st July 2025).

51. Wang, Y., Wang, Y., Wu, S., Xu, N., Zhang, Z., Ruan, Z., Wang, R., et al. (2024). Impact of volume indices in bioelectrical impedance measurement on the assessment of cardiac function indices by echocardiography in hemodialysis patients. *Renal Failure, 46*. https://www.semanticscholar.org/paper/26c7eb3d611071728155cb0338639136b5e75d27 (accessed on 1st July 2025).

52. Wei, P. F. (2020). Diagnosis and treatment protocol for novel coronavirus pneumonia (Trial Version 7). *Chinese Medical Journal, 133*, 1087–1095. https://doi.org/10.1097/cm9.0000000000000819 (accessed on 1st July 2025).

53. Wen, M., Zhao, S., Wang, H., Lv, Q., Liu, T., Han, J., Zhang, H., et al. (2025). Comparative analysis of perioperative renal function in patients undergoing heart transplantation and left ventricular assist device implantation: A multicenter retrospective study. *Journal of Thoracic Disease, 17*, 676–686. https://www.semanticscholar.org/paper/7a77984f162317d101b5b201a92098aadf025673 (accessed on 1st July 2025).

54. Xia, Z., & Rajak, R. (2023). OA10 Pregnancy-associated osteoporosis–A rare subset of bone disease. *Rheumatology Advances in Practice, 7*. https://www.semanticscholar.org/paper/4dd9685a93f917d49a8b22f167e45740c6935b2e (accessed on 1st July 2025).

55. Zhou, B., Hong, M., Jin, L., & Ling, K. (2024). Exploring the relationship between creatine supplementation and renal function: Insights from Mendelian randomization analysis. *Renal Failure, 46*. https://www.semanticscholar.org/paper/882ea9348d9dd77797fb74e30e5bc28e7f59d34d (accessed on 1st July 2025).

LIVER FUNCTION TESTS

9

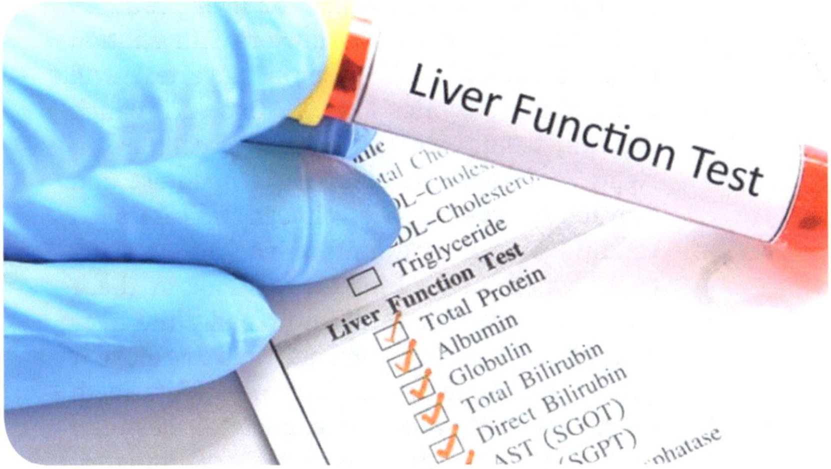

LEARNING OBJECTIVES

After studying this chapter, you will be able to:

1. Explain anatomy and physiology of the liver;
2. List the types of liver function tests;
3. Discuss the indications for liver function tests;
4. Describe interpretation of liver function test results;
5. Explore the common liver diseases detected by tests;
6. Focus on the limitations of liver function tests.

Introduction

Checking liver function is a critical step to actually know what's happening in the body. It's not just specifically about the liver—these tests, usually referred to as LFTs, provide information on everything from cell integrity to bile flow and whether the liver is functioning well to produce essential proteins. Doctors regularly check for such markers as AST, ALT, and ALP; these are markers that can indicate damage or problem even before the patient is aware of it. Look at, for example, the sudden changes sometimes seen after laparoscopic surgery (Sadia et al., 2025)—they encourage us to consider a lab result in context, as opposed to in isolation. In settings like surgery or where there are infections, the LFTs are even more important, necessitating a serious pre-op test and watchful eye post-op check-ups. Of late, it is more frequently observed that liver issues happen to patients fighting hard, and sometimes viral, diseases like COVID-19. Most of the time, research has shown that the majority of severe COVID-19 patients present with high liver enzyme levels on admission – a sign that their liver may already be stressed or damaged. More than 75% of COVID-19 admissions have been reported to have abnormal LFTs with AST and ALT levels through the roof (Himral et al., 2023). This complex interplay between liver function and overall health really makes the point: LFTs aren't just for identifying liver-specific problems, but they can monitor the convoluted paths of complex illness as well. These tests aren't necessarily easy to read.

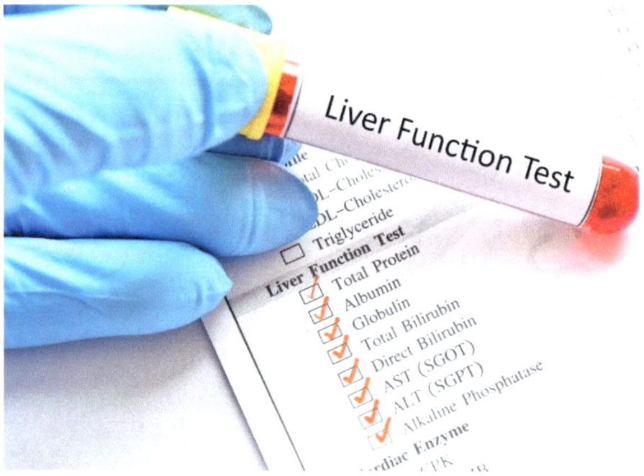

Figure 9.1. Liver function test.

Source: https://external-content.duckduckgo.com/iu/?u=https%3A%2F%2Fwww.thesouthafrican.com%2Fwp-content%2Fuploads%2F2021%2F01%2Fc8f60656-liverfunctiontest.jpeg.optimal.jpeg&f=1&nofb=1&ipt=2f0f1f68000756a82015ac1c46b3592d3dd997f713a9841869c5905d23e138f9.

Sometimes an elevated enzyme level doesn't mean the liver is in real danger at all—muscle injury, drug side effects, or even normal fluctuation after surgery can be involved. For instance, the post-operative changes of enzymes after laparoscopic procedures (Sadia et al., 2025) render it inevitable that the recent history of surgery and personal history of a patient must be taken into account. Physicians, most of the time, need to take a gentle, even a creative stance; unique findings demand careful scrutiny as well as a broader evaluation of one's overall health. This type of all-encompassing, somewhat disheveled grasp can directly inform treatment choices and, in the end, assist in guiding patients to improved outcomes (Figure 9.1).

Definition of Liver Function Tests

Liver function tests are a major deal in clinics, especially when there is liver problem. They basically analyze different enzymes, proteins, and other substances which the liver produces or secretes, and it provides doctors with a notion of the function of the liver. For instance, tests will likely check enzymes like ALT and AST, which basically tell us whether or not liver cells are all right. There are also alkaline phosphatase and bilirubin tests—those levels can indicate such conditions as bile flow issue or blockage. In many cases, when medical individuals look at these tests, they are able to tell how badly the liver might have been damaged and step in before it gets worse. Some populations of patients seem to show a special kind of correlation between liver tests and other disease. Take diabetes, for example; most diabetics will be found with elevated liver enzyme levels that may point to further complications. Studies have even found links between obesity, insulin resistance, and abnormal liver test results. High bilirubin and transaminase levels may mean that the liver is not functioning correctly and can even be disrupting blood sugar regulation—a two-way street, so to speak. This points toward why it is advisable to include liver tests in diabetic patient checkups from time to time, monitoring both blood glucose and liver function (Joseph et al., 2024). It's not just diabetes, though—liver problems are emerging in other conditions as well. During COVID-19 days, many of the patients had abnormal liver test results upon hospitalization, and abnormalities usually went hand in hand with a more challenging overall case. Some of the papers reported that elevated AST and ALT levels, along with low albumin, were quite common among hospitalized patients with COVID-19. This means the virus might make the liver do unusual things, risk on top of risk, and perhaps even warn of nastier things to follow. Ultimately, including liver tests as part of the formula when evaluating patients—especially during outbreaks of new diseases—ends up playing a major role in determining treatment (Himral et al., 2023).

Importance of Liver Health

The liver is absolutely vital to keeping us in working order—it has so many behind-the-scenes activities that, all in all, we can't help but take notice. It manages metabolism, removes toxins, and even helps whip up proteins we need. When things do go awry, even a small hiccup in the functioning of the liver can have a domino effect that ends in metabolic problems and a rise in infection dangers. Most studies now suggest that alcohol use, for instance, can really destabilize this balance, making liver function tests (LFTs) all the more important for people who drink heavily, including certain African communities (Mkhize et al., 2023). In many cases, spotting early signs of liver injury through these tests can stop more serious conditions from developing, so regular check-ups are a must if we're aiming for overall well-being. Viral outbreaks add a new layer of complexity to liver health. Sub-Saharan Africa sees hepatitis B and C infections occurring with frequency, and if HIV co-infection cases are seen, things get more complex. Alpha-fetoprotein (AFP) elevation has consistently been seen as markers—actually, not only indicating the worsening of the liver condition but also an early liver cancer (HCC). Hepatitis B patient studies, for example, have shown that patients with other infections have a notably raised AFP level, along with raised liver enzyme results; these are clear indicators that further tests might be necessary. The association observed between enzyme and AFP is typically reflective of the value of routine LFTs in groups with a higher risk (Tijani et al., 2024). Healthy livers are not merely a matter of one organ functioning on its own—it is linked to larger public health issues and even socio-economic issues. More instances of liver diseases, many of which are traceable back to the everyday habits we accumulate like what we eat or our drinking levels, necessitate innovative public health measures. In most cases, making individuals aware about the care of the liver and performing regular screenings can truly enable them to make better decisions for their own lives, even when sometimes the message seems dull. Meanwhile, ongoing joint research gradually reveals liver health inequalities, leading us towards improved healthcare policies and professional solutions. Therefore, promoting regular liver screening isn't a clinical ritual but an essential part of a thorough, whole-person care model across multicultural populations (Mkhize et al., 2023; Tijani et al., 2024) (Figure 9.2).

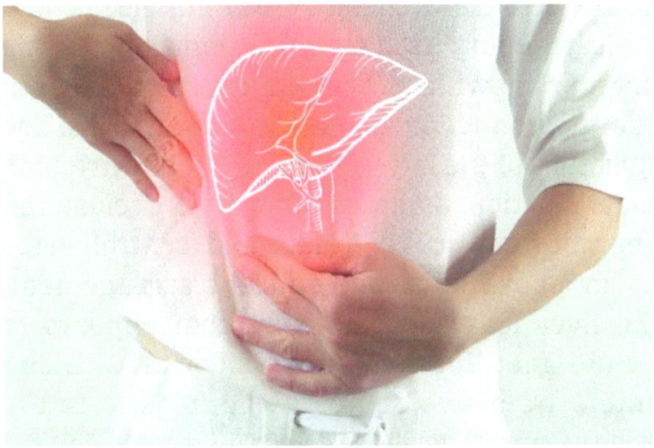

Figure 9.2. The importance of a healthy liver.

Source: https://external-content.duckduckgo.com/iu/?u=https%3A%2F%2Fwww.imcgrupo.com%2Fwp-content%2Fuploads%2F2022%2F11%2FThe-Importance-of-a-Healthy-Liver-01.jpeg&f=1&nofb=1&ipt=f47d7962d0093016ea9b4b80b401ecb4b2dffcc559f1fc8d80a64f103050786d.

9.1. Anatomy and Physiology of the Liver

Learning Outcome

- Location and size of the liver;
- Functions of the liver in metabolism;
- Role of the liver in detoxification.

The liver is at the center of our metabolism, essentially a busy workshop for many chemical reactions to keep our body's balance. It's where carbohydrates are turned into glucose—either quickly used as energy or glycogen storage. The organ also handles fats and proteins; excess amino acids are turned into urea, a process which is very important in detoxing. Most commonly, when doctors conduct tests for liver function, they monitor levels of enzymes and overall metabolism of nutrients. For example, an elevated transaminases (ALT and AST) could indicate injury to liver cells, pointing out the manner in which the liver coordinates both energy production and detoxification tasks. The structure of the liver, by the way, is as intriguing as its function. Composed of lobules of clustered hepatocytes, portal triads, and central veins in an unorthodox but efficient arrangement, the liver features a network that appears to be designed for continuous blood flow. Blood enters from two sources—the hepatic artery and the portal vein—and that mixture is critical to the process of nutrient metabolism and detoxification. The organ purifies blood, yes, but it also constructs proteins that are vital, like clotting factors. You can really visualize how its structure and function are one, how its form supports not only digestion but also immune status and overall metabolic balance. When the liver fails, the whole body suffers. Abnormalities here can potentially cause a cascade of problems, disrupting the body's metabolic balance. Liver function tests—such as the bilirubin, albumin, and coagulation studies—are important in detecting these abnormalities. For instance, hyperbilirubinemia might be suggestive of cholestasis, while hypoalbuminemia might be suggestive of diminished capacity for protein synthesis. All these tests, when conducted outside of the traditional laboratory setting, help doctors decide if conditions like hepatitis, cirrhosis, or fatty liver are present or not. In general, it is useful for doctors and scientists to understand how the liver's anatomy ties into its functions and the outcomes of tests as they create more efficient cures (Figure 9.3).

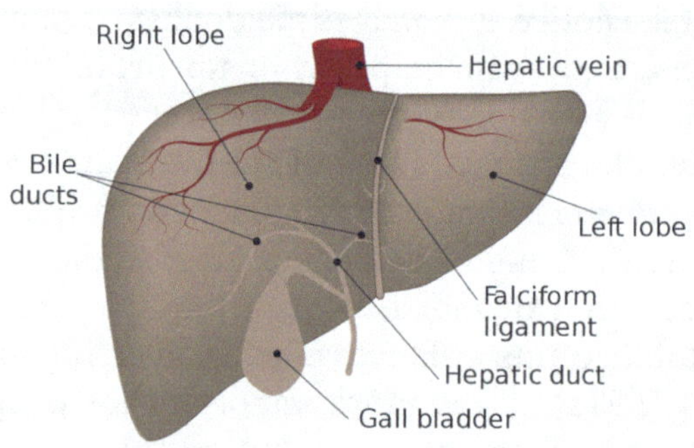

Figure 9.3. Human liver anatomy and physiology.

Source: https://external-content.duckduckgo.com/iu/?u=https%3A%2F%2Fonlinesciencenotes.com%2Fwp-content%2Fuploads%2F2021%2F03%2Fliver.png&f=1&nofb=1&ipt=4f47f97049a9d4280e128b6c40b0f367feb9172851d0c240629b2b1838d15be9.

9.1.1. Location and Size of the Liver

Understanding where the liver is located in our body is really crucial in everyday examinations. It mostly lives in the upper right-hand corner of the abdomen, but it extends a bit into the left side—a weird reminder of how massive it is. Livers in the majority of adults weigh around 1400 to 1800 grams, placing it as the largest gland overall and the largest mass of visceral tissue in that region in the peritoneum. This positioning, as well as this substantial weight, enables the liver to play an important role of drug metabolism and spitting out bile—both relatively key to digestion. Doctors, through palpation on a physical exam, should be able to sense any variations, so knowing approximately how big it is and where it's located really helps to understand liver tests and diagnosing disease. The liver is not great just because of its size; its blood supply is also complicated. Concealed deep inside the belly, it is nourished by not one, but two sources—the hepatic artery and the portal vein—and therefore it gets a kind of double whammy to play with. This means that the liver can be absorbing nutrients from the intestine and filtering out toxins simultaneously. Every now and then, results show levels of enzymes like ALT and AST to be raised, which can be an indirect clue that something's wrong—be it inflammation or damage. In most cases, these changes in enzymes remind us that observing both the organ's shape and its internal circulation is actually important in clinical exams (Daan et al., 2024). It's a complex mixture of form and function that renders each detail essential. For surgical procedures and transplants, the position and size of the liver become particularly critical. Its size is so big that it fills a big portion of the abdomen, but it is also endowed with an even greater ability for regeneration—partial transplants. Understanding exactly where the liver is located is critical to liver transplant patients, especially where complications such as cholangitis or other infections tend to develop suddenly. Indeed, even an instance of *Raoultella ornithinolytica* bacteremia in some transplant recipients was documented, sure to require extra caution (Daan et al., 2024). In general, understanding the liver's natural position and how large it is essential for healthcare professionals when they're reading tests of liver function and planning high-risk liver procedures.

9.1.2. Functions of the Liver in Metabolism

The liver is a busy metabolic factory that converts ordinary food into energy our bodies can use. It stores excess glucose in the form of glycogen during high blood sugar and releases those stores when blood sugar levels are low—keeping things humming even during fasting. It also works on fats by manufacturing fatty acids and cholesterol and by storing triglycerides for future use. If these processes go wrong, you can find things like steatosis or fatty liver disease developing, which seems to throw overall balance into chaos. Physicians will usually run liver function tests in the majority of patients in order to get a sense of how well this balancing process with nutrients is working. A massive part of what the liver has to deal with is proteins. It's where several critical proteins are made—albumin the most common one—and that, along with clotting factors, helps to manage blood pressure and transport hormones, drugs, and other things throughout the body. And the liver is getting overtime in breaking down ammonia (a byproduct of protein metabolism) into urea the kidneys can excrete. When these processes are not working quite properly, it can lead to protein imbalance like low albumin or even hepatic encephalopathy. Routine tests monitor this protein assembly lines, inspecting both the amount of albumin produced and the efficiency of ammonia detoxification. Lastly, the liver also acts to metabolize drugs and xenobiotics. It reverts fat-affined compounds into water-soluble types that the body is better able to eliminate via urine or bile. This process relies on a complete set of enzymes – like, for example, the cytochrome P450 system, which modifies drug molecules in manners that affect their overall behavior. When the liver begins to flag, drugs will be circulating longer than they should, raising the risk of toxicity or reducing their effectiveness. This is the reason why tests for liver function will also often examine such issues as enzyme activity and bilirubin levels, which offer a picture of how well detoxification is really taking place. In general, these results are significant to healthcare practitioners when they are formulating treatments and monitoring liver function (Choi et al., 2021; Jeon et al., 2023) (Figure 9.4).

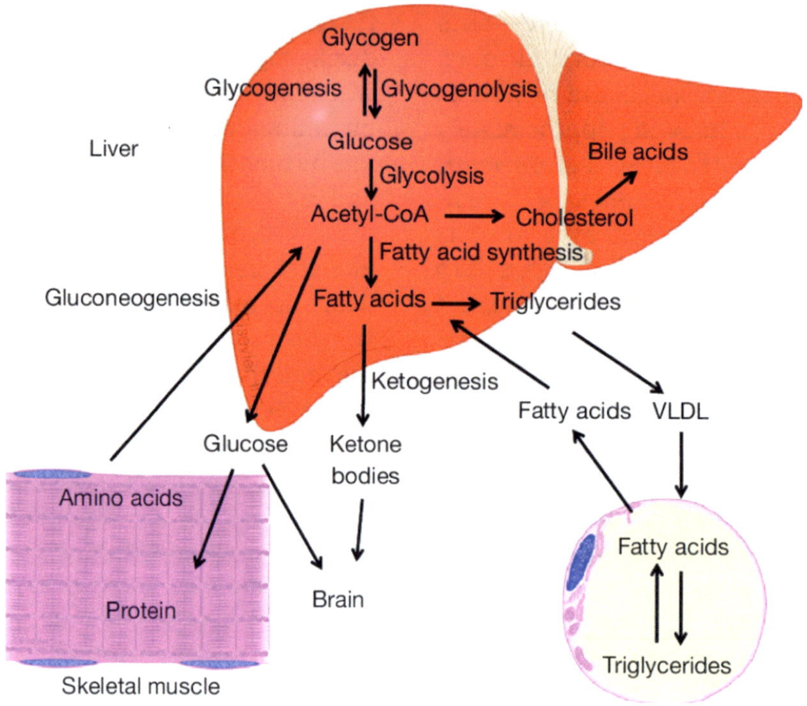

Figure 9.4. Major metabolic functions of the liver.

Source: https://external-content.duckduckgo.com/iu/?u=https%3A%2F%2Fwww.researchgate.net%2Fprofile%2FJohn_Chiang2%2Fpublication%2F271910276%2Ffigure%2Fdownload%2Ffig3%2FAS%3A667598400262156%401536179270549%2FMajor-metabolic-functions-of-the-liver-During-the-fed-state-glucose-is-stored-in-the.png&f=1&nofb=1&ipt=d45d287748ba72f96c2f9ee1ec9f9d3e42f78333c6ce34957eac4c765c709158.

9.1.3. Role of the Liver in Detoxification

The liver has a huge job—it's the major organ tasked with filtering out annoying toxins from our blood. Inside liver cells themselves, those tiny workhorses called hepatocytes handle a wacky set of chemical reactions. In essence, there is a two-step process at work. First, there's the oxidation and reduction (leaving most of it to the cytochrome P450 enzymes), and a secondary process whereby the byproducts get stamped with a water-friendly tag so they can be flushed out. It even converts that ugly ammonia from protein breakdown into urea, which eventually comes out of the body through the kidneys. These common steps, mostly, balance and protect us from the harmful actions of toxins, drugs, and general metabolic waste (Jennifer et al., 2021). Another facet of this detox industry is the way the liver metabolizes compounds both produced by our own bodies and compounds that come from the external world. It's not just about metabolizing pills and poisons; it's also keeping busy metabolizing hormones and nutrients in a way that, sincerely, keeps our system in check. Consider the way it metabolizes bile acids from cholesterol, for example—displaying its mettle while doing so, with the help of enabling fat absorption (Takahashi et al., 2016). Every once in a while, when these nice neat metabolic steps fall apart, it can cause issues ranging from drug toxicity all the way to hepatic encephalopathy. Liver function tests that check various enzymes and substances give us a glimpse of how well this balancing act is going. And there's more to it than just shuffling chemicals around. The liver's detoxing capabilities extend into recycling, as well. Once they've served their purpose in fat digestion in the intestine, all except a handful are reabsorbed and to the liver they return—a process that, while it can appear deceptively easy, is important to keep bile acids and metabolism at stable levels. Since these acids also signal changes in other metabolic routes, it's clear that their regulation is closely linked with the overall detox process of the liver (Takahashi et al., 2016). On that note, when liver function tests are run, they're not just ticking off the typical signs of good health but also nodding toward the fine-tuned balance of detox steps behind the scenes that keep our metabolism and cellular landscape rolling along (Figure 9.5).

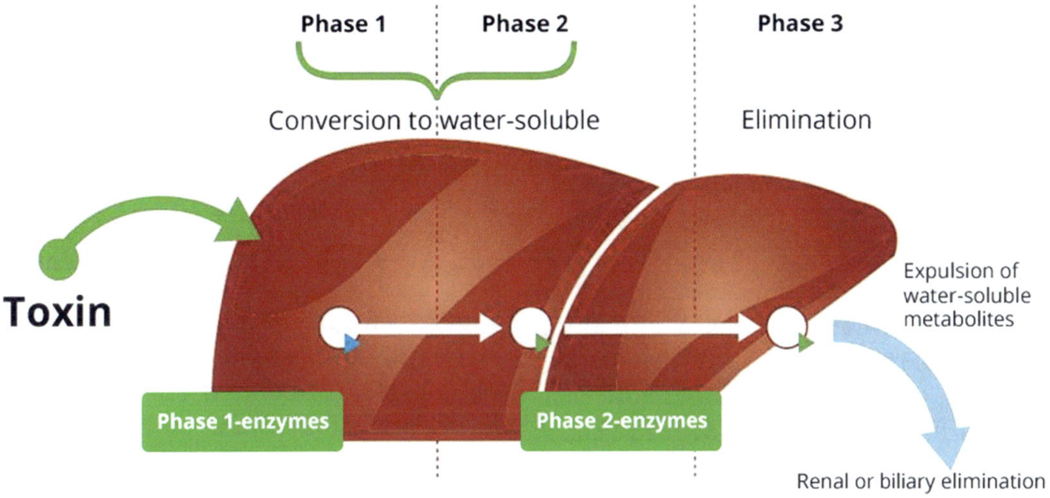

Figure 9.5. Detoxification.

Source: https://external-content.duckduckgo.com/iu/?u=https%3A%2F%2Fwww.pileje.com%2Fsites%2Fdefault%2Ffiles%2Fstyles%2Fnode_full%2Fpublic%2F2021-03%2Fliver%2520detoxication.png%3Fitok%3DJtsFIi3W&f=1&nofb=1&ipt=1ce662c68a1c5c2a1df9f7619902d110e332fc62a32fe73617f95bff6ed03a71.

Test Your Knowledge

1. What are the main lobes and structural units (lobules) of the liver, and how do they function?
2. How does the liver contribute to metabolism of carbohydrates, proteins, and lipids?

Learning Outcome

- Enzyme tests (ALT, AST);
- Bilirubin tests;
- Albumin and protein tests.

Liver testing is important in identifying liver problems. Physicians rely on these tests—a combination of various biochemical markers—to gauge how well the liver's doing. For instance, tests such as AST and ALT will increase when the liver cells are injured, suggesting conditions like hepatitis or even cirrhosis. Alkaline phosphatase (ALP) will surge when there is a bile duct blockage or cholestatic findings. Bilirubin, on the other hand, gives us signals about how well the liver is performing to break down and clear out the trash, occasionally repeating its message when something is not functioning properly. In the recent past, research has been pointing out lactate dehydrogenase (LDH) as an important marker, especially for hypertensive disorders during pregnancy. Generally, rising LDH levels—tactically often coupled with such tests as SGOT and SGPT—have been connected with more difficult prospects for both mother and child, suggesting that such elevated statistics might lead clinicians to handle such tricky situations differently. In most cases, determining cutoff points on such tests, as outlined by Shah et al. (2025), can actually refine expectations and improve care for liver conditions during pregnancy There is also a story to be shared on the infectious side. During the COVID-19 era, there was definitely a notch of patients who underwent liver function tests, with parameters such as albumin and total bilirubin showing very often in clinical notes. But the problem cannot be skirted—data for such tests sometimes comes with gaps or small inconsistencies, hinting at a larger requirement for improved lab data management (Ayad et al., 2025). More broadly, knowing what tests are significant and how they interrelate not only educates for the specific patient but also reveals hints about larger trends in health information that speak to our overall manner of evaluating liver status (Figure 9.6).

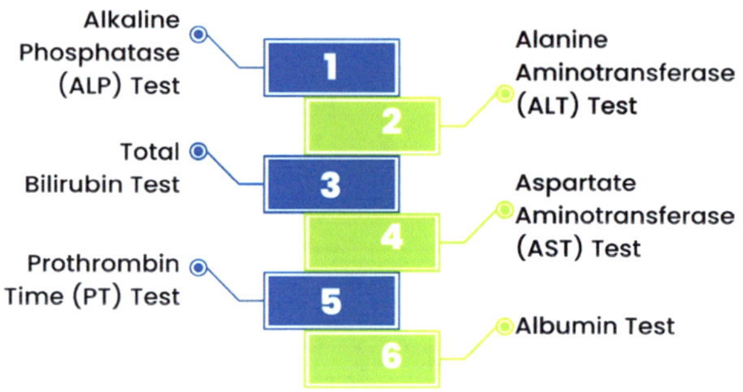

Figure 9.6. Types of liver function tests.

Source: https://external-content.duckduckgo.com/iu/?u=https%3A%2F%2Fdrmagnusjayaraj.com%2Fwp-content%2Fuploads%2F2023%2F02%2FInfographics-11-1024x655.webp&f=1&nofb=1&ipt=4428f1caa84dc907079f597db505772b36462cc2757f8a0186811c1d42416831.

9.2.1. Enzyme Tests (ALT, AST)

Enzyme studies have taken a place of precedence in how we track liver function—often as a critical diagnostic and monitoring tool in the case of liver disease. ALT (alanine aminotransferase) and AST (aspartate aminotransferase) have been discussed in so many instances since they also tend to reflect when liver cells are damaged. When these enzymes rise in the blood, it typically means inflammation or damage in the liver. Take hepatitis, fatty liver, or cirrhosis, for example; these conditions tend to result in elevated ALT and AST, which will guide treatment choices and even determine decisions about further action. While the tests seem straightforward, knowing their little details truly helps practitioners complete the larger picture of what the liver is doing. Recent research, in general, has examined the way that lifestyle adjustments may alter liver enzyme levels—and the results put a fascinating twist on our understanding of liver function. Intermittent fasting (IF) is one method that's gained attention as a potential method for increasing liver health. One systematic review even reported that IF caused significant decreases in both ALT and AST levels (Ranjbar et al., 2024). Such a result highlights why the combination of lifestyle change with standard medical care is of relevance in the management of liver disease. Aside from revealing potential pre-existing liver issues, such tests can on occasion prove useful as rapid indicators of whether or not lifestyle adjustment is indeed effective. On the other hand, experiments using nutritional supplements have provided a spottier set of results regarding altering liver enzyme levels. Resveratrol—take care to be wary of the hyperbole in its supposed health effects—did not have any real effect on ALT and AST levels in patients with nonalcoholic fatty liver disease (NAFLD) (Ebrahimpour et al., 2024).

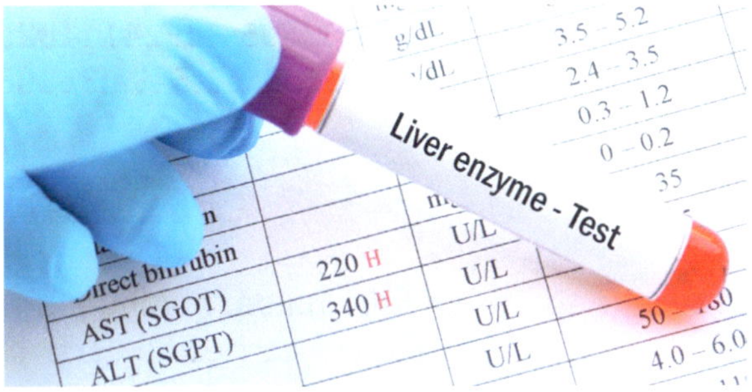

Figure 9.7. Enzyme tests.

Source: https://external-content.duckduckgo.com/iu/?u=https%3A%2F%2Fassets-global.website-files.com%2F5e066fbd0d37a10ebf1f4139%2F65af21c5a1068a628e586fae_Liver%2520Enzyme%2520Test.jpg&f=1&nofb=1&ipt=7983fb4ae9c15329a4931631278312d526e1ab138b134423d4e68d5042256575.

This finding, in most cases, comes as a reminder of the need for strict clinical trials before embracing new supplements as real avenues of therapy. Since there are so many variables involved in complicating enzyme levels and overall liver function, further research is needed to determine the most suitable treatments and prevention strategies, ultimately contributing to patient outcomes through evidence-based medical practice (Figure 9.7).

9.2.2. Bilirubin Tests

Monitoring of bilirubin levels has become the most crucial way of testing whether the liver is working or not. Elevated levels usually point toward possible liver illnesses or blockages – sometimes early signs can make a huge difference in a diagnosis course. In the average laboratory, they check total bilirubin and its two fractions, direct (conjugated) and indirect (unconjugated), to see how well the liver metabolizes and eliminates this hemoglobin breakdown product. If the indirect side is much higher than normal, it indicates conditions like hemolytic anemia; if the direct fraction is off the charts, that typically means cholestatic pathology. Having this information, even if it repeats in different forms, helps doctors with what other tests to perform on liver ailments. Bilirubin testing is not only performed to find the causes of ailments—it can also give information on how severe the sickness is. In the hospital, rising levels usually accompany worsening states. For instance, studies that were done on trauma patients recently found significant correlations between increased serum bilirubin levels and several conditions such as an increased need for mechanical ventilation and greater injury severity scores (Duswald et al., 1993). All the relationships in most cases seem to be telling us more than "liver trouble"; they are communicating a patient's condition overall. Most times, though, if physicians pay careful attention to these numbers, they complete a bigger picture that can signal a sudden decline in health if it is not addressed sooner. Furthermore, by tracking bilirubin levels over the course of some time, one can see if treatments are indeed fixing the problem. Ongoing observation could alert physicians if a therapy is working or if trouble occurs, even possibly liver failure. In the past, large increases in bilirubin have been correlated with specific liver disorders like obstructive jaundice or hepatitis and therefore need a clear analysis of other enzyme markers (Batta et al., 2011). In addition to other liver tests, these measurements in combination help to give a better, possibly messy picture of a patient's liver status. In total, in either diagnosing chronic problems or in keeping track of the progress of treatment, bilirubin levels remain the central piece in the liver function status puzzle (Figure 9.8).

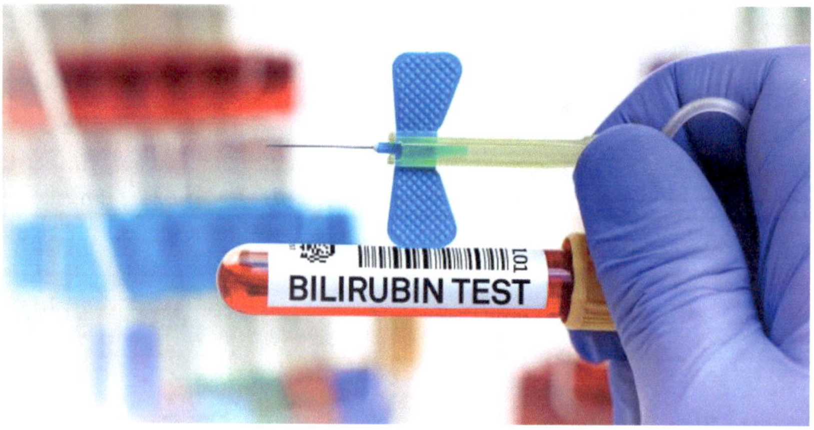

Figure 9.8. Bilirubin test.

Source: https://external-content.duckduckgo.com/iu/?u=https%3A%2F%2Fblog-images-1.pharmeasy.in%2Fblog%2Fproduction%2Fwp-content%2Fuploads%2F2023%2F05%2F24111826%2Fbilirubin.jpg&f=1&nofb=1&ipt=d6609dc021fda86500f0806dade08c21586e3ee2f549af3e80856168a5da6ecb.

9.2.3. Albumin and protein tests

Albumin and protein tests are a whopping' chunk of keeping an eye on liver function. Albumin is made in the liver – a main protein that keeps osmotic pressure balanced and carries all sorts of things around your body. When albumin falls, it's generally a sign that the liver isn't functioning properly; most of the time, this can be a sign of cirrhosis, some type of cancer, or even diseases like malnourishment. Most doctors supplement routine liver tests with an albumin test so that they can have a general idea of liver health and make appropriate changes in treatment. Checking the total proteins, including albumin and globulin together, gives a better indication of the liver's functioning. These tests essentially check whether the liver is sustaining normal protein output, an endeavor that's central to numerous body processes. Abnormalities in these numbers sometimes reveal disease elsewhere within the body too—e.g., inflammatory or infectious disease. Recent studies, in general, have reported that COVID-19 patients will present with markedly changed levels of protein (Dwivedi, 2024); such a finding speaks to the value of these tests in tracking disease progression and guiding therapy. There is a downside to this when considering the younger age group too. It has been found that obese adolescents will not only have higher levels of liver enzymes but also abnormal protein synthesis patterns compared to the leaner group (Shrivatsava et al., 2022). The link between obesity and metabolic derangement in the liver implies that incidental albumin and protein testing is a worthwhile tool, either for individual therapy or population-based public health intervention in youth. In general, understanding the association of these tests with global liver status can allow clinicians to treat early and potentially prevent long-term consequences related to dysfunction of the liver (Figure 9.9).

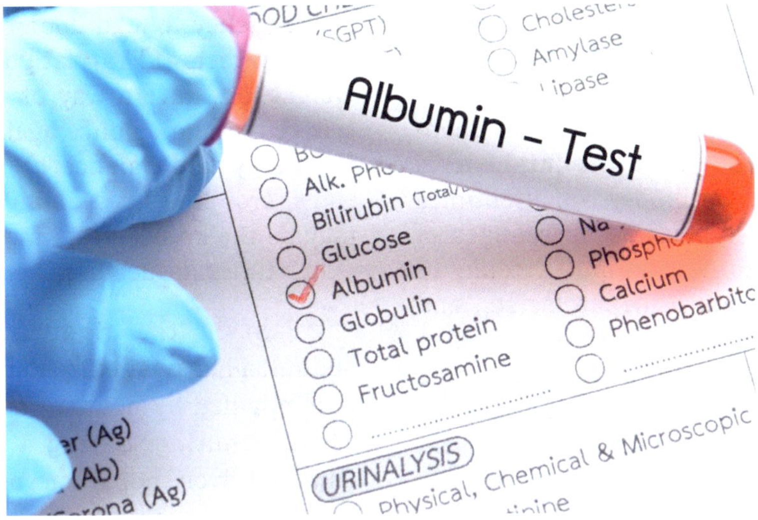

Figure 9.9. Albumin test.

Source: https://external-content.duckduckgo.com/iu/?u=https%3A%2F%2Fwww.emergency-live.com%2Fwp-content%2Fuploads%2F2022%2F07%2Falbumina-alta-albumin-test-1.jpeg&f=1&nofb=1&ipt=f2e450443824084c4140d055562dfa48738bf80321b5ae13dbc0fe4af7d669dc.

Test Your Knowledge

1. What biochemical parameters are commonly measured in liver function tests?
2. How do tests for bilirubin, ALT, AST, and ALP reflect different aspects of liver health?

9.3. Indications for Liver Function Tests

Learning Outcome

- Symptoms indicating liver dysfunction;
- Monitoring chronic liver diseases;
- Preoperative assessments.

Liver function tests (LFTs) are a first-line tool today for figuring out what's happening with the liver. They measure the liver's ability to filter out toxins, produce proteins, and even produce the chemicals needed to digest food—basically, everything an overworked organ does. NAFLD, or non-alcoholic fatty liver disease, often co-exists with unusual test results, and this may occur in roughly one in every four people in Western countries, mostly people with problems of obesity or type 2 diabetes. In most cases, the individuals with these conditions are classified as high-risk, and doctors therefore act proactively with a bit of added screening since if something does go wrong, complications like cirrhosis or even the need for a transplant could follow. Sometimes, however, the story is not quite so simple. It is hard to differentiate, for example, alcoholic liver disease from NAFLD on the basis of ratios of transaminases alone; an attentive probing of a patient's history and symptoms usually is needed, as a rule. For example, telling a person to quit drinking might be just what the doctor prescribed for alcoholic liver disease—but getting someone to quit isn't always easy for people with deep-seated dependencies. Where the initial tests leave some doubt, a liver biopsy will oftentimes end up proving the typical tissue changes of these diseases. Oftener, though, a team of experts—endocrinologists, hepatologists, and nutritionists—will end up working together, joined by the requirement to manage not just the liver illness but also the concomitant metabolic syndrome with which they so frequently present (Liguori et al., 2025). There is yet another twist: More and more patients, particularly those being treated with chemotherapy, are now getting LFTs on their visits. Doctors have begun identifying issues with the activity of dihydropyrimidine dehydrogenase (DPD), particularly in patients receiving 5-fluorouracil (5-FU)-based chemotherapy. Testing become routine sometimes, especially if a patient has undergone a liver transplant—here it is doubly crucial to investigate DPD activity in the transplanted liver to protect it. Standard protocols would then presumably not capture all the subtleties of liver function in such rare instances, thereby establishing an actual need for updated, case-specific guidelines. With changing modalities of treatment over time, the surveillance of LFTs continues to be at the core not only of the management of liver diseases but also of fine-tuning complex treatment protocols for patients with a complex medical history (Liguori et al., 2025).

9.3.1. Symptoms Indicating Liver Dysfunction

Liver health has a great deal to do with overall health, and you may realize whispers of difficulty way ahead of time. At times changes creep up slowly—such as a yellow color on the skin and eyes when there is too much bilirubin—by which many interpret as a silent warning sign. Jaundice, as it is correctly termed, has the tendency to lead doctors to prescribe liver function tests (LFTs); fatigue and spontaneous weight loss have a way of getting into the act too, reminding us once again of the liver's role in energy and balance of metabolism. These signs, cropping up seemingly out of nowhere, may be the body's first hint that all is not well. Other times, issues escalate abruptly.

Pain in the right upper part of the abdomen has the ability to hit all at once, often accompanied by bouts of nausea and, in some cases, vomiting. During a physical exam, an enlarged liver (hepatomegaly) can be found, a real indicator that the organ is not performing as it should be; in more advanced instances, fluid buildup in the stomach—ascites—can occur, along with bouts of confusion caused by hepatic encephalopathy. Overall, whenever these signs are present, doctors use a full battery of LFTs to assess the extent of the damage and to direct subsequent management. Identification of these signs does more than trigger early treatment—it also provides a framework for ongoing management.

Research would also mostly indicate that monitoring for liver-related signs is crucial in identifying more generalized systemic complications; e.g., some studies (Pooransari et al., 2024) have shown that abnormal enzyme levels correlate with severe cases of COVID-19 in patients such as pregnant ones. And then there is that co-possibility of liver failure happening along with other complications such as kidney in cirrhosis (Bhuyan et al., 2024). Overall, by combining accurate symptom screens with LFTs, physicians are better able to make decisions about interventions, which can improve patients' long-term outcomes (Figure 9.10).

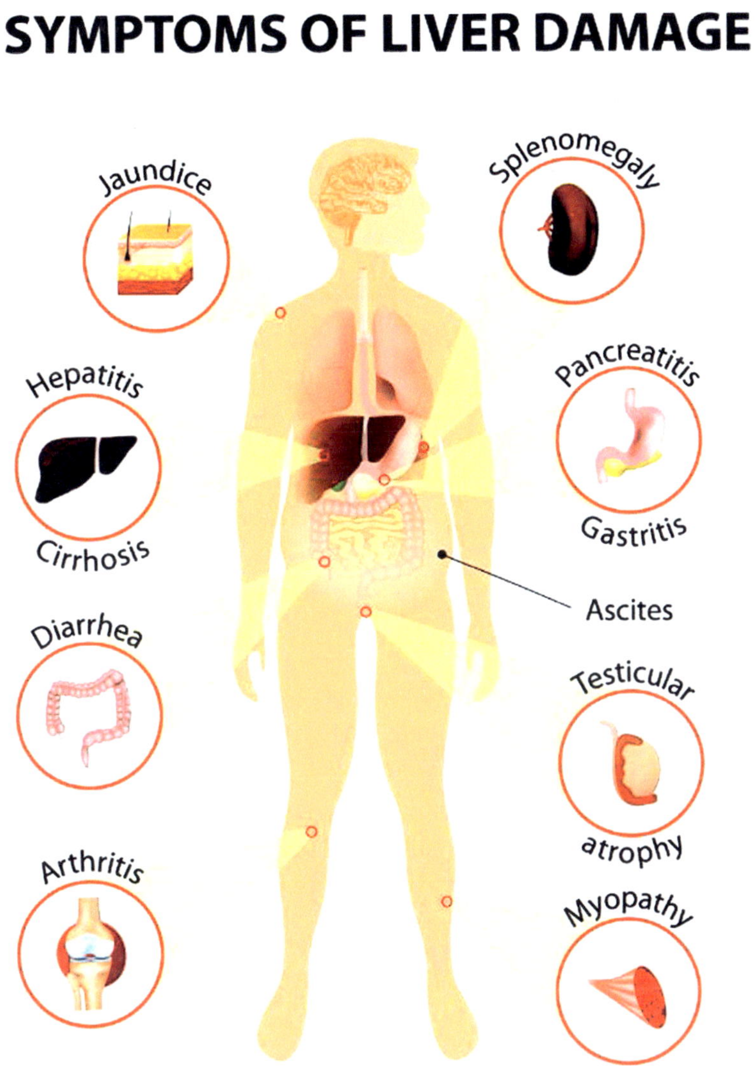

Figure 9.10. Symptoms indicating liver dysfunction.

Source: https://cdn.apollohospitals.com/health-library-prod/2021/01/Factors-May-Damage-the-Liver-scaled.jpg.

9.3.2. Monitoring chronic liver diseases

Chronic liver diseases require ongoing, careful monitoring to see how they are developing and if the therapies are effective. Regular liver function tests (LFTs) allow dentists—really, clinicians—to track important markers like ALT, AST, and total serum bilirubin (TSB). One research (Ali et al., 2025) found that such levels would be much higher in patients with chronic hepatitis B compared to others, demonstrating the tremendous value of such tests. Lower levels of albumin and prothrombin time also suggest a liver that's not running at its top speed; in most cases, this suggests the liver's ability to produce necessary compounds short. Overall, these trends alert physicians to craft treatment plans that suit each individual and determine whether additional tests may be necessary. Incorporating tumor markers into the standard arsenal can truly be a game changer for the treatment of chronic liver disease. For instance, incorporating alpha-fetoprotein (AFP) provides further information—especially since AFP is quite an important prognostic marker in the case of identifying hepatocellular carcinoma (HCC) at an early stage, a complication which usually comes with liver problems. Elevated AFP levels with abnormal LFTs can reflect an enhanced risk of malignancy (Poornima, 2023). Again and again, research has indicated correlations between rising AFP levels and abnormal LFT values and why repeated AFP testing is that critical added element in the care of liver disease. This combination strategy not only enhances monitoring precision but also paves the way for quicker, more targeted intervention when mistakes are made. Gender and age also subtly influence the way liver biomarkers present on laboratory tests. General research has also shown that the total serum bilirubin levels would decrease with age, and there are great differences between male and female patients in terms of AST levels (Ali et al., 2025). As was eventually discovered, sometimes these distinctions have less to do with variation in disease and more to do with variation in physiology. Modifying monitoring strategies to account for these demographic factors can offer a more nuanced characterization of liver health and help physicians optimize decision-making. Emphasizing this individualization—aside from a few minor errors here and there in the figures—can have the potential to enhance patient outcomes and our overall insight into chronic liver disease monitoring (Figure 9.11).

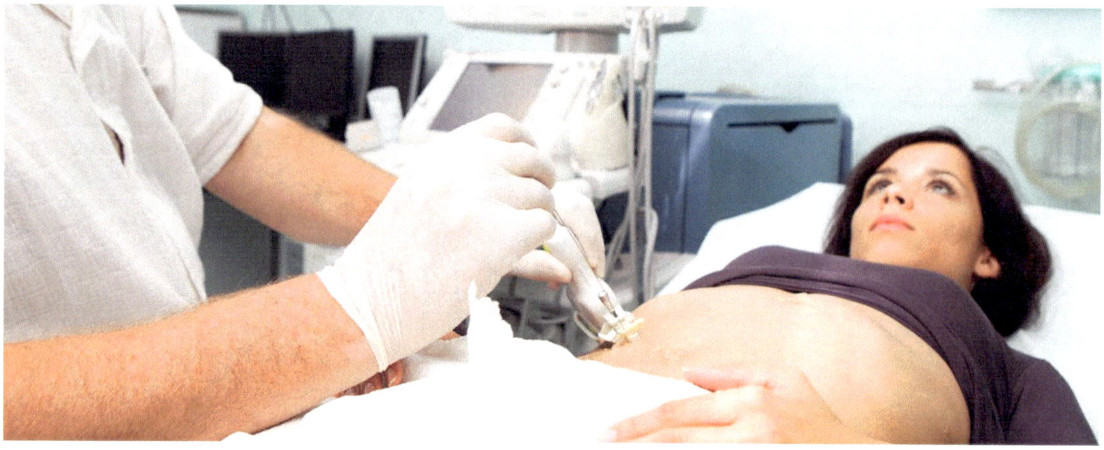

Figure 9.11. Monitoring chronic liver diseases.

Source: https://www.hopkinsmedicine.org/-/media/images/health/1_-conditions/liver-cancer/chronic-liver-disease-hero.jpg?h=500&iar=0&mh=500&mw=1300&w=1297&hash=BA095B82666F7E3AB7B76772783BEC65.

9.3.3. Preoperative Assessments

A liver test on a patient before surgery is really a big deal. Doctors usually prescribe a series of tests – like liver panels, imaging studies, and general health screening – to see if someone can have surgery safely. It is not a checklist; this procedure involves getting into the efficiency of the liver, and even subtle suggestions can dictate the game plan. In the majority of cases, knowing the liver's condition from the start enables the surgical team to adjust the method and the postoperative care, which, as you know, reduces risks and generally enhances patient safety (Oaknin et al., 2022).

Typically, the procedure is initiated with a series of liver function tests (LFTs) to check enzymes, bilirubin, and albumin levels – a snapshot of whether the liver is managing. Odd results might be pointing towards such issues like cholestasis, inflammation, or cirrhosis, making clinicians go a bit deeper. They might even encompass such studies as prothrombin time – that one sheds light on the efficiency with which the liver is handling clotting blood. In patients already suffering from liver complications, these studies are particularly crucial because their inherent reserve usually tends to be smaller (Jon et al., 2021). Sometimes imaging studies – ultrasounds, CT scans, or MRIs – weigh in to add a more vivid picture of the liver's shape and whether or not lumps or lesions are hiding in the background. Not only do the scans help chart how far along in the liver disease a patient is, but they guide surgeons on their next move. The integration of lab results, clinician examination, and imaging data offers a kind of holistic view which is helpful in risk stratification and decision-making. This kind of hands-on detail-oriented preparation, while spotty at times, is important to make the operation smooth and speed up recovery, illustrating how vitally essential thorough pre-op assessment is for liver surgery (Oaknin et al., 2022).

Test Your Knowledge

1. Why are LFTs commonly ordered in patients with jaundice or suspected hepatitis?
2. How are liver function tests used in monitoring drug toxicity or alcohol-related liver injury?

9.4. Interpretation of Liver Function Test Results

Learning Outcome

- Normal ranges for liver enzymes;
- Factors affecting test results;
- Implications of abnormal results.

Liver function tests (LFTs) give significant clues regarding the liver's storage capacity, especially where there is a suspicion of something being wrong with the health of the liver. Enzymes like ALT and AST come onto the scene as messengers; in case of injured liver cells, these enzymes spill into the blood, indicating damage. A grossly raised ALT value—e.g., in viral hepatitis—might point to acute inflammation, and on occasion an isolated AST elevation will make us consider other issues like alcohol use or indeed muscle damage. It's always a good idea to consider these numbers alongside a patient's presentation and history since what they are saying in context can differ significantly. And in the case of chronic liver disease—let's use hepatitis B as an example—LFTs are even more meaningful. In one series of patients with chronic HBV, there were extensive elevations in the ALP, ALT, and AST levels, which usually indicates some degree of inflammation of the liver and bile flow problem (cholestasis). The alterations one can see among chronic HBV patients and normal individuals point toward the reason we have to be extremely careful in interpreting these test results (Mohsen, 2023). In most cases, one has to look at even minute variations for the first diagnosis itself, as well as for whether or not treatment has to be started at all. Even slight seeming alterations in these enzymes may point toward serious underlying disorders, which is why monitoring has to be ongoing. Sometimes LFT interpretation isn't quite so black and white as it should be because different experts interpret them very slightly differently, especially if the case is a complicated knot of diagnostic possibilities. More recently, newer technology like automated imaging analysis caused a splash, helping standardize the way we perceive tests like MRCP—this is becoming quite trendy when LFTs come out somewhat unrealistically. In a study, direct MRCP was slightly quicker in identifying issues such as acute gallstones than conventional techniques, which would more than likely result in shorter hospital stays and medical costs (Novak et al., 2025). Overall, combining these laboratory values with cutting-edge imaging is emerging as the future of a less complex, more streamlined approach to determining liver disease over time (Figure 9.12).

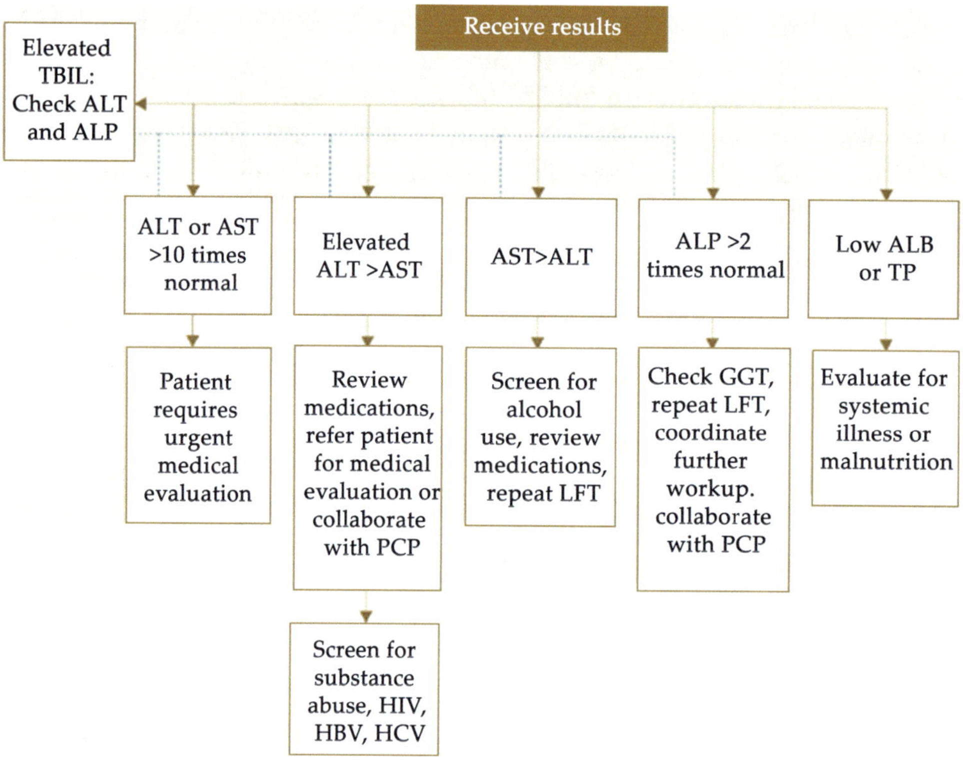

Figure 9.12. Interpreting liver function tests result.

Source: https://cdn.mdedge.com/files/s3fs-public/Image/September-2017/RTEmagicC_0adfcbe239.jpg.jpg.

9.4.1. Normal Ranges for Liver Enzymes

Tests of liver enzymes play an important role in monitoring how efficiently our liver works. Doctors usually also trust these tests since like ALT and AST they can tell them if anything is amiss. ALT would, for instance, be between 7 and 56 units per liter in most cases, while AST would usually range from 10 to 40 units per liter. These values must shift somewhat with age, sex, or overall health. Sometimes, if those enzyme levels soar, it may be an indication that liver cells are being battered about, while normal or decreased levels usually mean the liver is functioning in an adequate fashion. Overall, knowledge of these normal ranges is useful to health professionals on the front lines of patient care. There was also some research that took into account the stiffness of the liver, and researchers found that healthy patients in a population of Chinese patients ranged from 2.3 to

5.9 kPa (Chan et al., 2013). Information such as this is why having reference values tailored to specific populations is so important – after all, one size never quite fits all. It is also noteworthy that, occasionally, if enzyme concentrations such as alkaline phosphatase or gamma-glutamyl transferase appear abnormal, they may indicate biliary tract abnormalities or even evidence of liver cell injury. The combination of these studies really tugs a better detail when assessing liver function, especially when it comes to following up patients at risk. Besides that, it becomes increasingly hard to comprehend what liver enzyme tests are if you put medication and other health conditions into perspective. Think about children, for example – those receiving drugs for diseases like acute lymphoblastic leukemia will sometimes have unusual enzyme results because of their drug (Abid et al., 2005).

In most cases, a rise in serum aminotransferases in these situations is evidence that the liver is reacting to the therapy, so it may be drug-induced damage. So, doctors must be very cautious, not only thinking of the ranges but of all these additional factors. That is, how all normal values, patient history, and external variables get integrated just enhances how beneficial an in-depth liver test can be when it comes to making sure diagnoses and treatments are on target.

9.4.2. Factors Affecting Test Results

Liver function tests may be disturbed by an assortment of causes—some internal and some external. Diet, for example, plays a big part; unhealthy food could interfere with the liver's normal routine and lead to enzyme levels that don't tell the whole story. In some cases, malnutrition disturbed the liver's routine, so metabolic processes were altered as to change the readings on enzymes. Then there are of course things like antibiotics or anti-inflammatory drugs which can affect the manner in which the liver produces or clears enzymes—resulting in findings that can inappropriately suggest an issue. It so happens that uncovering in a patient's history deep down becomes extremely important when these are the case. And yet another thing, whatever one has just ingested, can change lab results, especially those for which one is screening for bilirubin or protein. All of these necessitate patient preparation in the correct way. Age and sex also affect LFT results.

All other things being equal, normal liver enzyme levels differ between the sexes, reflecting basic differences such as liver size and metabolic rate. With increasing age, liver function will also change; older patients will all tend to have lower enzyme levels than their younger counterparts, tending to obscure the issue. Also, conditions like diabetes or obesity can change test results further by modifying liver metabolism independently. For most scenarios, this type of health and demographic data is crucial for clinicians who wish to interpret the tests appropriately and offer a fair diagnosis. The lifestyle choice, particularly alcohol consumption, adds another dimension of complexity.

Excessive alcohol consumption is also causally linked with liver damage and can propel enzyme levels higher, sometimes generating the fallacious perception of desperately ill liver disease. Clearly, research has shown that excessively drinking patients are at significantly higher risk of death—not just from liver disease, but also from other life-threatening diseases like cancer or circulatory disease (Aithal et al., 2022; Morgan et al., 2022). This association means that doctors really do need to screen a patient's alcohol conduct as part of their general evaluation. Taking into account these life-style factors can lead to more tailored management strategies to each individual and ultimately improved health outcome (Figure 9.13).

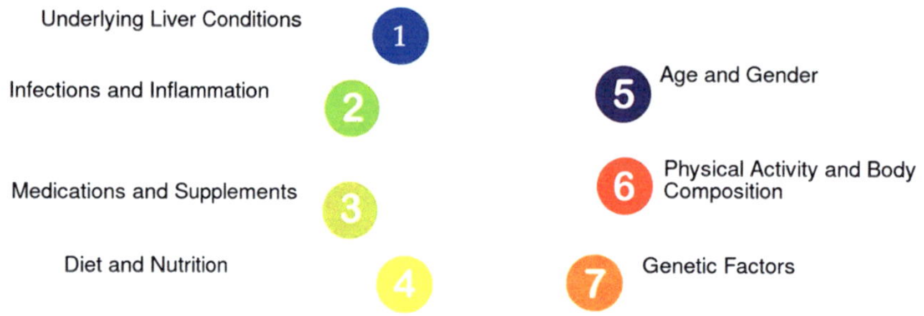

Figure 9.13. Factors affecting liver function test results.

Source: https://fastercapital.co/i/Liver-Function-Test-Center--How-Liver-Function-Test-Can-Measure-the-Enzymes-and-Substances-Produced-by-the-Liver--Factors-Affecting-Liver-Function-Test-Results.webp.

9.4.3. Implications of Abnormal Results

Unusual liver tests sometimes point to trouble percolating beneath the surface. When enzymes like aspartate aminotransferase (AST) and alanine aminotransferase (ALT) rise too high, it means liver cells might be being injured—a situation that can be caused by viral bugs, metabolic anomalies, or toxic exposures. Research among patients with dengue fever, for instance, indicated that as AST and ALT increased, the risk of mortality increased, especially in severe dengue shock syndrome (DSS) compared to uncomplicated disease (Jamil et al., 2025). This makes us track liver enzymes not only for the diagnosis but also to inform treatment. It is not infections that cause these alterations alone. Excessive drinking may also interfere with liver function, typically blurring the overall clinical presentation. Research in the aggregate demonstrates that heavy drinking is associated with elevated levels of liver enzymes—a risk factor to be balanced against other clinical signs. In statin patients, statin therapy would not necessarily result in a peak of liver tests by itself, but put a lot of booze drinking on statin therapy and lo and behold the ALT rises. That's an observation which shows that doctors should be checking a patient's alcohol intake as an everyday occurrence when they're reviewing LFT levels (Horne et al., 2022). Treatment of abnormal liver test results almost always involves a multidisciplinary approach. At times, it is literally just curtailing booze consumption in order for the liver to recover. As more is known now about how the liver is involved in overall metabolic well-being, an out-of-range test might be the starting point for further, more detailed testing—think tests for fatty liver or hepatitis. Ultimately, it's how to interpret these results as a middle ground between short-term, immediate treatment options and long-term lifestyle modifications that will only improve overall liver health. In a majority of instances, such an overall strategy is most important for minimizing the dangers of liver dysfunction.

Test Your Knowledge

1. What does an elevated ALT or AST suggest about hepatocellular damage?
2. How do ALP and GGT results help differentiate between hepatocellular and cholestatic disease?

9.5. Common Liver Diseases Detected by Tests

Learning Outcome

- Hepatitis (viral and autoimmune);
- Fatty liver disease;
- Cirrhosis and liver cancer.

Liver tests are becoming the norm for discovering how the liver actually is. They check things like enzyme levels, bilirubin, and protein output, and they can indicate things like chronic liver issues and metabolic hitches. And so it is that in all but a few cases, nearly 46.2% of children with high results for their liver tests may be dealing with long-term conditions, thereby indicating the critical importance of just such tests. In essence, doctors take these statistics to get an idea of what is occurring in the liver—they are able to detect hidden problems like glycogen storage problems that may otherwise wreak havoc if left undiagnosed. When the results are filtered through by clinicians, they can design treatment plans that address that particular issue at hand (Alvi et al., 2025). Sometimes a simple blood test is not enough and imaging studies come in to fill in the blanks. For instance, take choledocholithiasis—a condition defined by bile duct stones.

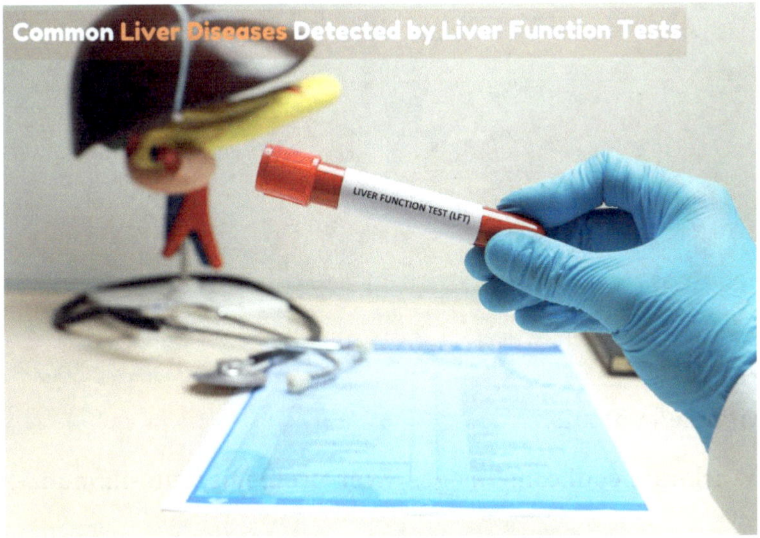

Figure 9.14. Common liver diseases detected by liver function tests.

Source: https://external-content.duckduckgo.com/iu/?u=https%3A%2F%2Fcontinentalhospitals.com%2Fimages%2Fblogs%2F7ce46c2365ba2c8984f75823af61f8d0.jpg&f=1&nofb=1&ipt=ddc6cd0d1da04b6dc898e16878629ab0ed068e36e3daa0554427392ff40c528d.

Here, the directions of liver tests rising and falling can direct treatment; it has been seen that the tests can even indicate whether stones are likely to pass on their own, thereby potentially reducing the need for invasive procedures such as endoscopic retrograde cholangiopancreatography (ERCP). Certainly, these tests do not paint the whole picture alone, but they do lay the initial platform for a more thorough investigation. A number of research studies have mentioned that while trends in liver test reports can be useful, they might not necessarily fit into place with the stone problem, reminding us that doctors must often mix and match different practices to get the complete picture (Bidarmaghz et al., 2023). It's not just a matter of catching issues in the first place—the most value in liver tests comes from tracking how the health of the liver is doing over time. As things in the liver progressively worsen or as new complications arise, changes in the results of tests can signal that treatment plans may need to be refined. Take hepatitis, for example; chronic diseases like that have a tendency to really unlevel enzyme levels, showing inflammation or even lasting damage. Monitoring such subtle changes throughout the course provides medical practitioners with a clearer picture of how the condition is progressing, which typically means improved patient outcomes. That very data even helps to spot potential complications in time for the initiation of timely interventions, which can radically change the course of the disease and enhance the well-being of the afflicted (Alvi et al., 2025) (Figure 9.14).

9.5.1. Hepatitis (Viral and Autoimmune)

Liver function tests are very much connected to the manner in which we acquire mastery over hepatitis types - whether it is the viral type like hepatitis A, B, or C or even the generally challenging autoimmune type.

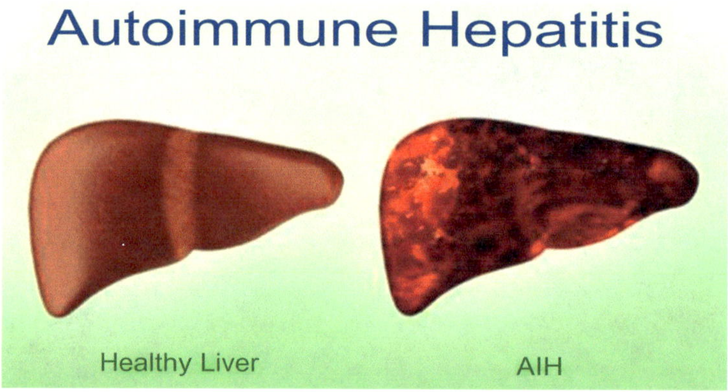

Figure 9.15. Autoimmune hepatitis.

Source: https://www.drkiranpeddi.com/images/liver-problems/auto-immune-hapatitis.jpg.

Viruses have a profound impact on the liver, and enzyme levels can swing wildly; the enzymes are continuously under scrutiny to measure the health of the liver. Take acute hepatitis A as an example: the laboratory tests will often show increased ALT and AST, which doctors use to decide if there's an extra layer, like an autoimmune process that's making things more complex. So, understanding these enzyme changes is crucial to choosing the proper clinical pathway even when the image gets cloudy. Autoimmune hepatitis (AIH) is an entirely different beast, usually leading clinicians down an alternate path to diagnosis and treatment. Even a case of viral hepatitis will sometimes elicit an autoimmune response - for instance, a patient with acute hepatitis A having rising levels of enzymes and presence of autoantibodies after an initial period of recovery. More often than not, these conditions reveal that close observation of liver function still remains pertinent even when all seems to be well. The correlation of laboratory values with a patient's clinical history is of value in helping doctors to more intuitively feel if autoimmune involvement is gaining the upper hand, and this can be of utmost significance in intervening before it is too late such that a liver transplant may become necessary (Kreimeyer et al., 2022). Stepping back to view things in the broader context, it's clear that liver function tests are not a universal diagnostic device—they're part of patient outcome management when hepatitis comes into play. Whether the problem is viral or autoimmune hepatitis, both can sufficiently impede liver function to require plans to be changed. In non-acetaminophen-induced acute liver failure (ALF), studies generally show that specialized tests such as the liver maximum capacity (LiMAx) test can predict outcomes reasonably well and help guide decision-making regarding transplantation (Kreimeyer et al., 2022). Liver stiffness measurement, mixed with a combination of coagulation values, also provides insight into the manner in which we assess risk for patients on their road to recovery. With a big toolkit of tests to call upon, health practitioners can balance all the variables that affect liver health and tailor their interventions in ways that intuitively just work, even when at times it seems more a matter of art than science (Figure 9.15).

9.5.2. Fatty Liver Disease

Metabolic disorders are upsetting the apple cart in the instance of non-alcoholic fatty liver disease (NAFLD). The liver begins storing fat—typically without warning—until suddenly it isn't doing very well. Catch it early; liver function tests (LFTs) leap into action as early warning signs by tracking enzyme levels that indicate something's not right. For instance, if serum glutamate pyruvate transaminase levels hit its ceiling and a couple of other lab tests look goofy, it could mean too much fat blocking the liver. Adding these tests to your routine checkup—again, not hard and fast, but as a preventive wink—nips likely issues in the bud and may even minimize other metabolic complications in the future (Ahmed et al., 2024). Fatty liver and metabolic syndrome have developed some sort of complex relationship these days. They appear to be working together in promoting the risk of NAFLD by means of obesity, dyslipidemia, and insulin resistance, rendering liver status assessment a bit of a mess. For example, Fatty Liver Index (FLI) is a non-invasive, if not straightforward, diagnostic marker that estimates the liver fat content approximately. When FLI values increase and enzyme levels fluctuate, it typically points to occult liver fat that's accumulating somewhere. In most instances, the implementation of LFTs in combination with the FLI will diagnose better and facilitate early interventions in patients at risk (Pouwels et al., 2022).

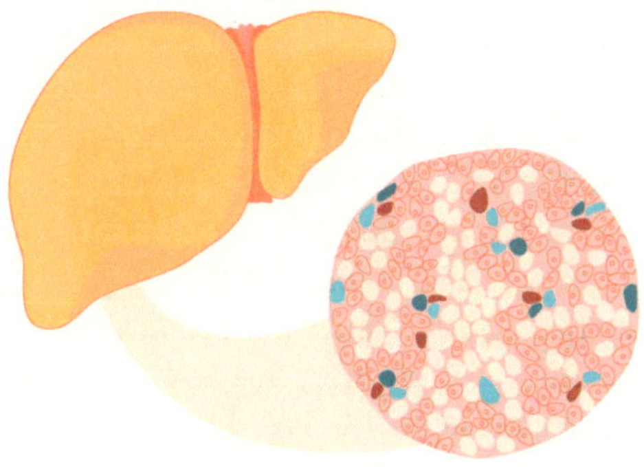

Figure 9.16. Fatty liver disease.

Source: https://media.post.rvohealth.io/wp-content/uploads/2020/09/12223-Everything_You_Need_to_Know_About_Fatty_Liver-thumb-732x549-1.jpg.

Uncovering more, a combination of marking off liver ailments is not just a diagnosis of fatty liver disease. While a liver biopsy remains the gold standard for nuance tissue data, not everyone is privileged to go down that invasive route. More recent, non-invasive technology – like FibroScan – has cropped up to give a glimpse into liver stiffness and fat load. LFTs, though, are more likely to signpost change, which triggers broader discussions around lifestyle change, from weight to facing metabolic syndrome head-on. For people who already have NAFLD, the treatments can range hugely from mild dietary modification to being put on medication, and following LFTs (even when they do change slightly in results) helps to determine whether or not the treatment is actually effective. Lastly, the inclusion of liver function tests in regular day-to-day clinical practice is quite significant in keeping the various aspects of fatty liver disease in sync (Ahmed et al., 2024; Pouwels et al., 2022) (Figure 9.16).

9.5.3. Cirrhosis and Liver Cancer

Cirrhosis sets off a series of liver abnormalities that, ultimately, lead to liver cancer. Damage builds slowly in the liver until fibrosis begins to replace healthy tissue, which in turn compromises the entire liver function. This slow, relentless breakdown creates the kind of setting on which hepatocellular carcinoma—the most common form of liver cancer—can develop. One strategy is to consider the relationship among these conditions as crucial for the early detection of issues and good control. Liver function tests, for example, are an effective tool for tracking the effectiveness of the liver in carrying out its function and for identifying the early indications of potential malignancies (Akbar et al., 2024; Chinnikatti et al., 2024). It is to be mentioned that liver cancer among cirrhotics has a very alarming incidence. Non-invasive diagnostic tests like routine liver function tests give doctors an idea of the chemical composition of the liver and help bring to notice disruptions in enzyme levels and synthesis activities that are conducive to detection by these tests. Imaging technologies, such as triphasic computed tomography scans, have further enhanced our ability to diagnose hepatocellular carcinoma at an early stage, which in the majority of cases means that the treatment will commence earlier and outcomes will improve. Such early detection not only guides the treatment protocols but literally changes lives by enhancing the overall quality of life, so periodic liver evaluations are essential in the management of cirrhosis (Akbar et al., 2024; Chinnikatti et al., 2024). Globally, solving the burden of cirrhosis and liver cancer needs a strategy that is not unidimensional. Furthermore, patient education and individualized treatment regimens also need to enter into the equation. Many of these liver conditions are due to modifiable risks like viral hepatitis or alcoholism, showing well-defined domains in which public health interventions could be effective. In most cases, close monitoring with liver function tests gives doctors the cues they require to monitor how heavily the liver is impaired and if complications like malignancy are imminent. Moreover, treatment plans must continue evolving in order to adapt to the peculiar challenges of cirrhosis and to deal with the ever-present risk of liver cancer. Lastly, with combining different specialists—from clinicians to researchers and public health supporters—comes the greatest promise of improved outcomes and a diminution of patients' burden (Akbar et al., 2024; Chinnikatti et al., 2024) (Figure 9.17).

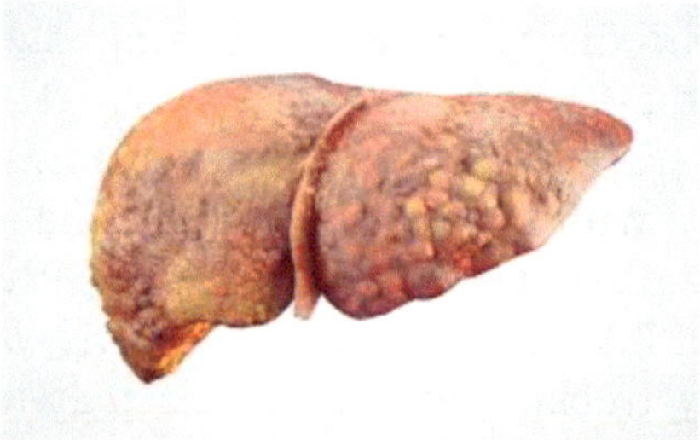

Figure 9.17. Cirrhosis and liver cancer.

Source: https://encrypted-tbn0.gstatic.com/images?q=tbn:ANd9GcQu-HBC5_jddePfASO0pkSXMYtJqNtzxPCuxQ&s.

Test Your Knowledge

1. How can LFTs aid in the diagnosis of viral hepatitis?
2. What abnormalities in LFTs are typically seen in alcoholic liver disease or cirrhosis?

9.6. Limitations of Liver Function Tests

Learning Outcome

- False positives and negatives;
- Variability in individual results;
- Need for additional diagnostic methods.

Liver function tests are very standard when keeping tabs on the health of the liver but by no means turn over every stone. We tend to count on them—basically, testing for enzymes like ALT and AST—to indicate damage to the liver cells, but these don't paint the entire picture. Take non-alcoholic fatty liver disease, for instance; more times than not, the tests come back within normal parameters despite the potential for the liver to be quietly being damaged. Age, gender, and other conditions tend to get the normal ranges all mixed up, so the numbers aren't as reliable as they look. In general, it's important to keep in mind that relying only on these tests can be hazardous, so most physicians find themselves complementing them with more comprehensive testing. Another turn-off is that these tests are not very specific. Sometimes, though, issues not with the liver itself—such as a heart attack or muscle disorder—will also increase enzyme levels, causing diagnosis to be misleading. The cross-over complicates it to try to ascertain if the problem truly begins in the liver or elsewhere, and generally takes more tests just to hazard a guess. Although LFTs are generally a useful first line of defense, their limitations often force the clinician to resort to other diagnostic tools in order to get a better picture and prevent errors in therapy. And let us not neglect how results can really get in a patient's head. Even slightly abnormal results might produce anxiety, especially if people are not frankly told precisely what these findings are supposed to indicate. Often, the people end up assuming that these results offer absolute answers—sometimes making them go into panic mode or even going ahead with unjustified procedures. In most cases, the patients and doctors themselves could have less anxiety if they were a bit more educated, so everyone could get a view of the real limits of the tests. Overall, integrating these conclusions into more stringent diagnostic protocols is central to an even-handed approach to liver care that yields better overall patient outcomes.

9.6.1. False Positives and Negatives

Liver function tests can significantly impact treatment, and a lot hinges on getting them right. A test can reveal evidence of liver trouble when there is none, causing further—and sometimes unwarranted—tests that create patient anxiety. On the flip side, not revealing a real issue with a false negative can postpone appropriate care to prevent complications. In the general instance, obtaining the balance right between identifying true cases (sensitivity) and not producing false alarms (specificity) is in effect the cornerstone of determining how reliable these tests are. Beyond the individual patient, the uncertainty in test results has wider ripple effects. Take, for instance, a study of liver fluke disease in red deer that created some puzzling differences in testing methods. The coproantigen ELISA (cELISA) later showed a higher rate of infection in frozen samples than in a fecal test; the overlap for single animals was, nonetheless, only moderate. The kind of finding makes sense to practitioners to drill more, juggling who's being tested and what tests are available. In the end, keeping disease estimates accurate for the whole population relies on choosing the right test to prevent misdiagnosis. Legal and ethical challenges add a layer of complexity to the issue because courts have a tendency to get mired in such diagnostic uncertainty. If unnecessary treatments are prescribed because of a false positive, legal mandates get intertwined with centuries-old tort law principles. As a general statement, most contemporary legal arguments currently emphasize how courts need to consider the mixture of solid evidence scientists use to arrive at healthcare decisions. Absent that sort of subtle knowledge, liability rules could become disconnected from actual scientific practice, stunting the development of diagnostic technology. Generally speaking, it's sorting out the aftermath of false positives and negatives in liver tests for real, both for the patients and for the credibility of our entire healthcare system.

9.6.2. Variability in Individual Results

Liver function tests (LFTs) can be pretty unpredictable—individual results often vary a lot. A mix of factors like how blood flows through the liver and the way test substances stick to plasma proteins all play a role. For example, when looking at indocyanine green (ICG) clearance, you'll notice that personal details such as body weight, age, and sex tend to sway the pharmacokinetic outcomes. Referring to these associations isn't just a neat piece of trivia; it actually enables doctors to better understand the test results and customize treatments for specific patients. In most cases, accepting this variability also enhances the validity of dynamic liver function tests (DLFTs), potentially opening the door to more bespoke treatment plans (Grzegorzewski et al., 2021). It gets even more complex when you factor in genetic and ethnic influences on these tests. Science generally is consistent in demonstrating that genetic elements can cause populations to respond differently to drugs and to diagnostic interventions. There was even a study that directly compared efavirenz pharmacokinetics between Ethiopian and Tanzanian populations, revealing considerable differences that were partially explained by genetic variants such as *CYP2B66** and *ABCB1 c.4036A>G*. These reminders underscore the importance of considering a person's genetic background when evaluating liver tests—metabolic variations can have actual effects on the safety and effectiveness of a drug. In most cases, integrating genetic data into assessments adds to our understanding of each patient's unique needs (Habtewold et al., 2013). All this complexity actually sets the stage for a shift toward precision medicine in liver testing. The interplay of everyday physiological quirks and underlying genetic traits has us likely in need of more advanced methods—maybe even computer models—to predict a person's response and to unscramble all the mysterious variables that affect liver tests. Attending to individual differences and how exactly these differences turn out pays dividends to clinicians, allowing them to hone diagnoses and treatment protocols. Ultimately, having a better grasp of why liver test results are so inconsistent could change clinical practice so that each patient is treated as unique as their own personal biological signature (Grzegorzewski et al., 2021).

9.6.3. Need for Additional Diagnostic Methods

Liver function can't be comprehended fully with routine tests alone. Routine liver function tests (LFTs) are okay for a snapshot, but they tend not to pick up on the nuances—especially when liver disease emerges gradually. In most cases, those old familiar assays won't detect what's really happening. Consider, for instance, in screening for diseases like NAFLD or chronic hepatitis. The routine biomarkers alone are not the whole story. Adding to the mix other means—such as more advanced imaging (e.g., elastography) and non-invasive serum biomarker panels—can identify issues earlier and quantify disease severity better, and allow for more accurate treatment. Disrupting our traditional testing, overall, is going to be the norm if we're to realize better results. Not everyone reacts to liver damage the same way. Metabolic quirks, hereditary predispositions, and even lifestyle factors merge into a very personal—and occasionally disordered—portrait of liver function. You may have two patients with nearly identical LFT results but with a very different disease course, each needing a very different approach to treatment. It's precisely because of this that it appears so crucial to look for new biomarkers—perhaps novel proteomic or genomic hints—that actually capture how every individual's liver is behaving. By relying on these sophisticated methods, doctors are better able to gauge risk and monitor disease advancement, eventually refining patient care. Obviously, "beefing up" our array of diagnostic tools isn't merely a choice; it's a necessity, forcing the medical community to innovate outside the box. Artificial intelligence has started to make its influence felt in this roundabout as well. AI platforms are able to search through complex sets of data—genetic information to imaging and serum markers—using a level of precision that tends to pick up on what older methods miss. Quite frequently, these intelligent algorithms recognize early warning signs of liver issues way before the classic markers would trigger any alarm. Using machine learning to guide decision-making can anticipate what will occur and direct therapy in ways unimaginable before. As hepatology and technology become more integrated, more and more apparent it becomes that we need an engaged, tiered strategy for assessment of the liver—one that addresses today's issues but prepares the way for tomorrow's breakthroughs.

Test Your Knowledge

1. Why do normal LFT results not always rule out significant liver disease?
2. How can extrahepatic conditions (e.g., bone disease) affect test interpretation?

Summary

Liver function is inseparable from the overall health of the organism and best shows why the likes of LFTs are absolutely essential in everyday clinical practice. In many scenarios, these tests are more than just confirming diagnosis – they diagnose root conditions, like the suggestion of diabetes mellitus. Several studies have indicated that when HbA1c is elevated, abnormal liver test results are likely to show up as well, which in turn will lead doctors to check both blood sugar and liver function in diabetic patients. This kind of holistic monitoring has a tendency to lead to smarter, more effective management strategies, better outcomes for patients, and intervention earlier when things start to go wrong (Joseph et al., 2024). The liver's stiffness and overall function can also be helpful in yielding further information, especially when it comes to liver fibrosis. Recent evidence suggests that LiMAx scores—a liver function test—have the tendency, in the majority of cases, to alter inversely to liver stiffness values. That is, one goes up and the other tends to go down. The reliance on the use of a single test will miss out on significant details; instead, the integration of LFTs with techniques such as ultrasound elastography gives healthcare professionals a broader understanding of liver dynamics and subtleties of insidious pathology (Senk et al., 2024). Finally, liver function tests are not simply run-of-the-mill lab results; they provide a multifaceted view of health through the integration of factors like glycemic control and overall systemic health. The evidence continues to point toward the very intimate relationship between blood sugar regulation and liver function, and it now appears likely that standard patient care practices will need to be reconsidered. As medicine continues its shift toward personalization, it is commonplace enough to include these tests as part of standard evaluation in the routine screening in the near future. Looking ahead, future research will probably have to further customize these test procedures and investigate other biomarkers that can inform us even further about how liver function affects the rest of the body's systems – paving the way for improved diagnostic and treatment strategies. Liver tests are not just a matter of checking boxes—it's balancing a mixture of techniques to capture the whole picture. Multiphase CT scans, performed at different times, have also been a significant help, especially if patients are being referred for significant liver surgery. Several research even name parameters like the iodine washout rate and the liver volume indexed for body surface area as good leads for recognizing severe dysfunction. In the majority of cases, these scans serve a two-for-one purpose by identifying both structural abnormalities and overall function, and subsequently, this directs treatment planning and patient prognosis (Nagayama et al., 2025). The evolution of liver function tests (LFTs) has literally revolutionized day-to-day care. The removal of the boxed warning for ambrisentan's liver risks marked the tipping point at which Risk Evaluation and Mitigation Strategies (REMS) guidelines underwent a significant revision. At night, ambrisentan began being administered to almost all patients, and tests taken at initiation of therapy or at refill plummeted. A switch so rapid in fact demonstrates the way practice guidelines can turn on a dime, reminding us of that drug performance and safety of patients always must be balanced (Feldman et al., 2024). It also helps to explain that an individual doesn't simply do one test or scan by itself—doctors actually have to keep on top of all of these changes. With real changes in prescribing habits following updates—as seen with both ambrisentan and bosentan—it is no surprise that staying up to date on liver function test (LFT) implications is essential. Better understanding of liver testing can enable a decrease in risk that comes with high-risk drugs so that liver health is not compromised in the process. Blending newer imaging techniques with revised guidelines is certain to make overall efficiency in liver testing, in the long run, benefit patients who undergo hepatobiliary disorders (Feldman et al., 2024).

KEY TERMS FROM THIS CHAPTER

- Albumin
- Ammonia
- Bilirubin
- Cirrhosis
- Gamma-glutamyl transferase (GGT)
- Indirect bilirubin
- Lactate dehydrogenase (LDH)
- Liver enzymes
- Serum globulins
- Alkaline phosphatase (ALP)
- Aspartate aminotransferase (AST)
- Cholestasis
- Direct bilirubin
- Hepatitis panel
- International normalized ratio (INR)
- Liver biopsy
- Prothrombin time (PT)
- Total bilirubin

Critical Thinking Questions

1. **Which of the following enzymes is most commonly measured to assess liver function?**
   a. Creatinine kinase
   b. Aspartate aminotransferase (AST)
   c. Lactate dehydrogenase (LDH)
   d. Amylase
2. **An elevated level of bilirubin in the blood is indicative of which of the following?**
   a. Kidney dysfunction
   b. Liver dysfunction
   c. Hyperglycemia
   d. Dehydration
3. **Which of the following liver function tests specifically measures liver cell injury or damage?**
   a. Albumin
   b. Prothrombin time (PT)
   c. Alanine aminotransferase (ALT)
   d. Bilirubin
4. **The liver function test known as "prothrombin time" (PT) evaluates:**
   a. The liver's ability to produce clotting factors
   b. The liver's ability to detoxify substances
   c. The kidney's ability to filter waste
   d. The heart's ability to pump blood
5. **An increase in serum albumin levels is most commonly associated with:**
   a. Acute liver disease
   b. Chronic liver cirrhosis
   c. Malnutrition or liver dysfunction
   d. Kidney failure

Answers to Critical Thinking Questions

1. (b); 2. (b); 3. (c); 4. (a); 5. (c)

Short Answer Questions

1. What is the purpose of liver function tests (LFTs), and what do they assess?
2. What are the key enzymes typically measured in LFTs?
3. How does serum bilirubin contribute to assessing liver function, and what can elevate levels indicate?
4. What is the role of alkaline phosphatase (ALP) in liver function tests, and what could an elevated level indicate?
5. How does gamma-glutamyl transferase (GGT) help in diagnosing liver and biliary tract disorders?
6. What is albumin, and how is its level used to assess liver function and synthesis ability?

References

1. Abid, H., Abid, A., Sohail, S., & Jawaid, S. (2025). Clinical and genetic analysis of methylmalonic aciduria in 60 patients from Southern China: A single center retrospective study. *Orphanet Journal of Rare Diseases, 20*. https://www.semanticscholar.org/paper/25ffc738d329624f21461309569c25bf9aae1ef6 (accessed on 1st July 2025).
2. Ahmed, M., Saeed, R., Kamani, L., Durrani, N., & Ahmed, F. (2024). Comparison of fatty liver index with fibro scan in non-alcoholic fatty liver disease. *Journal of Family Medicine and Primary Care, 13*, 1488–1495. https://www.semanticscholar.org/paper/426bfbec5572736cd07c58a215d64735289a239a (accessed on 1st July 2025).
3. Akbar, R., Ahmed, A., & Javid, S. (2024). Triphasic computed tomography for characterization of liver lesions identified on ultrasonography. *Journal of Bashir Institute of Health Sciences*. https://www.semanticscholar.org/paper/3d881d317354f09c22e43fbc1a66633c3adadac1 (accessed on 1st July 2025).
4. Ali, A. K., Baglivo, A., Govil, P., Gibbs, L. R., Bradley, M. C., Campbell, K. E., Chakravarty, A. G., et al. (2025). Characterization of SARS-CoV-2 diagnostic tests and liver function tests among patients with COVID-19 diagnosed in outpatient settings using administrative healthcare data and data from commercial laboratories. *Pharmacoepidemiology and Drug Safety, 34*(1), e70094. https://www.semanticscholar.org/paper/674cbb316029c8ef275e4dd056f579a3342da168 (accessed on 1st July 2025).
5. Ali, Z. A., Kadhim, H. M., Shammar, S. H., & Najm, Z. M. (2025). The assessment of serum cytokeratin 18 and liver function tests in chronic hepatitis B patients. *Journal of Kufa for Chemical Sciences*. https://www.semanticscholar.org/paper/89d8dcb7b0f990eeb8e937e4a27af060e37c653a (accessed on 1st July 2025).
6. Alvi, Q. A., & Parkash, A. (2025). Effectiveness of liver biopsy in diagnosing liver diseases using a five-point diagnostic scale among pediatric population. *The Professional Medical Journal*. https://www.semanticscholar.org/paper/d62915e7189c00ed25e3b000c491d113d5cfc398 (accessed on 1st July 2025).
7. Astirin, O. P., & Harini, M. (2009). Blood cholesterol levels of hypercholesterolemic rat (*Rattus norvegicus*) after VCO treatment. https://core.ac.uk/download/12346112.pdf (accessed on 1st July 2025).
8. Baksh, S. A., Muhammad, S., Parvez, U., Shirazi, B., & Khan, M. A. (2025). Impact of the laparoscopic approach on liver function tests: Comparison of elective biliary and non-biliary procedures. *Cureus, 17*. https://www.semanticscholar.org/paper/ee73dfde0a42828bf531c4b00ca634e45cea927d (accessed on 1st July 2025).
9. Balasubramanian, G., Hyngstrom, A., Kern, M., et al. (2016). Effects of laryngeal restriction on pharyngeal peristalsis and biomechanics: Clinical implications. https://core.ac.uk/download/213062275.pdf (accessed on 1st July 2025).
10. Batta, A. (2011). Cholecystitis & an enzyme study. *International Journal of Current Biomedical and Pharmaceutical Research*. https://core.ac.uk/download/pdf/14665.pdf (accessed on 1st July 2025).
11. Bhuyan, B., Das, J., Das, M., Bhattacharya, D. K., & Nath, C. (2024). Cystatin C as an early marker of renal dysfunction in patients with cirrhosis of liver: A cross-sectional study. *Journal*

of Clinical and Diagnostic Research. https://www.semanticscholar.org/paper/699005dcbce08db5f9793a67947a7fead4626b60 (accessed on 1st July 2025).

12. Bidarmaghz, B., Sabat, N., Sharma, A., McGregor, H., & Wong, J. (2023). Multicenter retrospective cohort study: Using trends in liver function tests to predict spontaneous passage of common bile duct stones in choledocholithiasis. *International Journal of Hepatobiliary and Pancreatic Diseases*. https://www.semanticscholar.org/paper/e5a97062fd41a0ab56b2854be0872b0fe2e99777 (accessed on 1st July 2025).
13. Cardoso, F., Senkus, E., Costa, A., Papadopoulos, E., Aapro, M., André, F., Harbeck, N., et al. (2018). 4th ESO–ESMO International Consensus Guidelines for advanced breast cancer (ABC 4). *Annals of Oncology, 29*, 1634–1657. https://doi.org/10.1093/annonc/mdy192 (accessed on 1st July 2025).
14. Chan, M., Fung, J. Y. Y., Lai, C. L., et al. (2013). Defining normal liver stiffness range in a normal healthy Chinese population without liver disease. https://core.ac.uk/download/38039640.pdf (accessed on 1st July 2025).
15. Chinnikatti, V. A., & Kulkarni, V. P. (2024). Cirrhosis of liver in Ayurveda with special reference to Yakrit Vikara. *International Journal of Ayurvedic and Herbal Medicine*. https://www.semanticscholar.org/paper/e4e5cf561345e8f99b0f8de5de65581f4eb2e3c6 (accessed on 1st July 2025).
16. Choi, J. H., Lee, J., Park, E., Bae, S., Kim, D., Kim, Y. H., & Choi, I. (2021). Nutrition and metabolism research abstracts. *JPEN. Journal of Parenteral and Enteral Nutrition, 45*(S1), 7–240. https://www.semanticscholar.org/paper/02cbd73c3bb6faeac33e59cc28bf6d9f1085eba0 (accessed on 1st July 2025).
17. Craine, A., French, A. S., Gibb, S. W., et al. (2016). Prevalence of liver fluke (*Fasciola hepatica*) in wild red deer (*Cervus elaphus*): Coproantigen ELISA is a practicable alternative to fecal egg counting for surveillance in remote populations. https://core.ac.uk/download/46559478.pdf (accessed on 1st July 2025).
18. Cranor, C. F., & Eastmond, D. A. (2001). Scientific ignorance and reliable patterns of evidence in toxic tort causation: Is there a need for liability reform? https://core.ac.uk/download/62568630.pdf (accessed on 1st July 2025).
19. Cruz-Jentoft, A. J., Bahat, G., Bauer, J. M., Boirie, Y., Bruyère, O., Cederholm, T., Cooper, C., et al. (2018). Sarcopenia: Revised European consensus on definition and diagnosis. *Age and Ageing, 48*, 16–31. https://doi.org/10.1093/ageing/afy169 (accessed on 1st July 2025).
20. De Coster, D. A., Carroll, M., Lavender, J., & Gibson, R. (2024). A case of *Raoultella ornithinolytica* cholangitis in a liver transplant recipient. *European Journal of Case Reports in Internal Medicine, 11*. https://www.semanticscholar.org/paper/28a33633a34f6288a754f2c3b1ba58ab0b79f864 (accessed on 1st July 2025).
21. Duswald, K. H., Jochum, M., Lenk, S., et al. (1993). Increased serum levels of procollagen type III peptide in severely injured patients. https://core.ac.uk/download/12170584.pdf (accessed on 1st July 2025).
22. Dwivedi, J. (2024). Comparative study of biochemical alteration in COVID-19 and non-COVID 19 patients: Association with liver function tests abnormalities. *Global Journal for Research Analysis*. https://www.semanticscholar.org/paper/22d884ac29e15868b831d5c905bce9dce3c4ebbc (accessed on 1st July 2025).

23. Ebrahimpour, P., Karamian, M., & Sharifi, A. (2024). Effects of resveratrol on liver function tests in patients with non-alcoholic fatty liver disease: A systematic review and meta-analysis of randomized controlled trials. *Russian Journal of Gastroenterology, Hepatology, Coloproctology*. https://www.semanticscholar.org/paper/caaee7a83ea2a1f8a8d3172865b1dad2e6e75645 (accessed on 1st July 2025).

24. Feldman, W., Mahesri, M., Sarpatwari, A., Huybrechts, K. F., Zhu, Y., Hwang, C. S., Lii, J., et al. (2024). Removing the FDA's boxed hepatotoxicity warning and liver function testing requirement for ambrisentan. *JAMA Network Open, 7*. https://www.semanticscholar.org/paper/680f31866da0a9246653c65a7f8265af555db2bc (accessed on 1st July 2025).

25. Firas, A. T., & Ilham, A. F. (2005). Effect of maintenance therapy for childhood with acute lymphoblastic leukemia by combination of methotrexate and 6-mercaptopurine on the liver. https://core.ac.uk/download/614657464.pdf (accessed on 1st July 2025).

26. Grzegorzewski, J., Köller, A., & König, M. (2021). Physiologically based modeling of the effect of physiological and anthropometric variability on indocyanine green based liver function tests. https://core.ac.uk/download/491202926.pdf (accessed on 1st July 2025).

27. Habtewold, A., Kassu, A., Tsegaye, A., Habtewold, A., Belanger, A. S., Ward, B. A., Schackman, B. R., et al. (2013). Importance of ethnicity, CYP2B6 and ABCB1 genotype for efavirenz pharmacokinetics and treatment outcomes: A parallel-group prospective cohort study in two sub-Saharan Africa populations. https://core.ac.uk/download/pdf/18410838.pdf (accessed on 1st July 2025).

28. He, H., Gao, H., Zhang, Y., Wang, Q., Li, Z., Wu, S., & Wen, C. (2025). Impact of non-alcoholic fatty liver disease on cognition and brain changes: A comprehensive review. *Reviews in the Neurosciences*. https://www.semanticscholar.org/paper/37477eb539860d1f7b40e93932a57d7407c7072e (accessed on 1st July 2025).

29. Himral, P., Bhawani, R., Bhardwaj, M., & Sharma, N. (2023). Liver function tests at admission as marker of severity and prognosis in COVID-19 patients–A retrospective analysis. *Journal of Family Medicine and Primary Care, 12*, 3108–3114. https://www.semanticscholar.org/paper/ccf361225a1efe064772dbeea06451bdef0e8071 (accessed on 1st July 2025).

30. Horne, B., Le, V., May, H., Knight, S., Bair, T., Muhlestein, J., Knowlton, K., et al. (2022). Abstract 11652: What is the relative risk for elevated liver function tests of single and combined statin and alcohol use and implications for management? *Circulation*. https://www.semanticscholar.org/paper/3c2a1f12647336568100d06d495eeab5e67f8b2e (accessed on 1st July 2025).

31. Jamil, M., Ahmed, T., Ali, M. M., Javed, H. J., Waheed, A., Ahmed, A., & Jamil, M. I. (2025). Assessment of abnormal liver function tests in dengue fever: Implications for disease severity and outcome. *Indus Journal of Bioscience Research*. https://www.semanticscholar.org/paper/50b8c390412b0d78631fcf7cd604e8bb95e3d850 (accessed on 1st July 2025).

32. Jeon, J., Lee, D., Kim, B., Park, B. Y., Oh, C. J., Kim, M. J., Jeon, J. H., et al. (2023). CycloZ improves hyperglycemia and lipid metabolism by modulating lysine acetylation in KK-Ay mice. *Diabetes & Metabolism Journal, 47*, 653–667. https://www.semanticscholar.org/paper/5e0d358486f370029cbde60d452f217c606bcfbb (accessed on 1st July 2025).

33. Jo, H. I., Kim, M., Yoo, J. J., Kim, S. G., Kim, Y. S., & Chin, S. (2022). Acute hepatitis A-induced autoimmune hepatitis: A case report and literature review. *Medicina, 58*. https://www.semanticscholar.org/paper/ef39823153fd69800aec85f2564964f5f4ba0d8f (accessed on 1st July 2025).

34. Joseph, K. I., Sivagami, K., Kumar, P. M., Aparnavi, P., & Jeevithan, S. (2024). Associations between HbA1c levels and liver function tests in diabetes: A comprehensive analysis. *Asian Journal of Pharmaceutical and Clinical Research.* https://www.semanticscholar.org/paper/fa1418c187206506021807977be35f8bf695587e (accessed on 1st July 2025).

35. Khan, J. U. A., Qaisar, A., & Sameen, D. E. (2023). Non-alcoholic fatty liver disease: Physician's worst nightmare. *Journal of Ayub Medical College, Abbottabad: JAMC, 35*(1), 1–2. https://www.semanticscholar.org/paper/e177d7db758d8c0b17f9eb85f6c5977fdeba634d (accessed on 1st July 2025).

36. Kreimeyer, H., Buechter, M., Best, J., Gieseler, R., Katsounas, A., Sowa, J. P., Gerken, G., et al. (2022). Performance of the Liver Maximum Function Capacity Test, fibrinogen, and transient elastography in patients with acute liver injury. *Digestive Diseases, 41*, 259–267. https://www.semanticscholar.org/paper/2f779d6516cadb486cdc05a6f05242879bfc5400 (accessed on 1st July 2025).

37. Lai, J. C., Tandon, P., Bernal, W., Tapper, E. B., Ekong, U. D., Dasarathy, S., & Carey, E. J. (2021). Malnutrition, frailty, and sarcopenia in patients with cirrhosis: 2021 Practice Guidance by the American Association for the Study of Liver Diseases. *Hepatology, 74*, 1611–1644. https://doi.org/10.1002/hep.32049 (accessed on 1st July 2025).

38. Liguori, C., Magi, S., Mandolesi, A., Agostini, A., Svegliati-Baroni, G., Benedetti Cacciaguerra, A., Parisi, A., et al. (2025). Adjuvant treatment with capecitabine in patients who received orthotopic liver transplantation with incidental diagnosis of intrahepatic cholangiocarcinoma. Implications on *DPYD* polymorphisms assessment: Report of two cases and review of the literature. *Cancer Chemotherapy and Pharmacology, 95.* https://www.semanticscholar.org/paper/482270fdb42c6f07e360f0730cccd4a833cc8239 (accessed on 1st July 2025).

39. Mkhize, N., & Thembane, N. (2023). Alcohol-induced liver injury: A retrospective study evaluating liver function tests in a South African population. https://core.ac.uk/download/560697404.pdf (accessed on 1st July 2025).

40. Mohsen, R. (2023). Receiver operating characteristic analysis of liver function tests in patients with chronic viral hepatitis B in Baghdad, Iraq. *Iraqi Journal of Industrial Research.* https://www.semanticscholar.org/paper/df89a86b6769f846544e9eb2b1bc5a8bb53f365e (accessed on 1st July 2025).

41. Morgan, T. R., Seth, D., & Whitfield, J. B. (2022). All-cause and liver-related mortality risk factors in excessive drinkers: Analysis of data from the UK Biobank. https://www.zora.uzh.ch/id/eprint/229249/1/Alcohol_Clin_Exp_Res___2022___Whitfield___All_cause_and_liver_related_mortality_risk_factors_in_excessive_drinkers_.pdf (accessed on 1st July 2025).

42. Nagayama, Y., Hokamura, M., Taguchi, N., Yokota, Y., Osaki, T., Ogasawara, K., Shiraishi, S., et al. (2025). Liver function estimation using multiphase hepatic CT: Diagnostic performance of iodine-uptake and volumetric parameters. *European Radiology.* https://www.semanticscholar.org/paper/d5c78fe5909ccd25d0491f3768e9035bfdb609b4 (accessed on 1st July 2025).

43. Novak, A., Acharya, A., Beer, S., Espinosa, A., Bond Smith, G., Saga, C., Andrews, J., et al. (2025). Pilot feasibility study to determine the utility of direct access and quantitative magnetic resonance cholangiopancreatography (MRCP) in the assessment of suspected acute biliary or ductal gallstone presentations. *BMC Gastroenterology, 25.* https://www.semanticscholar.org/paper/16480dc04ee7407b7f851c6b1f1e353f91796939 (accessed on 1st July 2025).

44. Oaknin, A., Bosse, T., Creutzberg, C. L., Giornelli, G., Harter, P., Joly, F., Lorusso, D., et al. (2022). Endometrial cancer: ESMO clinical practice guideline for diagnosis, treatment and follow-up. *Annals of Oncology, 33*, 860–877. https://doi.org/10.1016/j.annonc.2022.05.009 (accessed on 1st July 2025).

45. Pooransari, P., Pouransari, R., Gharib Laki, M., Abedi Asl, Z., Yavari, S., & Hosseiniara, R. (2024). Comparison of changes in liver function tests in pregnant women with mild and severe COVID-19. *Coronaviruses*. https://www.semanticscholar.org/paper/20e16760a6fa2ec4f9d56b465f83d5b8f0103981 (accessed on 1st July 2025).

46. Pouwels, S., Sakran, N., Graham, Y., Leal, A., Pintar, T., Yang, W., Kassir, R., et al. (2022). Non-alcoholic fatty liver disease (NAFLD): A review of pathophysiology, clinical management and effects of weight loss. *BMC Endocrine Disorders, 22*. https://www.semanticscholar.org/paper/2475ce6517e705ac214495d90ab4798cbd101c4c (accessed on 1st July 2025).

47. Ranjbar, M., Shab-Bidar, S., Mohammadi, H., & Djafarian, K. (2024). Effect of intermittent fasting on liver function tests: A systematic review and meta-analysis of randomized clinical trials. *Nutrition Reviews*. https://www.semanticscholar.org/paper/9990857ad89eae191fe788585c48faec46431fd8 (accessed on 1st July 2025).

48. Senk, K., Río Bártulos, C., Belkoura, J. M. C., Schmid, S., Schlosser-Hupf, S., Jung, E., Wiggermann, P., et al. (2024). LiMAx test and ultrasound elastography to measure biomarkers of declining liver function in patients with liver fibrosis: A correlation analysis. *Clinical Hemorheology and Microcirculation*. https://www.semanticscholar.org/paper/2b059225b62d6c67a860ac1199f596346c759a78 (accessed on 1st July 2025).

49. Shah, D., Saha, M., Uday, R., Mitra, R., & Fatima, M. (2025). Liver function tests as an indicator of adverse maternal and fetal outcomes in patients with hypertensive disorders of pregnancy. *International Journal of Reproduction, Contraception, Obstetrics and Gynecology*. https://www.semanticscholar.org/paper/b5df3e9eb0fd81dcf4aaa8b7f77e71a87a764f88 (accessed on 1st July 2025).

50. Shrivatsava, K., Sushma, B., & Lalwani, R. (2022). Assessment of liver function tests and bioelectrical impedance body fat analysis in obese adolescents. *International Journal of Health Sciences*. https://www.semanticscholar.org/paper/9b8d653a416e9f472b426eaf3077a7db40c02ef6 (accessed on 1st July 2025).

51. Sumadewi, K. T. (2023). Embryology, anatomy and physiology of the liver: Review. *Indian Journal of Clinical Anatomy and Physiology*. https://www.semanticscholar.org/paper/d9e85aba5eaeb77af1366b8b0d9afa5a69d39658 (accessed on 1st July 2025).

52. Takahashi, S., Fukami, T., Masuo, Y., Brocker, C., Xie, C., Krausz, K. W., Wolf, C. R., et al. (2016). Cyp2c70 is responsible for the species difference in bile acid metabolism between mice and humans. *Journal of Lipid Research, 57*, 2130–2137. https://doi.org/10.1194/jlr.m071183 (accessed on 1st July 2025).

53. Tijani, A. W., Ajiboye, K. F., Olaniyan, M. F., Apoyovwere, O. J., Odegbemi, O. B., Ochagu, O. R., Kanikwu, P. N., et al. (2024). Alpha-fetoprotein as a predictor of liver disease progression in HBV patients with HIV and HCV co-infections. https://core.ac.uk/download/630913289.pdf (accessed on 1st July 2025).

54. Varma, P. R. (2023). Association between serum alpha-fetoprotein level and liver function parameters in hepatocellular carcinoma patients: A case-control study. *International Journal*

of Clinical Biochemistry and Research. https://www.semanticscholar.org/paper/1d083950e46b37e4268a8f1bfa33bd0125665cf5 (accessed on 1st July 2025).

55. Vogel, J. D., Felder, S., Bhama, A. R., Hawkins, A. T., Langenfeld, S. J., Shaffer, V., Thorsen, A. J., et al. (2021). The American Society of Colon and Rectal Surgeons Clinical Practice Guidelines for the management of colon cancer. *Diseases of the Colon & Rectum, 65*, 148–177. https://doi.org/10.1097/dcr.0000000000002323 (accessed on 1st July 2025).

BLOOD GLUCOSE AND DIABETES MELLITUS

10

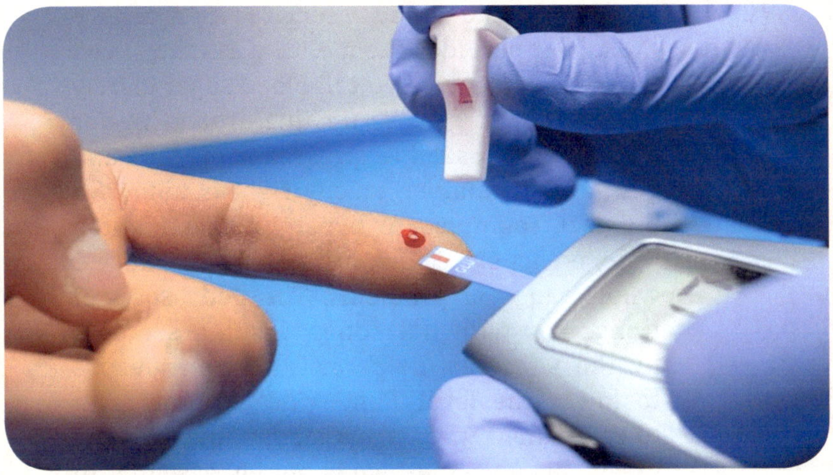

LEARNING OBJECTIVES

After studying this chapter, you will be able to:

1. Explain the types of diabetes mellitus;
2. Discuss about blood glucose regulation;
3. List the symptoms of diabetes mellitus;
4. Describe diagnosis of diabetes;
5. Illustration the management of blood glucose levels;
6. Explore the impact of diabetes on health.

Introduction

Diabetes mellitus is a difficult metabolic disease that weighs heavily on individuals and healthcare systems worldwide. The disease manifests as chronically elevated blood glucose because the body is either unable to make enough insulin or simply not using it correctly—basically, a double-whammy. You're looking at a couple of distinct faces here with type 1 and type 2 diabetes being the most common. It all has to do with how our bodies metabolize glucose; when that gets out of balance—most often due to lifestyle habits such as eating a poor diet and not exercising enough—it can lead to problems now as well as later in life, such as heart disease, nerve damage, and even vision issues. Overall, attempting to control blood sugar more efficiently, either by changing your diet or adding medicines to the mix, is more of a priority. When you look closer, diabetes isn't single-caused—it's just a jumble of genetic, environmental, and diet and lifestyle combined. In most Type 2 cases, the body starts to revolt against insulin, so blood sugar goes up and can be a path to other issues such as abnormal cholesterol or high blood pressure. There has been some fascinating research done more recently that looks at our gut bacteria and how they can affect insulin sensitivity and sugar metabolism. Other studies show that even small adjustments to the makeup of these gut microbes—like incorporating some aspects of diet such as those found in *Suaeda salsa*—could be enough to tilt the scales and change how the body reacts to sugar, opening the door to a whole new area of managing the disease (Yin et al., 2024).

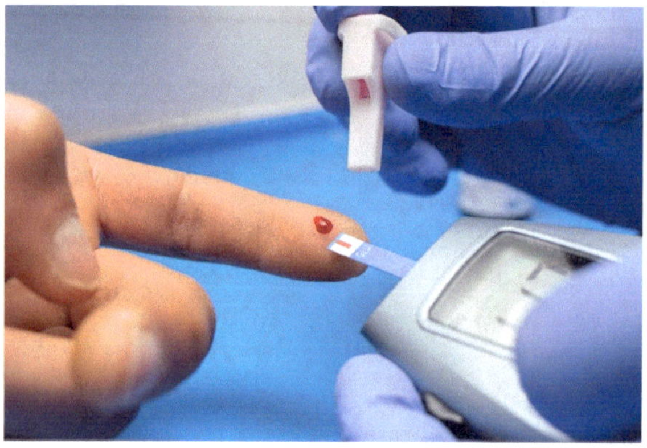

Figure 10.1. Blood sugar tests.

Source: https://www.yashodahealthcare.com/blogs/wp-content/uploads/2023/03/blood-sugar-test.jpg.

It's a field where gut health, nutrition, and diabetes all seem to dance in odd harmony together. Meanwhile, insulin therapy has changed the diabetes game in a big way. Insulin remains at the hub of evening out blood sugar levels, and now patients have many tools at their disposal to help smooth out those roller-coaster fluctuations. More novel approaches, like ultra-long-acting basal insulins, seem to reach goals like keeping HbA1c in check and lowering the rate of nasty low blood sugar events—this very much speaks to the beginning of personalized care. Scientists are essentially continually optimizing these treatments to be better suited to individual needs, such that an interplay between lifestyle changes, new medications, and an improved understanding of the inner workings of diabetes is the future (Aktas et al., 2024). On the whole, managing diabetes effectively seems to need a more multifaceted and versatile strategy, even when everything is not necessarily neatly so (Figure 10.1).

Definition of Blood Glucose

Glucose in the blood energizes our cells – literally, it provides them with what they need day after day. You could call blood sugar merely the amount of glucose floating around in our bloodstream (usually expressed in mg/dL), and getting that number exactly right is kind of a big deal. Too much, or hyperglycemia, and too little, or hypoglycemia, can actually produce a whole range of problems. The body sorts of things out with hormones; insulin, secreted by the pancreas, helps cells take in glucose to lower the levels, and glucagon comes in to raise them when they get too low. In most cases, this give-and-take is merely essential to keeping energy level steady, and if this balance is disrupted, it can instigate issues like diabetes mellitus, a condition that is increasingly proving challenging for health practitioners worldwide (François et al., 2019). The term blood sugar takes on more meaning when you consider diabetes – a condition which is defined by abnormally high levels, typically because the body is not producing enough insulin or because the cells simply are not responding in kind. You tend to hear about Type 1 and Type 2 diabetes a great deal in two general categories. Type 1, essentially, is when the immune system lashes out and destroys the cells which make insulin, so that there are very few to use; Type 2, on the other hand, is more of an insulin resistance, which is frequently mixed up. Having high blood sugar levels, as studies have shown, sets the stage for nerve damage (neuropathy), eye problems (retinopathy), even heart disease—complications that illustrate precisely why control of blood sugar is so critical in treatment strategies (Vos et al., 2017). Research into how best to keep blood sugar under control still holds new revelations on diabetes control. Today there's buzz about Continuous Glucose Monitoring (CGM) systems that provide immediate feedback on sugar swings, and then enable individuals to take their diet, exercise, and medications a bit more tailored. As diabetes is spreading all across the globe, the need for good education and smart clinical tactics aimed at glucose control grows. Broadly stated, this greater understanding not only directs personal choices but also molds more extensive public health strategies for mitigating the overall prevalence of diabetes in diverse populations (François et al., 2019; Vos et al., 2017).

Overview of Diabetes Mellitus

Diabetes is a monolithic worldwide issue that affects everything from the lives of individuals to national economies. It's not just about sugar in the blood—instead, it's a multifaceted illness that disrupts the body's normal balance in several ways. For example, what most of us call Type 1 comes when the immune system becomes invasive and annihilates the pancreas's beta cells that produce insulin—meaning individuals must take insulin for life. And then there's Type 2, which occurs in approximately 90–95% of the instances, where a mix of causes like obesity, too much sitting around, and the inability of the body to efficiently use insulin truly gets in the way. With obesity becoming more prevalent virtually everywhere, the incidence of type 2 diabetes puts an extreme strain on healthcare systems and requires enhanced prevention and control measures (Mary et al., 2023). Looking closer at diabetes, it essentially comes down to the body losing control over normal blood sugar regulation. When insulin isn't functioning quite right, glucose levels become out of control and that in turn beckons a host of other issues—heart problems, nerve damage, kidney stress, and even eye issues. The more time one has had diabetes and the less well it's controlled, the more severe these complications become. In most cases, modern recommendations for treatment require developing a strategy that is best suited to the individual. The therapy can include medication, changing a few habits, and constant monitoring of glucose to ultimately improve overall health outcomes and quality of life (Fiedorova et al., 2022). It should be added that diabetes does not always appear separately. Most people do wrestle with a cluster of conditions including insulin resistance, cholesterol levels that have been jacked up, and high blood pressure all at once—a team that together heightens the risk of significant heart events. The emergence of fatty liver disease in some patients illustrates how obesity, insulin issues, and liver function are so closely linked, and how it may require a more integrated, approach-oriented treatment plan to fix." Overall, managing all these interconnected variables is a collective effort of healthcare practitioners, patients, and caregivers, all coming together to mitigate the long-term public health implications of diabetes (Mary et al., 2023) (Figure 10.2).

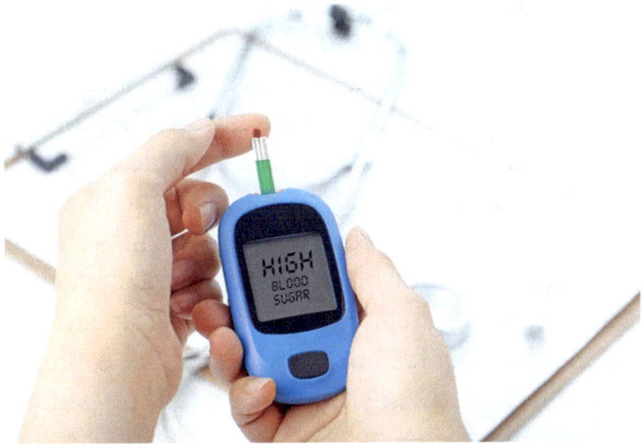

Figure 10.2. Diabetes mellitus.

Source: https://jsshospital.in/wp-content/uploads/2022/03/Blog.jpg.

Importance of Understanding Blood Glucose Levels

Diabetes management really begins with

understanding what your blood glucose level is. Elevated blood sugar is not a number, it can wreak havoc on your heart, nerves, and kidneys, so checking it frequently is quite a no-brainer. A few people have discovered that changing their eating habits and incorporating a small amount of exercise into the day can be a real lifesaver. Research, for example, shows that when patients enroll in self-help programs involving food changes and exercise, they have reductions in fasting blood glucose and even lower overall levels of cholesterol (Chinnawong et al., 2015). Providing people with the right tools and knowledge avoids ugly health issues down the line, resulting in a healthier future. It's also interesting to note that tracking blood sugar isn't just about personal care, it's about paying attention to how it relates to other health struggles. More people these days with chronic diseases—like HIV—seem to show signs of insulin resistance and inability to metabolize sugar, which only adds to the problems of diabetes management. For the most part, this places physicians in active modes of practice, especially when interventions like HAART (Wiwanitkit et al., 2007) are being done. When management of the blood sugar is integrated into overall health plans, practitioners are best able to protect against complications. In general, knowing that blood sugar is a complex issue is the most critical thing to bear in mind while creating care plans that work well in general. Also, knowing your blood sugar levels serves as a stimulus for educational programs for patients and medical professionals alike. There's plenty of research showing that just starting simple lifestyle changes—such as changing meals and exercising more—has a lot of impact. Some research even shows that self-managed diet and physical activity programs can greatly reduce fasting blood sugar levels (Chinnawong et al., 2015). When these lessons are integrated on a regular basis into day-to-day care routines, patients will be more likely to become invested in their own well-being. In most cases, blood sugar knowledge becomes the cornerstone of active diabetes management, influencing clinical decisions as well as daily practice.

10.1. Types of Diabetes Mellitus

Learning Outcome

- Type 1 diabetes;
- Type 2 diabetes;
- Gestational diabetes.

Diabetes is not one neat disease—it comes in a variety of flavors, and each has its unique features. Take Type 1, for instance: the body's immune system somehow gets out of whack and in a mistake lays siege to those insulin-making beta cells in the pancreas, so that the person essentially has no insulin and needs injections for life. And then there's Type 2, which typically shows up in older people (though rising obesity is driving it into a younger population) and happens when cells fail to get the message about insulin, say with declining insulin production over time as well. These two are quite different in how they interact with your blood sugars and your overall health, so how you manage them has to be distinct as well. Pregnancy adds another wrinkle. Gestational diabetes might strike when you least expect it—to wit, pregnancy—and while it usually resolves after delivery, it can cause real problems like glucose intolerance, macrosomia, or future risk of diabetes for both baby and mom. Secondary diabetes contributes to the confusion, arising as a complication of another disease or drug. Each has its own secrets, and cracking these secrets is the work of creating treatments that have an impact. New technology is coming in to assist as well. Machine learning is busy now sifting through enormous databases to forecast fluctuations in blood sugar and warn impending hypoglycemic attacks. Research, in most cases, shows that some models—neural networks, for example—are very sensitive to the work of forecasting these changes. This sort of forward-looking analysis gives patients an improved opportunity to customize care according to the response of the body. Overall, incorporating advanced algorithms into standard clinical practice seems a leap giant, reducing pressure on healthcare systems while improving the quality of life in diabetes mellitus patients (Adigun et al., 2022; Liu et al., 2023) (Figure 10.3).

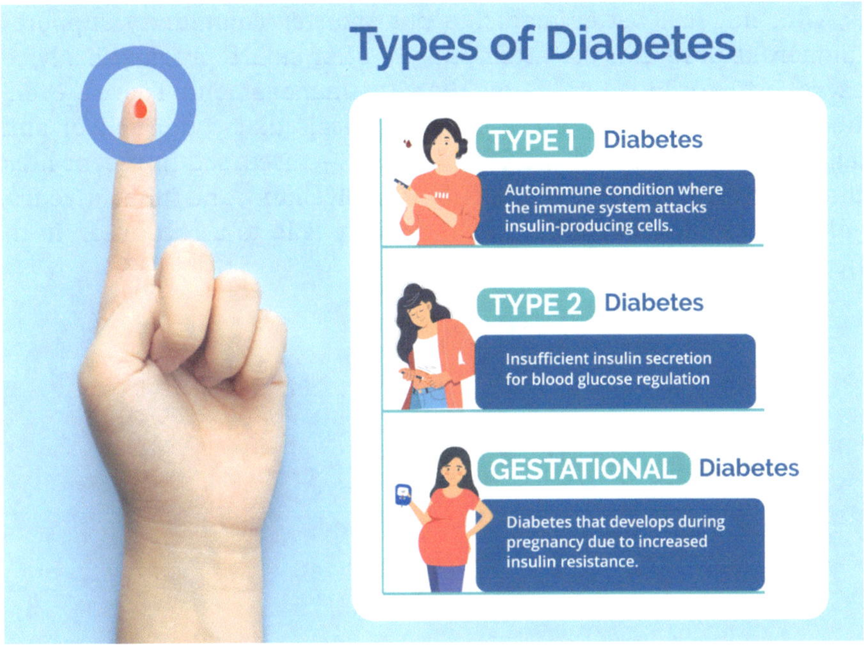

Figure 10.3. Types of diabetes mellitus.

Source: https://drshreyaendocrinologist.com/assets/img/treatment/diabetes-mellitus/diabetes-mellitus02.jpg.

10.1.1. Type 1 Diabetes

Genetics and the environment merge quite unexpectedly when dealing with Type 1 diabetes. At its core, the problem seems to start when the body targets the wrong cells within the pancreas—the ones that make insulin. If those cells are attacked, insulin is reduced, and blood sugar levels get out of hand. In most cases, scientists have found that well before any visible symptoms occur, the body is already sending out faint signals in the form of autoantibodies marking beta-cell issues. Faint biochemical signals sometimes serve as early indicators, offering a window to intervene sooner. And to make matters worse, our genetic constitution—namely, certain forms of human leukocyte antigen, for example—is significantly implicated, which implies that unravelling all those complicated factors could be the key to unlocking new treatments and prevention strategies. Keeping blood glucose levels stable in individuals with Type 1 diabetes is no picnic, mostly due to the fact that insulin treatment itself is a bit temperamental. Unlike type 2 diabetes, in which part of natural insulin still exists, type 1 individuals must rely completely on insulin derived from outside their bodies, either through multiple daily injections or insulin pumps. Such a routine is typically supplemented by devices that read blood sugar levels continuously, but despite all the technology, the problem remains. More recently, machines like the closed-loop systems have started to automate insulin dosing through real-time data, a promising spin. Yet even with these advances, the everyday anxiety and the perpetual risk of hypoglycemia reveal that managing the disease is not just about figures—it reaches body and mind. Type 1 diabetes goes far beyond the daily struggle with blood sugar; it also puts a burden on public health as a whole. The more that are diagnosed with the illness, regardless of which category, the more stressed the health care system becomes, with not just better medicine but smarter community support and education too. Nowadays, numerous programs are attempting to offer smart, pragmatic advice on everything from diet and exercise to social solutions for diabetes management. There's even more demand for natural products, including some of the phytochemicals that could deliver anti-inflammatory activity, potentially mitigating some of the complications—discussed in recent literature (Kong et al., 2020). Ultimately, synthesis of technology, public involvement, and innovative treatments seems to be the multi-disciplinary approach that might actually lead to a revolution in the treatment of this complex disease (Figure 10.4).

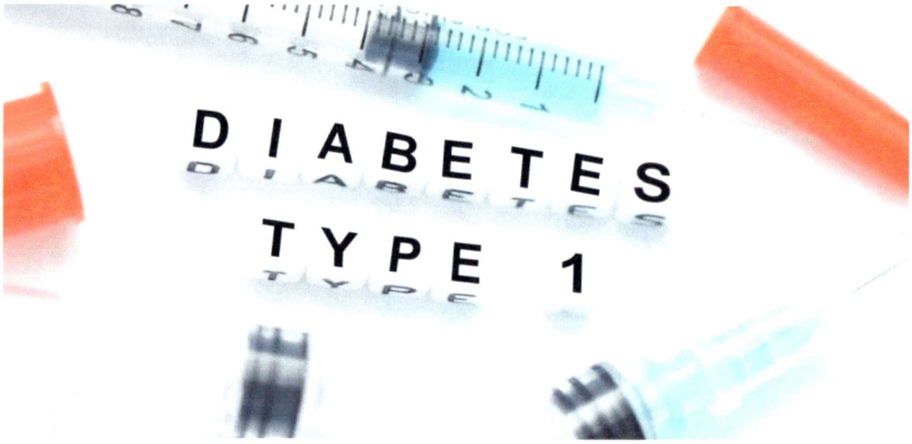

Figure 10.4. Type 1 diabetes.

Source: https://images.apollo247.in/pd-cms/cms/2023-06/Shutterstock_552738913.jpg.

10.1.2. Type 2 Diabetes

Blood sugar balancing in Type 2 diabetes is usually a tricky situation, especially where so many patients just can't seem to get their levels under control. Good self-care really stands out as a game-changer—science indicates that participants who practice good self-care have more stable sugar readings. Research was done at William Booth Hospital Polyclinic of Internal Medicine in Surabaya, which found that self-care individuals had healthier blood glucose levels. These results in general show the need to implement diabetes self-management enhancement so patients can reduce risks of complications (Dewi et al., 2023). In conclusion, building healthy self-care is integral to the whole plan for the management of T2DM. When patients try to manage their diabetes, day-to-day challenges they face can completely undermine their efforts. In fact, research among Chinese patients with uncontrolled Type 2 diabetes showed a mix of positive factors and actual challenges in controlling blood glucose levels. Yes, finding out about the risk for complications may encourage some, but mental illness has been found to suppress the creation of those lifestyle changes needed. And apart from that, possessing vague or imprecise information regarding diabetes merely adds to the misunderstanding, perpetuating myths as to what it means to be healthy. All of which clearly suggests a need for interventions addressing not only the health but also informational and psychological requirements of patients (Liu et al., 2022) – in short, giving them the information and know-how to actually get in control. Finally, controlling the many faces of Type 2 diabetes involves a mix of tough guidance and good support. Tailored lifestyle programs with added behavior change concepts can greatly improve patients' degree of participation in maintaining their blood sugar levels in check. It's also required—at least for most cases—that education on diabetes places greater emphasis on taking medication, checking blood glucose, and adjusting lifestyles when needed. These efforts, through building a support network behind healthy choices (with recurring inconsistency), can establish the ground for more effective care. Through integrating education and community support, professionals can build an organization that helps patients to better manage diabetes and ultimately reduce the complications that come with it (Dewi et al., 2023; Liu et al., 2022) (Figure 10.5).

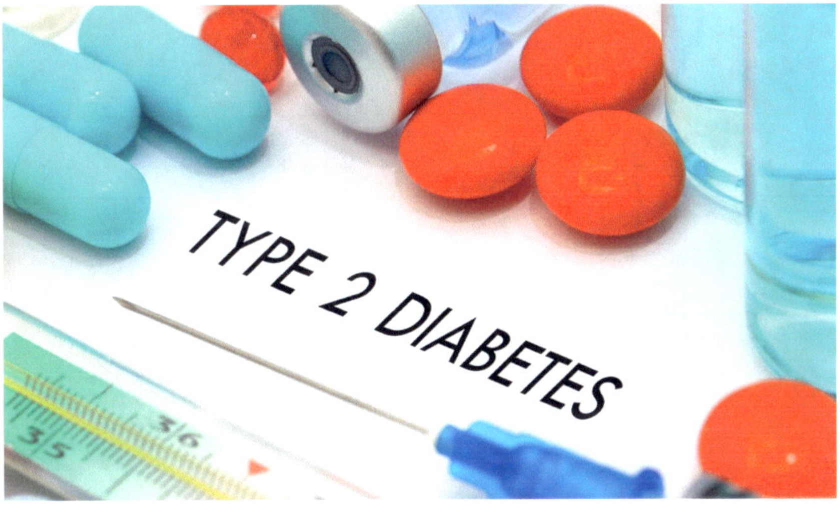

Figure 10.5. Type 2 diabetes.

Source: https://www.wshc.org/assets/Type-2-Diabetes-Nov-2022.jpg.

10.1.3. Gestational Diabetes

GDM is only harder to treat when psychological stress is a factor. Pregnant women with GDM have higher rates of depression and anxiety, and these mood shifts can wreak havoc on the balance of hormones in the body – especially in the mother and baby. Knowledge of these psychological issues is critical in most cases to allow for comprehensive, effective care. Scientists have attributed that addressing the emotional component not only maintains blood sugar stable but can also enhance the general result of pregnancy. Depression and anxiety screening and, subsequently, is thus an important measure to address GDM and take a holistic approach to maternal care (Ouyang et al., 2021). Family history, likewise, happens to play a surprisingly significant role in the way that gestational diabetes occurs. Growing evidence is that family history of diabetes (FHD) generally signifies higher risk for GDM, leading to complications like high fasting blood glucose and poor lipid profiles. According to one study, women with FHD were found to have significantly lower levels of

HDL at their third trimester and had greater glucose values at more than one location in the oral glucose tolerance test. These observations indicate that those with an inherited risk are subjected to further risks—e.g., preeclampsia and other complications in delivery—underlining the need for individualization of care based on personal risk factors, such as family history (Zhou et al., 2021). Education and small changes in lifestyle remain at the heart of successfully managing gestational diabetes. GDM women are usually advised to eat well and exercise regularly in an attempt to control their blood sugar levels. These actions not only treat the existing complication of GDM but also lower the risk of developing type 2 diabetes in the future. Specific nutrition guidance addressing the unique requirements of each pregnant woman helps to empower more informed choices, underscoring the need for self-care in the regulation of blood glucose. Additionally, being close to medical professionals offers ongoing support, monitoring, and availability of vital resources – a setting that genuinely promotes healthy pregnancies. It is still a matter of importance for clinicians and patients to be aware of GDM's long-term implications, creating advantages lasting well beyond pregnancy (Figure 10.6).

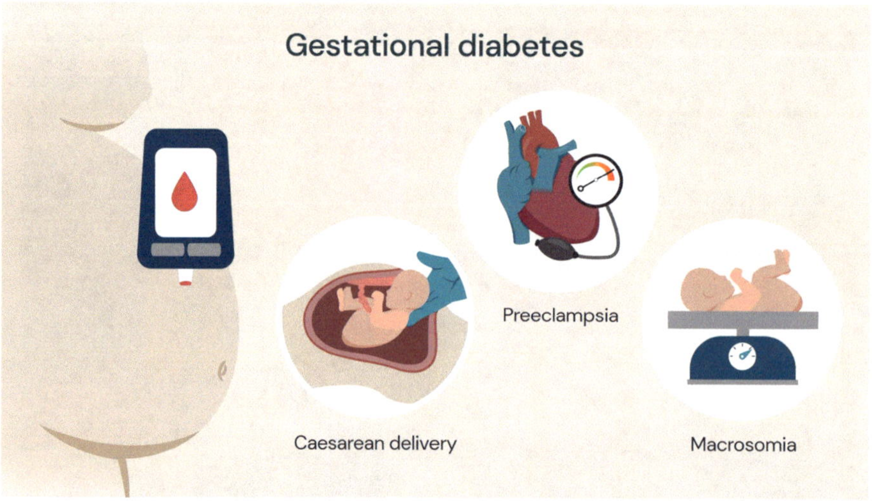

Figure 10.6. Gestational diabetes.

Source: https://guysandstthomasspecialistcare.co.uk/wp-content/uploads/2024/07/RS3716_259_RBH_Illustration_Gestational-Diabetes_v1.jpg.

Test Your Knowledge

1. What are the key differences between Type 1 and Type 2 diabetes mellitus in terms of pathophysiology?
2. How does gestational diabetes develop, and what risks does it pose for mother and child?

10.2. Blood Glucose Regulation

Learning Outcome

- Role of insulin in glucose metabolism;
- Mechanisms of blood glucose homeostasis;
- Impact of hormones on blood glucose levels.

Balanced blood sugar is the way to keep our bodies in line – particularly when diabetes enters the picture. The pancreas, through its beta cells, secretes insulin that assists in getting glucose into the cells for energy; when that doesn't happen as it should, as is so commonly the case with type 2 diabetes, managing blood sugar turns out to be a thorn in the side. Insulin resistance combined with lower insulin secretion exacerbates the issue, increasing levels in a manner that can harm the body over time. Increased blood sugar then has a tendency to lead to problems like heart disease and nerve damage, thus placing real significance on finding better management methods. There is growing recognition that multiple variables regulate blood sugar, and this has caused researchers to explore a whole range of treatment approaches – even taking a closer look at ancient Chinese medicine. Certain natural substances derived from these ancient remedies appear to offer some degree of kidney protection in diabetic patients. For the most part, by influencing the way that our body metabolizes both sugars and fats, these chemicals can potentially exert antioxidant, anti-inflammatory, and even reno-protective actions that might slow the course of the disease. In most cases, early research indicates that these strategies might be potent enough to justify further exploration into their unique molecular mechanisms (Guo-Tang et al., 2021). In other news, genetic and molecular advances have opened up new avenues for tackling blood sugar complications, particularly for gestational diabetes mellitus. One little but interesting player in this arena is microRNA – with miR-351 as a possible target. Studies have shown that by optimizing the PI3K/AKT pathway, central to insulin action and systemic glucose regulation, manipulating levels of miR-351 can reverse the insulin resistance that so commonly develops in pregnancy. In some model studies, upregulation of miR-351 seemed to increase insulin sensitivity and even dampen sugar production in the liver, implying a new strategy for controlling blood sugar (Chen et al., 2019) (Figure 10.7).

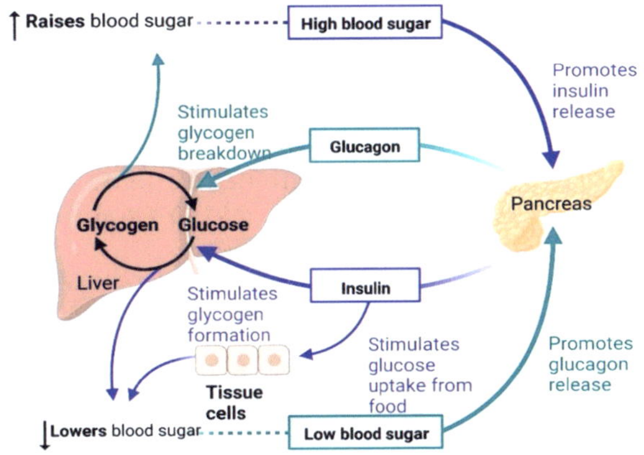

Figure 10.7. Regulation of blood glucose.

Source: https://www.researchgate.net/publication/365796836/figure/fig2/AS:11431281103421812@1669679602273/Regulation-of-blood-glucose-occurs-through-insulin-Regulation-of-blood-glucose-occurs.png.

10.2.1. Role of Insulin in Glucose Metabolism

Glucose metabolism actually hinges on insulin. When you eat carbohydrates, glucose floods into your blood, and your pancreas releases insulin rapidly—a hormone that basically tells your cells it's time to take in the sugar. Insulin then binds to receptors on cell membranes, especially on muscle and fat cells, which triggers the mobilization of transporters like GLUT4 to the cell surface. This mechanism, by which cells are able to trap glucose for energy, is necessary in order to keep blood sugar levels steady and prevent dangerous spikes. In most cases, insulin also results in further glucose to be converted to glycogen and stored in the liver and muscles so that energy can be saved for later use. It has the potential to be a mess when insulin signaling derails. In most cases, especially with Type 2 diabetes, cells start ignoring insulin's messages—a condition known as insulin resistance. Most commonly this occurs as a result of a combination of genetics and lifestyle, such as carrying extra weight or having a highly sedentary lifestyle. Insulin resistance is when cells do not grab glucose like they should, with excessive sugar lingering in the blood and typically leading to a chronic high blood sugar level. Having this persistent imbalance over time can lead to a multitude of complications, from heart and blood vessel disease to nerve damage, and even eye complications (The Society for Endocrinology Metabolism and Diabetes of South Africa, 2018). There has been some recent studies looking at approaches to enhance insulin sensitivity and keep glucose metabolism in check. For example, some studies suggest a moderate amount of red wine—specifically when combined with a Mediterranean diet—has some beneficial cardiovascular and sugar-controlling effects in Type 2 diabetes patients, although genetic factors can vary the results somewhat. In a single test, those who consumed one glass of red wine enhanced their lipid levels and blood glucose control, indicating that dietary choices, as well as other active ingredients in the wine, may help improve the body's handling of glucose. All in all, it would appear that a return to our meal patterns could be a beneficial component in the fight against insulin resistance and the numerous pitfalls of diabetic care (Gepner et al., 2015) (Figure 10.8).

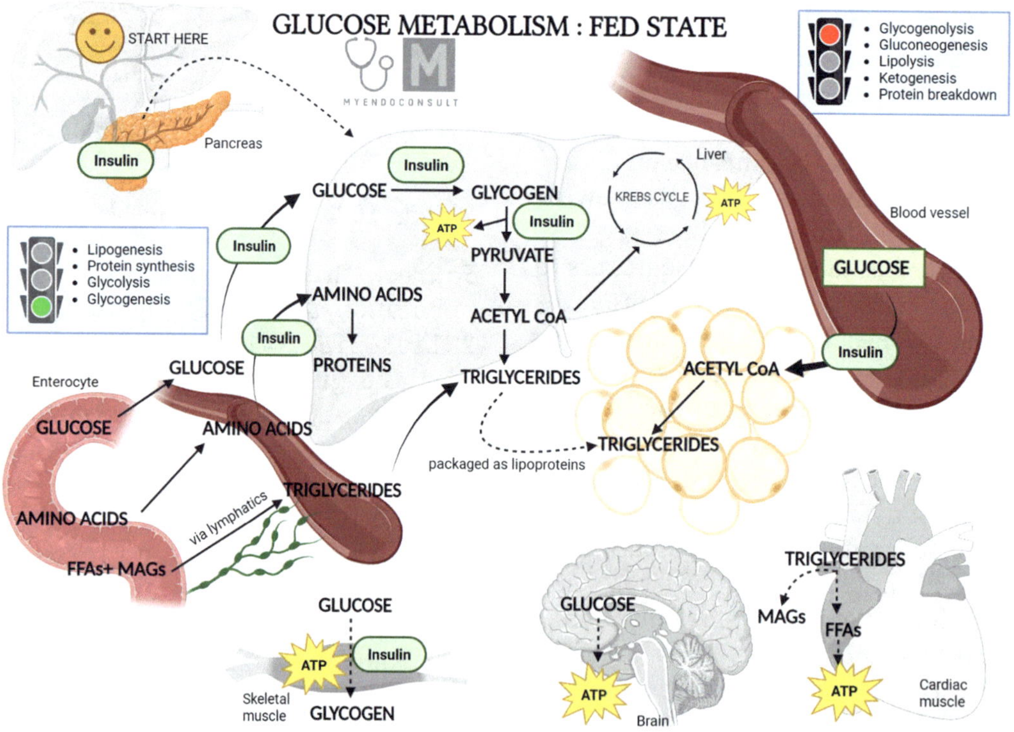

Figure 10.8. Role of insulin and glucagon in metabolism.

Source: https://endoconsult.b-cdn.net/wp-content/uploads/Glucose-Metabolism-Fed-State.png.

10.2.2. Mechanisms of Blood Glucose Homeostasis

Managing blood sugar isn't just a single-step deal—it's a layered mix of hormones and body processes all doing their part. Right in the thick of it, you've got insulin and glucagon from the pancreas, each doing its own contrary job. Insulin tells cells to grab sugar, pushing them to store it (boosting glycogenesis while slowing down new sugar production), which brings down sugar levels in the blood. On the other hand, when levels are low, glucagon calls on the liver to respond it breaks down stored glycogen and even creates sugar formation, counterbalancing the glucose around. That fine balancing act tallies a lot, in that it avoids both highs and lows of sugar occurrences that, in most cases, cause serious health complications—especially for diabetes mellitus patients (Unuofin et al., 2020). It's not just a matter of hormones, though; our cells and tissues get in on the act to control the sugar. Whether muscles and fat respond to insulin is crucial to making cells absorb and burn sugar as they're supposed to. When those tissues are less responsive—a frequent snag in type 2 diabetes—the system goes haywire, usually driving blood sugar higher. Inflammation and oxidative stress can aggravate this condition, rendering sugar control even worse. Mostly, knowledge of the balance between insulin sensitivity and blood sugar is basic to knowing diabetes, as it points to the need for treatment protocols that optimize insulin action and allow cell uptake of sugar (Sabir et al., 2019). The environment, too, has an insidious role to play here. These endocrine-disrupting chemicals have become a surprise set of villains in our sugar metabolism. Exposure to chemicals like cadmium and arsenic is associated with worse function of the critical enzymes that regulate both the creation of new sugar and breakdown of sugar. These toxins interfere with our hormonal homeostasis—altering insulin and glucagon release and provoking oxidative stress—and that interference with liver sugar metabolism too often underlies insulin resistance, the central impetus of diabetes. Meeting these environmental hurdles may well pave the way to novel strategies in prevention and management of this all-too-familiar metabolic challenge (Sabir et al., 2019; Unuofin et al., 2020) (Figure 10.9).

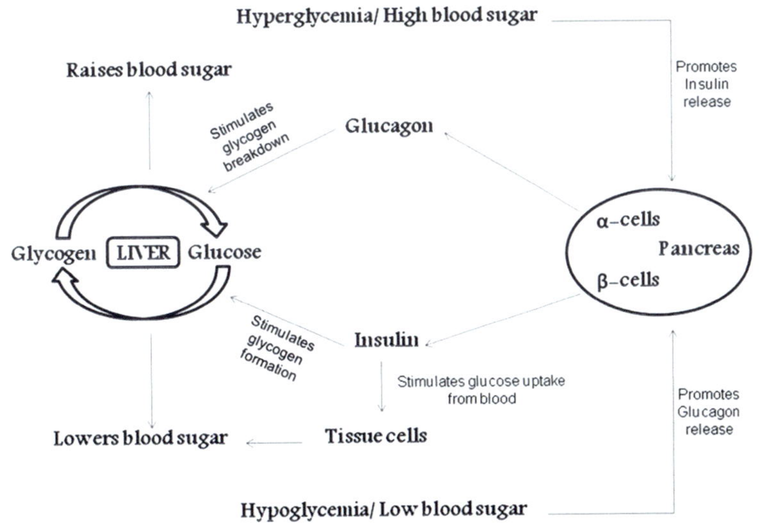

Figure 10.9. Mechanisms of blood glucose homeostasis.

Source: https://www.researchgate.net/profile/Amarchand-Murugan/publication/271711155/figure/fig1/AS:295009107628033@1447347060762/Mechanism-of-glucose-homeostasis.png.

10.2.3. Impact of Hormones on Blood Glucose Levels

Hormones actually control how our blood sugar behaves—even if at first glance it doesn't appear to. Insulin that the pancreas secretes is in the spotlight because it introduces glucose into tissues and makes it possible to reduce blood sugar. There are also hormones like glucagon and cortisol that step in during fasting or stressful times to drive sugar levels up. And when that balance gets upset, you can end up with hyperglycemia—a hugely trendy red flag in diabetes mellitus. Interesting, actually, the pull and push of those hormones not only dictating our overall metabolic tone but also guiding diabetes management; some case reports even suggest that determining that exact insulin dose can prevent disastrous complications such as long-term vascular injury and other metabolic complications (Sari et al., 2024).

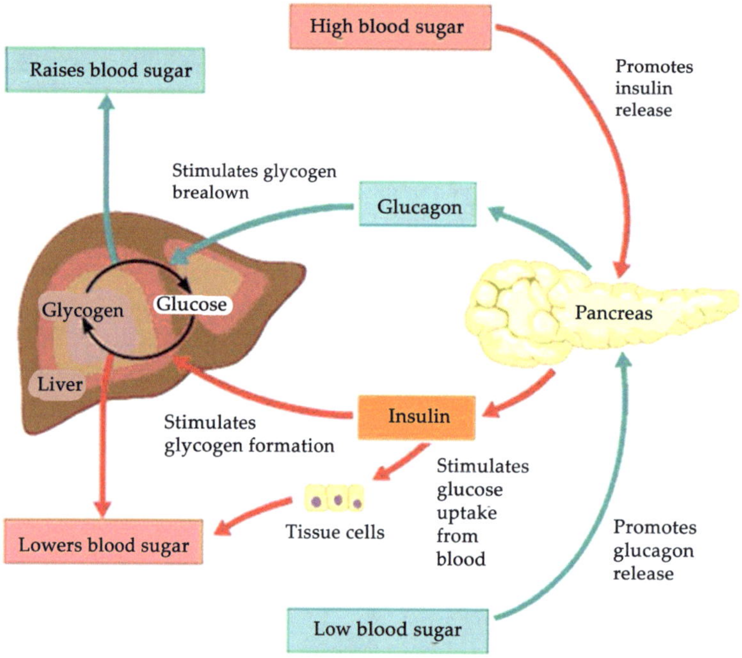

Figure 10.10. Hormonal regulation of blood glucose level.

Source: https://lh5.googleusercontent.com/NHmsljHBRKrb5JvLDouPC3gBq_e-FowMYtUJRcT4WgeY1kPXoFn26mCLZQItMFpEXHOl2EeQ2UC-Dxf1VVKsQenKLT5YdYvbM_Vr-5Rlgo_BzbydzvpMQBP0GhPEEKAX_-pe-D-V.

Thyroid hormones throw another curve into the mix. They affect our metabolic rate and seem to monkey with the efficiency with which insulin gets the job done. Abnormal thyroid function—either too much or too little—has a tendency to manipulate insulin sensitivity and obscures carbohydrate metabolism. The majority of studies seem to show that people who are having trouble with their thyroid have a more difficult time keeping their blood sugar under control. As an example, one instance of a 9-year-old girl presented with elevated blood glucose and unusual thyroid results, immediately demonstrating the degree to which thyroid hormones can play a role in diabetes control (Sari et al., 2024). Because of this, doctors find it necessary to check thyroid function when creating treatments and tracking blood sugar levels. Self-monitoring of blood glucose

(SMBG) has the effect of putting the whole story together, especially in insulin patients. When patients check their blood sugar regularly, they are more empowered to make lifestyle changes to their diet, exercise, and medication—most likely leading to better overall control. Evidence shows that a structured SMBG education program can improve compliance and reduce HbA1c values significantly, as some studies conducted in sub-Saharan Africa have shown. As patients become more aware of the effect their hormones have on their blood sugar, they actually manage their diabetes a bit more dramatically. This synergy of patient education, hormonal impact, and blood sugar regulation brings up new issues that need to be examined in greater detail in future models for the care of diabetes (Figure 10.10).

Test Your Knowledge

1. How do insulin and glucagon work together to maintain normal blood glucose levels?
2. What role does the liver play in glucose homeostasis through glycogenesis and gluconeogenesis?

10.3. Symptoms of Diabetes Mellitus

Learning Outcome

- Common symptoms of high blood glucose;
- Symptoms of low blood glucose;
- Long-term complications of uncontrolled diabetes.

Rolling blood sugars do more than just adjust a number on a lab report—they baffle an entire set of body markers that can have you with diabetes totally in the dark. You may find yourself dashing off to the bathroom much more frequently, with persistent thirst, or even struggling against relentless hunger. When blood sugar gets too high, the kidneys try to balance it out by dumping excess sugar along with water, which always leaves them dehydrated. People seek help because such symptoms are not just physical hiccups—these fill them with stress about being able to deal with everyday life and rigid diets. Most times, studies indicate that stress has the ability to exacerbate blood sugar swings, putting one on the road to a vicious cycle that both physically and mentally affects the body (Rahmad et al., 2024). High blood sugar isn't reserved for the infamous three of excessive thirst, increased urination, and hunger. It also opens the doors to tougher issues like diabetic neuropathy, where nerves actually get damaged. This sort of nerve damage would usually present itself in the form of pain, numbness, or even weakness in the legs and arms. For example, in one case study, a 58-year-old female patient who had type 2 diabetes for several years started experiencing sudden numbness and muscle weakness—a case which only turned more complicated when infection such as COVID-19 entered the scene. These episodes bring into view that prolonged high sugar levels are not just a question of transient distress but will also result in long-term nerve complications. On a larger scale, these complications are especially pertinent to highlighting the multi-faceted character of diabetes, pushing us towards caring plans that address both the body conditions as well as the psychosocial pressures (Bereda, 2024). And there is another aspect to this coin: stress and body mass index (BMI) seem to chat a great deal when diabetes symptoms are concerned. Increased stress has a tendency to prompt people toward unhealthy feeding habits, which ultimately lead to weight gain—a well-documented risk factor for type 2 diabetes. Overall, research indicates a relationship between stress, higher BMI, and even higher spikes in blood glucose levels, so managing stress is a key component in the diabetes equation. When physicians understand that emotional well-being is just as crucial to physical balance, they can formulate strategies that work for both. This form of care-whole body, mind and body-does not only help to counteract the symptoms-it also enhances overall well-being for those living with diabetes (Rahmad et al., 2024) (Figure 10.11).

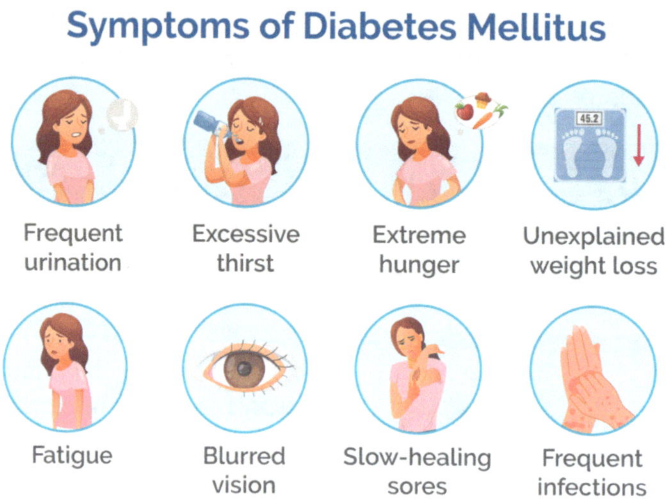

Figure 10.11. Symptoms of diabetes mellitus.

Source: https://drshreyaendocrinologist.com/assets/img/treatment/diabetes-mellitus/diabetes-mellitus03.jpg.

10.3.1. Common Symptoms of High Blood Glucose

Every now and then your body will provide you with hints that your blood sugar is increasing. You might notice yourself feeling abnormally thirsty all of a sudden, having to visit the bathroom more often, or even feeling weight loss that is a bit inexplicable. When there is excess sugar floating through your blood, your kidneys have to work double time to eliminate it, and that excess sugar goes out through your urine – causing dehydration and a never-ending need for more water. These alert signs can easily be brushed aside as normal fluctuations, but they are really subtle cues of metabolic alterations that are very important in the detection of diabetes at an early age before complications set in. If elevated blood sugar levels persistently become a norm, increasingly unusual manifestations begin to manifest. Fatigue, for example, can hit you hard – even if you're getting enough sleep – because cells are failing to absorb the sugar they need, and this robs you of enough energy. Your vision can start to blur as the lens inside your eye is displaced due to tiny fluid shifts generated by the deluge of sugar, and even the smallest cut can take seemingly forever to heal up. Impaired circulation, another consequence of long-term high glucose levels, complicates matters further by hindering healing and increasing the chances of infection (Vidya et al., 2024). In the worst-case situation, the body can enter a state known as ketoacidosis. This disease – marked by bouts of nausea, vomiting, and abdominal pain – arises when not enough insulin forces the body to break down fat too rapidly, leading it to excrete too many ketones that interfere with your body's natural balance, leading to metabolic acidosis. Overall, ketoacidosis is most common in Type 1 diabetes but can occasionally manifest in Type 2 as well under specific circumstances. Delays in seeking immediate medical attention become inevitable to prevent life-threatening complications, and early identification of them is not merely about controlling the acute symptoms—it also shows how elevated blood sugar levels over a long period of time can impair your health in the long term (Zhang et al., 2024) (Figure 10.12).

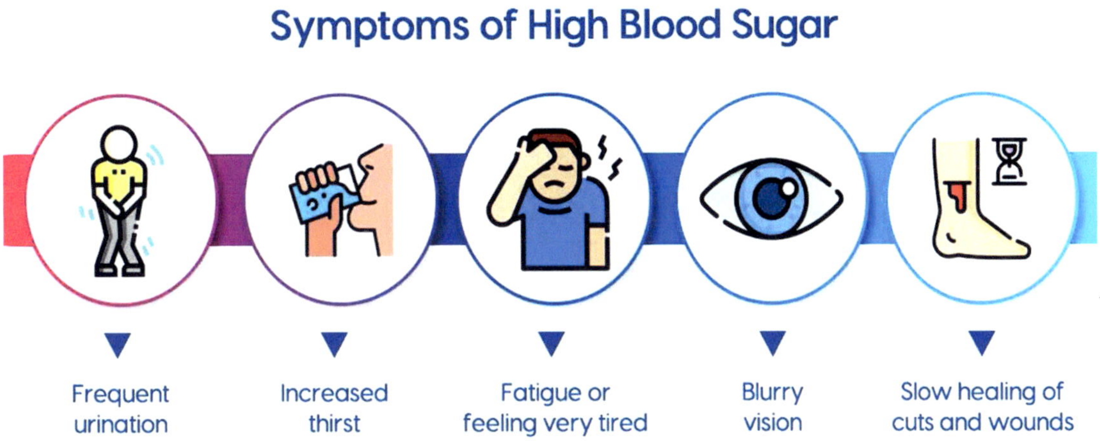

Figure 10.12. Common symptoms of high blood glucose.

Source: https://www.fitterfly.com/blog/wp-content/uploads/2024/10/Symptoms-of-High-Blood-Sugar.webp.

10.3.2. Symptoms of low blood glucose

Low blood sugar really puts a monkey wrench into things for diabetics. You'll catch yourself breaking out in a sweat, shaking, and having the sensation that your heart is racing away in your chest—like your body is trying to alert you hysterically. If these symptoms are not addressed, confusion can set in along with irritability, even leading individuals to pass out. The brain, remember, isn't operating on the fuel it needs, and that absence of fuel can muddle your mind. What's key is catching these warning signs early; if you don't, having diabetes is just that much harder. To understand hypoglycemia's impact, putting these symptoms alongside what's happening in your body offers a clearer picture. In general, when your blood sugar drops, your body secretes stress hormones like catecholamines, which tend to exacerbate feelings of anxiety and make your heart beat all the harder. It is natural that the individual confuses these symptoms with a panic attack, and such confusion aggravates the situation. Coupled with that, the brain's sensitivity to glucose level changes can cause dizziness and headaches. In most cases, if low blood sugar persists for a long time, people even stop being aware of warning signs altogether—a condition of hypoglycemia unawareness (Le et al., 2024). This serves to highlight the importance of regular monitoring of blood glucose levels. Discussion of hypoglycemia naturally leads on from that to the need for patient education. If the individual has some idea what to look out for, it is easier to take action beforehand—like understanding the taking of a glucose tablet or glass of sugar water before the situation spirals out of control. How interesting that symptoms differ from person to person, so treatment needs to be as individualized as the individual. Knowing how insulin affects you or what you eat controls your blood sugar is a balancing act of short-term fixes and long-term care in managing diabetes. And since spikes in blood sugar can have their own set of problems, vigilance is twice as important. In general terms, controlling low blood sugar is not merely a matter of handling crises—it's a component of an overall game plan for maintaining health (Sato et al., 2024) (Figure 10.13).

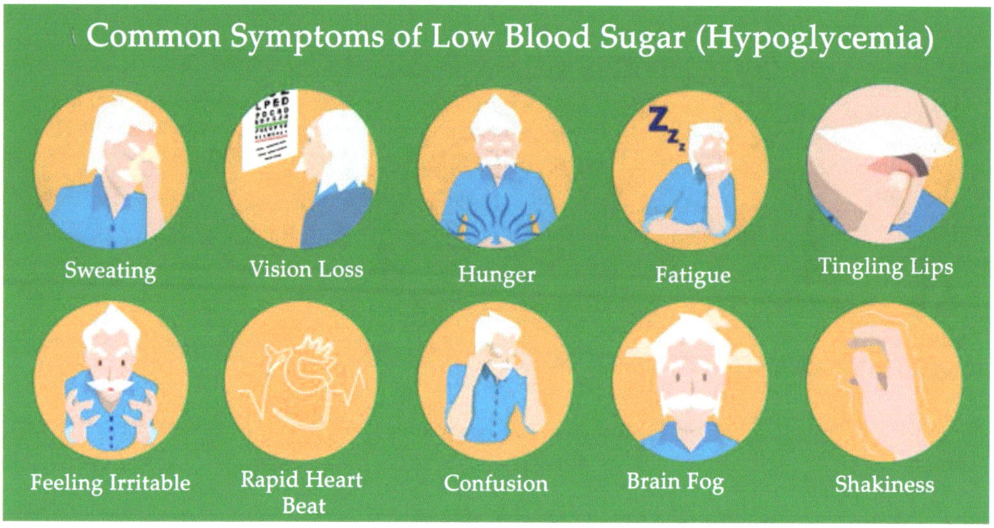

Figure 10.13. Symptoms of low blood glucose.

Source: https://www.bensnaturalhealth.com/blog/wp-content/uploads/2021/12/Low-Blood-Sugar-Symptoms-Infographic.jpg.

10.3.3. Long-Term Complications of Uncontrolled Diabetes

Uncontrolled diabetes not only brings on symptoms immediately—it creates havoc in the long run. If blood sugar stays elevated day after day, it has a tendency to bring on a combination of severe diseases. For example, constantly elevated readings can lead to heart disease, nerve damage that brings on pain and numbness in the limbs, kidney disease, and even blindness. High blood glucose levels tend to harden the arteries, increasing the chances of heart attacks or strokes. Consider this: every complication, ranging from nagging nerve damage to deteriorating circulation, is a sign that tighter control of the blood sugar level needs to exist. In most cases, glucose control just means lowering such risks, and honestly, proper education on controlling diabetes can be a long way. Diabetes, if not checked, starts wreaking havoc on almost every part of the body. One frightening thing is how the kidneys are affected. As blood sugar level rises, the filtering ability of the kidneys against poisons declines, and before you know it, there's an increase in noxious substance in the blood. Regular kidney tests—even if they're a minor hassle—may detect problems in time to delay the damage sometimes. And it's not just the kidneys; your eyes are at risk too. Diabetic retinopathy, for instance, can cause serious vision loss if it is not detected early. Daily eye exams, according to Visseren et al. (2021), are crucial in identifying and detecting such issues before they become more serious. It is not only the physical health that is affected. The ongoing battle against diabetes can also drain both a person's economic and mental strength. Chronic stress from trying to keep blood sugar in line may lead to bouts of depression or anxiety, complicating the treatment even more. In many cases, the split between physical and mental health is less clear than we'd like, which is why an approach that blends both can be so important. Add to that the enormous health care expense of treating long-term complications and you know right away why socio-economic factors come into play—affecting anything from access to care to everyday habits of health. Lifestyle modification and ongoing support, as proposed by Melanie et al. (2018), can help balance these problems. With all that in mind, addressing these disparate issues is the key to making individuals with uncontrolled diabetes have a brighter future.

Test Your Knowledge

1. What are the classic symptoms of diabetes known as the "three Ps"?
2. How do symptoms of uncontrolled hyperglycemia differ from those of hypoglycemia?

10.4. Diagnosis of Diabetes

Learning Outcome

- Blood tests for glucose levels;
- Criteria for diabetes diagnosis;
- Importance of early detection.

Diabetes detection is the key to managing it effectively and preventing further complications. One of the greatest tips at detecting it is blood sugar testing—which, essentially, tells us whether or not levels are too high, indicating insulin might be taking a break. When those numbers are high, generally speaking, it means the body's release or function of insulin isn't quite normal, which messes with metabolism in general. If not treated over time, high blood sugar continues to worsen the condition and can lead to severe complications like heart problems and kidney disease (Sameer et al., 2020). In the majority of cases, doctors combine and contrast a number of tests like fasting plasma glucose, the oral glucose tolerance test, and more and more, hemoglobin A1c level to gain an overall impression. Every test has its own contribution to knowing someone's metabolic health and helps physicians to design a treatment plan that actually fits. Receiving a closer look for diabetes diagnosis also involves checking many risk factors and personal history. Age, body mass index, family history, and daily lifestyle all play a role in how the body metabolizes sugar. For instance, an individual who has had gestational diabetes or is showing initial signs of insulin resistance may need to start screening earlier because they are usually more prone to developing type 2 diabetes (Wardani et al., 2019). Screening for symptoms such as frequent urination, thirst, and unexplained weight loss also puts information about clues. These markers, in addition to tests in the lab, help to narrow down whether it is type 1, type 2, or another type, and that—most of the time—ends up dictating the treatment that physicians provide. New technology and techniques have recently been upending the way diabetes is screened. Continuous glucose monitors and point-of-care testing now give a better overview of blood sugar oscillation, enabling repairs to be made more quickly. These innovations not only provide better management of sugar levels but also pave the way for more personalized care schemes. By alleviating the burden of traditional testing, these innovations promote patient involvement and even sometimes improve compliance with treatment. As the knowledge about the disease expands, the confluence of diagnostics and technology is set to unlock new methods for monitoring and controlling blood sugar, leading towards improved outcomes for diabetic mellitus patients (Sameer et al., 2020) (Figure 10.14).

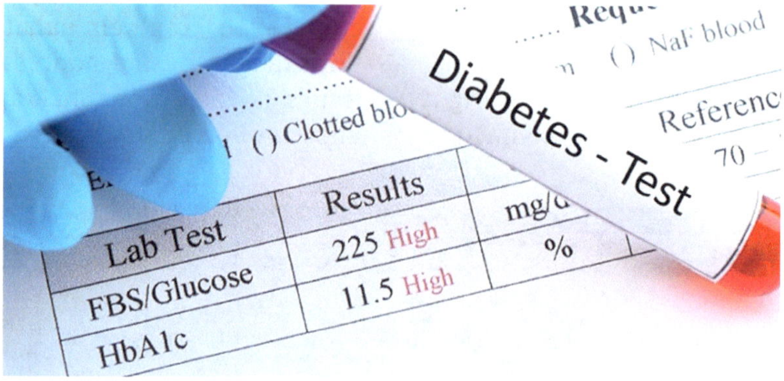

Figure 10.14. A blood sample labeled for diabetes testing rests on a laboratory report showing elevated fasting blood sugar (FBS) and HbA1c levels, indicating potential diabetes mellitus.

Source: https://lotusdiagnostic.com/wp-content/uploads/2023/03/Diabetes-Blood-Tests-1280x720-1.jpg.

10.4.1. Blood Tests for Glucose Levels

Understand blood sugar testing literally sets the stage on which to live with diabetes. One of the most important tests is the fasting plasma glucose test, usually done after an overnight fast; the test tells us if blood sugars fall within what one could call the range of normal or if they are creeping into prediabetes or diabetes on the basis of fairly accepted markers. And then there is the oral glucose tolerance test—there you drink a sweetened beverage and then your blood is drawn again—to see for yourself how your body metabolizes this burden of sugar. All of these aid in helping physicians to get a better, if sometimes partial, perspective on a person's overall condition of glycemia, which in turn helps guide the planning of treatment (Chalasani et al., 2017).

In contemporary times, the HbA1c test has finally realized its potential for tracking long-term blood sugar control. The test, by quantifying the level of sugar bound to hemoglobin for a period of roughly two to three months, yields a form of running average of blood glucose. Overall, such statistics aren't just statistics—they are indicators toward a patient's immediate management and can signal problems that could be around the corner. The tracking of this number every three months would appear to be optimal for most, whether adjustments demand changes in lifestyle, new medication, or even insulin changes. Close tracking of HbA1c avoids complications like eye and kidney disease (Chalasani et al., 2017). New technology devices have altered the landscape as well. Continuous glucose monitors now provide almost real-time feedback of day-long sugar fluctuations, a far cry from days of sporadic checking. Such monitors are more likely to pick up nuances in sugar direction that one test might miss, providing both patients and healthcare providers with an additional window when making decisions regarding diet or medications. In some cases, of course, pairing this blood glucose data with mobile health applications has actually encouraged more patient engagement in their own healthcare; technology and testing essentially colluded to redesign the playbook on how to manage diabetes (Weng et al., 2016).

10.4.2. Criteria for Diabetes Diagnosis

Diabetes is catching on fast, and that really makes creating clear, solid means of identifying it a priority. Catching individuals with pre-diabetes or full-blown diabetes is important—generally these diseases creep up stealthily undetected until problems become severe. Blood glucose levels measured by tests such as fasting plasma glucose (FPG) and the oral glucose tolerance test (OGTT) are the standard methods used to establish a baseline, enabling doctors to intervene early. Glucometer, a small device that is available for direct use by the patient, provides immediate accurate readings, which help make monitoring of the condition more convenient. For the majority, earlier diagnosis usually means better health and higher chances of disease management possibilities (Khan et al., 2019). Differences between diabetes types are not always distinct. Type 1 usually starts in childhood and basically happens when the body's own immune system strikes insulin-producing cells in the pancreas. On the other hand, type 2 diabetes strikes later, almost being coupled with lifestyle choices and sometimes with hereditary tendencies. Pre-diabetes, raising an unmistakable alarm, shows the reason why regular checks are really important for those who are at risk. Often, a timely identification of these warning signs is a chance to change lifestyle and treatment methods, offering healthcare personnel the possibility to create plans individualized for every single case (Khan et al., 2019). Scientists continue to discover other variables that could affect insulin sensitivity and how the body metabolizes sugar, further refining our diagnostic tools. While fasting glucose tests and OGTT remain the champions, latest research indicates that even simple interventions like magnesium intake could play a significant role. For instance, inadequate magnesium levels have been linked with insulin resistance, and certain studies suggest that a diet or supplement increase in magnesium will improve insulin sensitivity. These clues reflect the multifaceted relationship between diet and disease, which necessitates an integrated approach to diagnosis and therapy of diabetes (Figure 10.15).

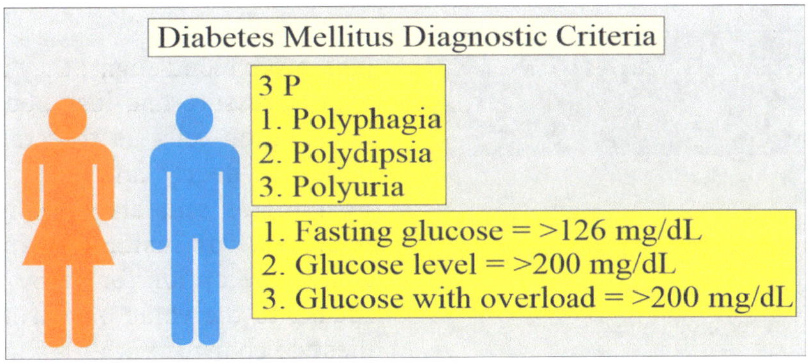

Figure 10.15. Criteria for diabetes diagnosis.

Source: https://labpedia.net/wp-content/uploads/2020/03/Diabetes-mellitus-criteria-1.jpg.

10.4.3. Importance of Early Detection

Diabetes, with its chronic high glucose levels, burdens us and our healthcare systems. Catching it early really does make a difference. When diabetes symptoms occur earlier in life instead of later, it enables us to step in sooner and lower the chances of devastating complications that come from years of elevated glucose. Several studies show that early diagnosis patients will mess up their lives somewhat and stick to treatment schedules, which usually makes them healthier in the long run. As such, when health practitioners diagnose the problem early, they are in a position to allocate their resources around more efficiently, enhancing community health and lowering total medical costs. Routine diabetes and prediabetes screenings open the door to prevent trouble before things get out of hand. Nowadays, with our improved understanding of diabetes and its many twists and turns, experts typically recommend initiating routine screening at age 45—or younger, in the event of risk factors like obesity or a family history of the disease. Routine tests like HbA1c screening demonstrate the average blood glucose over months and do a fine job of raising red flags. These focused screenings not only identify the disease earlier, but they also publicize to groups at risk why staying current with regular medical visits is important. It's often enough of an education in many instances to encourage folks to take more responsibility for their own health. There is also an extremely sincere money-saving benefit to early diagnosis, especially in communities where medical care is under siege. Diagnosing diabetes in its symptomless, silent phase can eliminate the heavy financial weight normally associated with full-blown complications such as heart disease or kidney disease. Early treatment even saves considerable amounts of direct medical expense as well as lost productivity, some studies say. For example, implementing an easy screening regimen for those who are at greatest risk will often mean not only better health returns but also a more efficient distribution of resources. Finally, finding diabetes early isn't just good medical sense—it's a good economic choice that gets lost in the big picture of both national and international health policy.

Test Your Knowledge

1. What are the standard diagnostic criteria for diabetes using fasting plasma glucose and HbA1c levels?
2. How is an oral glucose tolerance test (OGTT) used in diagnosing diabetes?

10.5. Management of Blood Glucose Levels

Learning Outcome

- Dietary recommendations for diabetics;
- Role of physical activity;
- Medication options for blood glucose control.

Glucose control is really crucial for diabetes patients, especially type 2 diabetes mellitus (T2DM). Diabetes isn't just about elevated sugar—it also carries a variety of serious threats and risks. One recent answer that has been in the limelight is the use of SGLT2 inhibitors, a new family of medicine that helps kidneys remove excess sugar. These medications don't just lower blood sugar; they also tend to lower blood pressure and lose body weight. Overall, information tells us that these drugs can be added at nearly any point in the treatment of diabetes and are usually extremely well tolerated. For instance, Dapagliflozin is now a first-line option for many physicians, which speaks to the value of pairing both drugs and lifestyle changes within an integrated diabetes regimen (Aldahash et al., 2025). Education of the patient also plays a massive role aside from putting another pill in the regime. A recent study actually took into account how well T2DM patients understand their disease—everything from what possible complications there can be to what blood glucose levels to aim for. What did they discover? A bit more than half of the patients actually had the fundamentals of diabetes control down pat, a wide knowledge gap.

Surprisingly enough, better-educated patients and younger individuals were more careful about what the correct targets are, including fasting and postprandial blood glucose levels. In all cases, these comments suggest that we need to enhance the diabetes education programs, marrying lifestyle change with complying with your medications (Alidrisi et al., 2024).

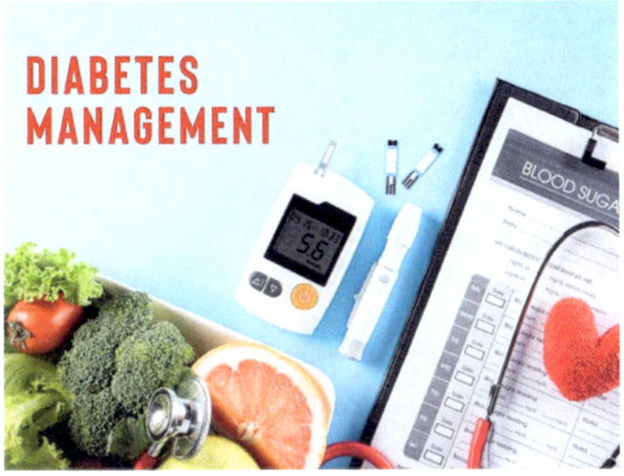

Figure 10.16. Management of blood glucose levels.

Source: https://images.onlymyhealth.com/imported/images/2022/January/25_Jan_2022/Big_dib.jpg.

Blood glucose management is not a one-size-fits-all proposition—it needs to be a plan that's every bit as flexible as it is inclusive. Continuous monitoring, accompanied by individually tailored modifications for every patient, is the key. Self-management by patients also goes a long way, especially when paired with clinician recommendations, but still much too many patients are not in the know about targets not only for glucose, but for dangers such as lipid measures and blood pressure. This lack of overall knowledge may very well undermine the effectiveness of both treatments and lifestyle advice prescribed. So, it's really crucial that healthcare professionals step in and provide wider education covering all aspects of diabetes care—ranging from the necessity of routine checks for associated complications. When patients are active in the loop, they are more likely to be responsible for their own care management, and this has a tendency to lead to better blood sugar control and general quality of life (Aldahash et al., 2025; Alidrisi et al., 2024) (Figure 10.16).

10.5.1. Dietary Recommendations for Diabetics

It starts with diet. For most who have this often-challenging disease, what and when they eat has a very real impact on the levels of blood glucose. A mix of whole grains, veggies, lean protein, and healthy fats can really do the trick to smooth out those spikes. The largest impact comes from carbohydrates, so paying attention to your carbs is a good place to start. In a few instances, simply switching over to high-fiber foods like legumes, nuts, or whole grains delays the absorption of sugar, which, by the way, keeps it level all day long. Eating at regular daily mealtimes may be simple, but it controls blood sugar levels, too. Generally speaking, these dietary habits not only regulate sugar, but they also help with overall well-being and lower the risk for complications (Mary et al., 2023). Portion sizes are also part of the calculation. Even healthy foods consumed in excess can lead to too many calories and a little extra weight that makes insulin resistance worse. A clean trick is to visualize your meal broken down into portions—perhaps half your plate is packed with non-starchy veggies, a quarter is populated with lean protein, and the remaining quarter is whole grains. A gimmick such as this, in combination with keeping a food diary or utilizing an app, can help identify patterns between your food intake and changes in blood sugar. This kind of cautious surveillance enables diabetics to make more informed choices and has a tendency to lead to more stable metabolism and healthier daily life (Livingston et al., 2020). Exercise does its job, too. Regular training improves the ability of muscles to absorb glucose and keeps weight healthy, which is crucial because excess weight might increase cardiovascular risks. It usually does not hurt for patients with diabetes to discuss things with their doctors first, to discover an exercise routine that is suitable to their capabilities and interests. A brisk walk or a small amount of cycling incorporated into daily activities can do wonders in combination with a balanced diet. Lastly, the combination of healthy food habits with exercise can increase insulin sensitivity, regulate blood glucose levels, normalize blood glucose levels, and reduce the likelihood of long-term diabetes complications (Mary et al., 2023) (Figure 10.17).

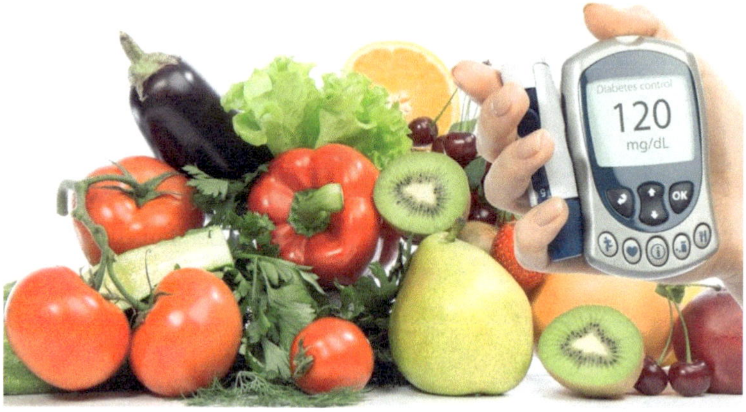

Figure 10.17. The importance of diet in managing diabetes.

Source: https://external-content.duckduckgo.com/iu/?u=https%3A%2F%2Fhealthacharya.com%2Fwp-content%2Fuploads%2F2020%2F09%2FUntitled17.jpg&f=1&nofb=1&ipt=7eb42a7542fca85977ab8cc4a930e829d792706f4eeb5ce4c9987b741bf2adb5.

10.5.2. Role of Physical Activity

Diabetes management is highly linked with daily choices, and taking up activity seems to matter more than we might first believe. Exercise in normal exercise helps the body use insulin more efficiently and handle sugars more comfortably – very significant for individuals with diabetes. Evidence usually shows that a routine built around planned exercise can lower blood glucose levels, with some lowering HbA1c, for example, one study on children subjected to social distancing had the outcome that more daily activity-controlled sugars, especially in children who started with super-high HbA1c readings (Cho et al., 2025). In short, exercise is a preventative, much being incorporated into the care routine. Structured exercise programs have a long history of being beneficial in the management of diabetes. Individualized approaches – better known as Structured Physical Exercise Programs (SPEP) – and other types of such programs have repeatedly yielded positive results in blood glucose management and general well-being. Such regimens always combine aerobics, strength training, and stretching, all combined to increase endurance and optimize the body's energy system. For the majority of people, sticking to these regimens translates into lower capillary blood sugar values and even eases other type 2 diabetes complications (Sharna et al., 2025). With an ongoing exercise routine, people not only improve their control over sugar, but also improve their overall everyday life. It is also worth noting that regular movement does well for the mind, not only the body. Regular exercise is also usually associated with less stress, a better mood, and that added bit of motivation to stick to diabetes care. A little extra confidence from success in small exercise goals can encourage someone to check blood glucose more often and stick to diet guidelines. And sometimes, being in a group exercise setting is with social support—small but critical—that helps promote healthier habits. In general, adding more movement to daily routines does not just manifest itself in improved physical outcomes but also in mental advantages, and as such, it is a major factor in the overall management of diabetes.

10.5.3. Medication options for blood glucose control

Managing blood sugar in diabetics is a delicate balance that involves a mix of methods, and a great many meds are included in the combination. There are no one-fits-all treatments – they are chosen based on the type of diabetes and individual idiosyncrasy. Take type 2 diabetes, for example; well-known oral medications like metformin, sulfonylureas, and DPP-4 inhibitors all have their own unique mechanisms. They raise your body's sensitivity to insulin, and others make your body release more of it, both lowering blood sugar levels but in different ways. The individual choice most often depends on how well a patient follows plan, other health conditions, and lifestyle habits, all of which result in treatment regimens that somehow feel especially tailored to one's own life. Keeping to a prescribed drug regimen is crucial – research overall shows that patients who remain on their drug regimen are much more likely to achieve their blood sugar targets. One study reported 92.6% of individuals who kept to the regimen had good fasting blood sugar levels, while all who did not persist with high levels. This acerbic contrast reminds us why patient education and support systems really do make a difference. It highlights why it is helpful for healthcare providers to include tailored aid, gentle reminders, and other educational information so patients feel empowered to manage their diabetes effectively (Permatasari et al., 2025). In the case of pregnant women with gestational diabetes, things are more complicated. They might not need any meds at all, but when they do, the rollercoaster of motivation at various stages of pregnancy adds a challenge. Current research brings to light that stress factors like age, income, and even pregnancy complications can affect how motivated a woman is to manage her blood sugar – that is, these motivations do not trace a smooth curve. In most cases, tailoring intervention to these very specific motivational patterns is critical. The detection and engagement with these unique drives can potentially improve both adherence and diabetes care as a whole, setting both mother and infant on an improved path (Gao et al., 2025) (Figure 10.18).

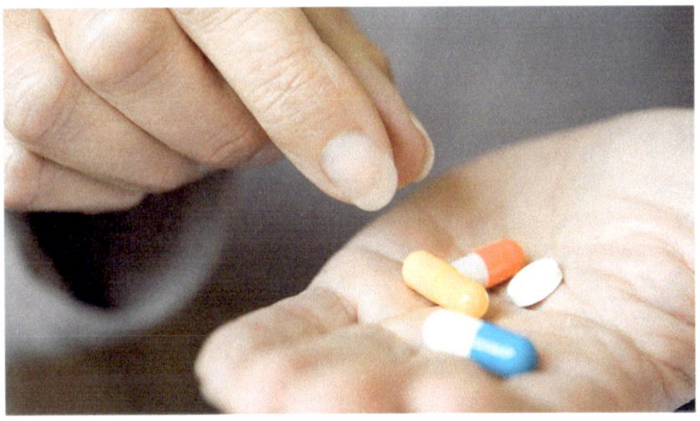

Figure 10.18. Medication options for blood glucose control.

Source: https://external-content.duckduckgo.com/iu/?u=https%3A%2F%2Fimages.everydayhealth.com%2Fimages%2Fdiabetes%2Ftype-2-diabetes%2Fcommon-medications-that-can-affect-blood-sugar-control-rm-1440x810.jpg%3Fsfvrsn%3D34041c40_0&f=1&nofb=1&ipt=29749cba39c847b25264b3d16633f723f1cc9065f0873eb3f9b1cd27611d66cc.

Test Your Knowledge

1. What lifestyle modifications are recommended for effective blood glucose control?
2. How do oral hypoglycemic agents differ from insulin therapy in managing diabetes?

10.6. Impact of Diabetes on Health

Learning Outcome

- Cardiovascular complications;
- Neuropathy and its effects;
- Kidney damage and diabetes.

Diabetes isn't just about managing blood sugar—it turns the whole body around in ways you might not expect. The disease, in which blood is too filled with sugar, wreaks havoc on a variety of systems and causes serious health issues. Studies have shown that most people who have diabetes encounter issues like cardiovascular issues, kidney failure, and even eye problems. In the majority of cases, prolonged elevation of blood sugar levels seems to set off a cascade of effects—such as a breakdown of the inner lining of blood vessels and a reduction of normal regulation of inflammation—that together clear the way for secondary complications.

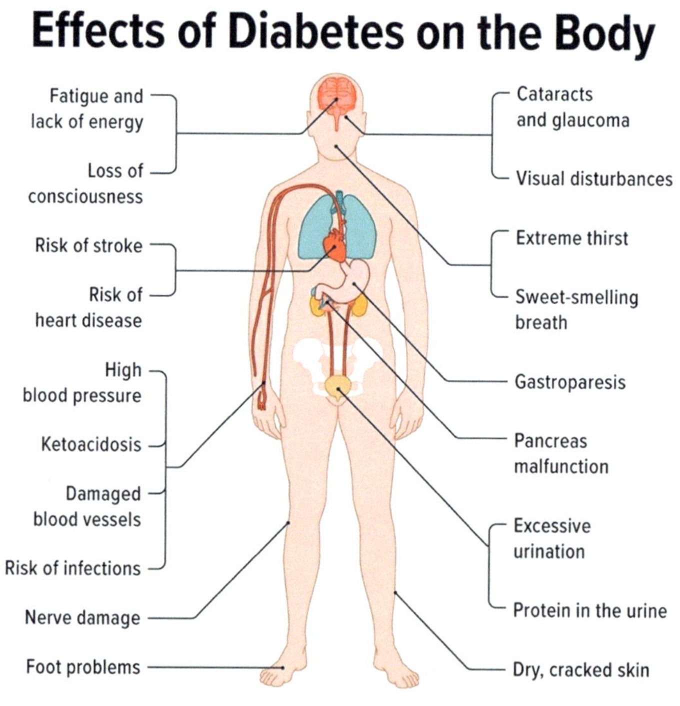

Figure 10.19. Impact of diabetes on health.

Source: https://encrypted-tbn0.gstatic.com/images?q=tbn:ANd9GcQHvAl8VumyVO3ovUHN6UALZTrIY3-66_8PeA&s.

These problems not only eat into the quality of life but also increase healthcare expenses, and the need for wise day-to-day strategies to level out sugar levels and reduce health risks is glaringly obvious. Once the problem of mental health is brought up, diabetes has baggage that people may overlook. Having the disease can initiate chronic stress, periods of anxiety, or depression—problems that really impact how an individual feels on a daily basis. The manner in which an individual feels is deeply linked to following treatment protocols, taking care of oneself, and staying active, and it can further make complicated the disease course. In general, when psychological barriers do appear, they tend to lead to inadequate coping and worsen the physical condition. As some experts have noted, integrating mental health care into standard diabetes care offers a more comprehensive view, one that works to improve outcomes more effectively and enhance quality of life. Lack of exercise also plays a significant role in this situation. Most adults today are getting less physical activity than they really need, and that inactivity greatly contributes to the aggregate burden of such diseases as diabetes. The chronic sitting lowers the body's ability to control sugar and fats to a level that it brings direct complications to diabetes control. For example, the American Heart Association says that more daily activity can decrease the chances of getting into trouble with diabetes. When activity drops, on the other hand, health takes a downturn in the wrong direction, another wave is fueled to mobilize Americans. By adding exercise to the routine in combination with diet and medication, we might be able to find a healthier and more well-rounded approach to assisting diabetes patients in moving towards a healthier state of being (Figure 10.19).

10.6.1. Cardiovascular complications

Blood sugar and cardiac health bear an unexpected relationship, especially in diabetics. High sugar can start a complex process in the body with no such instruction manual, so to speak. When blood sugar is constantly high for a long time, it seems to weaken the inner lining of blood vessels, and that weakening subsequently enables plaque to build up over time. This build-up, driven by an inflammatory response high blood sugar levels cause, accelerates the danger for nasty heart problems—and, in most cases, even mortality. It truly demonstrates the exact reason why it's so crucial to maintain blood sugar levels in check for a patient with diabetes. Getting more specific, it's discovered that diabetic heart disease has little to do with raised blood pressure or narrowing of the arteries. Others are left to cope with heart failure or blockage due to the fact that the excess glucose provides fuel to processes like oxidative stress and inflammation that silently remodel the heart's architecture. The heart operates harder, and occasionally nerve damage—the kind diabetes can cause—couples with the chaos to make it even harder for doctors to untangle. In general, managing these complications also means not only attacking high sugar but adopting a more holistic approach, i.e., changing your diet and lifestyle to protect overall cardiovascular health. There are even new treatment ideas on the horizon that might calm or even reverse these complications in the heart that occur with diabetes. Sodium butyrate is one such compound that has been found to be a potential helper by reducing inflammation and combat oxidative stress. It seems to make the body more responsive to insulin and lower the nasty fats at the same time—a double benefit as regards treating diabetes and its secondary effects on the heart. Such breakthroughs herald the coming of newer treatments that move beyond the conventional pill-and-dose routine. Blending sodium butyrate with diabetes therapy may prove revolutionary for susceptible patients, and increased research into these substances—as emphasized by Gusenbekova et al. (2023) and Sarlak et al. (2024)—remains instrumental in informing a more holistic treatment strategy tailored to the unique conditions of diabetes patients.

10.6.2. Neuropathy and Its Effects

Diabetes and nerve issues have a complex, but necessary, association—managing blood sugar levels is very important. It is unremittingly high glucose that causes nerve damage in the long term, which may express itself as loss of sensation or weak muscles. Such changes are usually realized when minor foot injuries or pressure sores go unnoticed, sometimes leading to infections or, worse still, even amputations. In all but the most exceptional situations, careless lifestyle habits serve to add fuel to the fire, heightening vulnerability in nerves even more. In general, it's clear that controlling diabetes holistically—by tracking and evening out blood sugar—strongly protects against undesirable knock-on harm to nerves.

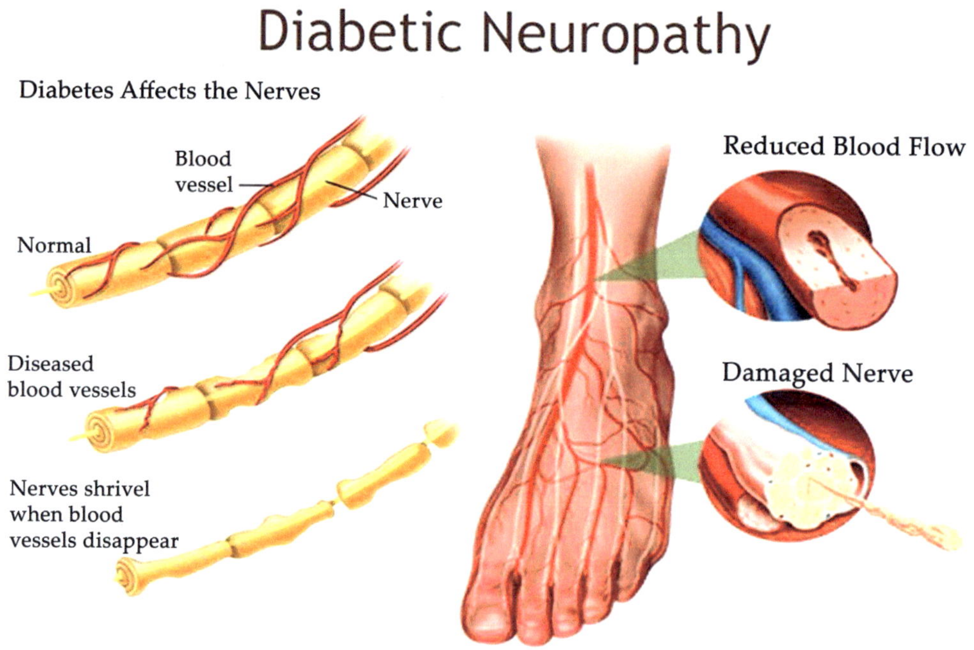

Figure 10.20. Diabetic neuropathy.

Source: https://www.bethaniyaclinic.com/media/services/Diabetic_Neuropathy_PiFV9OL.jpg.

In regard to nerve damage in type 2 diabetes (T2DM), it's usually important to track glycosylated hemoglobin (HbA1c) levels. Experiments show that variations in red blood cell (RBC) lifespan may actually interfere with HbA1c measurements; occasionally, when RBCs don't live as long as they should, high blood glucose levels become masked, fooling the actual extent of the condition. Most often, such an underestimation welcomes cardiovascular complications and other nerve problems. Others advocate the use of adjustment formulas to correct for less-than-ideal RBC lifespan, which could then give a more realistic picture of actual blood sugar control. Adjustment, in most instances, could avert both incidence and severity of diabetic nerve issues (Zhang et al., 2025). It needs to be stated here as well that hands-on therapy and lifestyle modification help towards symptom relief of neuropathy. Research—and sense—indicates that brief, focused exercises coupled with practical day-to-day adjustments will maintain blood sugar more stable and enhance nerve sensitivity. Thus, aqua therapy, for example, has been hailed as an effective one: using water-based exercise routines leveled off blood sugar and enhanced sensory response, a real benefit for T2DM patients seeking to prevent further complications. By adding regular exercise to targeted treatment, managing those unwanted neuropathic side effects becomes a more feasible one. Complete, holistic treatment that combines these methods treats not only the blood sugar rollercoaster, but the matted nerve issues that usually trail along behind diabetes (Susanti et al., 2024) (Figure 10.20).

10.6.3. Kidney Damage and Diabetes

Diabetes comes with a multitude of chronic complications that loom over everyday life and even survival itself. At the head of the list is destruction of the kidneys - informally known as diabetic nephropathy - that takes place when surplus blood sugar slowly alters kidney structure and function, decreasing their capacity to flush out waste. Increased pressure in the filtration units and extra load to those tiny nephrons can further spread the damage. In most cases, a complex interaction of body inflammation and metabolic disturbances leads to scarring that gradually impairs kidney function. As this illness goes on, patients can start developing symptoms like protein in the urine; by the end of it, things might get as severe as end-stage renal disease, where dialysis or even a transplant becomes an option. Diabetes combined with high blood pressure totally makes things tricky. Evidence suggests that people with diabetes will also struggle with high blood pressure—something else that makes kidney problems more complicated. When these conditions co-exist, it is a different ball game altogether to treat them. Hypertension strains the glomeruli, which speeds up kidney degradation and exposes them to cardiovascular disease complications. In addition, conditions like obesity and dyslipidemia are usually accompanied by them, creating a cycle that exacerbates hypertension as well as kidney injury. It is evident, then, that doctors must control blood sugar and blood pressure at the same time to keep complications at a distance (John et al., 2017). New therapies have opened up more pathways to manage kidney damage in diabetic patients. For example, recent research shows that medications like ACE inhibitors lower blood pressure as well as protect the kidneys. Likewise, certain SGLT2 inhibitors can tame blood sugar levels while reducing the risk of kidney damage. As a general rule, these developments indicate that a dual treatment approach—tackling sugar control and heart health—is the direction to take. More often than not, detecting problems early and responding promptly are the keys to slowing kidney deterioration. With such advancements, healthcare workers can significantly improve outcomes for individuals suffering from both kidney and diabetes problems (François et al., 2019).

Test Your Knowledge

1. How does poorly controlled diabetes increase the risk of cardiovascular diseases?
2. What complications can arise from long-term damage to the kidneys, eyes, and nerves in diabetes?

Summary

Diabetes management is not a one-dimensional task—it's a mix of direct care, in-the-field education, and daily habits that patients create for themselves. Studies have a tendency to discover a clear link between self-care and overall positive emotions. When patients check their blood sugar, take medications, and make everyday choices that foster good health, results improve dramatically. It appears that being interested in your own health—whatever form that takes—actually does make a difference, something that has been highlighted by several studies (Kurnia et al., 2024). There actually has been a clear shift in the monitoring of blood glucose. While those time-tested lab tests still remain very meaningful, more recent options like point-of-care testing offer patients a means of rapid checking of their numbers, at minimal inconvenience. In most cases, the findings from such portable tools match the results in the regular lab work, making home monitoring convenient as well as a tool to act in a timely fashion when there is a change, ultimately reducing the workload on our healthcare system (Yousaf et al., 2024). When you think about it in the bigger sense, maintaining blood glucose in check is more about public health. As diabetes is rising everywhere, more emphasis on personal care and innovative monitoring ideas may help alleviate some of the public health challenges that we currently experience. Sustained pressure for diabetes education will make people more at ease with managing their own blood levels, potentially even diminishing the risk of serious complications in the long term. Since research is always in favor of the implementation of both patient engagement and new technology in monitoring, it seems wise that medical professionals implement these processes as a standard practice—most times leading to better results and a better life for patients with diabetes mellitus (Kurnia et al., 2024; Yousaf et al., 2024).

Mixed signals from gut bacteria and diabetes make for a complex story. Long-standing Type 2 diabetes has a tendency to come with a decrease in helpful gut bacteria—like Bacteroides and Faecalibacter—that can raise inflammation. In the majority of cases, studies suggest that when these helpful microbes decline, it can trigger the retinoic acid-inducible gene-I-like receptors (RLR) pathway, which will trigger the nuclear factor kappa-B (NF-κB) pathway, leading to inflammation eventually (Liu et al., 2024). Therefore, gut health care can not only cure your microbial imbalance but also treat inflammatory disease, recalling the interconnectedness of metabolism and immune response in T2DM. Shared care is becoming a healthy way of approaching diabetes care, challenging patients to take things into their own hands. One research that tracked a cohort of patients from a shared care clinic found that, at around six months, individuals became more skilled at daily self-management—specifically, at monitoring blood sugar and even inspecting their own feet (Zhang et al., 2018). The majority of participants indicated a marked increase in capacity to perform daily health tasks. Also, staying in touch with healthcare providers appeared to enhance overall psychological adjustment, which is crucial when managing the emotional roller coaster of a chronic illness like diabetes. It would appear that putting patients at the center of their care truly does pay off when it comes to managing blood glucose levels. Putting together what you eat, how you feel, and your gut condition into one diabetes plan can reap long-term rewards. For example, the interplay between low levels of bacteria in the gut and impairment in glucose control proves that what you eat can affect your gut environment—and that in turn affects your blood sugars (Liu et al., 2024). Besides that, shared care plans improve individual self-management, in addition to establishing a teamwork-based support system among healthcare professionals (Zhang et al., 2018). Lastly, this overall process makes it easier to have customized plans that address physical as well as emotional problems, ultimately leading to more predictable blood sugar control and improved general well-being.

KEY TERMS FROM THIS CHAPTER

Blood glucose
Continuous glucose monitoring (CGM)
Diabetic neuropathy
Fasting blood glucose (FBG)
Glycated hemoglobin (HbA1c)
Hypoglycemia
Insulin
Insulin resistance
Oral glucose tolerance test (OGTT)
Carbohydrate counting
Diabetic ketoacidosis (DKA)
Diabetic retinopathy
Gestational diabetes
Hyperglycemia
Hypoglycemic agents
Insulin pump
Non-insulin dependent diabetes
Pre-diabetes

Critical Thinking Questions

1. **Which of the following is the most common cause of hyperglycemia in patients?**
   a. Exercise
   b. Insulin deficiency
   c. Low-carbohydrate diet
   d. Vitamin C deficiency
2. **Which of the following blood glucose levels is considered the diagnostic threshold for diabetes mellitus during a fasting plasma glucose test?**
   a. 100 mg/dL
   b. 126 mg/dL
   c. 140 mg/dL
   d. 180 mg/dL
3. **What is the primary function of insulin in the body?**
   a. Increase blood glucose levels
   b. Stimulate the breakdown of fat
   c. Facilitate the uptake of glucose into cells
   d. Increase urination
4. **Which type of diabetes is most commonly diagnosed in childhood and requires insulin therapy for management?**
   a. Type 1 diabetes
   b. Type 2 diabetes
   c. Gestational diabetes
   d. Latent autoimmune diabetes in adults (LADA)
5. **Which of the following is a common symptom of untreated diabetes mellitus?**
   a. Weight gain
   b. Frequent urination and excessive thirst
   c. Decreased appetite
   d. Severe fatigue

Answers to Critical Thinking Questions

1. (b); 2. (b); 3. (c); 4. (a); 5. (b)

Short Answer Questions

1. What is the normal range for fasting blood glucose levels in adults?
2. Define diabetes mellitus and differentiate between Type 1 and Type 2 diabetes.
3. What is the role of insulin in regulating blood glucose levels?
4. What is the glycemic index, and how does it relate to blood sugar control in diabetes?
5. How does the oral glucose tolerance test (OGTT) work, and what does it diagnose?

References

1. Adigun, O., Okikiola, F., Yekini, N., & Babatunde, R. (2022). Classification of diabetes types using machine learning. *International Journal of Advanced Computer Science and Applications*. https://www.semanticscholar.org/paper/0c73fa0df54c129f681eacf874581d8f3064a9e6 (accessed on 1st July 2025).

2. Aga Syed Sameer, Banday, M. Z., & Nissar, S. (2020). Pathophysiology of diabetes: An overview. *Avicenna Journal of Medicine, 10*, 174–174. https://doi.org/10.4103/ajm.ajm_53_20 (accessed on 1st July 2025).

3. Aktas, G., & Taslamacıoğlu Duman, T. (2024). Current usage of long-acting insulin analogs in patients with type 2 diabetes mellitus. *Expert Review of Endocrinology & Metabolism, 19*, 155–161. https://www.semanticscholar.org/paper/08385950ba56dd07f284dcd0de64c0840dea1de0 (accessed on 1st July 2025).

4. Aldahash, R., Aldossari, K., Aljohanni, N., Alsabaan, F., Alzahrani, W., Alwabel, A., & Alhendi, A. M. N. (2025). Type 2 diabetes mellitus in Saudi Arabia: Prevalence, risk factors, and management strategies: A review. *Endocrine, Metabolic & Immune Disorders Drug Targets*. https://www.semanticscholar.org/paper/78f9b554565be361c83d31fe3538203cfd2a4f89 (accessed on 1st July 2025).

5. Alidrisi, H., Hammoud, M. M., Abd Ali, H. Y., & Radhi, M. E. (2024). Type 2 diabetes mellitus patients' knowledge about disease complications and management targets for glucose, lipids, blood pressure, and body weight. *Cureus, 16*. https://www.semanticscholar.org/paper/33b1cd28ccea2925ebfa77ed58dd2c739f11c4e9 (accessed on 1st July 2025).

6. Bereda, G. (2024). COVID-19 is associated with high blood glucose levels: Diabetic neuropathy during the SARS-CoV-2 pandemic: A case report. *Annals of Medicine and Surgery, 86*, 7318–7321. https://www.semanticscholar.org/paper/29c12ac36f17b113a423fbb838ad373360e63c90 (accessed on 1st July 2025).

7. Chalasani, N., Younossi, Z. M., Lavine, J. E., Charlton, M., Cusi, K., Rinella, M. E., Harrison, S. A., et al. (2017). The diagnosis and management of nonalcoholic fatty liver disease: Practice guidance from the American Association for the Study of Liver Diseases. *Hepatology, 67*, 328–357. https://doi.org/10.1002/hep.29367 (accessed on 1st July 2025).

8. Chen, S., Liu, X.-N., & Peng, Y. (2019). MicroRNA-351 eases insulin resistance and liver gluconeogenesis via the PI3K/AKT pathway by inhibiting FLOT2 in mice of gestational diabetes mellitus. *Journal of Cellular and Molecular Medicine, 23*, 5895–5906. https://doi.org/10.1111/jcmm.14079 (accessed on 1st July 2025).

9. Chinnawong, T., Kritpracha, C., & Pamungkas, R. A. (2015). The effect of dietary and exercise self-management support program on dietary behavior, exercise behavior, and clinical outcomes in Muslim patients with poorly controlled type 2 DM in a community setting in Indonesia. https://media.neliti.com/media/publications/154630-EN-the-effect-of-dietary-and-exercise-self.pdf (accessed on 1st July 2025).

10. Cho, M. H., Shim, Y., & Lee, H. (2025). Impact of COVID-19 lockdown on blood glucose levels in pediatric patients with type 1 diabetes mellitus. *Annals of Pediatric Endocrinology & Metabolism, 30*, 25–30. https://www.semanticscholar.org/paper/140257d4798f3d7e70b7d420ff7fe3403f495b22 (accessed on 1st July 2025).

11. Davies, M. J., D'Alessio, D. A., Fradkin, J., Kernan, W. N., Mathieu, C., Mingrone, G., Rossing, P., et al. (2018). Management of hyperglycemia in type 2 diabetes, 2018. A consensus report by the American Diabetes Association (ADA) and the European Association for the Study of Diabetes (EASD). *Diabetes Care, 41*, 2669–2701. https://doi.org/10.2337/dci18-0033 (accessed on 1st July 2025).

12. Dewi, E., Widari, N. P., Nursalam, N., Mahmudah, M., Sari, E. Y., & Susiana, Y. F. N. (2023). The relationship between diabetes self-care management and blood glucose level among type 2 diabetes mellitus patients. *International Journal of Public Health Science (IJPHS)*. https://www.semanticscholar.org/paper/5f3c7aef1c4cc49222ca8cea0827fe7b7412e3b3 (accessed on 1st July 2025).

13. Fiedorova, K., Augustýnek, M., Kubíček, J., Kudrna, P., & Bibbo, D. (2022). Review of present method of glucose from human blood and body fluids assessment. *Biosensors and Bioelectronics, 211*, 114348–114348. https://doi.org/10.1016/j.bios.2022.114348 (accessed on 1st July 2025).

14. Gao, Y., Liu, J., Zhu, Q., Zhang, Z., Dai, Q., Guo, Y., Zhang, W., et al. (2025). Blood glucose management protection motivation trajectory and its associated factors in pregnant women with gestational diabetes mellitus: A longitudinal study. *Patient Preference and Adherence, 19*, 809–821. https://www.semanticscholar.org/paper/779f14d04bb47323b688eff05a2b76c99f57fa13 (accessed on 1st July 2025).

15. Gepner, Y., Golan, R., Harman-Boehm, I., Henkin, Y., Schwarzfuchs, D., Shelef, I., Durst, R., et al. (2015). Effects of initiating moderate alcohol intake on cardiometabolic risk in adults with type 2 diabetes: A 2-year randomized, controlled trial. *Annals of Internal Medicine, 163*(8), 569–579. https://www.semanticscholar.org/paper/43670e077e598b6ec5450bdaa40b8ff1f88ea3f2 (accessed on 1st July 2025).

16. Gusenbekova, D., & Ostroumova, O. D. (2023). Cardiovascular risk and self-monitoring of blood glucose in patients with diabetes mellitus. *Clinical Review for General Practice*. https://www.semanticscholar.org/paper/a0b0662b98570b99f8cc23e84a1e924bc7e8854a (accessed on 1st July 2025).

17. Khan, R., Chua, Z. J. Y., Tan, J., Yang, Y., Liao, Z., & Zhao, Y. (2019). From pre-diabetes to diabetes: Diagnosis, treatments and translational research. *Medicina, 55*, 546–546. https://doi.org/10.3390/medicina55090546 (accessed on 1st July 2025).

18. Kong, M., Xie, K., Lv, M., Li, J., Yao, J., Yan, K., Wu, X., et al. (2020). Anti-inflammatory phytochemicals for the treatment of diabetes and its complications: Lessons learned and future promise. *Biomedicine & Pharmacotherapy, 133*, 110975–110975. https://doi.org/10.1016/j.biopha.2020.110975 (accessed on 1st July 2025).

19. Kurnia, E., Desi, K., Trijayanti, N., Idris, R., & Rahmat, R., et al. (2024). Self-management and life quality of diabetes mellitus patients: A literature review. *DIAGNOSA: Journal Ilma Kesehatan dan Keperawatan*. https://www.semanticscholar.org/paper/e5ff3c8d3848a285297b93d200dab337f0f6bcc4 (accessed on 1st July 2025).

20. Le, Y., Zhang, J., Hong, T., & Yang, J. (2024). Coexistence of type 2 diabetes mellitus, arginine vasopressin deficiency, and Marfan syndrome: A case report. *Journal of Diabetes Investigation, 15*, 964–967. https://www.semanticscholar.org/paper/4c8e136a359aba8cbc83213ec5eef6ff508e6914 (accessed on 1st July 2025).

21. Liu, K., Li, L., Ma, Y., Jiang, J., Liu, Z., Ye, Z., Liu, S., et al. (2023). Machine learning models for blood glucose level prediction in patients with diabetes mellitus: Systematic review and network meta-analysis. *JMIR Medical Informatics, 11*. https://www.semanticscholar.org/paper/f0217cb9f5d065fcdc50ec67ba5931f1441c074c (accessed on 1st July 2025).

22. Liu, N., Yan, X., Lv, B., Wu, Y., Hu, X., Zheng, C., Tao, S., et al. (2024). A study on the association between gut microbiota, inflammation, and type 2 diabetes. *Applied Microbiology and Biotechnology, 108*. https://www.semanticscholar.org/paper/8cc76f293efb51e04fe79e8526a60db565e28f03 (accessed on 1st July 2025).

23. Liu, Y., Jiang, J., You, W., Gong, D., Ma, X., Wu, M., & Li, F. (2022). Exploring facilitators and barriers to self-management engagement of Chinese people with type 2 diabetes mellitus and poor blood glucose control: A descriptive qualitative study. *BMC Endocrine Disorders, 22*. https://www.semanticscholar.org/paper/d560260329842ca2d2496beb55c0f904c1781771 (accessed on 1st July 2025).

24. Livingston, G., Huntley, J., Sommerlad, A., Ames, D., Ballard, C., Banerjee, S., Brayne, C., et al. (2020). Dementia prevention, intervention, and care: 2020 report of the Lancet Commission. *The Lancet, 396*, 413–446. https://doi.org/10.1016/s0140-6736(20)30367-6 (accessed on 1st July 2025).

25. Lobelo, F., Young, D. R., Sallis, R. E., Garber, M. D., Billinger, S. A., Duperly, J., Hutber, A., et al. (2018). Routine assessment and promotion of physical activity in healthcare settings: A scientific statement from the American Heart Association. *Circulation, 137*. https://doi.org/10.1161/cir.0000000000000559 (accessed on 1st July 2025).

26. Mach, F., Baigent, C., Catapano, A. L., Koskinas, K. C., Casula, M., Badimón, L., Chapman, M. J., et al. (2019). 2019 ESC/EAS guidelines for the management of dyslipidemias: Lipid modification to reduce cardiovascular risk. *European Heart Journal, 41*, 111–188. https://doi.org/10.1093/eurheartj/ehz455 (accessed on 1st July 2025).

27. Madhu, S. V., Chawla, R., Makkar, B. M., Ghosh, S., Saboo, B., & Kalra, S. (2020). RSSDI-ESI clinical practice recommendations for the management of type 2 diabetes mellitus 2020. *Indian Journal of Endocrinology and Metabolism, 24*, 1–1. https://doi.org/10.4103/ijem.ijem_225_20 (accessed on 1st July 2025).

28. Muhali, S. S., Muhali, F. S., Mfinanga, S., Sadiq, A. M., Marandu, A. A., Kyala, N. J., Said, F. H., et al. (2024). Impact of self-monitoring blood glucose on glycemic control among insulin-treated patients with diabetes mellitus in Northeastern Tanzania: A randomized controlled trial. *Journal of Diabetes Research, 2024*. https://www.semanticscholar.org/paper/a168b90b8cd130422aadbe105aa15031c4e89d64 (accessed on 1st July 2025).

29. Ouyang, H., Chen, B., Al-Mureish, A., Li, L., & Wu, N. (2021). Associations between gestational diabetes and anxiety or depression: A systematic review. *Journal of Diabetes Research, 2021*, 1–10. https://doi.org/10.1155/2021/9959779 (accessed on 1st July 2025).

30. Park, J. H., Moon, J. H., Kim, H. J., Kong, M. H., & Oh, Y. H. (2020). Sedentary lifestyle: Overview of updated evidence of potential health risks. *Korean Journal of Family Medicine, 41*, 365–373. https://doi.org/10.4082/kjfm.20.0165 (accessed on 1st July 2025).

31. Permatasari, P., & Sutanto, H. (2025). The relationship between adherence to oral antidiabetic medication and fasting blood glucose control in type 2 diabetes mellitus patients at Palmerah District Health Center in 2024. *International Journal of Social Health*. https://

www.semanticscholar.org/paper/c4891a2ddfbef0708a4d1a4268826b13e1f7b903 (accessed on 1st July 2025).

32. Petrie, J. R., Guzik, T. J., & Touyz, R. M. (2017). Diabetes, hypertension, and cardiovascular disease: Clinical insights and vascular mechanisms. *Canadian Journal of Cardiology, 34*, 575–584. https://doi.org/10.1016/j.cjca.2017.12.005 (accessed on 1st July 2025).
33. Rahmad, M. N. R., Pratiwi, P., & Suryandari, D. (2024). Relationship between stress levels and body mass index on blood sugar levels in type 2 diabetes mellitus patients in the working area of Puskesmas Gemarang. *Blambangan Journal of Nursing and Health Sciences (BJNHS)*. https://www.semanticscholar.org/paper/109be0e401e75952b325b81303f7b003a14e9997 (accessed on 1st July 2025).
34. Rinella, M. E., Neuschwander-Tetri, B. A., Siddiqui, M. S., Abdelmalek, M. F., Caldwell, S. H., Barb, D., Kleiner, D. E., et al. (2023). AASLD practice guidance on the clinical assessment and management of nonalcoholic fatty liver disease. *Hepatology, 77*, 1797–1835. https://doi.org/10.1097/hep.0000000000000323 (accessed on 1st July 2025).
35. Sabir, S., Akash, M. S. H., Fiayyaz, F., Saleem, U., Mehmood, M. H., & Rehman, K. (2019). Role of cadmium and arsenic as endocrine disruptors in the metabolism of carbohydrates: Inserting the association into perspectives. *Biomedicine & Pharmacotherapy, 114*, 108802–108802. https://doi.org/10.1016/j.biopha.2019.108802 (accessed on 1st July 2025).
36. Sari, N. K. P., Mulyantari, N., Herawati, S., & Lestari, A. A. W. (2024). A-9-years-old female with diabetes mellitus type 1 with hyperthyroidism. *Indonesian Journal of Clinical Pathology and Medical Laboratory*. https://www.semanticscholar.org/paper/35ab8644c055ee720ee4fdcfe5420e7ccdc191c5 (accessed on 1st July 2025).
37. Sarlak, Z., Naderi, N., Amidi, B., & Ghorbanzadeh, V. (2024). Sodium butyrate, a gut microbiota derived metabolite, in type 2 diabetes mellitus and cardiovascular disease: A review. *Cardiovascular & Hematological Agents in Medicinal Chemistry*. https://www.semanticscholar.org/paper/c7035e183533e295569adec0c5b26f2728c0aa45 (accessed on 1st July 2025).
38. Sato, M., Otsuki, M., Mori, T., Yanagida, J., Yamamoto, T., & Nakagami, T. (2024). Remission of insulin-dependent diabetes mellitus in multiple endocrine neoplasia type 2A after adrenalectomy. *JCEM Case Reports, 3*. https://www.semanticscholar.org/paper/9c22b78397dd2a1f01cee3ff93af30975f346e7b (accessed on 1st July 2025).
39. Sharna, S. Y., Hossain, K. M. A., Kabir, F., Hossain, M. Z., Jahan, S., Rahman, E., Agarwal, S., et al. (2025). Multicenter randomized controlled trial protocol comparing structured physical exercise programmed (SPEP) and medication versus conventional care for glycemic control in type 2 diabetes mellitus. *BMJ Open Sport & Exercise Medicine, 11*. https://www.semanticscholar.org/paper/8d450e070d4b70854dbc0f79ee4b2f4cadf95549 (accessed on 1st July 2025).
40. Susanti, S., & Bistara, D. N. (2024). The impact of foot solus per aqua (SPA) on blood sugar levels and paresthesia sensitivity in patients with diabetes mellitus type 2. *Journal Keperawatan Respite Yogyakarta*. https://www.semanticscholar.org/paper/9d13de254a4cb4bbecf89fec9a4f67f4538f43a9 (accessed on 1st July 2025).
41. Tang, G. Y., Li, S., Zhang, C., Chen, H., Wang, N., & Feng, Y. (2021). Clinical efficacies, underlying mechanisms and molecular targets of Chinese medicines for diabetic nephropathy treatment and management. *Acta Pharmaceutica Sinica B, 11*, 2749–2767. https://doi.org/10.1016/j.apsb.2020.12.020 (accessed on 1st July 2025).

42. The Society for Endocrinology Metabolism and Diabetes of South Africa. (2018). Chapter 11: The approach to achieving glycemic control. *South African Family Practice*. https://www.semanticscholar.org/paper/d84cca25f0a3f925d3c428c6547498194a9d23b6 (accessed on 1st July 2025).

43. Toprak, Ö., Kurt, H., Sarı, Y., Şarkış, C., Us, H., & Kırık, A. (2017). Magnesium replacement improves the metabolic profile in obese and pre-diabetic patients with mild-to-moderate chronic kidney disease: A 3-month, randomized, double-blind, placebo-controlled study. *Kidney & Blood Pressure Research, 42*, 33–42. https://doi.org/10.1159/000468530 (accessed on 1st July 2025).

44. Unuofin, J. O., & Lebelo, S. L. (2020). Antioxidant effects and mechanisms of medicinal plants and their bioactive compounds for the prevention and treatment of type 2 diabetes: An updated review. *Oxidative Medicine and Cellular Longevity, 2020*, 1–36. https://doi.org/10.1155/2020/1356893 (accessed on 1st July 2025).

45. Vidya, S. G. V., Veda, S. M., & Suchethakumari, N. (2024). Evaluation of lipid profile and uric acid level in type II diabetes mellitus. *Research Journal of Biotechnology*. https://www.semanticscholar.org/paper/eee2deca188733954fe570637f76e7048354601a (accessed on 1st July 2025).

46. Visseren, F. L. J., Mach, F., Smulders, Y. M., Carballo, D., Koskinas, K. C., Bäck, M., Bénétos, A., et al. (2021). 2021 ESC guidelines on cardiovascular disease prevention in clinical practice. *European Heart Journal, 42*, 3227–3337. https://doi.org/10.1093/eurheartj/ehab484 (accessed on 1st July 2025).

47. Vos, T., Abajobir, A. A., Abate, K. H., Abbafati, C., Abbas, K., Abd-Allah, F., Abdulkader, R. S., et al. (2017). Global, regional, and national incidence, prevalence, and years lived with disability for 328 diseases and injuries for 195 countries, 1990–2016: A systematic analysis for the Global Burden of Disease Study 2016. *The Lancet, 390*, 1211–1259. https://doi.org/10.1016/s0140-6736(17)32154-2 (accessed on 1st July 2025).

48. Wardani, E. M., Zahroh, C., & Ainiyah, N. (2019). Diabetic foot spa implementation in early neuropathy diagnosis based on blood glucose levels, foot sensitivity and the ankle brachial index in patients with diabetes mellitus. *Journal NERS, 14*, 106–110. https://doi.org/10.20473/jn.v14i1.9950 (accessed on 1st July 2025).

49. Weng, J., Ji, L., Jia, W., Lu, J., Zhou, Z., Zou, D., Zhu, D., et al. (2016). Standards of care for type 2 diabetes in China. *Diabetes/Metabolism Research and Reviews, 32*, 442–458. https://doi.org/10.1002/dmrr.2827 (accessed on 1st July 2025).

50. Wiwanitkit, V. (2007). Primary care for diabetes in HIV-infected patients. https://core.ac.uk/download/pdf/86947.pdf (accessed on 1st July 2025).

51. Yin, X., Sui, Y., Chu, Z., Han, S., Ge, X., Liu, T., Zeng, F., et al. (2024). Regulation of intestinal flora by *Suaeda salsa* extract ameliorates hyperglycemia in a mouse model of type 2 diabetes mellitus. *Frontiers in Nutrition, 11*. https://www.semanticscholar.org/paper/188ebafb941d4fcdd609e543dbddef0f7a9706f3 (accessed on 1st July 2025).

52. Yousaf, Z., Ahmed, S., Raza, M., Rashid, S., Qasim, S., & Hanif, M. T. (2024). Role of pathology and point of care testing in the estimation of fasting blood glucose levels in type 2 diabetes mellitus patients. *Journal of Health and Rehabilitation Research*. https://www.semanticscholar.org/paper/955bdfce4ace7ec1b90952a63192fec3b080d59f (accessed on 1st July 2025).

53. Zhang, D., Li, A., Jing, L., & Zhang, J. (2018). Effect evaluation of shared care-based diabetes management in tertiary hospital. *10*, 322–326. https://www.semanticscholar.org/paper/3d2b7a871f8669d996e120153a8d75114f716d60 (accessed on 1st July 2025).

54. Zhang, L., Gao, X., Meng, X., Ma, G., Li, J., Wang, W., Chen, S., et al. (2025). Rectify the impact of shorter red blood cell lifespan upon HbA1c detection values in T2DM patients: Modeling and internal-external verification. *Frontiers in Endocrinology*. https://www.semanticscholar.org/paper/bf4a546dfb1697a385501d77272e28256c20076d (accessed on 1st July 2025).

55. Zhang, Y., Wang, M., Li, P., Lv, G., Yao, J., & Zhao, L. (2024). Hypoglycemic effect of polysaccharides from *Physalis alkekengi* L. in type 2 diabetes mellitus mice. *Biology, 13*. https://www.semanticscholar.org/paper/3a03a269818641d13c8d8f5ae1528e7e512e2aee (accessed on 1st July 2025).

56. Zhou, Y., Xie, N., Zhang, L., & Chen, D. (2021). Impact of family history of diabetes on blood glucose, lipid levels and perinatal outcomes in pregnant women with gestational diabetes mellitus. *Journal of Zhejiang University (Medical Sciences), 50*, 329–334. https://doi.org/10.3724/zdxbyxb-2021-0193 (accessed on 1st July 2025).

LIPID PROFILE AND CARDIOVASCULAR RISK

11

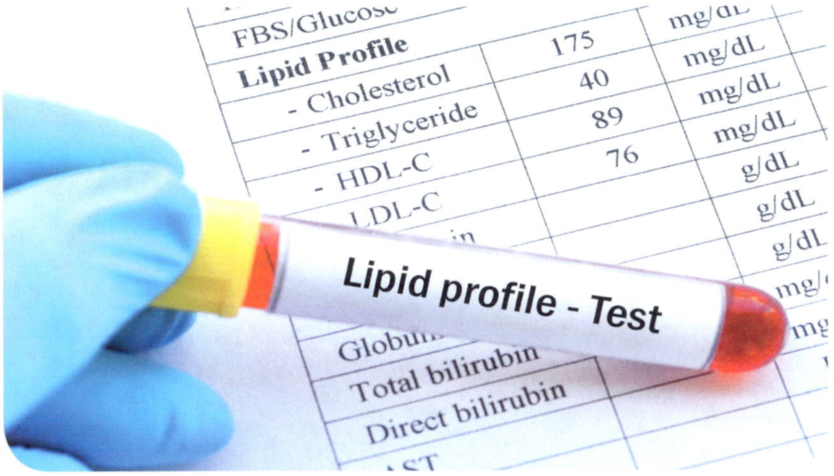

LEARNING OBJECTIVES

After studying this chapter, you will be able to:

1. Discuss the components of lipid profile;
2. Define the role of lipids in the body;
3. Explain lipid profile and cardiovascular disease;
4. Identify the risk assessment and management;
5. Explore the population variability in lipid profiles;
6. Identify the emerging research and trends.

Introduction

Lipid levels and heart risk go hand in hand, especially since global health issues are on the rise. Recent studies on the manner in which our body metabolizes fat show that even slight alterations in lipid levels can really make a significant difference in how our hearts function. Much of the research points to high LDL cholesterol as a warning to avoid impending heart occurrences, while higher HDL levels seem to be beneficial. And naturally, there's a role for genes and lifestyle as well, and when you put it all together, the interplay of factors all plays into a sense of just how useful lipid testing can be to identify risk—given that conditions like obesity and insulin resistance are only becoming more common. A more fascinating spin is to look at how the activity of belly fat—so-called visceral adiposity—affects lipid results. Literature has a tendency to suggest that visceral fat excess is accompanied by dyslipidemia, which may raise cardiac risk. This makes advanced imaging, like Dual-Energy Computed Tomography (DECT), very important for having the correct picture of where the fat is settling and how it disrupts lipid metabolism. In a second study in which they looked at both visceral fat and lipid function tests, there were clear correlations with over-abundant visceral fat and elevated levels of total cholesterol and triglycerides (Sam et al., 2024). Even counting up lipid statistics does not seem to be the full story when cardiac risk is concerned. The story doesn't end there—genetics and the way our bodies react to drugs complicate matters further. As an example, genetic variations in genes such as GSTT1 seem to affect how people respond to drugs like metformin, a commonly used drug in treating type 2 diabetes. Although current findings have a tendency to show that the correlation isn't exactly black and white regarding metformin's role in heart risk through such gene variations, the entire scenario does suggest the need for further research. Careful analysis of drug responses and cardiac outcomes may eventually lead to more individualized management of dyslipidemia and complications (Dewi, 2025). In most cases, such data not only improves what we currently know but also provides an avenue for personalized treatment (Figure 11.1).

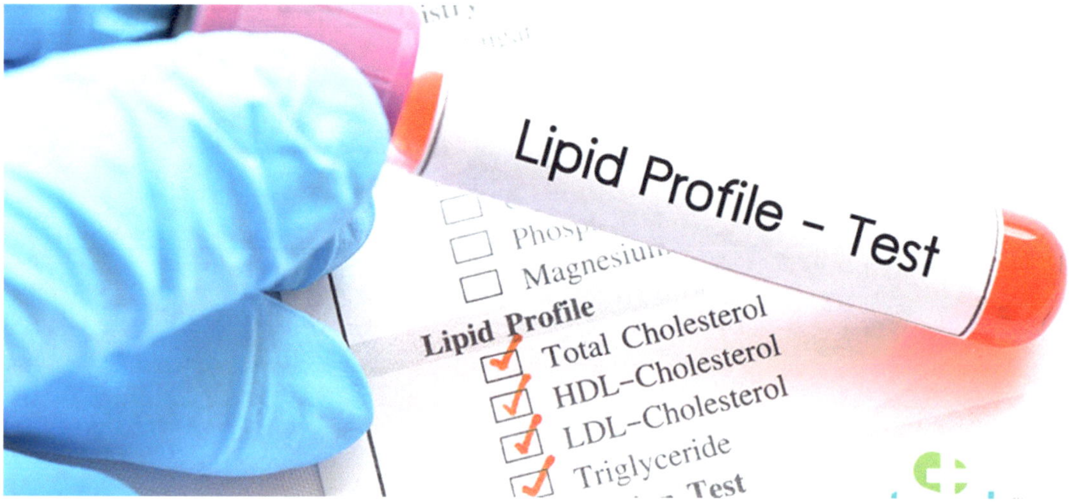

Figure 11.1. Lipid profile test.

Source: https://external-content.duckduckgo.com/iu/?u=https%3A%2F%2Fwww.netmeds.com%2Fimages%2Fcms%2Fwysiwyg%2Fblog%2F2021%2F02%2F1613636799_Lipid_big_450.jpg&f=1&nofb=1&ipt=c794180763f2c127a0a291ef82febff09ab0e28e8bc6d7f4c847871272ef66c7.

Definition of Lipid Profile

Heart health these days is typically quantified by one's lipid profile. Most commonly this is screening for total cholesterol, the so-called "bad" LDL, the "good" HDL, and triglycerides. Increased levels of LDL and triglycerides will typically signal plaque deposition—something that can lead to atherosclerosis—while HDL will typically serve as a type of safety net for the heart. Doctors generally monitor these figures to classify patients based on risk and recommend initial interventions to prevent complications. Since the way lipids work is very complex, studying them isn't exactly numerology—it's monitoring how different fats interact with each other in our cells, something that's essential in handling heart risks. Recent research largely points to the fact that context has a lot to do with reading these profiles. Your age, sex, genetic characteristics, and even any underlying health issues that you might have can alter those figures in some fairly unexpected ways. For example, there are some gene variations that will push someone towards dyslipidemia, adding to the risk scenario. Everyday habits—the food you eat, how much you move, and whether or not you smoke—have a big impact on your lipids, and by extension your cardiac risk. Overall, how we combine all these elements is what we must do to develop individualized treatment plans. In the majority of cases, this individualized plan is actually what we need to deal with the growing problem of heart disease, so guidelines currently aim to cover all these different aspects (Visseren et al., 2021). There is also controversy over using non-invasive tests—like some imaging procedures and highly advanced blood tests—along with standard lipid tests to better predict heart risk. These procedures provide us with a clearer view of how our bodies process fats, at times revealing issues that standard tests might miss. Unbeknownst to many, linkage between levels of lipids and conditions like non-alcoholic fatty liver disease (NAFLD) demonstrates just how intricate our metabolic process can be when relating to cardiovascular health. The more science that emerges, incorporating these new facts into everyday practice, seems not only logical but necessary in an effort to perform more educated risk assessment and improve patient management (Mary et al., 2023).

Importance of Lipid Profile in Cardiovascular Health

Cardiovascular health actually hinges a lot on your overall lipid profile—these numbers create a picture of how likely it is that someone will have heart problems. Consideration of total cholesterol, LDL (that "bad" type), HDL (the "good" type) and triglycerides gives doctors a glimpse into whether or not plaque might be accumulating.

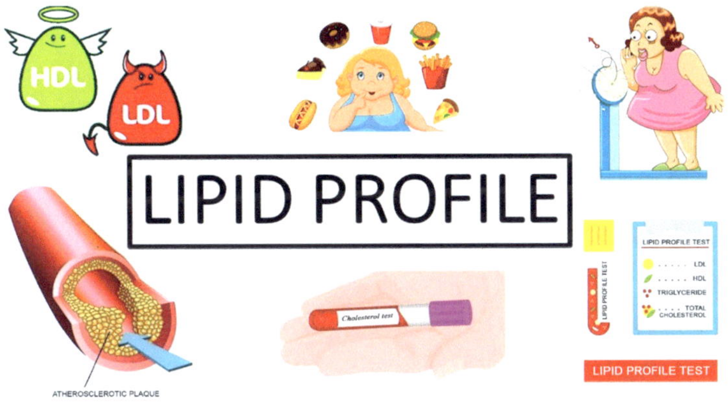

Figure 11.2. Lipid profile in cardiovascular health.

Source: https://external-content.duckduckgo.com/iu/?u=https%3A%2F%2Frapidlaboratory.in%2Fwp-content%2Fuploads%2F2024%2F02%2FLipid-Profile-Testing.png&f=1&nofb=1&ipt=7eeeacc58bdbe27f3ebc4e29f46943678ba8b54b94ec77ee8d4216ff16dac908.

Raised LDL levels can spark plaque growth, raising the risk of heart attack or stroke, whereas HDL sweeps cholesterol out of your system like a cleaning crew. So, a full lipid test isn't just a diagnostic procedure—it helps determine the game plan for preventing and treating heart disease on an individual basis. Monitoring your lipids is the key thing—especially now that more people are aging and lifestyle issues come into play. Regular screenings can identify dyslipidemia (i.e., when your lipids get somewhat derailed), which quite literally means opening the door to early treatment.

Physicians in most cases are incentivized to incorporate these screenings within routine visits so they can offer individualized advice about dietary changes, exercise, and other changes. These early measures can reduce the risks of high cholesterol and enable patients to learn more about maintaining healthy hearts; this not only enhances personal health but also reduces the general pressure on our healthcare systems. With heart disease on the rise, there is a growing trend to incorporate lipid screening into more general health programs. Spreading the word about what your numbers mean can help rally communities around better heart health. Local campaigns may focus on the connections between diet, exercise, and managing your lipids. As mentioned in the ESC/EAS Guidelines, healthcare pros play a big role in guiding patients through all this—always keeping in mind each person's unique situation. If we can create a setting in which individuals are getting educated and motivated to undergo regular lipid tests, then there is a real chance to decrease total heart risks as well as enhance public health outcomes (François et al., 2019; Livingston et al., 2020) (Figure 11.2).

Overview of Cardiovascular Risk Factors

Cardiovascular wellness is a complex interrelationship between elements that converge in unexpected combinations. Hypertension is one of the chief villains - in 2019, it accounted for approximately 55.5% of disability-adjusted life years due to stroke, a number that indicates just how stealthy chronic, often asymptomatic hypertension can be. It's not just pressure, though; a high body mass index (BMI) and raised fasting plasma glucose also push the risk higher. Looking back from 1990 to 2019, global trends even hint that strokes have risen and weight issues have become the fastest-growing problem. Essentially, grasping these complex issues is crucial if we're to design effective, targeted strategies to reduce heart problems and save lives. Lifestyle and environmental factors, too, really merge into this equation. Smoking by itself, for example, accounts for up to 17.6% of DALYs for stroke, which speaks volumes about being more than an unpleasant habit—more of a health hazard. Air pollution does not take second place either; particulate air pollution exacts its own burden on vascular health, especially in smog-girt areas. Individuals who reside in constant air pollution most likely have a higher chance of heart disease, which is evidence that our lifestyle and surroundings are more related than we realize. Quitting smoking and embracing better habits can be as easy as a piece of cake, but they're significant actions that could ease these dangers significantly. In most cases, even little adjustments to daily habits might cause greater, healthier alterations. Social and financial issues also bear heavily on heart health. 2019 statistics generally point towards death rates for strokes being substantially higher in low-income populations compared to more prosperous communities. Lack of access to quality medical care, limited educational experiences, and poor diet all contribute to worsening conditions such as high blood pressure and diabetes within those communities. For example, areas where there is bad medical care are likely to experience a rise in preventable cases, and concerns such as high fasting plasma glucose need interventions that target, specifically these economic inequities. In general, ensuring equal access to healthcare and redistributing resources more equally matters if we really want to decline cardiovascular disease—and narrow the health gap that still remains between groups.

11.1. Components of Lipid Profile

Learning Outcome

- Total cholesterol;
- Low-density lipoprotein (LDL);
- High-density lipoprotein (HDL).

Cardiovascular health literally depends on your lipid levels. Total cholesterol, LDL, HDL, and triglycerides all factor in—each contributes its share to the story. Total cholesterol gives a general overview of your fat balance, both good and bad. When LDL—bad in character—is up, there's usually a greater likelihood of atherosclerosis, which in most instances primes the pump for heart problems. At the same time, HDL (the so-called good cholesterol) helps ferry excess cholesterol from your arteries over to the liver for processing. Simply put, keeping these measurements in balance matters greatly not just for you, but for our collective health too. Food choices are a surprising force behind these numbers. The connection between your regular diet and your lipid profile is not always straightforward; nonetheless, studies have again and again shown that the Mediterranean-style diet makes a difference. People who continue to be more consistent with this kind of diet will see triglycerides decrease and, in some instances, HDL increase. This synergy of nutrients—fiber, unsaturated fats, and other nutrients—seems to work synergistically to naturally keep those lipid levels in check, and ultimately lower cardiovascular risk. For most individuals, embracing this kind of balanced diet plan is a healthy thought for heart health (Vitale et al., 2018). Doctors and healthcare professionals also depend on these measures when making treatment suggestions. For example, guidelines from the European Society of Cardiology and European Atherosclerosis Society (ESC/EAS) are useful in learning how to take these numbers into account (François et al., 2019). Generally speaking, they recommend that one not compare lipid readings with such things as a person's age, sex, and any condition they may have. Using these guidelines, clinicians can then usually tailor their approach to best maximize lipids and more or less eliminate heart disease risk over time. Finally, being well informed about your lipid profile gives you the foundation for prevention and personalized treatment, placing you on a healthier long-term path of health (Figure 11.3).

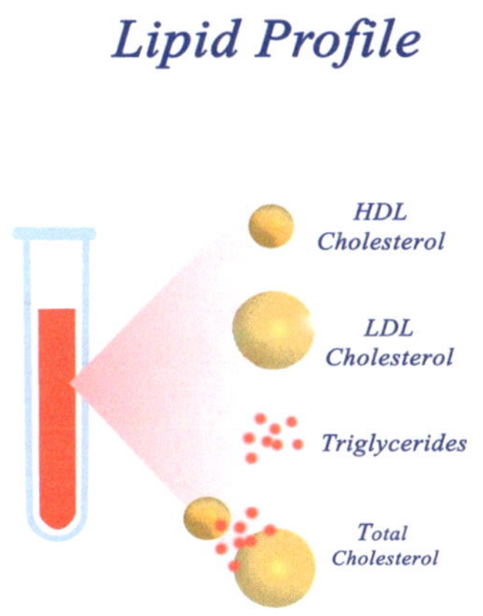

Figure 11.3. Components of lipid profile.

Source: https://external-content.duckduckgo.com/iu/?u=https%3A%2F%2Fthumbs.dreamstime.com%2Fb%2Ffour-components-lipid-profile-152245560.jpg&f=1&nofb=1&ipt=e486dec90eb237b4f51a0dc4991272b1dc6ec6d11e38a5a870692fcb25fbf3c7.

11.1.1. Total Cholesterol

Total cholesterol is a matter of concern when heart risks are being determined. Doctors keep an eye on your lipid levels - that total cholesterol reading - because higher numbers can mean something is amiss with the functioning of your arteries. High numbers can imply processes that lead to deposits of plaques within your blood vessel walls, which in some instances ends up causing heart attacks or strokes. They check cholesterol in clinics together with some other indicators of fat to obtain a fuller but occasionally messy picture of cardiac well-being. Studies seem to suggest that, by modifying your diet, exercising, or taking certain drugs, it is possible to lower these numbers and consequently reduce your risk. It's all about controlling cholesterol before it becomes more of a problem. Some new studies, in most cases, suggest that the manner in which your cholesterol behaves long-term can actually pen your heart's history – and it's not just an adult phenomenon. For example, scientists have found that teens with high levels are more likely to have thicker artery walls as adults—basically early signs that the arteries might be clogging up. That longer picture indicates that early monitoring and management of cholesterol can actually show a payoff. A decrease in cholesterol in those early years of development is typically associated with fewer threats of detrimental alterations in the blood vessels, and that does help affirm the value in monitoring cholesterol at an early age as a long-term strategy for heart protection. There's also an interesting connection between cholesterol and our body's inflammation. As it turns out, when overall cholesterol levels are high, there typically is a spike in markers such as high-sensitivity C-reactive protein (hs-CRP), another indication that the heart is stressed. Some studies—typically a heterogeneous group of evidence—suggest that weight loss and lipid level reduction (occasionally following procedures like laparoscopic sleeve gastrectomy) tend to have a positive effect on both the cholesterol and inflammatory aspects. To some extent, lowering cholesterol and losing a small amount of weight typically accompany lowering inflammation, highlighting the close relationship between the two. In general, a strategy that treats both high cholesterol and inflammation would seem to be very much needed to decrease the risk factors of heart disease (Figure 11.4).

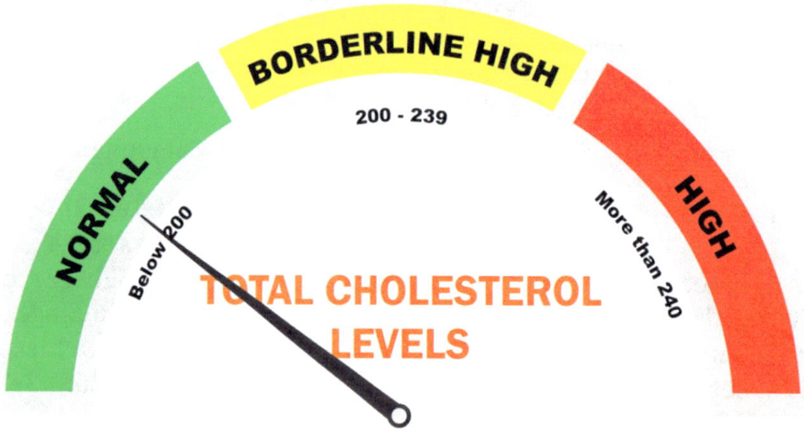

Figure 11.4. Total cholesterol levels.

Source: https://cdn4.vectorstock.com/i/1000x1000/51/78/total-cholesterol-levels-vector-50115178.jpg.

11.1.2. Low-Density Lipoprotein (LDL)

LDL is closely associated with heart issues—a discovery that keeps appearing and reappearing in medical studies. Elevated levels of LDL, or bad cholesterol, tend to build up in arterial walls and cause atherosclerosis; such buildup eventually leads to heart attacks, strokes and other cardiovascular alerts. People with dyslipidemia, especially those whose levels of LDL are elevated, are at a very much greater risk. Everyday habits—like missing out on a proper diet and lacking sufficient exercise—can actually push these levels up. Research conducted on Indonesian working women found that almost 80% of them had high levels of LDL, highlighting a serious risk for heart problems (Yani et al., 2025). Not all LDL particles are alike, though. Overall, the denser and smaller particles tend to migrate into the arterial walls and cause plaque formation more readily, while the larger, heavier ones do not seem as harmful.

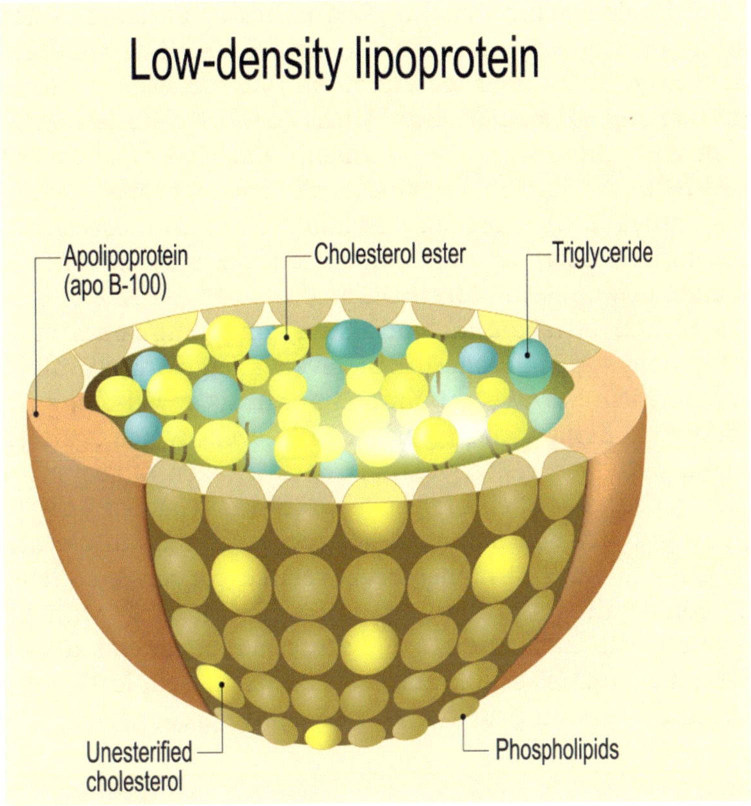

Figure 11.5. Low-density lipoprotein (LDL).

Source: https://external-content.duckduckgo.com/iu/?u=https%3A%2F%2Fas2.ftcdn.net%2Fv2%2Fjpg%2F01%2F96%2F37%2F09%2F1000_F_196370998_DvJCTyyqvbyNfuN0dWMJbmXUIxrv3Mr7.jpg&f=1&nofb=1&ipt=eba55f125b537843b0c71594418753fe4e16a92d8029a5f99228f13b8c48e101.

This difference definitely points to a total evaluation of the lipid profile, as opposed to just a look at overall figures, but also to a comprehension of particle size and type. Recent research even suggests that LDL may be doing more than merely serving as a marker; it may actually be playing an active role in creating inflammation and modulating the immune response. For example, patients with infections like tuberculosis are found to have typical alterations in their profiles of LDL with an added cardiovascular risk (Karolína et al., 2025). Lowering LDL is important when it comes to avoiding heart disease. Shaking up your lifestyle—more fiber, fewer saturated fats, a bit of omega-3—can reduce LDL levels, and statins are often thrown into the regimen for high-risk individuals. Regular monitoring of lipid levels, along with these lifestyle and drug changes, works well in keeping LDL in equilibrium and reducing occurrences of large heart events. In most cases, combining a bit of day-to-day management with sound clinical advice is the best option given that dyslipidemia is on the rise in severity, particularly in those who are most at risk. To understand exactly how LDL carries out its role is very critical to enhancing overall heart health (Yani et al., 2025) (Figure 11.5).

11.1.3. High-Density Lipoprotein (HDL)

Healthy HDL cholesterol levels usually signal a good indicator of heart health. It is considered a good shield against heart problems by most individuals because HDL removes surplus cholesterol from the body and delivers it to the liver for excretion. One recent study, for instance, found that those who underwent one-anastomosis gastric bypass (OAGB) were left with much greater HDL levels afterward, which were more likely to be linked with lower cardiovascular risk (Torija et al., 2020). Having good HDL isn't just about cholesterol control, though—it's part of a grand plan to minimize heart-related death. HDL doesn't just idle around. In most cases, it performs a busy role by displaying anti-inflammatory and antioxidant effects. Studies generally point to the fact that a healthier lipid composition with more HDL might lower the risk of atherosclerosis as well as other coronary complications. Take a look at a study on young South Indian male athletes; it showed that elements of body type influenced HDL levels along with overall lipid profiles, hinting at a pretty tangled link between how we're built and our heart's well-being (Andrew et al., 2024). It seems burning calories and being active can shift HDL levels, which again shows lifestyle really does matter when it comes to heart risk. Doctors have now taken to keeping a closer eye on HDL when assessing whether a person is at risk for heart problems. That said, they also track other fats like LDL cholesterol and triglycerides. Some studies recognize that an elevated total cholesterol-to-HDL ratio is more likely to warn of higher heart-related concerns, so it would be prudent to track these figures in combination. Through the study of HDL along with the remainder of the lipid data, clinicians can typically make dietary and exercise recommendations more specifically. In the end, HDL is not so much a passive indicator—it is a leading indicator of personal and public heart health trends, even if everything isn't always so neatly predictable.

Test Your Knowledge

1. What are the key components measured in a standard lipid profile test?
2. How do LDL, HDL, and triglycerides differ in structure and function?

11.2. Role of Lipids in the Body

Learning Outcome

- Energy storage and metabolism;
- Cell membrane structure;
- Hormone production.

Lipids actually count for our well-being—they're responsible for energy storage, cell structure formation, and even hormone regulation. Consider this: triglycerides are an energy dense package, and phospholipids and cholesterol provide the framework for our cell membranes to remain fluid and operational. In most instances, these facts are also the building blocks of our hormone production and other signaling molecules, so our metabolism works smoothly. But when lipids become unbalanced, nastiness can ensue, especially for the heart; elevated LDL-C and high triglycerides have long been recognized as potential culprits of coronary maladies, so checking your lipid profile might be more important than you know. Researchers have examined how our lipid pairs relate to cardiovascular health, and evidence appears to be persuasive. For example, to have excess levels of low-density lipoprotein cholesterol (LDL-C), also known as the "bad cholesterol," is firmly established to be a risk factor for atherosclerosis, a disease in which plaque builds up in artery walls. Elevated levels of high-density lipoprotein cholesterol (HDL-C), that "good cholesterol," on the other hand, are found to offer some protection. In fact, more contemporary studies suggest that the apoB/apoA-1 ratio is an even better measure of cardiac events, demonstrating that it's not so much the amount of fat that it's a question of, but rather what types are present in the mix.

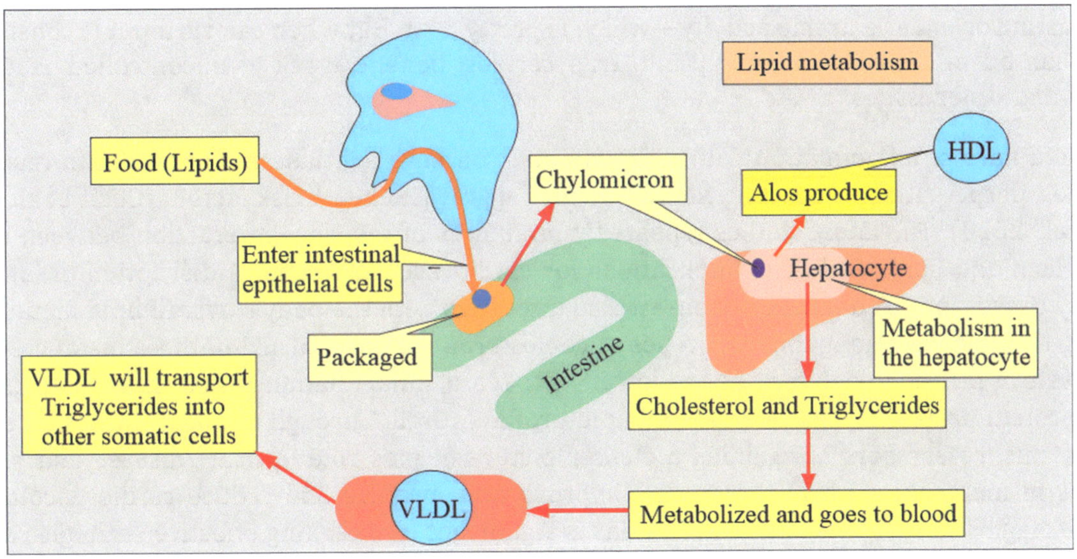

Figure 11.6. Lipids role in our body.

Source: https://external-content.duckduckgo.com/iu/?u=https%3A%2F%2Flabpedia.net%2Fwp-content%2Fuploads%2F2020%2F01%2FLipid-metabolism.jpg&f=1&nofb=1&ipt=c7afb95030b0456f2bebd0e9c4981e08379d4627239eb6fba31ad790a99a200b.

Diets, lifestyle habits, and even a normal day can have an effect upon these balances in quite unexpected manners. It's interesting to observe how some fats are a part of the pregnancy process as well. Overweight pregnant women, for example, often present signs of vitamin D deficiency, which might flip their bodies' management of lipids on its head – a phenomenon whose effects might extend to both mother and child. Current trials of vitamin D3 supplementation tend to say that while levels of vitamin D rise, there is no visible difference in maternal or fetal lipid levels, for example, levels of triglycerides or cholesterol (Harreiter et al., 2022). Also, research on apolipoproteins such as apoB and apoA-1 appears promising for the identification of future cardiovascular events in pregnant women with pre-existing conditions and that would be prudent to monitor these markers (Holme et al., 2008) (Figure 11.6).

11.2.1. Energy storage and metabolism

Fat tissue and energy regulation intersect in unexpected ways that determine our lipid composition and, ultimately, impact heart risk. When all is well, fat cells store excess energy and release it as needed, regulating our metabolism. But in obesity, the equation is thrown off—fat tissue begins to behave badly with an excess of lipids and a sort of chronic, low-grade inflammation. This. This alteration makes our bodies less responsive to insulin, usually resulting in diabetes type 2 and elevating cardiovascular risk. Interestingly, fat cells also release a variety of bioactive signals called adipokines, and when signaling molecules become deranged, they might well set the stage for metabolic disease. Clearly, getting a grip on this messy relationship is key to crafting ways to better manage lipid profiles and lower heart risks (Chait et al., 2020; Tilg et al., 2020). Look a little closer and you'll see that how fat adapts to too much energy is central to keeping overall metabolism steady. In everyday life, the lipids of fat tissue are a readily available energy reserve when fasting or under extreme activity—which is pretty neat. But when caloric input is consistently more than burnt off, calories pile up into triglycerides; beneficial but, if uncontrolled, leading to NAFLD and other issues.

Add a flare of inflammation within the fat, and you have a situation where insulin resistance increases, perpetuating a vicious cycle that further aggravates heart risk factors (Chait et al., 2020; Tilg et al., 2020). The latest studies repeatedly remind us of the close interaction between energy metabolism and lipids and their implications for cardiovascular health. A disruption of fat tissue not only causes localized inflammation—it also interferes with the body's overall lipid metabolism, altering the balance among different types of cholesterol. It's not unusual in these instances to see high levels of LDL and triglycerides and lower HDL. More, inflammation is associated with changes in lipoprotein processing that worsen the lipid profile overall. Through the deconstruction of such mechanisms, researchers are gaining a clearer picture of fat's role in heart disease and probing changes in metabolic pathways that may improve lipid profiles and reduce cardiovascular risk. Overall, digging deeper into such correlations is significant in designing effective strategies against heart disease (Chait et al., 2020; Tilg et al., 2020).

11.2.2. Cell membrane structure

Cell membranes are not just physical barriers—there is a fundamental role they play in how cells communicate. Their structure, basically a double bilayer of phospholipids to which are added proteins, cholesterol, and carbs, plays a crucial role in keeping the cell's internal balance. In fluid mosaic model, lipids and proteins will be floating around more freely, facilitating the transport of nutrients and the delivery of signals. This is a form of flexibility that is usually crucial; when disturbed, metabolic processes may go wrong and at times lead to ailments like type 2 diabetes mellitus (T2DM). Since insulin signaling heavily depends on the membrane being strong and responsive, it thus dictates cardiovascular risk in patients with metabolic afflictions (Galicia-Garc et al., 2020). The lipid composition in the membrane largely dictates how it behaves. Think about lipid rafts-tiny microdomains crammed with cholesterol and sphingolipids-as informal social sites that focus signaling molecules and enhance interactions, triggering a range of biological responses. On other occasions, alterations in these lipid profiles can foster insulin resistance, another defining feature of T2DM, thus linking membrane architecture to cardiovascular well-being.

In addition, higher levels of saturated fatty acids, to which you are more likely to be exposed in processed foods, have been shown to disrupt membrane fluidity and worsen the risk of atherosclerosis and other cardiovascular disease. It seems that not only having particular lipids, but how they are allocated and interact among themselves, is important to preserve metabolic homeostasis (Sharifi et al., 2020). Oxidative stress also makes things more complicated in the vicinity of cell membranes. Sustained exposure to oxidative substances has the potential to trigger lipid peroxidation—a process by which membrane integrity and function are slowly compromised. This deterioration has the potential to alter normal signaling mechanisms, especially those involving insulin action, which in turn increases the vulnerability of T2DM and sets the stage for other cardiovascular complications. In the majority of cases, everyday choices like diet and exercise contentedly regulate levels of oxidative stress, thus linking food lipid profiles, membrane integrity, and heart risk. Elucidation of these complex relationships is important for developing interventions that can lessen the impact of metabolic diseases and their associated cardiovascular outcomes (Galicia-García et al., 2020) (Figure 11.7).

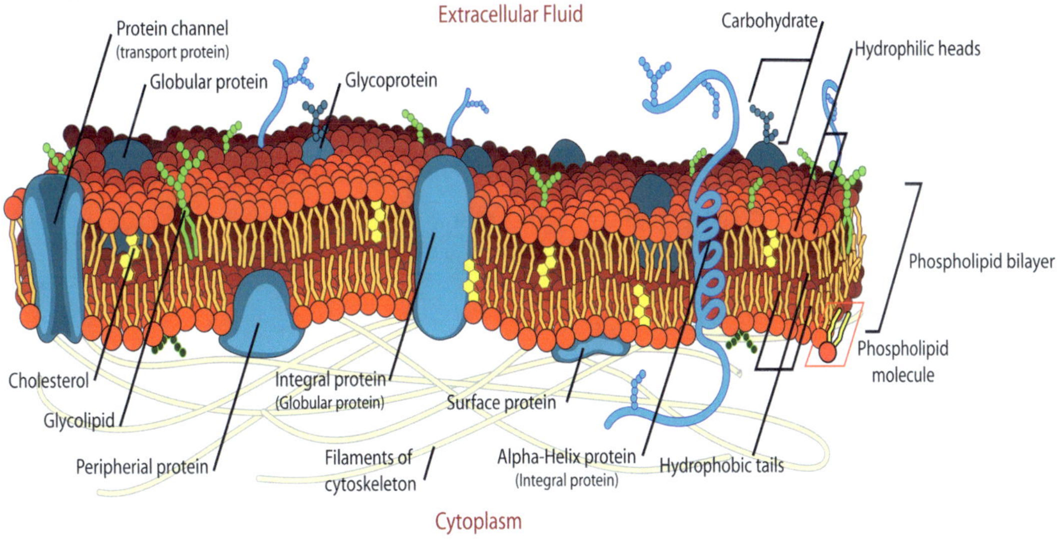

Figure 11.7. Lipids and cell membrane structure.

Source: https://external-content.duckduckgo.com/iu/?u=https%3A%2F%2Fimage4.slideserve.com%2F329176%2Flipids-and-cell-membrane-structure-l.jpg&f=1&nofb=1&ipt=b15396717709925cce69209f35649b4dee8d907b907c0320baa6f150bab00b96.

11.2.3. Hormone Production

Fat tissue and cardiovascular well-being mix in a rather complex way – hormones are front and center. Fat does not just hold energy; it secretes hormones like adiponectin, which, in most cases, regulates our lipid level. You typically find that when one is obese, adiponectin is reduced, and this reduction typically accompanies lipid modification: triglycerides go up whereas the "good" HDL goes down, moving heart disease risks in a positive direction (Elvita et al., 2025). It's kind of interesting how understanding this link between adiponectin and lipid metabolism becomes pretty crucial if we're trying to improve overall metabolic health and lower the risk to our cardiovascular system. Other hormones from fat tissue play their own roles too—leptin, for example, wields considerable influence over both energy balance and appetite. Most frequently, high leptin (a common occurrence in the overweight) is not so benevolent; it's accompanied by further fat deposition and has even been known to set the stage for dyslipidemia by increasing levels of LDL cholesterol. And then insulin resistance; that metabolic quirk, which often develops alongside obesity, only serves to worsen these hormonal abnormalities. Generally, the relationship between leptin and insulin shows us how hormone production by fat tissue directly affects lipid profiles, something we really need to keep in mind when analyzing cardiovascular health problems. Diet, too, can stir up this complicated cocktail. Nutrient constituents, sometimes in the form of nutraceuticals like *Centella asiatica* or even cayenne pepper, have been shown to influence hormone secretion and lipid metabolism in various quite unexpected ways. When these substances are incorporated into standard meals, they can increase insulin sensitivity and reduce inflammation – effects that many see as a move toward better metabolic well-being. Research even shows that these supplements not only contribute to body weight reduction but also regulate hormone levels, such as insulin and leptin, resulting in improved lipid profiles. For the most part, implementing these dietary changes personalized to a person's own genetic makeup can quite possibly make them function even more effectively in eliminating cardiovascular risks, another reminder that diet, hormone physiology, and heart health are all very interlinked (Oganija et al., 2024).

Test Your Knowledge

1. What functions do lipids serve in cell membranes and hormone production?
2. How do triglycerides act as an energy storage form in the body?

11.3. Lipid Profile and Cardiovascular Disease

Learning Outcome

- Correlation between lipid levels and heart disease;
- Mechanisms of atherosclerosis;
- Impact of triglycerides on cardiovascular risk.

Lipid levels and cardiovascular health are quite directly related. Different fats in our blood seem to be involved with the state of our arteries, and knowing how each of them behaves is really significant. LDL, which most people call "bad" cholesterol, has a tendency to pool in the arteries, possibly forming plaques that could eventually lead to obstruction, heart attack, or stroke. HDL, on the other hand, does a form of cleaning by picking up excess cholesterol and carrying it away from the arteries. For most cases, having these two in equilibrium accounts for a lot since any extreme shift in their levels—either way—will lead to harm to the heart. This is the reason doctors often stress the importance of full lipid tests, especially in people who come in with the presentation of metabolic syndrome (Simkiene et al., 2025). New studies have been bringing out the point that what we eat actually can alter our lipid profiles, and therefore our risk for heart problems.

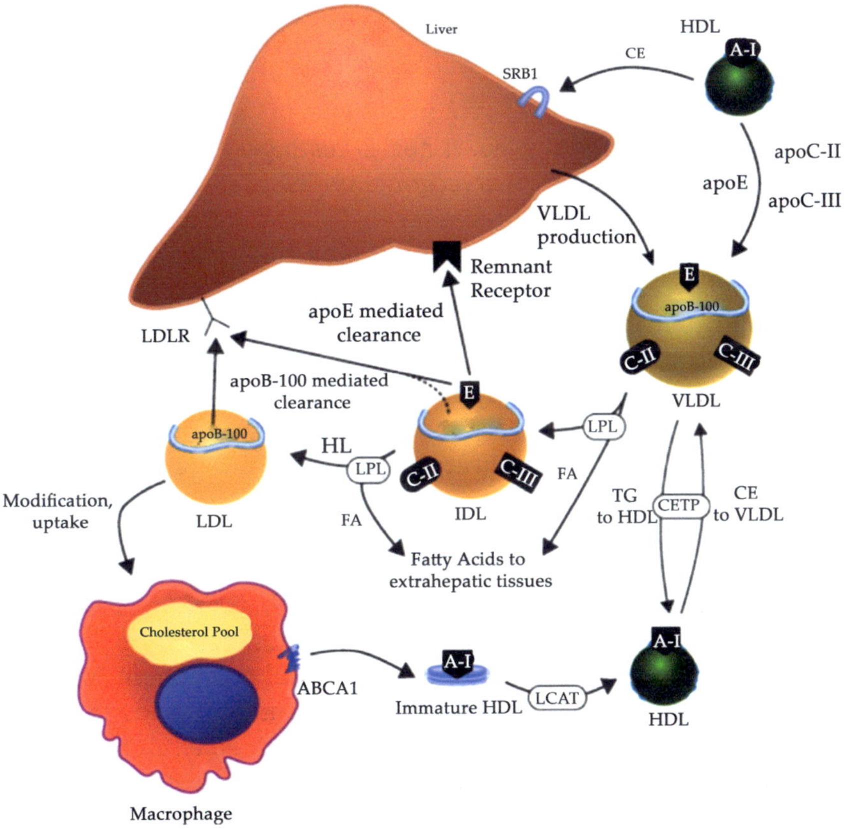

Figure 11.8. Lipid profile and cardiovascular disease.

Source: https://external-content.duckduckgo.com/iu/?u=https%3A%2F%2Fwww.creative-diagnostics.com%2Fupload%2Fimage%2FLipid-Cholesterol-Metabolism-and%2520Cardiovascular.png&f=1&nofb=1&ipt=1d9e862c30d06945450b9b2e38d676d4279e33720bf4cc3a8c826ece9ce758a3.

For example, foods with a high burden of omega-3 fatty acids—fatty fish or even certain nuts are examples that come to mind—can actually lower triglycerides and raise HDL levels, which many consider a benefit to heart health. A fascinating study also noted that subjects who ate a well-balanced diet including some unique ingredients like wolfberry had improved lipid profiles that could decrease heart risk. It was discovered that HDL levels specifically increased along with certain forms of phosphatidylcholines, which suggests that our daily dietary habits can contribute significantly to our lipid composition (Toh et al., 2024). Apparently, modifying what you consume can be quite an effective mechanism for managing those fat-based risks. And in addition, understanding the underlying biology of how such fats affect the heart can open doors to more effective prevention. For instance, higher levels of certain fats, like ceramides, appear to go along with higher total cholesterol and other cardiovascular risk factors. Various bits of information from diet and lipid research remind us that a one-trick panacea just won't work—instead, the addition of lifestyle changes to the regimen with occasional tweaks of lipid levels seems to be necessary. The inclusion of inflammation and oxidative stress in the mix as villains that interfere with lipid metabolism offers the potential for treatments on the horizon for health. In general, an accurate comprehension of these interactions is key to the prevention of heart disease, and that's why repeated lipid screening remains an important part of evaluating overall cardiovascular risk (Simkiene et al., 2025) (Figure 11.8).

11.3.1. Correlation Between Lipid Levels and Heart Disease

Lipid levels are a doozy when it comes to heart health testing—they actually have a pretty strong correlation with risk for heart trouble. You've got this disorder dyslipidemia that shows up as abnormal blood fats; basically, it clogs up the arteries so they can get clogged. For instance, patients with Type 2 diabetes are likely to have elevated total cholesterol, elevated low-density lipoproteins (LDL) and triglycerides, and declining high-density lipoprotein (HDL) levels. Such a metabolic imbalance in the body is likely to elevate the risk of cardiovascular disease, and for this reason, doctors are advised to keenly check these levels during routine check-ups (Abebe et al., 2017). Tracing these lipid levels will identify those who are at risk, and there is the opportunity to treat them in advance and prevent heart disease complications. Research substantiates this evidence that blood fat levels are an accurate predictor of heart trouble. A single study, for example, found that patients with Type 2 diabetes had far greater cholesterol levels, larger levels of LDL and triglycerides, and, on the other hand, their HDL was lower than in healthier patients. In most cases, being triglyceride-rich typically implies a higher threat of heart disease, which means a relatively clear-cut connection between these fat imbalances and heart threats (Abebe et al., 2017). This trend means that surveillance and even modulation of lipid levels isn't just about reducing risk factors—potentially, it will become an essential component of treatment design for individuals already battling metabolic disease. All this information leads us to wonder how lipid profile screening can shake up the practice of public health in general. Health care professionals truly need to prioritize lipid screening, particularly for patients who are already afflicted with conditions such as diabetes. Even studies and clinical practice both seem to substantiate the notion that by integrating evidence-based practices with standard lipid screening, the way we prevent heart disease is likely to change. Ultimately, acting early, even if it involves catching a few small flaws along the way, is paramount for reducing heart disease occurrences and alleviating its impact over the long term (Figure 11.9).

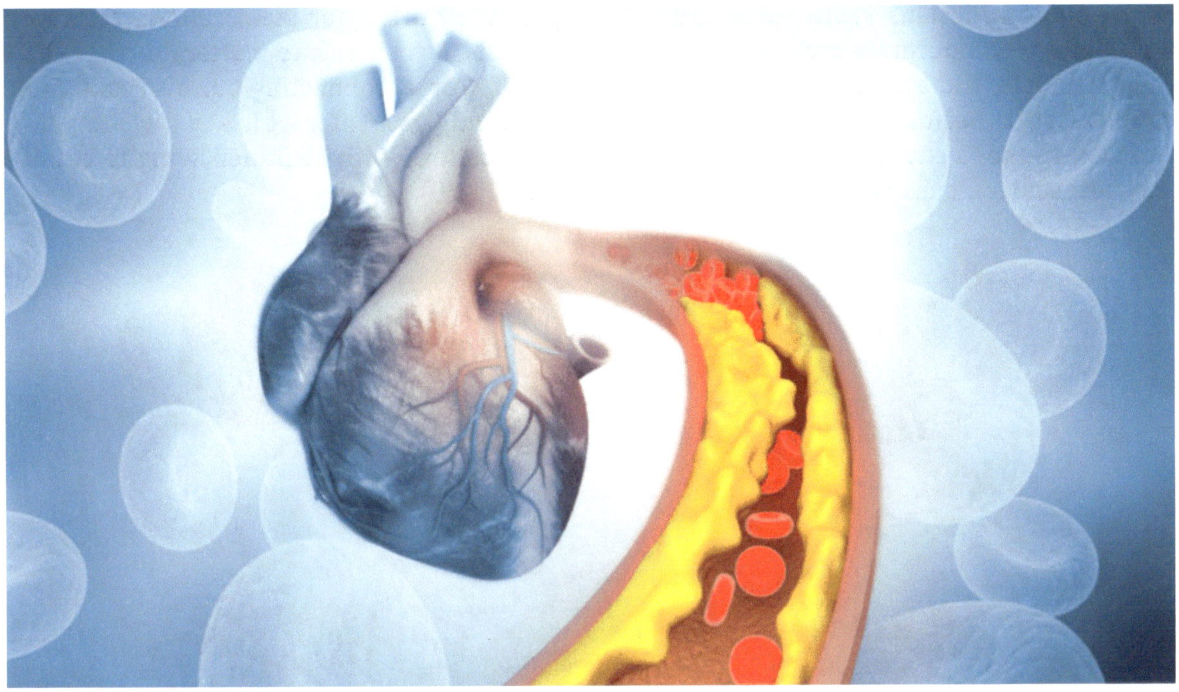

Figure 11.9. Conceptual illustration showing the buildup of plaque (yellow) in an artery leading to the heart, representing the link between high cholesterol and cardiovascular disease.

Source: https://sugunahospital.com/wp-content/uploads/2023/10/What-is-the-link-between-Cholesterol-and-Heart-Diseases.jpg.

11.3.2. Mechanisms of atherosclerosis

Atherosclerosis accumulates haphazardly, at the whim of whatever rubbish remains in the way. Inert waste like apolipoprotein-B-containing lipoproteins gets stuck way back in the wall of arteries. If they stick to it, they kind of act as red flags—waving before the body and signaling the immune cells (monocytes and macrophages come to mind) to rush over. This sets off a cascade that piles up foam cells, gradually building up plaque and narrowing the bloodstream. Chronic inflammation prefers to stick around too, slowly making the arterial injury worse and raising heart risk. All of these show us how our lipid levels and the body's inflammatory responses are all interconnected, indicating where new treatments may, in most cases, slow things down. As the disease progresses, there comes to be a delicate equilibrium between different types of macrophages. Inflammatory macrophages tend to proliferate, causing plaques to enlarge and even rendering them vulnerable—especially when they are involved in thinning of that fibrous cap. They are able to convert the surrounding environment into one of relentless, if not always useful, inflammation. Resolving macrophages meanwhile perform their part by clearing dead cells and secreting collagen, which maintains plaques stable and keeps catastrophic clotting events less likely. Effectively, this push and pull between cell types actually organizes plaque formation and even regression, sometimes, and that's why it's so important to treat both fats and inflammation when dealing with cardiovascular risk (François et al., 2019). It's not just fat accumulation, either; lifestyle habits or genetics get thrown in as well. High cholesterol, for example, brings more monocytes into the game, increasing inflammation and lesions growing. Excess blood lipids even drive our stem cells to create even more monocytes, inducing a cycle of chronic inflammation. To complicate matters further, factors like age, lifestyle, and a touch of daily stress make things worse, connecting our everyday choices to cardiovascular health. Recognizing how all these bits and pieces interact is key if we're going to create well-rounded strategies that combine smart lipid control with healthier living to cut down on cardiovascular issues (François et al., 2019) (Figure 11.10).

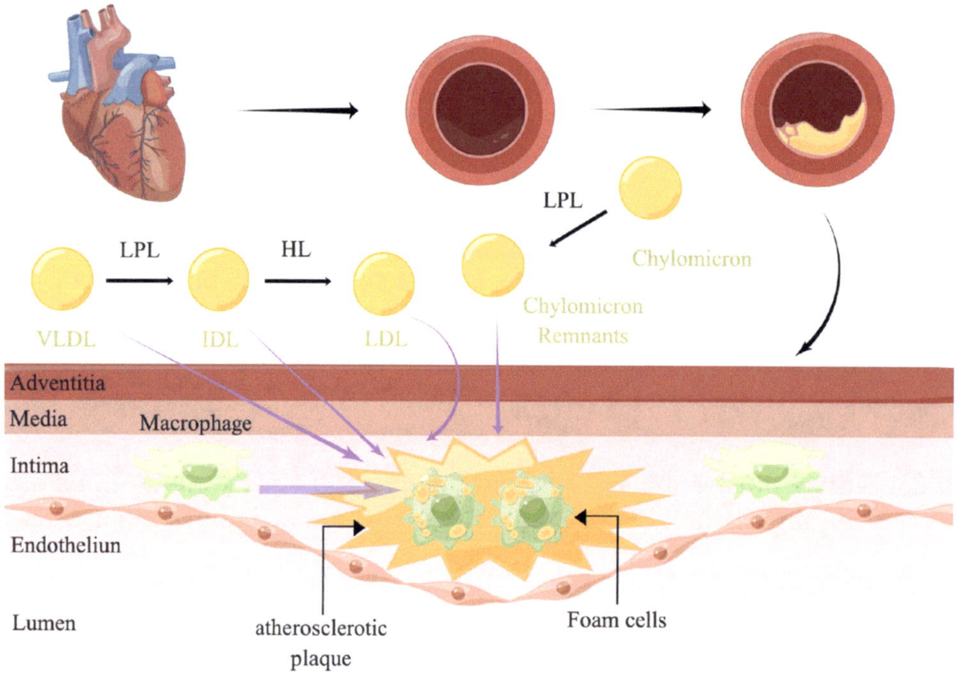

Figure 11.10. The mechanism of atherosclerosis.

Source: https://www.researchgate.net/publication/364442676/figure/fig3/AS:11431281187248279@1694168522951/The-mechanism-of-atherosclerosis-LPL-along-the-capillary-lumen-surface-hydrolyzed-VLDL.tif.

11.3.3. Impact of Triglycerides on Cardiovascular Risk

Lipid tests do a lot of the legwork for heart health—triglycerides, for instance, get all the credit. And that's because high triglycerides can be a sign, a signal that your heart might be troubled in the future by issues like obesity or insulin resistance. You know what they say: what goes up must come down; what goes up is triglycerides, and what comes down is heart health. Tracking those levels isn't just routine; it's a significant component of the whole cardiovascular risk formula. Mostly, it all just comes down to the complex mix between what our bodies metabolically accomplish and how the fats in blood interact, calling for solutions to counter both aspects without overcomplicating the matter. Triglycerides do play a significant role in our overall blood fat story. When they're intoxicated, they can induce inflammatory reactions that injure the lining of the blood vessel—essentially the first step in heart disease. Levels that are too high, or hypertriglyceridemia, seem to set the stage for plaque buildup that can eventually result in events like a heart attack or stroke. Guidelines in more recent times have started stressing the need to keep these levels in check, especially if someone is also under medication for diabetes or hypertension. This sort of comprehension permits physicians the room to develop more specific, and sometimes unexpected, ways to lower cardiovascular risk. Current research brings even more nuance to the equation, proposing that it's not simply a matter of having too many triglycerides, but also the character of the triglyceride-rich lipoproteins in the water in your veins. Different forms of these particles, including small, dense LDL particles—which tend to manifest when triglycerides are imbalanced—appear to be more trouble than their bigger, less dense cousins. Notably, studies have found that consuming a small amount of vitamin D can indeed lower the level of triglycerides, potentially lowering cardiovascular risk (Daniel, 2019; Mary et al., 2023). In general, these findings suggest that a flexible, multi-component framework for the interpretation of lipid profiles can be at the center of developing individualized strategies to the prevention and treatment of heart disease.

Test Your Knowledge

1. How does elevated LDL cholesterol contribute to atherosclerosis?
2. What is the relationship between high triglycerides and cardiovascular disease?

11.4. Risk Assessment and Management

Learning Outcome

- Guidelines for lipid level assessment;
- Lifestyle modifications to improve lipid profiles;
- Pharmacological interventions.

Risk assessment from lipid profiles is critical in order to determine cardiovascular issues. A significant majority of people come in with lipid problems that actually make it more probable to contract ASCVD to a considerable degree. A research study conducted on a mixed population demonstrated that about 31.6% of the patients were in the high-risk category – an unmistakable sign that problematic lipid levels are all too common and do bear concrete consequences on the heart. The cholesterol and LDL values seem to shoot through the roof in these patients, which ties those values very strongly to ASCVD risk (Parikh et al., 2024). These results are apt to encourage frequent follow-ups and smart fixes—whether lifestyle changes or even meds—to steer high-risk groups towards better overall results. Other than the routine check-ups, linking dots between different types of lipids and heart threats is what can really sharpen the way we treat these risks. Research shows that when HDL goes down, the risk for ASCVD also rises, therefore having a proper level of HDL is important. Individuals with low HDL are at increased risk of heart events, so that simple changes, like modifying their diet or exercising more, can have an impact. Concurrently, there is a discernible pattern wherein age and total cholesterol increase together with the risk of ASCVD, indicating that managing risk factors usually requires a combination of approaches (Parikh et al., 2024). Since there is not much one can do to prevent aging, it's sensible to focus more on therapies for the elderly in order to reduce the weight of heart disease. There is a new buzz developing on new dietary approaches that seem to optimize both cardiovascular health and lipid profiles. Time-restricted fasting (TRF) has recently been much in the spotlight due to its potential to bring different risk factors into alignment, including lipids. A couple of recent studies indicate that individuals who try TRF lose body fat and weight – a change that typically accompanies improved lipid parameters and a lower overall cardiac risk. As more researchers investigate these eating habits, TRF may be a valuable tool for the management of lipid disorders, an alternative for those going down the path to drugs. Blending these nutrition-focused strategies with standard screening protocols could lead, in most cases, to care that really prioritizes the patient and tackles cardiovascular disease from multiple fronts (Figure 11.11).

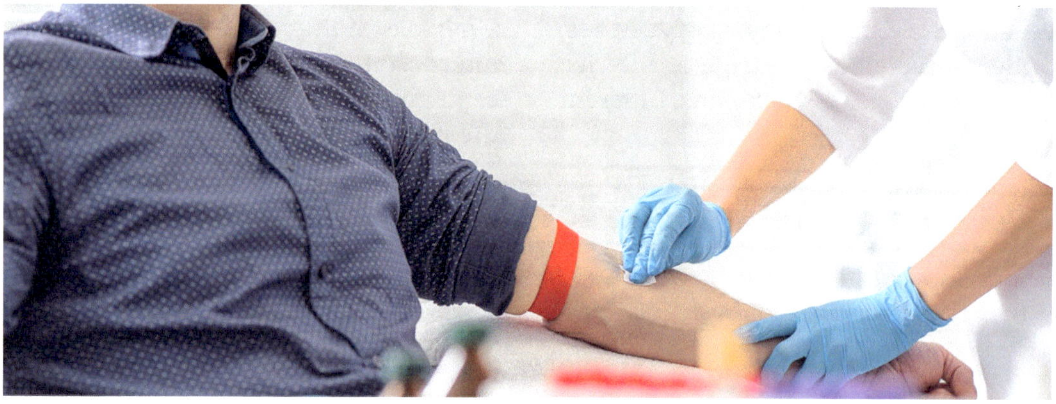

Figure 11.11. A healthcare professional prepares a patient for a blood draw; a common procedure used for lipid profile testing and other diagnostic evaluations.

Source: https://www.hopkinsmedicine.org/-/media/images/health/_-images-to-be-filed/lipidtesthero.jpg?h=500&iar=0&mh=500&mw=1300&w=1295&hash=DB0C666C7EC015FD402A2F3FD5710285.

11.4.1. Guidelines for Lipid Level Assessment

Lipid measurement is a basis for studying heart health. Doctors may begin by measuring a set of numbers—total cholesterol, LDL (the so-called "bad" one), HDL (typically referred to as "good"), and triglycerides—all of which are designed to spot imbalances. Most often, these imbalances, known as dyslipidemia, signal an increased threat to heart problems. Today's advice stresses that if an individual has family history of heart disease, is overweight, or carries other risk factors, extra focus on these figures is on order. It's not only the test itself; marrying it with a look at the way a person lives can better drive personalized treatment plans. New data are fueling updated guidelines for testing lipids at just the right time. Overall, the European Society of Cardiology (ESC) has issued new guidelines for managing lipid testing across different patient groups. Generally, adults 40 years and older are urged to get tested routinely, and even younger persons with other risk factors are not excluded. ESC seems to lead clinicians into a careful, multi-dimensional approach by taking into account each patient's unique circumstances. This integration of hard science and personalized care will definitely lead to a more personalized strategy, one that scales evidence-based medicine and in-the-trenches realities equally. Following these guidelines is in fact most crucial to both better outcomes as well as minimized heart-related complications. The WHO, for instance, shows how physical exercise corresponds directly with healthier lipid profiles (Bull et al., 2020). Plain old-fashioned customs—a combination of aerobic exercise and strength training—also can significantly improve lipid profiles, reducing overall risk. Doctors are thus encouraged to include these lifestyle lessons in patient conversation, sometimes even highlighting the advantages in unconventional but riveting terms. Lastly, integrating regular lipid screening with a healthy regime of living and exercise presents an all-inclusive plan that promotes long-term cardiovascular well-being and overall wellness (Visseren et al., 2021) (Figure 11.12).

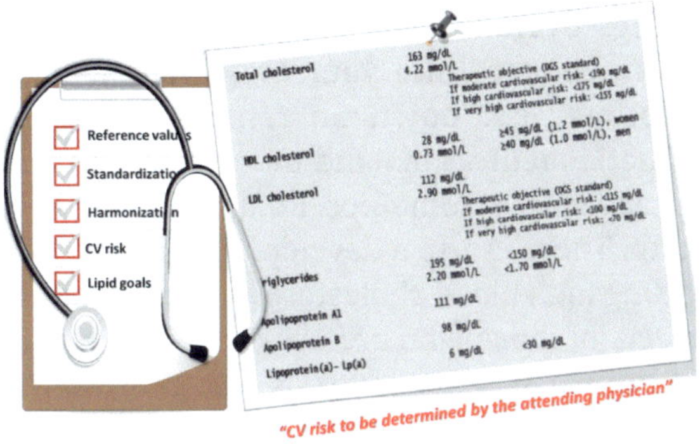

Figure 11.12. Standardization of laboratory lipid profile assessment.

Source: https://www.revportcardiol.org/pt-standardization-laboratory-lipid-profile-assessment-articulo-S0870255117302184

11.4.2. Lifestyle Modifications to Improve Lipid Profiles

Lifestyle modifications can work wonders, particularly in keeping your lipid profile in check. It may sound a tad disorganized, but changing your diet to a healthier one—less saturated fats, less trans-fat, lower cholesterol—can lower those annoying LDL levels, which are commonly referred to as the "bad" type of cholesterol. Many people do battle on a daily basis with this, and it can actually result in serious illness. A simple swap, such as adding on the fruits, vegetables, whole grains, and lean proteins, can do the trick. Some diets, like the Mediterranean diet, have been shown to decrease inflammation (a definite villain in my book) and lipid levels, especially if you throw in some exercise here and there. Getting in gear is another key part of the puzzle—no daily marathons in the gym, but 150 minutes of moderate exercise a week gets the job done. Brisk walking, biking, or playing in the pool all work to raise your HDL, which is a cleanup crew for excess cholesterol. It also helps in weight control and has your heart in a better place, lowering dangers like coronary problems. Typically, a mix of many aerobic exercises distributed throughout your week seems to make a notable impact, giving the overall body a bit more resilient and less susceptible to heart problems. Then there's the whole issue of stress and sleeping—two things that can mess with your lipid levels without even realizing it.

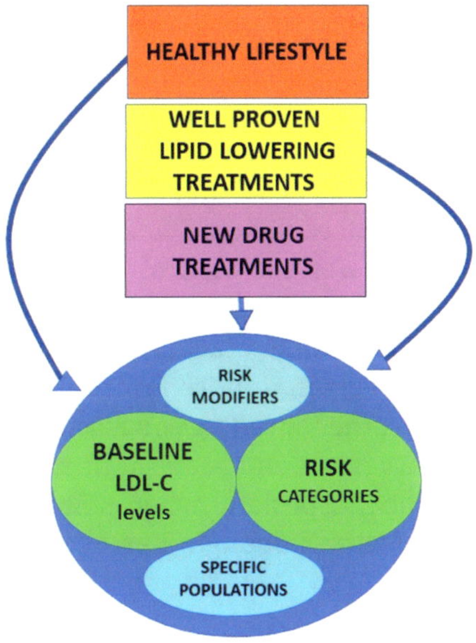

Figure 11.13. Lifestyle modifications to improve lipid profiles.

Source: https://www.escardio.org/static-file/Escardio/Medias/337_Guasti_FINAL%20FOR%20PUBLICATION_Central%20illustration_escardio-hPhotoLarge.jpg.

Chronic stress, by raising cortisol levels, can cause further fat storage and wreak havoc on your body's balance. Trying things like mindfulness, yoga, or even just deep breathing can put that tension at bay. And while we're on the topic, don't forget sleep; poor or erratic sleep patterns have been linked to not-so-great changes in lipid metabolism. A regular sleep routine—with bedtimes that aren't always perfectly on schedule—can support better overall heart and lipid health. In the end, integrating healthy eating, regular exercise, stress management (even when things get a bit hectic occasionally), and solid, consistent sleep can add up to a healthier, better-balanced life (Figure 11.13).

11.4.3. Pharmacological interventions

Medications now play an important role in controlling heart risks. Many experts have learned that the use of cholesterol-lowering drugs—statins, for instance—is helpful to lower bad cholesterol. These medications target to correct imbalances in blood fats, and therefore it seems to lower the risk of serious events like heart attack and stroke. Research tends to demonstrate that statins not only place cholesterol levels in a more favorable position but also have other advantages, such as improved lining of the vessels and reduced inflammation. This approach, especially when small lifestyle changes just aren't enough, has become quite crucial. Examining high blood pressure, more recent evidence suggests that combining natural therapies with standard medication will yield additional benefit. Some recent research has attempted to use natural products—ginger is a good example—along with standard antihypertensive medication. Consumption of ginger tea appears to lower both the upper and lower readings of blood pressure, and enhance the lipid profile—lowering total cholesterol and raising the "good" HDL cholesterol. These findings overall validate the idea that adding dietary changes into your drug treatment can sometimes cut down on reliance on totally synthetic medication, and overall, this blended strategy shows some potential for better heart health. There is also a developing challenge with tackling high blood cholesterol levels in children, especially those who are obese. Early discovery of atypical lipid profiles is far greater than important since genetic factors combined with everyday lifestyle decisions can increase future dangers. While a healthier way of life is usually the first to be suggested, doctors often come to comprehend that medication becomes inevitable when it involves safeguarding these high-risk adolescents from serious cardiovascular disease. Interestingly, recent AI advancements indicate the potential for a future in which screenings and treatments become better than ever before (Taskeen et al., 2025; Zaheer et al., 2024).

Test Your Knowledge

1. How is a lipid profile used in assessing overall cardiovascular risk?
2. What lifestyle interventions are recommended for patients with abnormal lipid levels?

11.5. Population Variability in Lipid Profiles

Learning Outcome

- Genetic factors influencing lipid levels;
- Impact of age and gender on lipid profiles;
- Ethnic and cultural differences in lipid metabolism.

Genetics, daily habits, and where people reside all become entangled to affect lipid levels we see among various groups. Divergence in food, socioeconomic status, and even the ease with which someone might have access to health care – sometimes in ways we'd not anticipate – all enter the mix to explain why lipid levels are not the same. Take, for instance, nations like India and Kyrgyzstan; studies show that people in Kyrgyzstan have higher levels of low-density lipoprotein (LDL), high-density lipoprotein (HDL), and overall cholesterol compared to Indians (Kamal et al., 2024). In most cases, awareness of such specific trends is key to designing interventions to reduce the risk for heart disease. Abnormal lipid levels, or dyslipidemia, also occur commonly in individuals who are coping with other illnesses, like serious mental illness. Research usually discovers that they are at higher risk of cardiovascular issues due to conditions like obesity, hypertension, and lack of exercise compounding each other. For example, those patients who are on medications like clozapine develop unexpected alterations in lipid profiles, necessitating follow-up visits on a regular basis to keep heart risk factors in check (Shahzad, 2024). Recognition of such group-specific problems enables clinicians to initiate targeted interventions that do not only tackle dyslipidemia but also aim to improve overall cardiac well-being, finally optimizing outcomes in risk-prone settings. Considering differences in lipid levels across populations is also a matter of gaining some control over the diverse means through which health care is addressed around the world. In certain instances, variation in public health policy, cultural notions of staying healthy, and the availability of treatments can lead to lack of consistent follow-up on lipid-lowering regimens. Areas that move towards prevention – recall routine screenings and community outreach campaigns – manage cardiovascular threats much better. Meanwhile, others, lacking such precautions, end up with worse outcomes, added to the lack of good access to quality healthcare (Kamal et al., 2024). For the most part, improved health care and education tailored to the specific needs of individual communities could quite possibly make a very serious impact on the prevalence of heart disease related to abnormal lipid profiles, and direct us towards a healthier world view.

11.5.1. Genetic Factors Influencing Lipid Levels

Learning about how our bodies process fats has taught us that genetics does indeed play a role in lipid levels. Scientists found that even small DNA tweaks—alterations to the enzymes that break down and move fats—can radically change an individual's fat profile. Take the case of the PNPLA3 gene, for example; a variation in one there has been linked to extra fat building up in the liver, which goes and derails triglyceride levels and heightens the risk of NAFLD. Gene variation like this can even put more pressure on liver cells, the very ones working in overtime mode to keep our blood fats in check. In short, if you inherit certain genetic predispositions, you may also be more susceptible to heart issues because of these imbalanced lipids. In general, knowing these gene impacts is the key to developing personalized diets and treatments that address the root causes rather than just messing around with the numbers (Mary et al., 2023). Adding fuel to the fire, a full complement of genes seems to have jobs in fat processing and storage that you would never dream. Genes such as MBOAT7 and TM6SF2 have shown to be key participants here. Just to name an example, in the TM6SF2 case, certain variants are capable of preventing the exportation of triglycerides by the liver—i.e., more fat staying on the premises. These genetics not only control overall amounts of fat but may also cause more serious liver illnesses like cirrhosis or even liver cancer (Tilg et al., 2020). When the everyday factors like diet and physical activity are completely amplified by these genetics, they can push heart disease risk to extremely divergent levels. Clearly, the whole scenario needs to incorporate genetic data into our general approach for cardiovascular care in a way that therapy becomes more tailored to each person's unique configuration. The same goes for lifestyle decisions and everyday milieu that can fortify or diminish the effects of these genetic tendencies on lipid levels and cardiac well-being. Many individuals, even if they're genetically predisposed to elevated lipids, can escape problems if they have a healthy diet and regular exercise. On the other hand, a high-fat, high-calorie diet might even intensify the most undesirable of these innate hazards, leading to the creation of imbalances in the body's fat. It's because it would seem so crucial to know which kinds of lifestyle changes can offset such built-in dangers. Some practitioners now depend on genetic screening as a component of their strategy for regulating amounts of fat and heart risk—offering a form of preventive care that is science-driven. Using both genetics and lifestyle, healthcare providers can better respond to heart care more holistically, and eventually optimize patient outcomes (Mary et al., 2023) (Figure 11.14).

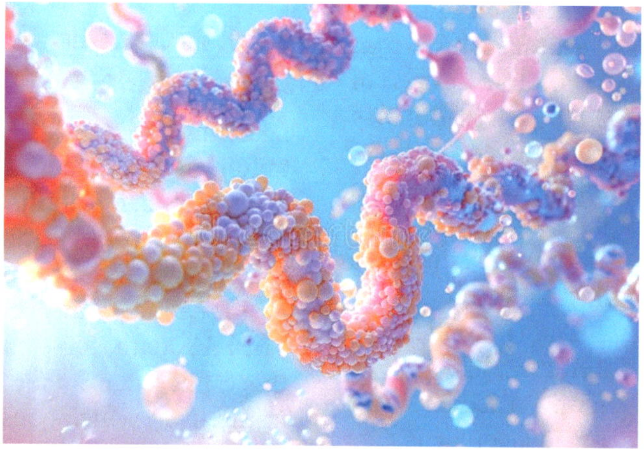

Figure 11.14. Artistic 3D representation of genetic structures influencing lipid metabolism, illustrating the molecular complexity of gene-lipid interactions and their relevance in personalized healthcare.

Source: https://external-content.duckduckgo.com/iu/?u=https%3A%2F%2Fthumbs.dreamstime.com%2Fb%2Fd-visual-explanation-genetic-factors-influencing-lipid-metabolism-their-implications-personal-health-care-332101867.jpg%3Fw%3D768&f=1&nofb=1&ipt=5be4419088b4224afd6b0d5ab3378c123dbf7d378b2c6964777558b021682655.

11.5.2. Impact of Age and Gender on Lipid Profiles

Age, sex, and the way our bodies process fats all seem to be very connected to heart health. With age, our physiology can change in subtle ways, and it can affect the way we process fats, so you might notice a different fat pattern now than you did when you were younger. You often find that overall cholesterol levels go up with age—likely because physical activity slows down and eating habits change along the way—putting some folks at extra risk for heart issues. Looking at age-adjusted data, it's clear that men and women don't follow exactly the same pattern; age mixes with gender in unique ways. For example, after menopause, the majority of women show changes in their fat compositions that can increase risks to the heart and make them more vulnerable (Apte et al., 2017). If you compare between gender differences, studies are likely to show that lipid patterns vary considerably across women and men. Women carry higher amounts of HDL cholesterol—the kind that usually protects against heart problems—during those years but when menopause comes along and hormone levels shift, that advantage can be lost. Men are more likely to produce increased triglycerides, which is a sign that the risks of heart disease might be rising. An East African study, for example, discovered that not only did women have higher chances of getting metabolic syndrome (with elevated triglycerides) but also accumulated more belly fat—a big red flag for cardiovascular risks (Motala et al., 2009). It seems like both age and gender actually determine the way these fats end up, so one-size-fits-all interventions simply won't cut it. Understanding how gender, age, and fat metabolism overlap is crucial if we're to lower heart disease in general. Acknowledging these factors may even boost our prevention and screening efforts. Take older women, for example—they experience more issues after menopause because unconstructive changes in their lipids start to reveal themselves. Public health initiatives encouraging better diet and exercise could do much to stem this here. Also, in light of how much difference in fat storage—specifically in the waist area—seems to matter, there is a need for more targeted research and interventions (Apte et al., 2017). With the exception of very few cases, by taking these complex interactions into consideration, health professionals can help people regulate their fat levels and reduce their overall cardiovascular risk (Figure 11.15).

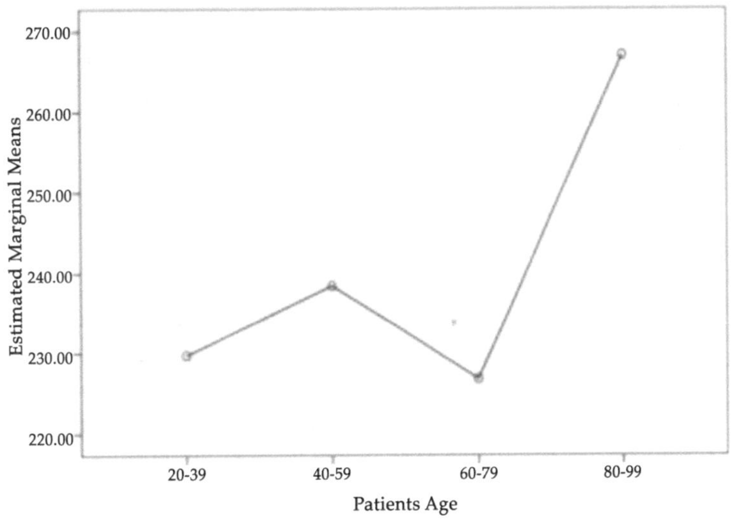

Figure 11.15. Effect of age on lipid profile.

Source: https://www.researchgate.net/profile/Murwan-Sabahelkhier/publication/310314505/figure/fig3/AS:429019528208386@1479297634211/Figure9-9-Effect-of-age-on-lipid-profile-for-Figure-10-Effect-of-gender-on-lipid.png.

11.5.3. Ethnic and Cultural Differences in Lipid Metabolism

Different populations metabolize fat differently, and that can indeed make a significant difference in how susceptible an individual is to heart disease. Genetics has a way of affecting lipid processing, so people from one background may store and use fats in a different manner than others. For example, some populations have an unusual reaction to some dietary fats, and therefore the typical lipid management strategies won't work equally well for everyone. It is a reminder that even tiny variations in how metabolism occurs might necessitate a more customized strategy for the prevention and treatment of heart disease—again, frequently by listening to cultural nuances. Lifestyle factors also mix into this picture, with diet and exercise taking center stage. Many communities pass down eating habits over generations, which in turn shapes what ends up on our plates. Certain persons would eat diets with high levels of saturated fats and refined carbs that tend to increase LDL levels, while others like to have lots of whole grain, fruits, and vegetables on their plates—possibly giving them a bit of a heart-health benefit. When diet merges with genetic traits, certain groups are more vulnerable to diseases like dyslipidemia. All in all, it appears that dietary changes in familiar cultural habits could well help reduce heart risks. And then there is the whole matter of day-to-day circumstances that affect health. Accessibility to quality medical care, proper education on keeping a healthy heart, and even financial hardship can all affect peoples' capacity to manage lipids. In other communities, folks simply don't know they are at risk because they don't get enough information or timely care. Local programs and community health initiatives—sometimes designed with the culture in mind—are what truly get people to take charge of their heart health. In the end, grappling with this intricate mix of genetics, daily habits, and social factors is the key to closing the heart health gap between ethnically diverse groups.

Test Your Knowledge

1. How do genetic factors influence lipid levels among different populations?
2. What role do diet and lifestyle play in population differences in lipid profiles?

11.6. Emerging Research and Trends

Learning Outcome

- New biomarkers for cardiovascular risk;
- Advances in lipid-lowering therapies;
- The role of inflammation in lipid metabolism.

Lipid testing has finally turned the corner in recent times, with new markers coming on to sort out heart risks in ways older tests simply cannot. Researchers noticed that standard lipid tests might be lacking, so they set about studying such things as non-HDL cholesterol, ApoB, and lipoprotein(a) [Lp(a)] as more precise measures of cardiovascular health. More recent studies even show—generally speaking—that these less common markers are better at distinguishing risk, especially among those with metabolic disorders. It seems the older tests don't predict as accurately as they should, and that is prompting researchers to look into these newer markers (Mehmood et al., 2023). All this evidence points to us combining old tests with these new markers, which could give us more personalized care when dealing with heart risks. Along with these new biomarkers, measures like lipidomic profiling are also on the rise in heart research. New high-throughput devices enable scientists to plot complex lipid profiles without concern for just one factor. This approach offers a wider, close-to-shocking, view of how lipids contribute to heart disease as well as other diseases such as obesity, diabetes, and atherosclerosis. Through vast databases obtained from online sites like PubMed, scientists are identifying principal lipid–protein interactions that illuminate the mechanisms of cardiovascular disease (Anyaegbunam et al., 2023). In a way, this shift in strategy is nudging us toward a gentler, more subtle view of lipid metabolism that may eventually guide more specific treatment. With further advancement of the lipid sciences, incorporating these trends into everyday clinical practice remains necessary. Unraveling the intricate dance among different lipids and what they mean for heart disease is actually transforming how doctors evaluate risk. For example, research on lowering LDL cholesterol with novel drugs like PCSK9 inhibitors—and even omega-3 fatty acids—illustrates practical approaches these emerging results are influencing treatment practices (Mehmood et al., 2023). The continued in-depth investigation of lipid profiles, in addition to technological advancements, assures us that managing cardiovascular risk today is an interdisciplinary effort. In the long run, these changes could open up the way to care that is more personalized, combining both the traditional and new indicators to better judge heart health.

11.6.1. New Biomarkers for Cardiovascular Risk

Cardiovascular risk screening remains a highly challenging area, which has encouraged researchers to search for novel biomarkers that provide us with a better perception of lipid profiles. Traditional tests—those basic lipid profiles—are often not sufficient to predict heart complications, and this has led researchers to look at other indicators. One such idea is to look at the apolipoprotein ratio, specifically ApoB and ApoA1, to shed further light on heart hazards linked with lipoproteins. ApoB generally tracks the number of harmful, atherogenic particles, while ApoA1 plays a role in helping high-density lipoprotein (HDL) to do its job. Double consideration here gives a better idea about a person's potential for the onset of coronary heart disease, particularly since rising ApoB levels indicate more floating low-density lipoprotein (LDL) with atherogenetic potential. In the majority of cases, the inclusion of these markers in standard clinical practice would more accurately refine risk stratification and lead to therapy regimens that more precisely predict an individual's personalized lipid metabolism (Mary et al., 2023). Emerging evidence also suggests that NAFLD-associated markers might be the solution to filling out our portrait of cardiovascular risk. Inflammation in NAFLD is, in most cases, associated with atherosclerosis as well as more broad heart disease. For instance, non-invasive fibrosis tests can yield more information about cardiovascular health—even if it looks like a sudden plot twist. Being able to identify patients with high-risk NASH (those with biopsy-proven nonalcoholic steatohepatitis and significant fibrosis) enables medical practitioners to make more informed estimates about the interconnectedness of liver problems and heart risk. This multidimensional, multilayered approach really emphasizes the need to detect metabolic dysregulation, which is often associated with unusual lipid profiles and heightened cardiovascular risk (Mary et al., 2023). Lipidomic profiling is now occupying center stage for the estimation of heart risk in one more step towards personalized care. Rather than using only a handful of traditional markers, this method investigates the entire lipidome—considering various lipid subclasses and their functions in unprecedented depth. It is able to identify certain lipid species that are involved in inflammation and even influence plaque stability, thereby increasing our ability to forecast adverse cardiac events. Incorporating these measures with conventional biomarkers offers a better overall evaluation of cardiovascular well-being, allowing for the tailoring of interventions targeted to an individual patient's lipid profile. Ultimately, the inclusion of these advanced markers into routine clinical practice may usher in the use of more subtle risk assessments and more tailored treatments (Muscella et al., 2020) (Figure 11.16).

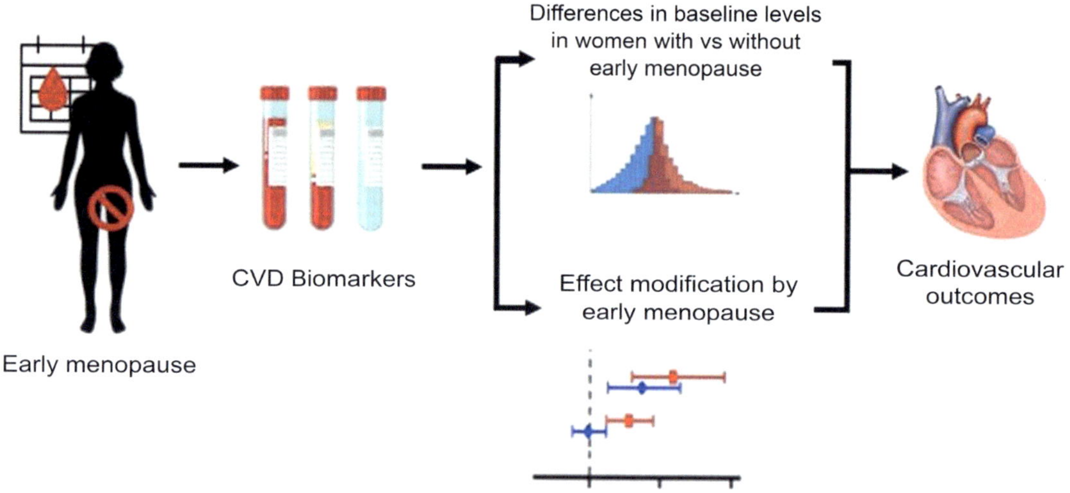

Figure 11.16. New biomarkers for cardiovascular risk.

Source: https://external-content.duckduckgo.com/iu/?u=https%3A%2F%2Fwww.ahajournals.org%2Fcms%2Fasset%2F3d509fe1-ea6f-416c-aaba-219e9d04d666%2Fjah38637-fig-0003.png&f=1&nofb=1&ipt=3937f80417f79ef83b82f8b0a16a4d3bfa182708b04a6dd28f20cb3a7fc65d5f.

11.6.2. Advances in Lipid-Lowering Therapies

Lipid-lowering drugs have accomplished this quietly in flipping the script on heart risk management, especially for patients at increased risk for atherosclerosis. Statins emerged and set the bar higher for reducing LDL cholesterol and mitigating overall cardiovascular issues. They've provided real-world benefits—reducing major adverse cardiovascular events (MACEs) and reducing mortality in patients with challenging lipid profiles and coronary artery disease (CAD). These drugs, in effect serving as the groundwork in treatment, set the stage for others like ezetimibe; though its impact is in a way narrow in scope, adding to statin treatment with it does lower risks. This blend of approaches kind of showcases how optimizing treatments to individual demand can result in better results when it comes to managing lipid profiles. More recent treatments are starting to gain notice, especially for familial hypercholesterolemia or individuals who just don't respond to the standard meds. PCSK9 inhibitors are one such example, and they can reduce LDL levels way below what statins alone usually achieve. In one recent patient study on individuals with homozygous familial hypercholesterolemia, these drugs knocked the LDL levels way down, and it seems to have a significant impact on long-term heart outcomes. A multi-med approach seems to be finally gaining traction as a way to aim for those lipid targets—clinical practice is shifting away from one-size-fits-all approaches to complicated dyslipidemias. The whole specialty of lipid management is moving, so further research and continued messing around with treatment modalities is clearly indicated.

More advanced lipid therapies are not all about lowering cholesterol; they could well revolutionize the overall heart risk profile in patients already at risk. Future options like bempedoic acid and inclisiran are the focus now, and preliminary results are that they induce improved lipid profiles and reduced cardiovascular events. Of course, long-standing therapies like statins and PCSK9 inhibitors have been the workhorses for decades, but these new agents are offering more choices for managing patients. As treatment of diabetic dyslipidemia continues to advance as well, more and more effort is being focused on how all these treatments interact on cardiovascular health overall. Clinical trials persist and will soon offer valuable information, eventually unraveling the long-term benefit of intensive lowering of lipids—especially in patients with concurrent conditions like diabetes (Erasmo et al., 2024; Velidakis et al., 2024) (Figure 11.17).

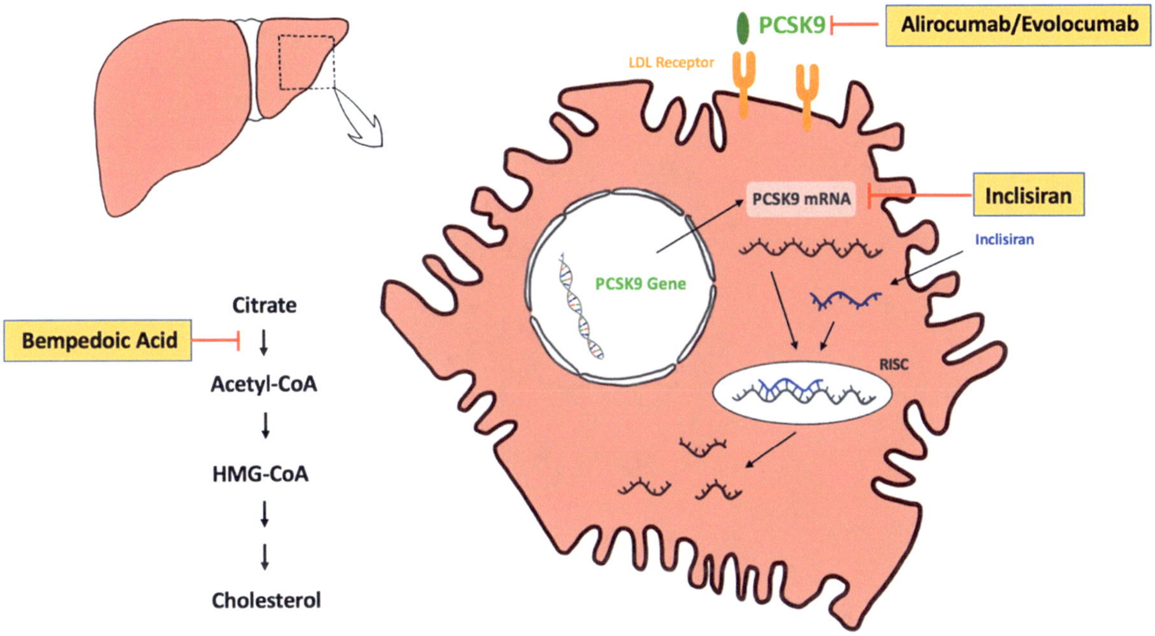

Figure 11.17. New treatment targets and innovative lipid-lowering.

Source: https://www.mdpi.com/biomedicines/biomedicines-10-00970/article_deploy/html/images/biomedicines-10-00970-g001.png.

11.6.3. The Role of Inflammation in Lipid Metabolism

Chronic inflammation changes the way our bodies process fats – and that can have very bad consequences for heart health. When the body flares up, it prefers to produce a whole bunch of pro-inflammatory signals that mess with the usual fat profiles. High levels of these signals seem to bump excess free fatty acids out of the way and alter the function of lipoproteins, typically causing dyslipidemia. In diseases like rheumatoid arthritis, not only does this systemic inflammation speed up fat oxidation, but it also seems to make lipoproteins more prone to be in the position to cause plaque formation, thus making them susceptible to cardiovascular complications. All of this can explain why chronic inflammatory diseases induce irregularities in fat metabolism and cause more heart attacks for those who have it. Sometimes, the use of therapies like immunosuppressive therapy might address these metabolic flaws and lessen heart risk (Ancuta et al., 2018). Inflammation's function in fats does not only involve deranging cholesterol concentration – it also involves how fat is stored and how it engages with the body's larger inflammatory systems. For example, obesity—traditionally considered a condition of low-grade inflammation—has been linked to changes in fat storage and enhanced inflammatory signals released by adipose tissue. These extra signals can serve to potentiate insulin resistance, making management of the fat even more challenging and putting individuals at a heightened risk for type 2 diabetes and cardiovascular disease. Clearly, this link points to treatment with a multi-faceted approach to both managing inflammation and fat levels. With evidence piling up that couples increased inflammatory markers with poorer fat profiles, a balanced solution that incorporates dietary change and regular exercise is the solution—not just for fat management, but also for reducing the inflammatory heart risks (Agarwal et al., 2018).

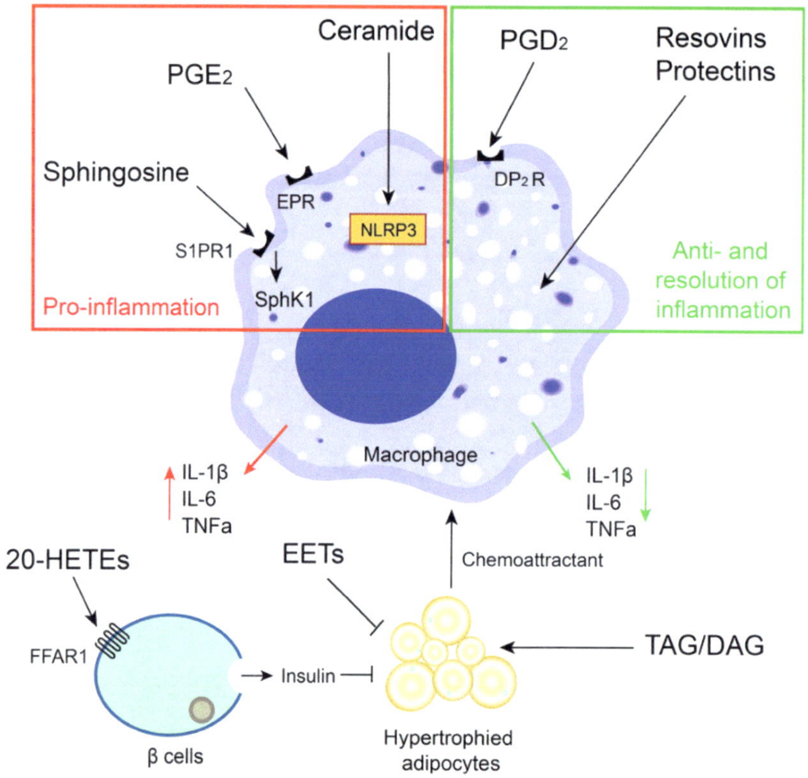

Figure 11.18. Lipid metabolism in inflammation.

Source: https://pubs.rsc.org/image/article/2018/AN/c8an01046c/c8an01046c-f4_hi-res.gif.

The dialogue between fat metabolism and inflammation really brings into perspective how much more important it is to take cardiovascular risk factors into account more broadly and comprehensively, especially for people who have ongoing inflammation. Ongoing studies are finally starting to dissect the ways in which inflammation can result in changes to fat behavior, indicating there may be targets to treat both issues at once. For instance, some anti-inflammatory medications have shown promise by helping to increase fat profiles and even inhibit the natural inflammatory processes. And then there's lifestyle change—such as adopting an anti-inflammatory diet plan and staying consistently active—whose effect on the way the body metabolizes fats can be substantial.

The more that scientists discover about these interacting pathways, the more it becomes clear that effective treatment of heart risk requires treating both inflammation and fat metabolism as key, interlinked features of treatment (Ancuta et al., 2018) (Figure 11.18).

Test Your Knowledge

1. What new biomarkers beyond traditional lipids are being studied for cardiovascular risk assessment?
2. How is personalized medicine influencing lipid management strategies?

Summary

Exploring the connection between lipid levels and heart problems reveals a multitude of intricacies that call for a more personalized approach to heart health. Research has a tendency to determine that dyslipidemia occurs quite often in groups like kidney transplant patients—suggesting our usual ways of measuring heart risk are missing some pertinent detail. For example, one paper pointed out that even though dyslipidemia was very common among such patients, it was not very strongly related to such classic issues as high blood pressure and diabetes (Ali et al., 2025). That means that models like the Framingham Risk Score may not represent all aspects of heart risk for various individuals. Clearly, personalized lipid management based on risk factors is the key if we are to improve outcomes after transplants as well as overall heart health. When you put metabolic risk and cardiovascular risk together, it's obvious that what we require is a system where all of that comes together. Evidence in individuals with type 2 diabetes, for instance, is that when metabolic complications occur—think high HbA1C, dyslipidemia, and elevated inflammatory markers (Kanagala et al., 2024)—they usually are accompanied by cardiovascular control problems in the body. In most cases, heart risk is not simply a matter of lipids; it's also driven by how the body processes metabolism and inflammation. Therefore, investment in fixing these metabolic glitches is truly a requirement, especially for patients who are battling diabetes. By focusing on metabolic equilibrium as well as lipid profiles, physicians can design care plans that not only nicely cover all the bases but enhance cardiovascular outcomes. Finally, the growing body of evidence compels us to rethink our conventional way of quantifying heart risk. It happens that our conventional checks may lose some significant risk bits, especially in populations with distinctive health histories. And the finding that dyslipidemia does not always correlate with traditional risk factors introduces an intriguing possibility for researchers and clinicians alike—it's the opportunity to refine the way they stratify individuals by risk. If we start adding more varied mixes of metabolic and inflammation markers to these tests, we will potentially have a more comprehensive, realistic sense of worldwide heart risk. It would be a new way of thinking that would make prevention and control potentially more effective, reminding us that our tools must keep pace with the refined, real-world demands of cardiovascular management.

Cardiovascular health is often hanging in the balance on something as picky as the ratio of fats in your bloodstream. Take LDL, HDL, and triglycerides, for example—each plays its own role within the grand scheme. Having too much LDL has a tendency to lay the groundwork for unwanted plaque buildup in the arteries, while having lots of HDL has a tendency to offer some protection. When you combine other medical issues or even your personal family history, it just makes clear the way that a full check-up of your lipid levels can be significant. Regular tests and some well-thought-out adjustments in lifestyle or treatment can really cut the risk of future heart issues down quite considerably. Prevention-wise, managing these lipid numbers is as much a matter of being smart as it is science. These and other organizations like the European Society of Cardiology and the European Atherosclerosis Society publish guidelines that, in large measure, doctors try to tailor to each patient's unique situation. On a general level, the approach is to combine new scientific information with a considered assessment of individual needs, even as the process can get a little dotty at times. It also fares better where these recommendations are balanced by frequent updates from public health officials (François et al., 2019). Beyond individual therapy, screening for lipid levels has the potential to cascade to a healthier-for-all community impact. With cardiovascular disease on the rise, extended screening and targeted intervention initiatives may make a tangible difference for public health. Educating people about healthier food options, some increase in physical exercise, and adherence to their prescription routines instills a culture where prevention is natural. And when community outreach brings up the issue of how lipid levels might even be related to conditions such as dementia, it invokes the need for health measures addressing both cardiovascular and long-term brain well-being (Livingston et al., 2020).

KEY TERMS FROM THIS CHAPTER

Apolipoprotein A1 (ApoA1)
Apolipoproteins
Cardiovascular disease (CVD)
Coronary artery disease (CAD)
High sensitivity C-reactive protein
LDL/HDL ratio
Low-density lipoprotein (LDL)
Plaque formation
Statins
Total cholesterol/HDL ratio
Apolipoprotein B (ApoB)
Atherosclerosis
Cholesterol-lowering drugs
Fasting lipid profile
High-density lipoprotein (HDL)
Lipoprotein(a)
Non-HDL cholesterol
Risk factors for CVD
Total cholesterol
Triglycerides

Critical Thinking Questions

1. **Which of the following components of a lipid profile is most commonly associated with an increased risk of cardiovascular disease?**
   a. High-density lipoprotein (HDL)
   b. Low-density lipoprotein (LDL)
   c. Triglycerides
   d. Total cholesterol
2. **What is the desirable level of total cholesterol according to most guidelines for cardiovascular risk management?**
   a. Less than 240 mg/dL
   b. Less than 200 mg/dL
   c. Less than 100 mg/dL
   d. Less than 150 mg/dL
3. **Which of the following lipid profile components is considered "good cholesterol" and is protective against cardiovascular diseases?**
   a. LDL
   b. HDL
   c. Triglycerides
   d. Very low-density lipoprotein (VLDL)
4. **A high level of triglycerides in the blood is most strongly associated with which of the following?**
   a. Increased risk of diabetes
   b. Increased risk of cardiovascular disease
   c. Decreased risk of cardiovascular disease
   d. No association with cardiovascular disease
5. **What is the role of LDL cholesterol in cardiovascular disease development?**
   a. It helps to remove excess cholesterol from arteries.
   b. It transports cholesterol to cells for energy use.
   c. It contributes to the formation of plaques in the arteries.
   d. It is a major anti-inflammatory agent in the blood.

Answers to Critical Thinking Questions

1. (b); 2. (b); 3. (b); 4. (b); 5. (c)

Short Answer Questions

1. What are the key components of a lipid profile?
2. How is total cholesterol calculated, and what are the desirable levels for adults?
3. What is the role of low-density lipoprotein (LDL) cholesterol in cardiovascular risk?
4. What does high-density lipoprotein (HDL) cholesterol indicate, and why is it considered "good" cholesterol?
5. How does an elevated LDL cholesterol level contribute to the development of atherosclerosis?
6. What is the atherogenic index of plasma (AIP), and how does it relate to cardiovascular risk?

References

1. Abebe, M., Abebe, S. M., Alemu, A., Baynes, H. W., et al. (2017). Correlation between serum lipid profile with anthropometric and clinical variables in patients with type 2 diabetes mellitus. https://core.ac.uk/download/478439415.pdf (accessed on 1st July 2025).
2. Agarwal, S., Gangaram, D., & Saleem, M. (2018). Periodontitis in patients with type 2 diabetes mellitus. https://core.ac.uk/download/215353402.pdf (accessed on 1st July 2025).
3. Ali, M., Prodhan, M. J. A., Salauddin, S. M., Mukerrama, S. M., & Al-Amin, M. (2025). Association of dyslipidemia with traditional cardiovascular risk factors and Framingham risk scoring. *Saudi Journal of Medical and Pharmaceutical Sciences*. https://www.semanticscholar.org/paper/0f8b888fac28c782dbb434cee51910a902c9cc78 (accessed on 1st July 2025).
4. Ancuta, C., Ancuta, E., & Mihailov, C. (2018). Cardiovascular safety of anti-TNF and non-TNF biological therapy in patients with rheumatoid arthritis. https://core.ac.uk/download/322437067.pdf (accessed on 1st July 2025).
5. Andrew, N., Chokkalingam, M., Niren, S., Raj, R., et al. (2024). Influence of lipid profile and somatotype on aerobic capacity in athletes. https://core.ac.uk/download/640070061.pdf (accessed on 1st July 2025).
6. Anyaegbunam, U. A., More, P., Fontaine, J. F., ten Cate, V., Bauer, K., Distler, U., Araldi, E., et al. (2023). A systematic review of lipid-focused cardiovascular disease research: Trends and opportunities. *Current Issues in Molecular Biology, 45*, 9904–9916. https://www.semanticscholar.org/paper/e19ad9bf9d1080d47bd9d8fa34fb726c4de0c75f (accessed on 1st July 2025).
7. Apte, R. S., Chee, M. L., Cheng, C. Y., Fan, Q., et al. (2017). Plasma lipoprotein subfraction concentrations are associated with lipid metabolism and age-related macular degeneration. https://core.ac.uk/download/129070096.pdf (accessed on 1st July 2025).
8. Bull, F., Al-Ansari, S. S., Biddle, S., Borodulin, K., Buman, M. P., Cardon, G., Carty, C., et al. (2020). World Health Organization 2020 guidelines on physical activity and sedentary behavior. *British Journal of Sports Medicine, 54*, 1451–1462. https://doi.org/10.1136/bjsports-2020-102955 (accessed on 1st July 2025).
9. Cavero-Redondo, I., Saz-Lara, A., Martínez-García, I., Otero-Luis, I., & Martínez-Rodrigo, A. (2024). Validation of an early vascular aging construct model for comprehensive cardiovascular risk assessment using external risk indicators for improved clinical utility: Data from the EVasCu study. *Cardiovascular Diabetology, 23*. https://www.semanticscholar.org/paper/809047a2c177ad9f1919f1ab082610cd5751a84a (accessed on 1st July 2025).
10. Chait, A., & den Hartigh, L. J. (2020). Adipose tissue distribution, inflammation and its metabolic consequences, including diabetes and cardiovascular disease. *Frontiers in Cardiovascular Medicine, 7*. https://doi.org/10.3389/fcvm.2020.00022 (accessed on 1st July 2025).
11. D'Erasmo, L., Bini, S., Casula, M., Gazzotti, M., Bertolini, S., Calandra, S., Tarugi, P., et al. (2024). Contemporary lipid-lowering management and risk of cardiovascular events in homozygous familial hypercholesterolaemia: Insights from the Italian LIPIGEN Registry. *European Journal of Preventive Cardiology*. https://www.semanticscholar.org/paper/ecd2d4d52c8ee8d3493d731d2bab7eb75fa035b0 (accessed on 1st July 2025).
12. Dewi, N. L. M. N. (2025). Dual impact analysis of *GSTT1* polymorphisms on the metformin

response and cardiovascular risk: A novel integrated approach in type 2 diabetes mellitus management. *Svāsthya: Trends in General Medicine and Public Health*. https://www.semanticscholar.org/paper/18fef9063de43590bd8a0f0f4417c84615b3b38d (accessed on 1st July 2025).

13. Dibaba, D. T. (2019). Effect of vitamin D supplementation on serum lipid profiles: A systematic review and meta-analysis. *Nutrition Reviews, 77*, 890–902. https://doi.org/10.1093/nutrit/nuz037 (accessed on 1st July 2025).

14. Eliopoulos, A. G., Gkouskou, K., Tsioufis, K., & Sanoudou, D. (2025). A perspective on intermittent fasting and cardiovascular risk in the era of obesity pharmacotherapy. *Frontiers in Nutrition, 12*. https://www.semanticscholar.org/paper/a80a48b05977112653135f156e8cbd83c9c0c293 (accessed on 1st July 2025).

15. Elvita, A., Desmawati, D., & Lipoeto, N. I. (2025). The role of adiponectin in lipid profile of adults with obesity: Implications for cardiovascular health. *World Journal of Advanced Research and Reviews*. https://www.semanticscholar.org/paper/ac505388b14a7a39dec8c768151fdfddfe88cbca (accessed on 1st July 2025).

16. Esmaeili, F., Tohidi, M., Khalili, D., Valizadeh, M., Momeni Moghaddam, A., Abdi, A., Azizi, F., et al. (2024). Trajectories of lipid profile during adolescence and risk of subclinical atherosclerosis in early adulthood: A two-decade population-based study. *European Heart Journal*. https://www.semanticscholar.org/paper/56cf499ad66007400696dc243d093e884a74d48d (accessed on 1st July 2025).

17. Feigin, V. L., Stark, B., Johnson, C. O., Roth, G. A., Bisignano, C., Gebreheat, G., Abbasifard, M., et al. (2021). Global, regional, and national burden of stroke and its risk factors, 1990–2019: A systematic analysis for the Global Burden of Disease Study 2019. *The Lancet Neurology, 20*, 795–820. https://doi.org/10.1016/s1474-4422(21)00252-0 (accessed on 1st July 2025).

18. Gaddi, A. V. (2009). Non pharmacological control of plasma cholesterol. https://core.ac.uk/download/11167892.pdf (accessed on 1st July 2025).

19. Galicia-García, U., Benito-Vicente, A., Jebari, S., Larrea-Sebal, A., Siddiqi, H., Uribe, K. B., Ostolaza, H., et al. (2020). Pathophysiology of type 2 diabetes mellitus. *International Journal of Molecular Sciences, 21*, 6275–6275. https://doi.org/10.3390/ijms21176275 (accessed on 1st July 2025).

20. Hany, M., Demerdash, H. M., Abouelnasr, A. A., Agayby, A., Ibrahim, M., Arida, R. E., & Torensma, B. (2024). Relationship between weight loss, changes in serum hs-CRP levels and apo A-1 lipoprotein, and high-density lipoprotein-cholesterol ratios as predictors for improved cardiovascular risk factors after laparoscopic sleeve gastrectomy. *Obesity Surgery, 34*, 3401–3411. https://www.semanticscholar.org/paper/df243a494d978782b70b0b9d9b9c45cd7aa68fcd (accessed on 1st July 2025).

21. Harreiter, J., Mendoza, L. C., Simmons, D., Desoye, G., Devlieger, R., Galjaard, S., Damm, P., et al. (2022). Vitamin D3 supplementation in overweight/obese pregnant women: No effects on the maternal or fetal lipid profile and body fat distribution—A secondary analysis of the multicentric, randomized, controlled vitamin D and lifestyle for gestational diabetes prevention trial (DALI). *Nutrients, 14*. https://www.semanticscholar.org/paper/608a548d61479979999751e491b2c15ea7caf85f (accessed on 1st July 2025).

22. Holme, I., Cater, N., Faergeman, O., Kastelein, J., Olsson, A., Tikkanen, M., Lytken Larsen,

M., et al. (2008). Lipoprotein predictors of cardiovascular events in statin-treated patients with coronary heart disease: Insights from the Incremental Decrease in End-points through Aggressive Lipid-lowering Trial (IDEAL). *Annals of Medicine, 40*, 456–464. https://www.semanticscholar.org/paper/912b34a31ffcb3ee682086d39b3930f85255631c (accessed on 1st July 2025).

23. Imbalzano, E., Ilardi, F., Orlando, L., Pintaudi, B., Savarese, G., & Rosano, G. (2023). The efficacy of PCSK9 inhibitors on major cardiovascular events and lipid profile in patients with diabetes: A systematic review and meta-analysis of randomized controlled trials. *European Heart Journal. Cardiovascular Pharmacotherapy*. https://www.semanticscholar.org/paper/3913235a6120b0ae5c1d97eca4f11abfea329092 (accessed on 1st July 2025).

24. Kanagala, A., & Harsoda, J. M. (2024). Metabolic dysregulation and its multifaceted impact on cardiovascular autonomic control in type 2 diabetes mellitus: Insights from comprehensive assessment. *Cureus, 16*. https://www.semanticscholar.org/paper/607e1c559a2b9f8643d5a808629d583f57d15cb1 (accessed on 1st July 2025).

25. Kelly, K., Curley, M., & Webber, A. (2025). Combining clinician skills, patient empowerment and AI tools to predict and prevent cardiovascular risk factors and events: A case study. *International Journal of Integrated Care*. https://www.semanticscholar.org/paper/8b29dafe63ca9dc3d242684c568ea0414f356699 (accessed on 1st July 2025).

26. Kubalová, K., Porvazník, I., Majherová, M., Demková, L., Piotrowska, A., & Mydlárová Blaščáková, M. (2025). Lipid levels and atherogenic indices as important predictive parameters in the assessment of cardiovascular risk in patients with pulmonary tuberculosis—Slovak pilot study. *Medicina, 61*. https://www.semanticscholar.org/paper/10f6152987bab4760f89b37f2913f647e491c75d (accessed on 1st July 2025).

27. Livingston, G., Huntley, J., Sommerlad, A., Ames, D., Ballard, C., Banerjee, S., Brayne, C., et al. (2020). Dementia prevention, intervention, and care: 2020 report of the Lancet Commission. *The Lancet, 396*, 413–446. https://doi.org/10.1016/s0140-6736(20)30367-6 (accessed on 1st July 2025).

28. Mach, F., Baigent, C., Catapano, A. L., Koskinas, K. C., Casula, M., Badimón, L., Chapman, M. J., et al. (2019). 2019 ESC/EAS guidelines for the management of dyslipidemias: Lipid modification to reduce cardiovascular risk. *European Heart Journal, 41*, 111–188. https://doi.org/10.1093/eurheartj/ehz455 (accessed on 1st July 2025).

29. Mehmood, A., Hafeez, S., Wassan, S. M., Kadir, S., Akram, S., & Shah, T. Z. (2023). Evaluation of lipid profile alterations for early diagnosis and therapeutic management of cardiovascular and metabolic disorders. *Pakistan Journal of Medical and Health Sciences*. https://www.semanticscholar.org/paper/3f5bdfed02b659d175e847c41977d4ebb8a9e47d (accessed on 1st July 2025).

30. Motala, A. A., Swai, A. B., Perry, A. C., Muhihi, A., Walker, A. R., Filmer, D., Hu, D., et al. (2009). Gender-related differences in the prevalence of cardiovascular disease risk factors and their correlates in urban Tanzania. https://core.ac.uk/download/pdf/11307378.pdf (accessed on 1st July 2025).

31. Muscella, A., Stefàno, E., & Marsigliante, S. (2020). The effects of exercise training on lipid metabolism and coronary heart disease. *AJP Heart and Circulatory Physiology, 319*, H76–H88. https://doi.org/10.1152/ajpheart.00708.2019 (accessed on 1st July 2025).

32. Oganija, K. Y., Badmos, A. H. A., Alli, O. O., & Toye, A. A. (2024). Nutrigenetic effect of *Centella asiatica* and *Capsicum annum* on body weight and cardiovascular risk in chickens. *Nigerian Journal of Animal Production.* https://www.semanticscholar.org/paper/26245f57985211a74a6b7d1ea9d2e0e3141ab73d (accessed on 1st July 2025).

33. Parikh, R., Chougule, N., Deore, R., Suryawanshi, S., G, G., Cleetus, N., & Revankar, S. (2024). Assessment of lipid profile and its correlation with ASCVD risk in the general population. *World Journal of Advanced Research and Reviews.* https://www.semanticscholar.org/paper/4b06b177def3c50bbd02d7415f9c3820d7416c46 (accessed on 1st July 2025).

34. Qiu, Z., Huang, E. Y. Z., Li, Y., Xiao, Y., Fu, Y., Du, J., & Kan, J. (2024). Beneficial effects of time-restricted fasting on cardiovascular disease risk factors: A meta-analysis. *BMC Cardiovascular Disorders, 24.* https://www.semanticscholar.org/paper/67142f2dd1cc06ba91ccf0137a266963c1ce239a (accessed on 1st July 2025).

35. Rinella, M. E., Neuschwander-Tetri, B. A., Siddiqui, M. S., Abdelmalek, M. F., Caldwell, S. H., Barb, D., Kleiner, D. E., et al. (2023). AASLD practice guidance on the clinical assessment and management of nonalcoholic fatty liver disease. *Hepatology, 77,* 1797–1835. https://doi.org/10.1097/hep.0000000000000323 (accessed on 1st July 2025).

36. Sam, A., Mohideen, A. B. K., Buhari, M. A. S., Ramakrishnan, K., & Haritha, S. P. (2024). Dual-energy computed tomography-guided assessment of visceral adiposity and its correlation with lipid function test: A retrospective study. *Cureus, 16.* https://www.semanticscholar.org/paper/adb86138db396c0b664ff312b1252a762a930f51 (accessed on 1st July 2025).

37. Shahzad, A. (2024). Lipid profile and cardiovascular risk monitoring in patients on clozapine–An audit at a community mental health resource center in Scotland. *BJPsych Open, 10,* S260–S261. https://www.semanticscholar.org/paper/18fa42d1c572c4792daab0ec2aa860369f5324ae (accessed on 1st July 2025).

38. Sharifi-Rad, M., Kumar, N. V. A., Zucca, P., Varoni, E. M., Dini, L., Panzarini, E., Rajković, J., et al. (2020). Lifestyle, oxidative stress, and antioxidants: Back and forth in the pathophysiology of chronic diseases. *Frontiers in Physiology, 11.* https://doi.org/10.3389/fphys.2020.00694 (accessed on 1st July 2025).

39. Sharma, K. H., Mohan, S., Shah, S., Konat, A., Shah, K., Mehta, S., Tavethia, J. J., et al. (2024). Prevalence of traditional cardiovascular risk factors in high-risk Kyrgyzstan population as compared to Indians – An Indo-Kyrgyz cardiometabolic study. *Journal of Family Medicine and Primary Care, 13,* 5621–5625. https://www.semanticscholar.org/paper/43490b1ddf5514b3baf50703e92b97a56b18215d (accessed on 1st July 2025).

40. Tabas, I., & Lichtman, A. H. (2017). Monocyte-macrophages and T cells in atherosclerosis. *Immunity, 47,* 621–634. https://doi.org/10.1016/j.immuni.2017.09.008 (accessed on 1st July 2025).

41. Taskeen, S., Hafeez, M. A., & Ikram, I. (2025). Investigating the role of ginger tea ORAC value in hypertension management. *Insights–Journal of Health and Rehabilitation.* https://www.semanticscholar.org/paper/4e9200724a68c3f5f68603f9be7c25b88660d8cf (accessed on 1st July 2025).

42. Tilg, H., Adolph, T. E., & Moschen, A. R. (2020). Multiple parallel hits hypothesis in nonalcoholic fatty liver disease: Revisited after a decade. *Hepatology, 73,* 833–842. https://doi.org/10.1002/hep.31518 (accessed on 1st July 2025).

43. Toh, D. W. K., Zhou, H., Cazenave-Gassiot, A., Choi, H., Burla, B., Bendt, A. K., Wenk, M., et al. (2024). Effects of wolfberry (*Lycium barbarum*) consumption on the human plasma lipidome and its association with cardiovascular disease risk factors: A randomized controlled trial of middle-aged and older adults. *Frontiers in Nutrition, 11*. https://www.semanticscholar.org/paper/5606c72ccf1472c9d391906c2b624bfb279f7a10 (accessed on 1st July 2025).

44. Torija, M. J. C., Caballero, M. Á. C., Alija, M. J. C., García Villanueva, M. J., et al. (2020). Changes in lipid profile, body weight variables and cardiovascular risk in obese patients undergoing one-anastomosis gastric bypass. https://core.ac.uk/download/560815060.pdf (accessed on 1st July 2025).

45. Velidakis, N., Stachteas, P., Gkougkoudi, E., Papadopoulos, C., & Kadoglou, N. (2024). Classical and novel lipid-lowering therapies for diabetic patients with established coronary artery disease or high risk of coronary artery disease—A narrative clinical review. *Pharmaceuticals, 17*. https://www.semanticscholar.org/paper/0e1a89b2076d0db4a45402c2bb765734603 7f908 (accessed on 1st July 2025).

46. Visseren, F. L. J., Mach, F., Smulders, Y. M., Carballo, D., Koskinas, K. C., Bäck, M., Bénétos, A., et al. (2021). 2021 ESC guidelines on cardiovascular disease prevention in clinical practice. *European Heart Journal, 42*, 3227–3337. https://doi.org/10.1093/eurheartj/ehab484 (accessed on 1st July 2025).

47. Vitale, M., Masulli, M., Calabrese, I., Rivellese, A. A., Bonora, E., Signorini, S., Perriello, G., et al. (2018). Impact of a Mediterranean dietary pattern and its components on cardiovascular risk factors, glucose control, and body weight in people with type 2 diabetes: A real-life study. *Nutrients, 10*, 1067–1067. https://doi.org/10.3390/nu10081067 (accessed on 1st July 2025).

48. Yani, A., Patricia, V., & Meilana, S. R. (2025). Assessment of cardiovascular disease risk based on lipid profile in productive-age women. *Journal of Noncommunicable Diseases Prevention and Control*. https://www.semanticscholar.org/paper/ae7e94fb330491d6d2f624aa1b058015c7379a7a (accessed on 1st July 2025).

49. Zaheer, A., Saeed, H., Arshad, M. K., Iftikhar, U., Abid, A., Khan, M. H., Khan, A. S., et al. (2024). Managing dyslipidemia in children: Current approaches and the potential of artificial intelligence. *Cardiology in Review*. https://www.semanticscholar.org/paper/0f58143d95cd6f 119255f1d10f25aa80fcf6b8fa (accessed on 1st July 2025).

URINALYSIS

12

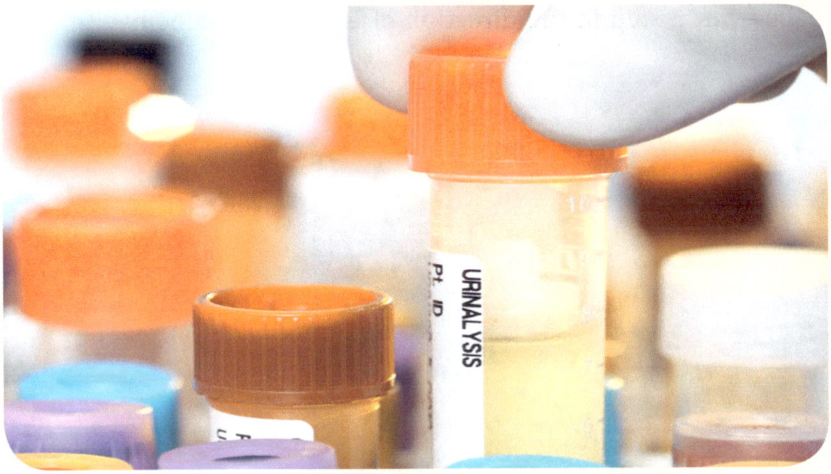

LEARNING OBJECTIVES

After studying this chapter, you will be able to:

1. Give history of urinalysis;
2. Explain the types of urinalysis;
3. Discuss the procedures for conducting urinalysis;
4. Identify the common conditions diagnosed by urinalysis;
5. Explore advances in urinalysis technology;
6. Focus on the limitations and challenges of urinalysis.

Introduction

Developing fast and trustworthy tests is something you can't help but notice when it comes to health care. Testing urine, for instance, isn't just another lab test—it's sometimes the first thing to help diagnose a wide range of conditions. New technology has made detection and sensitivity higher, and practitioners can discover issues that otherwise may have been missed. Take the rise in carbapenem-resistant Enterobacteriaceae (CRE) infections, for example; this is one which clearly demonstrates the need for rapid diagnostics when deciding what form of treatment is called for. To a large extent, scientists are now testing out such technologies as polymerase-accessibility antibiotic susceptibility testing (pol-aAST) in the expectation of lowering the time it takes for actionable results (Garner et al., 2020). Diagnostic devices have evolved a lot from the traditional types, marking a line of innovative devices for better results. Paper microfluidic devices, for example, have come up as cost-effective and handy but still delivering pin-point results. They not only make urine tests handy but also make the testing process even simpler. Today, plain dipsticks and lateral-flow arrangements are a testament to fundamental bioengineering concepts made practical. For the most part, as devices improve over time, they may well become increasingly prevalent in clinics – providing health professionals with the speed required without compromising standards (Martinez et al., 2017). Savvy to note the practice of urinalysis evolution, because it actually does seem like an evolution in the way that we provide patient care. Quick turnaround times enable doctors to act sooner – which is important when waiting could essentially make a patient sicker. Moreover, these innovations do not merely enhance what we currently do; they open up new paths to finish what past methods were unable to. By linking laboratory science to the patterns of daily care, these advances are allowing everyone to make improved, more informed decisions about treatment. In general, the future of urinalysis isn't just a case of refining medical science—but a step in the direction of enhanced public health results (Figure 12.1).

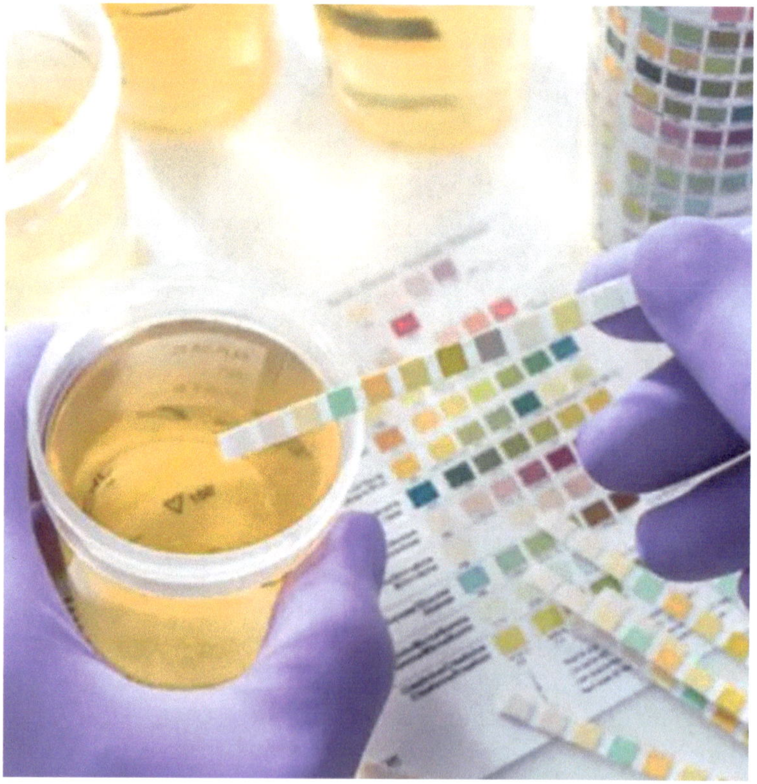

Figure 12.1. Urinalysis.

Source: https://i0.wp.com/www.elevatedhealth.md/wp-content/uploads/2022/11/urinalysis.jpg?fit=500%2C500&ssl=1.

Definition of Urinalysis

Urinalysis provides us with a window into general health through the examination of what is in the urine. The makeup of the urine – its color, clarity, concentration, and pH, along with the makeup of the cells and metabolites contained within – can tell us much about a person's metabolic and systemic status. Physicians frequently depend on this speedy, painless check to identify problems such as UTIs, diabetes, or even kidney disease, and, in most instances, to guide clinical choices. By examining the physical, chemical, and even microscopic characteristics of urine, health professionals make concrete conclusions regarding body functions; it's something that, to be honest, works in a number of ways. In urinary tract infection diagnosis and the understanding of the urinary microbiome, urinalysis has come a long way beyond its original function. Science continues to demonstrate that the urinary environment is much more complex than we initially imagined – sometimes the culprits of the past, such as the traditional uropathogens, simply don't act as they should, or, occasionally, the bacterial load is so minimal that it disrupts traditional diagnostics. Improved methods, such as metagenomic sequencing, now give us a better picture of the urinary world, highlighting symptomatic as well as asymptomatic disease. Studies show that conventional culture methods prefer the normal, expected causative agents, so there is merit in refining and updating our test methods (Adu-Oppong et al., 2022). There is more to it, too. Urinalysis is not only a matter of identifying infection; it's also a matter of how urinary health relates to overall well-being. New science indicates that identifying inflammation in the urine does not always mean there's an imbalance of microbes – so most of the time, a simple read will need some reappraisal. Clinicians now have to take into account both the presence (or absence) of pathogens and the broader, frequently anarchic, mix of microbes and their activities. This evolving mindset gives merit to the idea of combining traditional tests with fresh microbiome information ultimately benefits patient care and outcomes as a whole (Chew et al., 2012).

Importance in Medical Diagnostics

Diagnostics have come a long way—what used to be an unsophisticated practice of watching has become married to old wisdom with cutting-edge science. Recall that Ayurveda folks really enjoyed getting a good look at pee; they'd examine its color, smell, even tiny sediments floating around, believing these clues pierced the natural balance of the body. Before, it was all one whole picture, a sort of general sense of bodily balance. Today, however, a quick visual check is just the first step—labs now include chemical testing and microscopic examinations to get lots of information. More often than not, combining this old-fashioned gut feeling with modern technology shows us that going back can in fact help improve patient care, adding depth and detail to our health assessment (Mansoria et al., 2023). Better modern testing has made urinalysis a much more reliable tool. New lab methods are able to pick up on compounds such as glucose, protein, and even red blood cells—tiny details that diagnose illnesses such as diabetes or kidney disease. Rapid tests, for instance, have nipped response times so that doctors get instant feedback almost in the blink of an eye. And there is also this thrilling method—polymerase-accessibility antibiotic susceptibility testing (pol-aAST)—which not only speeds up the detection of stubborn infections but also fine-tunes treatments by catching cues missed by earlier tests. It's like having a double guarantee, and firmly cementing just how vital urine analysis remains to be addressing the healthcare issues of the day while improving patient outcomes (Garner et al., 2020). Merging centuries-old visions with present-day diagnostic tools is an optimistic outlook for the future of medicine. As urinalysis technology improves, it's becoming increasingly clear that one-size-fits-all just won't work—every person's health story needs its own customized examination. There is a gradual shift, overall, towards combining holistic intuition with hard evidence-driven information, though reconciling these disparate methodologies can sometimes be tricky. That challenge only confirms the need for greater interdiscipline coordination. When old experience and new approaches are combined, doctors develop a diagnosis system that's robust and tailored to individual treatment. By doing so, not only does one pay homage to the prosperous history of urine testing but it also brings the profession to new solutions, eventually contributing to better overall health outcomes (Garner et al., 2020; Mansoria et al., 2023).

12.1. History of Urinalysis

Learning Outcome

- Ancient practices in urine examination;
- Development of urinalysis techniques over time;
- Key figures in the history of urinalysis.

Medicine has been digging around the body's garbage for clues for ages, even when ancient civilizations were trying to get used to life. Ages ago, human beings were aware that even as ordinary a substance as urine had something to tell them about health, ages before modern science came along. Ancient Egyptians, for instance, physicians carefully monitored the color and texture of urine, writing down their findings on scrolls of papyrus like recording an everyday mystery. This was not haphazard trial and error but actually provided the foundation for linking body fluids with overall health. As populations developed through the ages and communities changed, so did knowledge of urine. In medieval Europe, a combination of observation with pragmatism gradually made urinalysis a routine instrument for doctors, demonstrating observation and knowledge were often complementary. By the 17th century, chemistry was rewriting the rules in a big way. Inventors like Thomas Sydenham and Robert Boyle were beginning to apply more systematic approaches rather than just experimenting with what they could see. They began extracting chemicals like glucose and bile pigments from the secret locations in urine, which compelled doctors to go from mere opinions to actual measurements. Most of the time, that transformation helped to detect diseases such as diabetes and liver disease. And, surprisingly, this melding of chemistry and medicine wasn't all about medical innovation; it pushed public-health ideas forward, encouraging societies to heed what a urine test might reveal. And then, in the 19th century, the creation of microscopy flipped the script once more. Suddenly, minute structures like cells, casts, and crystals were seen, and the entire new depth of insight into what was actually happening inside the body was observed. Detection of causative agents in urine specimen extended its use further, and it helped detect conditions like urinary tract infections and other renal disorders. Over time, something that had begun as a peculiar test became a standard component of routine checks—a step that rendered patient care more targeted. Now, studies still depend upon urinalysis in extensive medical plans for early prevention and detection, demonstrating that the long, serpentine journey of urine analysis is a testament to its long-lasting impact on medicine (Figure 12.2).

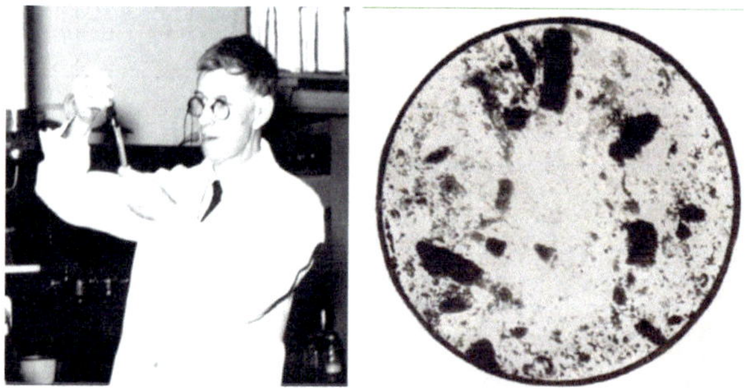

Figure 12.2. A history of urine microscopy.

Source: https://www.degruyterbrill.com/document/doi/10.1515/cclm-2015-0479/asset/graphic/j_cclm-2015-0479_fig_006.jpg.

12.1.1. Ancient Practices in Urine Examination

Throughout the centuries, civilizations have

relied on urine analysis as a convenient method to identify health issues. In old writings from Mesopotamia, Egypt, and Greece, you'll find that people took a good, hard look at urine as a window into one's well-being. Take ancient Greece, for instance—Hippocrates and his peers were watchful for color, texture, and the occurrence or lack of sediment particles in urine as a way of determining imbalances in the body. They'd note these features and use them to guide treatment, linking observations with the humoral theory under which, with exceptions being few, what occurred in the body was associated with changing conditions out in the world and changes happening within. In a sense, these early methods weren't blind guesses; they created a form of utilitarian paradigm that resonated into the past and to current medical methods, even if the logic at the time wasn't nearly as sophisticated as that which we expect today. Traveling to another part of the world brings us to Indian Ayurvedic medicine, where urine testing became some serious business. Ayurvedic doctors, guided by the concept of Tridosha—which categorizes an individual's constitution into Vata, Pitta, and Kapha—examined urine with utmost care. They did not just rely on color; they examined smell and even, in extremely rare situations, taste to detect medical issues. By linking these qualities of the urine with the types of energy, they developed treatment plans to meet the individual condition of each individual. This holistic, at times even global, strategy is the antithesis of the more limited, reductionist models so common today. But those ancient Indian procedures were not simply pathology-based; they worked towards a more global view of the interrelatedness of body and mind, an inspiration that remains real today among integrative health practitioners. Even today, prints of those ancient urine analysis methods remain in the management of urinalysis in modern medicine. Today's tests integrate visual examination, chemical reactions, and microscopic viewing in order to quantify overall health. However, the basic approach—watching details closely and distinguishing them from each other—is much the same. Despite all the technological advances, the basic principle that urine yields useful health information continues to hold true. Looking back at these old methods evokes a conversation between old wisdom and new scientific inquiry. By investing the time to explore these rich, if at times quirky, traditions, professionals not only establish the long-standing history of their profession but also establish the path for the integration of old knowledge with new research all in the name of further enhancing patient care (Figure 12.3).

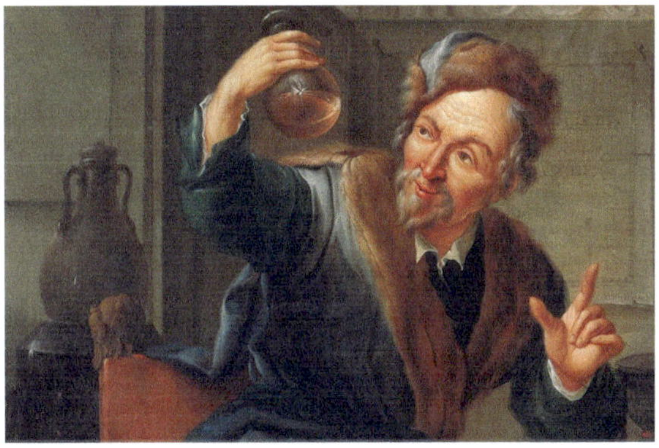

Figure 12.3. Early doctors diagnosed disease by looking at urine.

Source: https://daily.jstor.org/wp-content/uploads/2023/03/early_doctors_diagnosed_disease_by_looking_at_urine_1_1050.jpg.

12.1.2. Development of Urinalysis Techniques Over Time

Urinalysis is the story of a long and convoluted past that started off in ways few would suspect. Early individuals like the Greeks and Egyptians noticed that merely looking at urine—how it appeared, whether it was clear or not—could imply medical issues. They utilized simple visual checks to determine health, a method that in its time was very clever. Subsequently, things became more of a turn when people began looking beyond appearances, but actually chemical makeup and sediment in the liquid. This gentler progression from random observation into more critical examination was likely to improve diagnostic accuracy and aid in developing treatments for specific conditions. In most cases, integrating some raw observation with new science really set up a foundation for modern medical testing. Urinalysis in the modern age is founded on a wave of technological advances. Dipstick urines, for instance, now allow professionals to immediately detect such variables as pH, glucose, and protein level with ease. These rapid tests have placed urine analysis within easier reach for clinics and even outpatient departments. Automated laboratory systems have redesigned the typical process—increasing throughput and, admittedly, reducing man-made mistakes. These kinds of quick developments always play a significant role in controlling problems from diabetes to kidney stones and also guide preventive health care efforts in the correct direction. The capacity to detect even subtle biochemical abnormalities in urine not only helps indicate what's amiss at the moment but also provides hints for preventing problems in the future. Mixing old-school with modern innovation is what lends urinalysis its special flair. Old ways, such as Ayurvedic medicine that focused on an extremely personal analysis of urine, still retain their applicability when compared side by side with today's science. The old knowledge sometimes works well in tandem with new techniques, especially when it comes to interpreting metabolic illness and refining patient treatment. Increasing numbers of experts are welcoming the idea of bringing together different methods—teaming ancient intuition with advanced technology may even enhance diagnostic capabilities in challenging cases, such as urolithiasis, where metabolic pathways abound in useful clues (Bartosiński et al., 2025). All such cooperation between ancient and modern, by no means always neat and well-behaved, continues to propel urinalysis into new territories on our evolving medical map.

12.1.3. Key Figures in the History of Urinalysis

Throughout the ages, a handful of great minds have pushed our knowledge of health by researching something as ubiquitous as urine. Consider Thomas B. Barlow—practicing during the late 1800s—who developed established methods to examine urine samples. He thought that testing both the appearance of urine and its chemical composition could identify disorders such as diabetes or infections. Barlow's research, in a way, broke the centuries-old speculation and set the stage for rapid testing and treatment. His curiosity about what our waste can reveal transformed the medical scene and showed remarkable just how important this body fluid is. The scene transformed again in mid-century when Howard L. McCray integrated modern technology into the picture. He experimented with microscopic sight and chemical analyses used together in his time to help detect infections and metabolic derangements sooner and more precisely. He promoted laboratory quality control and regulation that incorporated urinalysis as a standard diagnostic procedure; equipment that developed later took his idea and transported testing to the bedside itself, significantly more conveniently. McCray's fresh insight not only advanced our knowledge of what urine could tell us but also completely overhauled everyday clinical practice. To this day, researchers continue to enhance the analysis of cells in urine, keeping the science on the move. New label-free detection methods and even electrical property tests for urine are being explored to quickly detect red and white blood cells—markers of issues like hematuria or kidney stones. This is a move that, in some sense, illustrates how, for the most part, urinalysis continues to be at the center of modern medicine and preventive health. Through the detection of tiny alterations in urine, these developments could potentially allow us to diagnose diseases before they are born, remembering that the inheritance of groundbreaking research undertaken by early urinalysis scientists is very much alive in our clinics (Nasir et al., 2020; Summers et al., 2017).

Test Your Knowledge

1. How was urine first used in ancient medicine for diagnosing disease?
2. What role did the practice of uroscopy play in medieval healthcare?

12.2. Types of Urinalysis

Learning Outcome

- Physical examination of urine;
- Chemical analysis of urine;
- Microscopic examination of urine.

Urinalysis has more than one trick up its sleeve. Several techniques come to mind when examining urine, and dipstick testing is still widely used. You simply place a chemical strip in the specimen and—plain magic—it lights up to reveal such things as glucose, protein, or blood. A Belgian occupational physicians' survey revealed that roughly 69% utilize dipsticks on a regular basis, despite global guidelines not supporting regular testing for hematuria or proteinuria in asymptomatic individuals (Braeckman et al., 2012). The divergence between everyday practice and strict evidence-based guidelines indicates whether habits are drifting away from being reinforced by robust research.

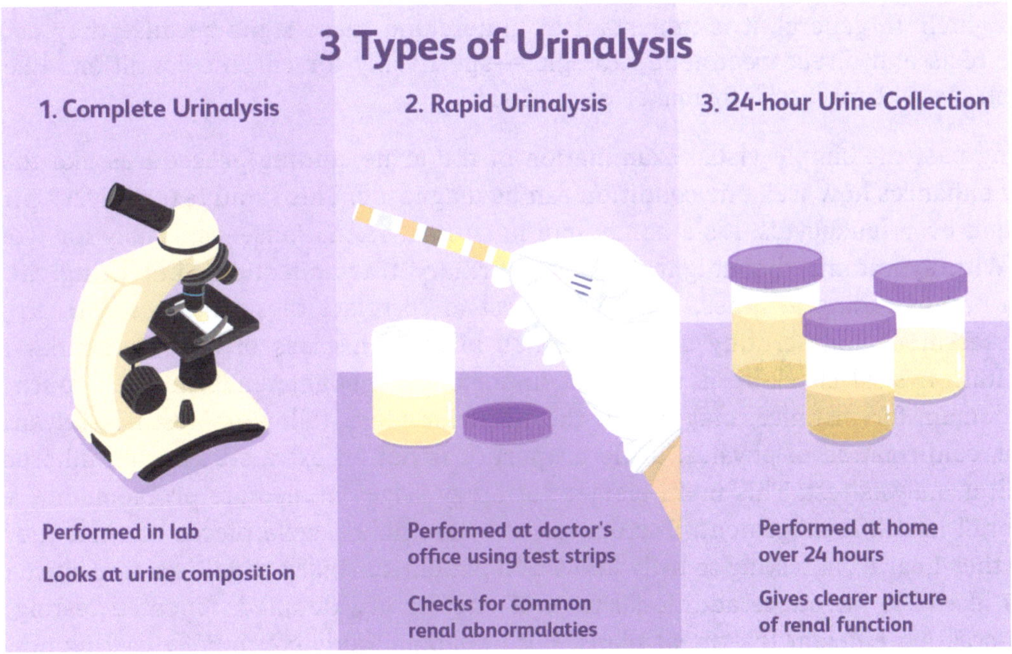

Figure 12.4. Types of urinalysis.

Source: https://www.verywellhealth.com/thmb/1CSy-NkV6JJb8uiD6wO3FdENyzs=/1500x0/filters:no_upscale():max_bytes(150000):strip_icc()/3156950_color-5ba560b4c9e77c008233667f.png.

Following that, there's the approach of getting more specific with quantitative urine analysis. This approach goes a little deeper, often adding to the dipstick to confirm results. For example, equipment like the Sysmex UF-5000 analyzer has been shown to precisely measure kidney cell fragments—RTECs and TECs—in samples (Boelens et al., 2020). These automated systems have a tendency to simplify the process compared to out-of-date manual microscopy; in most cases, selecting the right type of test is actually what makes a diagnosis accurate even if the process occasionally seems lopsided. Microscopic examination is still a vital component as well, giving a second dimension that chemical tests sometimes cannot provide. You see up close the cells, the crystals, and other small things that can be a sign of something like an upper urinary tract infection—a hint that things may have to be approached differently than a lower tract issue (Boelens et al., 2020). Combining these old-school techniques with new technology creates a sort of toolkit that allows clinicians, uh, to make better decisions in the moment. Every test has its subtleties and utility, and all of them together constitute a useful, if somewhat unkempt, manual of patient care (Figure 12.4).

12.2.1. Physical Examination of Urine

Urinalysis is not just one test—it's actually a series of checks that can reveal a great deal about an individual's general health. The routine physical examination of urine is one such test that stands out from the rest. It starts with general indications like its color, whether it's clear or slightly cloudy, its smell, and even its heft (that certain gravity business). Each detail might hint at dehydration, an infection, or even hidden metabolic issues. For instance, dark or murky urine can mean you're not getting enough water or perhaps hints at an infection, and a strange odor might point to a metabolic glitch. In general, it is important to understand these signs because they usually lead to further tests and direct treatment strategies—specifically for chronic conditions like rUTI, as reflected in present research (Brubaker et al., 2018).

Moving past the simple visual examination of the urine, adding procedures like the dipstick test really enhances how well one condition can be diagnosed. This rapid test analyzes pH, protein, ketones, and even leukocytes. It's a handy tool in so many situations—especially for women who come in with symptoms that might suggest a urinary tract infection—but using the dipstick alone can be misleading at times. It's usually best to correlate these findings with an adequate clinical assessment and scrutiny of the patient's history. In cases of rUTI or similar recurring issues, a full physical check-up is of utmost importance; a slight tenderness on touch near the lower abdomen, for instance, may reveal the need for more follow-up testing (Edward, 2017). In general, confirmation of physical urine properties is not an extra step but an inherent part of the overall urinalysis test. This multi-element strategy seizes immediate problems but also helps direct overall health management. Doctors have to assemble puzzle pieces of what they observe and what they hear from testing to truly know of a patient's urinary condition. And since recurrent infections like rUTI introduce additional tiers of uncertainty, detailed, repeated testing becomes crucial in creating efficient treatment plans. With ongoing study continually casting new light on urinary dysfunction, practitioners are now confronted with the task of integrating these results into everyday examination, underlining again the importance of urine analysis in modern practice (Brubaker et al., 2018) (Figure 12.5).

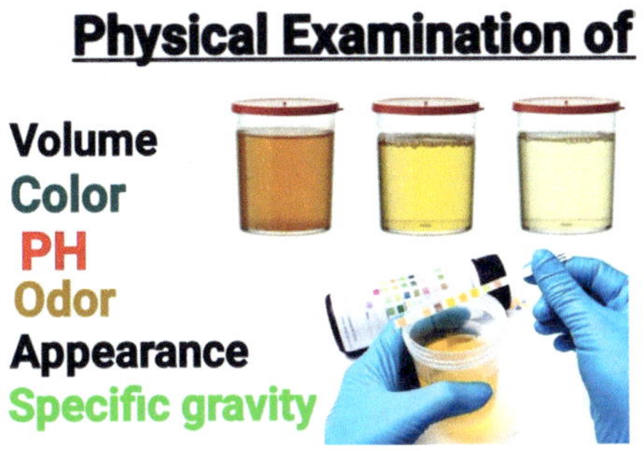

Figure 12.5. Physical examination of urine.

Source: https://i.ytimg.com/vi/LL231AQ5E5U/maxresdefault.jpg.

12.2.2. Chemical Analysis of Urine

Urine is a complex cocktail, and its chemical purification is extremely important. Instead of a neat checklist, many things are read through in the different elements to check if the body of a person is running smoothly or there's some hidden issue. You might seek signs in something like glucose, protein, or ketones—each one hinting at the overall health scenario. For example, traces of glucose in the mixture could be a sign of glycosuria, a condition most often seen with diabetes mellitus, while added protein can be a sign of kidney disease or other serious conditions. Dipstick tests, as they are quick and inexpensive, are usually the first resort, and in many cases, more specialized methods enter the picture to refine the results—especially when working with children, where the getting of the numbers right is indeed imperative. This series of tests demonstrates how chemical analysis aids in early detection and monitoring of ongoing processes, as reports on urinary tract infections among children suggest (Doley et al., 2005). Not satisfied with mere suspects, newer urine tests also analyze such items as non-protein nitrogen-containing substances and electrolytes. These are quite significant when monitoring metabolic function and checking in on how the kidneys are doing. Urea and creatinine measurement, for instance, is important if you want to know whether the kidneys are filtering waste properly, a sort of baseline to measure the glomerular filtration rate (GFR). More recent studies on biomarkers like cystatin C have broadened our evidence base for diagnosing kidney disease, hoping that it will pick up chronic kidney disease early—although, as a whole, more cross-validation between groups is still needed (Abrahamson et al., 2016). On the whole, this general chemical screening offers clinicians the essential information they need to create effective treatment regimens that truly make significant differences in patients' lives. In addition to examining individual chemical markers on their own, combining a variety of test results significantly enhances the diagnostic potential of urinalysis.

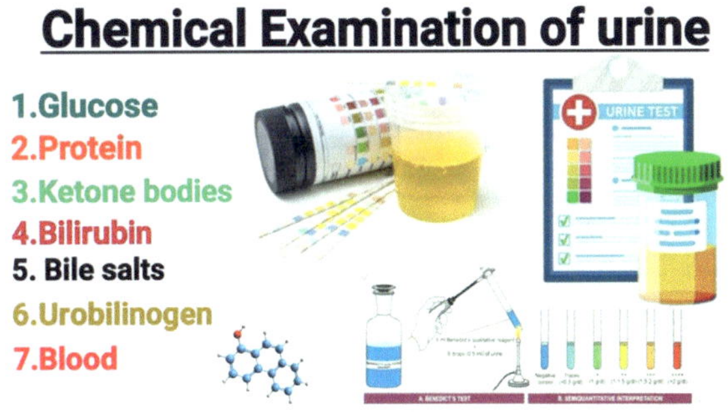

Figure 12.6. Chemical analysis of urine.

Source: https://i.ytimg.com/vi/vgZ3PDj4TT8/maxresdefault.jpg.

When multiple chemical clues are paired together, sometimes it reveals complicated health issues that might be hidden if you only had one exam. One such example is when dipstick examinations show both leukocyte esterase and nitrites—a pair that has proven very reliable for identifying urinary tract infections and can minimize the need for further cultures in children (Doley et al., 2005). This sort of layered approach not only rationalizes clinical decision-making but also avoids putting patients through unwarranted further testing. And as testing technology gets better and better, it's only a matter of time before further studies are needed to further hone these protocols and increase the clinical uses of urine chemical analysis, so treatments reach both exactly and in time for those with multiple health problems to deal with (Figure 12.6).

12.2.3. Microscopic examination of urine

Microscopic examination of urine is a critical diagnostic test that helps to confirm the diagnosis of various urinary tract ailments. New evidence emphasizes that even the presence of red cells, white cells, and even crystals is a probable sign of diseases like UTIs or kidney disorders. In many cases, samples are spun on a centrifuge and examined under an optical microscope—this manual technique more often than not reveals information that may be overlooked by automated testing. In the majority of cases, evaluation has revealed seemingly differential differences between women and men as well as seasonal fluctuations affecting urinary states (Abdullah et al., 2024). In essence, this intimate analysis not only improves diagnostic accuracy but also compels clinicians towards more personalized treatment regimes. Urine analysis has an ancient pedigree that spans from treatments in antiquity through to modern laboratory techniques. In such systems as Ayurveda, for example, professionals would carefully note color, sediment, and overall look of urine to assess imbalances and guide therapies. In those times, basic observations were common and served as an essential guide to patient health. Even as the technology of the day is considerably more advanced, the integration of these centuries-old findings with quantifiable accuracy—like glucose, protein, and crystal concentrations (Mansoria et al., 2023)—creates an unexpected synergy. Overall, this marriage of age-old wisdom and modern data provides a more holistic understanding and allows for closing the gap between tradition and evidence-based practice. Imaging advances have also reshaped our practice of diagnosing urinary ailments. New techniques not only speed the process, but they also provide a more complete picture of the arrangement of the urinary tract, something that plays nicely as an adjunct to the older microscopic examination. The antiquated manual examination is nonetheless unavoidable; its ability to identify minute nuances—like wacky crystalline precipitates or pesky pathogens—is the difference between life and death, even when high-tech systems are used. With advances in clinical practice, combining these tried-and-true techniques with the latest imaging promises the deeper understanding of urinary disorders, ultimately leading to improved patient outcomes (Abdullah et al., 2024) (Figure 12.7).

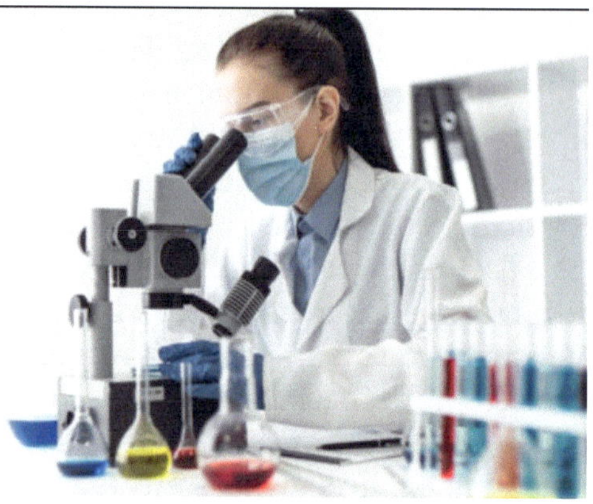

Figure 12.7. A laboratory scientist examines samples under a microscope, surrounded by various reagents and test tubes, as part of diagnostic and biomedical research procedures.

Source: https://www.bioscience.com.pk/media/zoo/images/293_a1b8a3455506e00fc2218b4a6002777d.jpg.

Test Your Knowledge

1. What are the main types of urinalysis: physical, chemical, and microscopic examination?
2. How does dipstick testing differ from microscopic urinalysis?

12.3. Procedures for Conducting Urinalysis

Learning Outcome

- Sample collection methods;
- Laboratory processing techniques;
- Interpretation of results.

Urinalysis is not very important as far as determining several health issues and checking the overall well-being of a patient is concerned. It all starts with the whole procedure of urine collection—usually by collecting a midstream, clean-catch sample in order to exclude any extra contaminants. A sterile sample container is mandatory in this case, and the sample is supposed to be examined relatively soon after it was collected, or else its quality may deteriorate. Sometimes, if the collection is not properly carried out, the outcome can quite easily be off the track, so the training is actually required by everyone who is involved. The sample is then subjected to a mixture of physical, chemical, and even microscopic examinations; all these different appearances help outline the state of the kidney and indicate any problems with the overall body. How the sample is handled once you get your hands on it matters as well. If you can't possibly test it immediately, refrigeration is best and see if you can have the tests done within 24 hours—this helps its properties not degrade. The test itself checks for various parameters, including color, clarity, pH, specific gravity, and proteins, glucose, and ketones present. In effect, using these normal techniques (with a slight variation now and then) not only makes it simpler to spot any abnormality but also boosts one's confidence with the final results, which in most cases actually goes quite a distance towards guiding clinical decisions. But reading the results needs an excellent appreciation of how normal should look. When everything comes back off, it could mean things like urinary tract infections, kidney problems, or even metabolic disorder. It definitely helps to remember other details, like the history of the patient and any other symptoms that they're exhibiting, so the numbers don't just hover by themselves. In recent times, increasingly sophisticated equipment like automated urine analyzers has been adopted to give speed and correct touch to the testing. Overall, compliance with good quality control procedures and compliance with issued clinical guidelines, such as those of professional organizations, remains a top priority for better patient outcomes and better standards of healthcare (Dean et al., 2016; Omuro, 2013) (Figure 12.8).

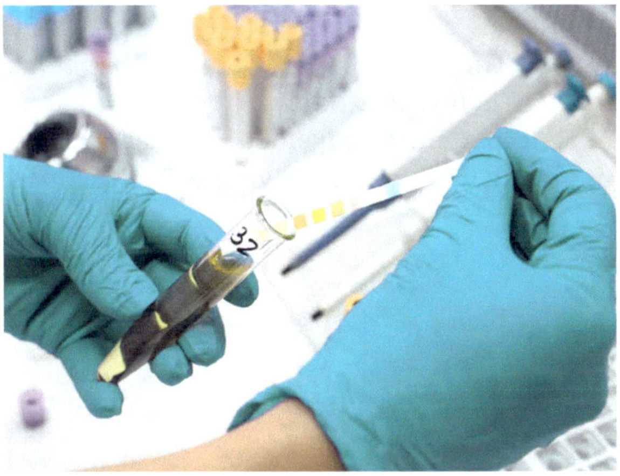

Figure 12.8. Procedures for conducting urinalysis.

Source: https://media.post.rvohealth.io/wp-content/uploads/2023/07/urine-sample-testing-732-549-feature-thumb-1-732x549.jpg.

12.3.1. Sample collection methods

Urinalysis really hinges on getting the sample of urine in the first place, since even a marginal difference in technique can tilt the final results. There are many different methods for drawing a sample—midstream clean-catch, catheterization, and even suprapubic aspirate are only a few. The midstream clean-catch method is most clinics' method of choice because it reduces contamination from the genital skin it is surrounded by, providing more precise screening and diagnosis. Of course, the process actually depends on the patient being receptive to the process and well informed about it. And also, if the sample is not shifted or transported a bit too flawlessly, errors have a tendency to creep in and spoil the analysis. Sticking to established protocols, as seen in Delanghe et al. (2014), is how these preanalytical errors are avoided and the overall reliability of the diagnosis is improved. While the clean-catch method is everybody's first choice, there are those times when the alternative is in order. When patients, due to some medical problem or anatomical peculiarity, can't handle a neat sample collection, a catheterized sample might be best. Sure, it's more invasive, but it's got sterility that makes a big difference in cutting down the risk of infection—especially convenient to use in isolating urinary tract infections. In another turn, the suprapubic aspiration drains urine from the bladder straight out, something that's particularly handy with neonates or whenever getting the sample that cleaner is absolutely necessary. Overall, it largely depends on clinical situation; using the wrong technique could just as easily lead to misdiagnosis or incorrect treatment. It is not just a question of reaching diagnostic accuracy but also impacts patient safety, treatment success, and even health care cost-effectiveness. For instance, diagnosing UTIs in a timely manner is generally most important as long as they are so common and complications arise (Lamond et al., 2006). The way you obtain the sample can actually speed up—or slow down—how quickly you get to a diagnosis, and thus how quickly the treatment begins. If the specimen is obtained poorly, you'll be held back or have to redo tests that will cost you more money. When you do it all correctly by what is properly established routines, the risk of errors gets less, and patient management is much simpler. In short, scrupulous attention to the way samples are obtained is absolutely vital to proper urinalysis and overall quality patient care (Figure 12.9).

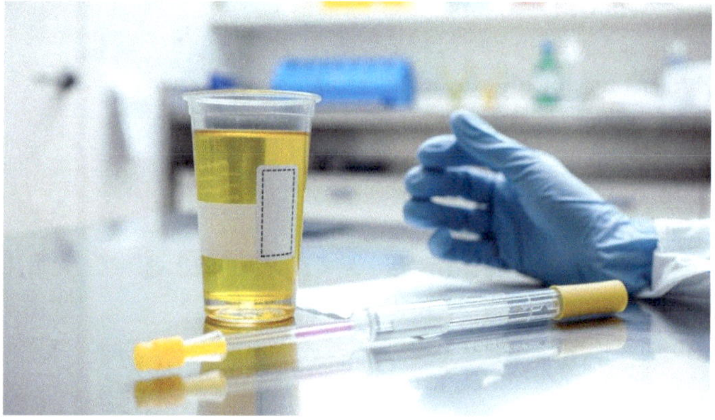

Figure 12.9. Urine sample collection.

Source: https://referrallabs.in/wp-content/uploads/2024/12/image-2-1024x585.jpeg.

12.3.2. Laboratory Processing Techniques

Diagnostic medicine really relies on the management of lab samples, especially when it comes to analyzing urine. Accurate results don't magically happen in the lab—they are more a function of what happens first, as in collecting, shipping, and even specimen handling. Many times, patients collect their own specimens, which for the most part leaves the field open for mistake. Incautious sampling or faulty shipping can quickly spoil the quality, and that taints the test. New technology has pushed labs in the direction of more regulation on these initial steps in recent times, so standard procedures are more crucial than ever to keep things consistent. In the majority of cases, resolution of these matters is at the forefront of maximizing the use of urinary tests and, in the long term, enhancing patient care, especially as areas such as metabolomics keep getting discovered (Delanghe et al., 2014). In the meantime, laboratories are embracing automation and it's actually changing the game for urine tests. Fast and accurate screening technology is now a requirement, particularly when screening for something like urinary tract infections, which—let's be honest—are a prevalent problem with a lot of people. Back-bench urine culture, taking as long as 24 hours, has the ability to delay treatment effectively unnecessarily; but with such technologies as the Sysmex OF-1000i and FUS200 systems, quicker solutions are now available. Research indicates that these newer systems decrease the number of plates required in cultures, reducing the load on the lab while keeping their sensitivity and specificity absolutely astronomical. This not only simplifies the process as a whole but also assists doctors in deciding treatment a bit more quickly, which could be a gigantic win for patient outcomes (Aldeal et al., 2018). Lab procedures aren't standing still, either. As processing technologies go forward, it's not really that difficult to understand that maintaining current technology is a must. Computerized systems now give a much better idea of what is in urine, with time-saving advantages to boot. Some even believe that machine-learning software will soon initiate more accurate predictions and even tailor treatment options based on patients. Ensuring each pre-test process is performed properly—along with advances in technology—positions laboratories to better meet the growing demand for quick and precise urine testing. In general, the future goal seems to be the continuous improvement of urine diagnostics through a marriage of today's scientific innovation and the demands of clinical practice tomorrow (Delanghe et al., 2014) (Figure 12.10).

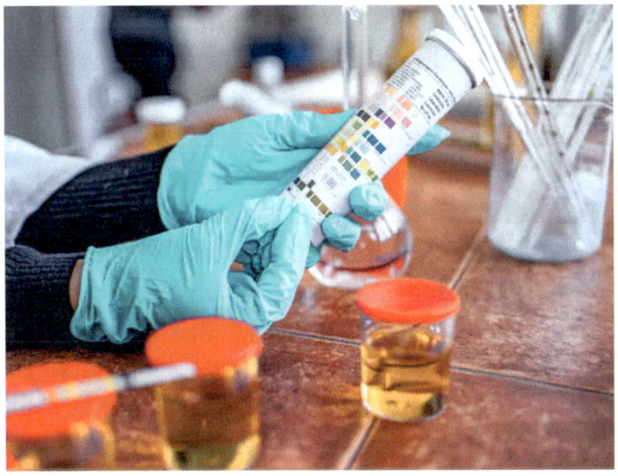

Figure 12.10. Laboratory processing techniques.

Source: https://media.post.rvohealth.io/wp-content/uploads/2021/08/Practitioner-measuring-pH-test-strips-of-urine-sample-732x549-thumbnail-732x549.jpg.

12.3.3. Interpretation of Results

Urinalysis is not all about numbers—it takes a sound knowledge of what these tests are measuring. There is new technology, such as photometric analyzers employing a dry chemistry method, which has improved urine information to be more comprehensive and precise. But this development is accompanied by its own set of challenges. Overall, while these new techniques are more accurate, they are not infallible; i.e., when a routine microscope screen of urine sediment yields results that aren't always reliable, they can direct decisions off course. That's why practitioners must be aware of the nuts and bolts of the techniques so they know how internal and external factors are playing out in the larger picture (Dugusheva et al., 2025). Beyond the technicalities, physicians simply need to weigh what these urinalysis results actually mean in the patient's life. A patient's history, hydration level, and even diet can all send the results into abnormal directions—a lone abnormal value, after all, doesn't really scream disease. In most cases, doctors end up combining this lab data with other clinical data to get a fuller picture of a person's health. For instance, a bit more protein in the urine might be due to nothing more than a strenuous workout or even a day without water, not necessarily any sign of some underlying condition. This is how combining these different pieces remains a complex, but essential, factor in arriving at an actual diagnosis (Qiao et al., 2024). Even as technology continues its relentless march forward in the area of urinalysis, keeping an unadulterated, analytical eye on how things are interpreted is most important. New technologies like artificial intelligence are now coming into play, allowing lab data to be seen in vibrant new language—machine learning unravels patterns and can at times even predict outcomes with jaw-dropping accuracy. But it is also the case that in bringing such benefits, they bring new issues of intelligibility and transparency. Physicians, for their part, must be watchful not just to the numbers that such systems spew forth, but to assumptions upon which they are founded. Most of the time, continuous learning and a dash of critical thinking are quite indispensable if we are to keep clinical decisions as well-informed and as reliable as possible (Dugusheva et al., 2025).

Test Your Knowledge

1. What are the standard steps for proper urine collection and handling before testing?
2. How is a chemical dipstick urinalysis performed and interpreted?

12.4. Common Conditions Diagnosed by Urinalysis

Learning Outcome

- Urinary tract infections (UTIs);
- Kidney diseases;
- Diabetes mellitus.

Interpreting a urinalysis test can uncover a whole load of hidden health secrets, often leading to faster, accurate diagnoses. Sugar in the urine—glucosuria, to use the medical term—is usually a sign of high blood sugar present in diabetes mellitus; this happens when blood sugar levels are higher than what the kidneys can eliminate, so more glucose is passed. Sometimes you even get a mix of ketone bodies with the sugar, which in most cases is an indicator of a poor metabolic occurrence like diabetic ketoacidosis. There is also the matter of too much protein in the urine, or proteinuria, which may be a sign of kidney illness like glomerulonephritis or even nephrotic syndrome. While this is not an invasive or complicated test, it has the effect of making healthcare professionals drill deeper, which allows them to rationalize patient care and maximize outcomes. Urinalysis is at its best when identifying urinary tract infections (UTIs), especially in groups who are more likely to be at risk. Those who have a burning sensation upon urination or suddenly feel compelled to go right away are most often steered into further investigation. It's interesting, however—the results can be misleading at times. Take, for instance, renal transplant recipients (RTR); one may have a situation where routine tests cannot identify infection; studies show that over half of RTRs can develop at least one UTI within the first year, and this puts them at risk of developing long-term complications such as loss of graft (Contreras-Sanz et al., 2014). Often screen for leukocyte esterase and nitrite, but occasionally the patient needs additional markers to actually reach the issue. This really addresses a conflict of clinical practice in that more test protocols may be what saves high-risk patients. Outside of diabetes and UTI, urinalysis also shows signs of liver and renal function. Hepatitis or cirrhosis will put additional bilirubin and urobilinogen into the picture, in broad terms, suggesting that the liver is not working well. In addition, if the urine itself has an unusual color or lack of clarity—sometimes slightly untypical—it will commonly suggest dehydration or other systemic issue worth pursuing. A look at the urine sediment will also reveal small casts or crystals; the presence of these can point towards kidney ailments ranging from an acute insult to a chronic long-standing process. All of these signs, as meager as they are, warrant thorough patient evaluation and highlight the importance of urinalysis as a critical component of the total diagnosis.

12.4.1. Urinary Tract Infections (UTIs)

Urinary tract infections hit clinical practice hard—especially in already-at-risk patients, including kidney transplant recipients. More than half of these patients will have at least one UTI during the first year after their transplant, which is pretty surprising. Standard tests, such as leukocyte esterase and nitrite dipstick screening, are not always capability-for-work; sometimes they miss infections that later lead to chronic illness or even jeopardize a graft. For the most part, research illustrates that conventional methods fail miserably in identifying bacteria sheltered within urinary cells.

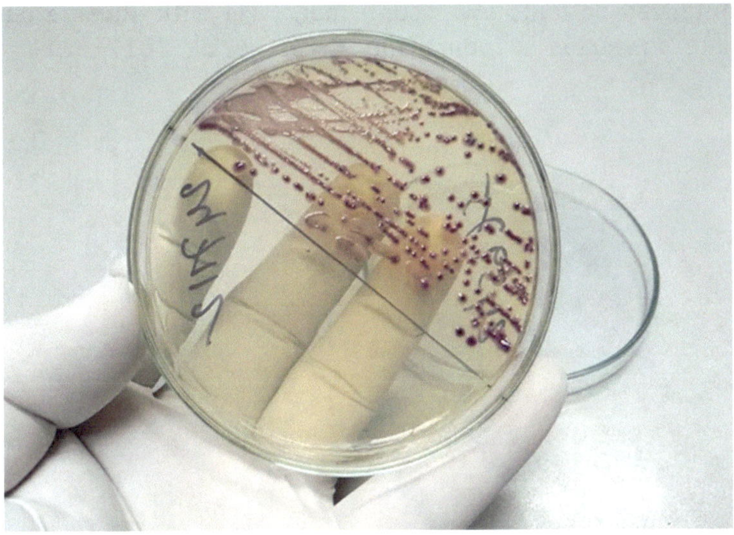

Figure 12.11. Urinary tract infections (UTIs).

Source: https://assets.clevelandclinic.org/transform/32ab1d5f-1d98-4b5e-952d-e9727ab97d94/23-URL-3524809-CQD-650x450-A_jpg.

So, in short, examining alternative approaches—like measuring urinary ATP levels—might simply offer a more sensitive way to identify those sneaky infections (Contreras-Sanz et al., 2014). The same is true in veterinary medicine. Veterinarians managing uncomplicated UTIs in pets are often presented with circumstances not vastly different from those of human infections, even though treatment recipes might differ somewhat. In broad terms, this suggests that a briefer, more concentrated antibiotic course might not only be effective but could even enhance owner compliance and avoid the speeding up of antimicrobial resistance. Measurement of various treatment lengths seems to make important observations that will eventually make waves in human medicine as well (Chew et al., 2012). The tie between precise urinalysis and strong treatment results can't be stressed enough. Understanding a good sense of how urinary pathogens are uncovered takes the path toward more targeted care, which in turn greatly improves outcomes in patients. Most of the time, diagnosing a UTI correctly doesn't just help one person—it helps formulate public health guidelines used to stem the tide of antibiotic-resistant bacteria as well. As guidelines evolve and new techniques gradually gain traction, adding advanced diagnostic techniques may polish our urinalysis modus operandi as a whole and prevent complications due to delayed or misdirected treatments. Ongoing research is still important to maintaining both human and animal health practice as effective as possible when diagnosing and treating UTIs (Chew et al., 2012; Contreras-Sanz et al., 2014) (Figure 12.11).

12.4.2. Kidney Diseases

Kidney diseases affect your health in ways you just can't ignore, especially when urine pathology comes into play. Doctors will often turn to urinalysis – a painless, swift test – to identify early signs of kidney disease. It may pick up glomerulonephritis or even a UTI. At times, the presence of protein in the urine suggests glomerular injury or chronic inflammation. In a different research, solitary urine culture in hospitalized patients often confirmed UTIs with adverse outcomes, particularly in patients with catheters inserted in their urine (Carson et al., 2017).

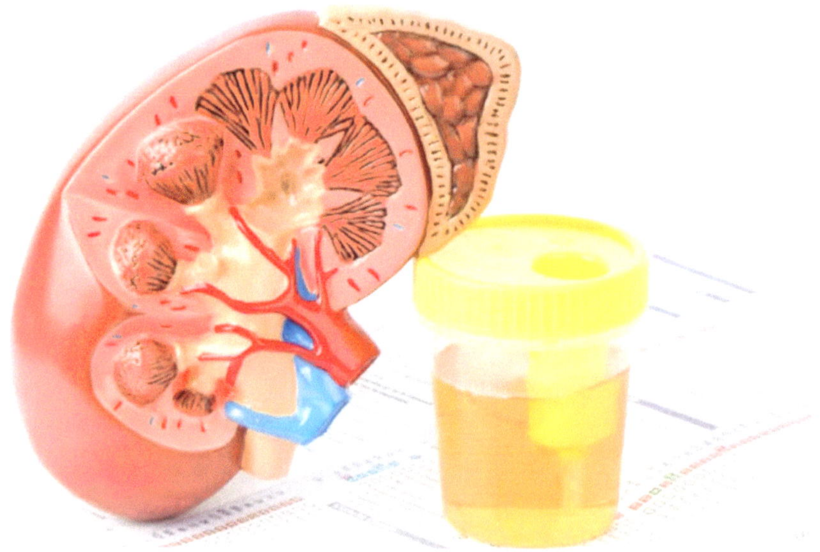

Figure 12.12. Kidney diseases.

Source: https://img.mlo-online.com/files/base/ebm/mlo/image/2023/11/6564fb8a8d242b001ecb3ef1-dreamstime_xxl_38866186.png?auto=format,compress&fit=max&q=45&w=640&width=640.

Finding these changes in urine enables health workers to intervene earlier so that they can avoid additional damage to kidneys. Proteinuria is another spin in the story. There exists a condition, commonly known as protein-losing nephropathy, which occurs in some cases and shows how important monitoring the urine is. For example, in the case of coccidioidomycosis, research generally established that infected dogs showed a great level of proteinuria, demonstrating that systemic infection has the potential to completely impair the nephrons and interfere with urine composition (Mehrkens et al., 2016). When protein levels are consistently high in the long term, it is an early warning sign for glomerular issues, so routine urinalysis is quite imperative for diagnosing these types of issues before they get worsened. Urinalysis is capable of doing more than just proving kidney complications – it enables clinicians to measure if treatment is effective as well. Clinicians monitor variations in urine parameters to observe if patients with chronic kidney disease or acute kidney injuries are responding appropriately. Decrease in protein after treatment is a sign that everything is on the right track. And this test also tends to pick up other complications, including infection or even metabolic disturbances spreading with kidney problems. Generally, this is the kind of thing that means an adequate urinalysis gives not only a snapshot of renal status but also guides decision-making in-patient management, even if occasionally the fine detail is rather woolly (Figure 12.12).

12.4.3. Diabetes Mellitus

Diabetes is not just about regulating blood sugar—it turns out to affect a whole lot more of the body than you'd imagine. When blood sugar levels get too high, the kidneys are overwhelmed, and excess glucose spills into the urine—a state individuals call glycosuria. This excess sugar in the urine is not just a sign that metabolism is imbalanced; it also gives an easier chance for urinary tract infection to develop. Diabetics commonly have more UTIs partly because neuropathy disrupts normal bladder mechanics so that urine residue gives bacteria a chance to establish themselves. Regular screenings, like urinalysis, can actually help catch these complications before they have a chance to develop and get things under control (Jennifer et al., 2019). Urinalysis is crucial to diabetes care because it provides an overall profile of internal health that goes beyond blood glucose levels alone. Testing the urine can reveal signs of issues like kidney problems or underlying infections. For instance, finding even minute levels of protein or ketones can suggest that diabetic nephropathy or other imbalances are in the future. Persistent protein in the urine, usually showing up as small, almost undetectable amounts initially, generally requires closer follow-up and, in certain situations, earlier intervention. And detecting something like asymptomatic bacteriuria can cause doctors to take action before it becomes a full-blown UTI. In general, the inclusion of urinalysis within routine care allows for modulation of therapies as needed and can play a crucial role in overall health outcomes (Steven et al., 2017). Diabetes and urinary health share a close relationship that all health care providers ought to keep in mind. A patient with diabetes may not always know something is wrong until symptoms such as urination frequency, urgency, or pain signal a problem to them. These presentations must necessitate an early urinalysis, since infection can be detected early and may mean the difference between avoiding crises such as diabetic ketoacidosis or facing them. Education of patients in general regarding taking these symptoms seriously and being tested regularly enables them to act earlier than they would otherwise. Withdrawing regular urine tests from routine diabetes care can eventually lead to refined control of blood sugar and an increase in quality of life (Jennifer et al., 2019).

Test Your Knowledge

1. How is urinalysis used in detecting urinary tract infections (UTIs)?
2. What findings in urinalysis suggest kidney disease or glomerular disorders?

12.5. Advances in Urinalysis Technology

Learning Outcome

- Automated urinalysis systems;
- Use of biomarkers in urinalysis;
- Integration of urinalysis with digital health technologies.

Urinalysis is a long way from that now. For decades, doctors just used a simple urine test to track the function of the kidneys and warn them of more systemic issues in the body. Today, though, all of that is much different—with simpler chemical testing and even more sophisticated microscopes on the table, labs can now detect sneaky, antibiotic-resistant urinary tract infections that need more concentrated care for better results. Thani et al. (2019) highlights that the new molecular tests, with which one can quickly identify bugs from a urine sample, restrict the use of time-consuming traditional culture methods. In the majority of cases, this shift speeds up diagnosis and also deals with the increasingly problematic problem of antibiotic resistance. Urine microscopy, before just being a crude diagnostic tool, has started to yield hints about acute kidney injury that were not so obvious before. The old custom of just looking at urine sediment has progressed far; more recent studies show that what the microscope shows—like granular casts—on some occasions can predict how a patient will fare. Peter et al. (2011) goes as far as stating that counts of such casts and other microscopy scores have strong correlations with worse outcomes, leading them to imply they might give important hints for prediction. Overall, incorporating these emerging findings into routine testing provides a more comprehensive view and aids in personalizing patient care a step further. In the years to come, urinalysis is riding the wave of cutting-edge technologies. Such smart machines process humongous amounts of data, often detecting infinitesimal patterns that can easily go unnoticed by humans, and thus enhance how urine samples are interpreted. This innovation has real promise for early detection of conditions and starting appropriate intervention. Basing care on automated systems and intelligent algorithms (which sometimes run a bit unpredictably), health workers can work faster without sacrificing quality. With the discipline continuing to develop, embracing these technological innovations is certain to sharpen diagnosis and enhance patient care in general (Figure 12.13).

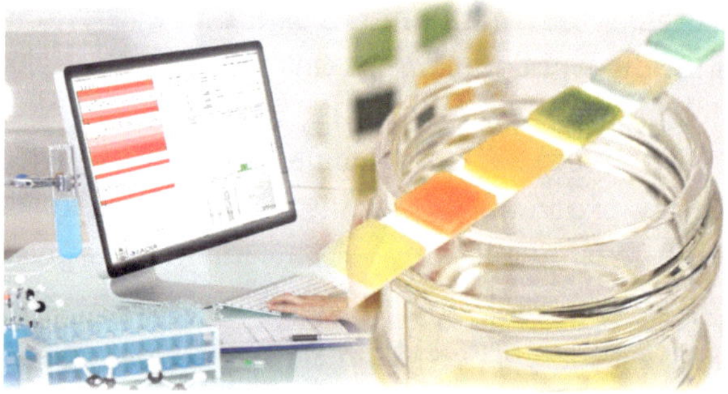

Figure 12.13. Technology advances transform urinalysis.

Source: https://medicalbuyer.co.in/wp-content/uploads/2019/12/Urinalysis_Instruments_July-2019.png.

12.5.1. Automated Urinalysis Systems

Automation of urinalysis is finding acceptance in laboratories worldwide. Time-consuming, often irregular conventional methods simply weren't up to meeting the growing demands. Advanced systems now take care of the heavy work by speeding up processes and enhancing accuracy. A sample of an advanced technology, a microscopic tool founded on acoustofluidic theory, promises high throughput with more accurate concentration control. It keenly incorporates machine learning for imaging analysis, typically capturing erythrocyte and leukocyte detection rates of 94.6% and 95.1%, respectively (He et al., 2024). In addition to boosting diagnostic certainty, this novel approach propels urinalysis in the direction of point-of-care use, increasing its utility in healthcare. When contrasting the manner in which such intelligent systems compare with the conventional manual method, researchers conventionally find a robust agreement in results. For instance, in a clinical study in Ghana, a fully automated urine analyzer was compared with standard methods like urine color, appearance, and pH, and they were found to be very close (Gyamfi et al., 2024).

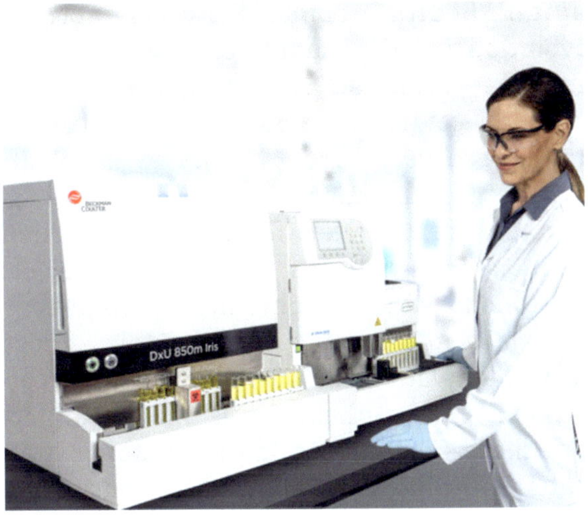

Figure 12.14. Automated urinalysis systems.

Source: https://media.beckmancoulter.com/-/media/diagnostics/products/urinalysis/dxu-iris/us/dxu-iris-workcell-us-micrscopy-focus-568-480.jpg?rev=922549fb618a4ab29d7e867ce30fc1af&h=480&w=568&la=en&hash=254D9E239C70E1C484D1C4E1541F789B.

Correlations for cell count and specific gravity were extremely good, with really emphasizing how effective automation is practically. In spite of this, there remains a place for manual microscopy for accurate sediment screening, which suggests that both systems can coexist rather than one being a replacement for the other. In spite of all these benefits, transitioning entirely to automated urinalysis is not without its glitches. There are still impediments like high cost, availability in only certain areas, and an astronomical learning curve for laboratory workers. For the most part, however, automation does well with the physical and chemical analysis but still relies on experts to decode enigmatic sediment issues that could elude technology (Gyamfi et al., 2024). For the future, improvements should target these hindrance areas. Collaborative work between technology developers and clinicians will be critical to make these systems more sophisticated such that they can meet a wide range of diagnostic needs while keeping patient care at its best (Figure 12.14).

12.5.2. Use of Biomarkers in Urinalysis

New biomarker identification has indeed revolutionized the operation of urinalysis today. Instead of clinging on to those old culturing methods—which, come on, can be slow and sometimes leave patients waiting for treatment—markers like lactoferrin now come as early signs of infection. Practitioners can, in a sense, interpret these inflammation and immune response indicators faster. This advancement not only reduces the need for additional rounds of antibiotics (which, in most cases, helps combat antimicrobial resistance) but also supports a broader trend toward more personalized and targeted diagnostics. And as an aside, new technologies that screen for pathogens along with biomarkers at the same time have stealthily turned around the fortunes of urinalysis. Take, for example, integrated biosensor platforms built by methods such as sandwich hybridization coupled with electrochemical assays. These systems can quantify both immune markers and uropathogens at the same time. Research generally shows they rate highly for sensitivity and specificity—crucial data for obtaining accurate clinical readings. To begin with, studies establish a strongly persuasive correlation between lactoferrin levels and leukocyte esterase, an indication that these multi-faceted methods can really streamline the manner in which we diagnose infections. In practice, such developments alleviate pressure from over-stretched health care systems and help to streamline patient management plans to their optimum.

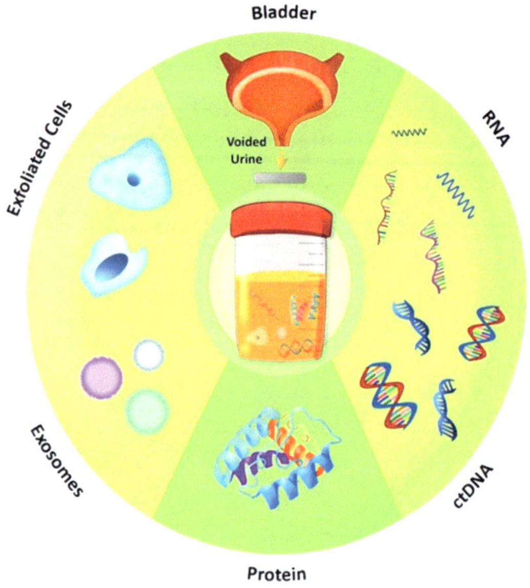

Figure 12.15. Use of biomarkers in urinalysis.

Source: https://www.researchgate.net/publication/361231780/figure/fig5/AS:11431281210574969@1702053611149/Urine-based-biomarkers-A-schematic-representation-of-the-various-materials-in-urine.tif.

Where high-technology laboratory facilities are not available, point-of-care (POC) testing for biomarkers is a useful alternative. Here, POC tests designed to detect bacterial invaders and quantify host immunological responses have shown promise—most notably in sub-Saharan Africa, a region beset by high antimicrobial resistance. By leveraging the newer technologies like real-time PCR and microfluidics, these tests frequently yield quicker diagnoses, thereby complementing antimicrobial stewardship. It's especially critical where traditional diagnostics simply can't keep up. According to the literature, incorporating biomarker-directed POC testing into daily practice not only increases diagnostic accuracy but also gives healthcare practitioners a better picture when making choices, ultimately resulting in enhanced patient outcomes and supporting the effort against the AMR crisis (Bonaconsa et al., 2024; Ruz et al., 2011) (Figure 12.15).

12.5.3. Integration of Urinalysis with Digital Health Technologies

Digital health technology has actually revolutionized the manner in which we treat medicine—urinalysis, say, now gets a new spin. Presently, combining mobile applications with digital records enables doctors to keep tabs on patients much more closely, usually cutting short the time it takes to diagnose. A patient can even forward their urine sample by way of a smartphone with no inconvenience; this not only decongests the data pipeline but also boosts patient activation and compliance with care regimens. Telehealth platforms, when combined with these results, give the practitioner more context in the moment, rendering the consultation more data-informed. Overall, these shifts are responsible for quality enhancement, increased accessibility, and overall increased efficiency in healthcare. At the same time, the combination of urinalysis with advanced digital tools starts to address certain monumental issues in public health, especially in low- and-middle-income nations. Current advancements reveal that underinvestment in laboratory resources has amplified healthcare inequalities and, in the majority of cases, prematurely resulted in too many avoidable deaths from untreated diseases. With the integration of smart diagnostic platforms, neighborhood clinics are able to catch suspects like urinary tract infections or other quirks sooner than they would have before. This practice, in large part, not only speeds up treatment, but also introduces greater parity to communities that might otherwise fall through the cracks. There's more to it than personalized patient care, either. When digital technology is married to urinalysis, it produces a steady stream of information that can be used to inform public health policy. Consolidated findings can shape policy and determine where resources should be shifted at any given time, sometimes even identifying trends or predicting epidemics. Essentially, this information-based strategy allows for mobilization of medical care precisely where—and when—it's most required, thereby enabling close monitoring of emergent health hazards. Finally, the integration of urinalysis with technological innovations holds the promise not only of better individualized care, but also of wiser, more flexible health policy.

Test Your Knowledge

1. How have automated urine analyzers improved accuracy and efficiency?
2. What role do biosensors and point-of-care urinalysis devices play in modern diagnostics?

12.6. Limitations and Challenges of Urinalysis

Learning Outcome

- Factors affecting accuracy of results;
- Misinterpretation of findings;
- Ethical considerations in urinalysis.

Urinalysis in medical practice is linked with various problems that have the potential to greatly affect diagnostic accuracy. Most practitioners remain wedded to dipstick testing even when firm evidence for their application in screening symptom-free individuals is lacking. In a survey of Belgian occupational physicians, approximately 69% reported frequently using dipstick urinalysis to screen for protein and blood—something international guidelines tend to discourage in healthy adults (Braeckman et al., 2012). This disconnection between clinical practice and evidence-based recommendations can generate unwarranted patient anxiety and set in motion well-meaning but incorrect treatment courses; it further illustrates why we need improved, more effective educational programs to bridge the gap. The test results themselves might be as unreliable as they are intriguing. False-positive and false-negative results often obscure the question because water, food, and medication can unpredictably alter urine composition. Sometimes the compounds in the urine will pretend to be protein or glucose and could trigger unnecessary alarms on tests. Existing techniques are always subject to the challenge of sensitivity, especially concerning challenging cases or toxins. Take the case with the detection of Orellanine toxin: current tissue-based techniques simply don't cut it—they are usually nonspecific and unsensitive (Anantharam et al., 2016). In all but a few cases, they require new technologies and improved testing techniques to actually refine the precision of urinalysis.

And then there is the hurdle of interpretation itself. Without a standardized protocol, interpreting results can vary wildly among physicians, which in turn facilitates unequal patient care. Not every practitioner catches the subtleties hidden within a urinalysis, particularly when guidelines have not been clearly strengthened or uniformly taught. This dis-equilibrium, coupled with inhomogeneous training, sometimes means out-of-date or off-topic information continues to guide decisions—information that can substantially harm patient results. Clearly, more regular training and up-to-date material are needed so urinalysis can finally fulfill its potential as a trusted clinical decision-making tool (Braeckman et al., 2012).

12.6.1. Factors Affecting Accuracy of Results

When you're considering urinalysis, quality of application of how methods and accuracy in results the most crucial aspect in is getting a solid diagnosis. A lot of what's executed with urinalysis—especially when you're working with UTIs—suggests that the degree of attention to detail in setting tests will actually weigh the scale when it comes to results. Some of these studies, for example, which utilized the QUADAS tool merely comment that most reports stumble over poor details and imprecise descriptions of methods. Not only are these errors making it harder to estimate actual diagnostic accuracy, but they are also making it harder to combine findings across multiple studies. Reviewing every QUADAS item, you can notice that careful, quasi-more stringent examination of the test phases is what truly counts; basically, you need high-quality primary studies as a solid base for diagnostic meta-analyses (Biggi et al., 2005). Sample selection and sample manipulation are another giant piece of the puzzle in getting proper urinalysis outcomes. Miscollecting, delayed before processing, or even alteration of storage conditions can all lead to off results. Such mishaps are often tragic ones in most clinical laboratories—even where antibiotics are used regularly on a bit of guesswork. Studies in pyelonephritis patients, for instance, have often found that results from urine dips in the dipstick fail to match culture results, representing poor sampling actually generating diagnostic doubt. Such uncertainty not just obscures treatment choices but also underscores the necessity of standardizing the management of samples to improve precision and overall patient care (Bergstrom et al., 2017). Finally, excelling at interpreting urinalysis results ultimately depends on the clinician's experience and understanding of pitfalls of the test. Misreads can result from a combination of thinking shortcuts, excessive reliance on experience, or insufficient training to grasp all the test subtleties. Since both technical and interpretation mistakes detract from diagnostic accuracy, ongoing education for physicians in most cases is absolutely necessary. It makes sense to place a focus on training that covers it all—from the importance of good method and handling of samples to the subtleties of test result interpretation. Over time, covering all of these will tighten diagnostic accuracy and lead to more thought-through clinical decisions and better patient results (Bergstrom et al., 2017; Biggi et al., 2005) (Figure 12.16).

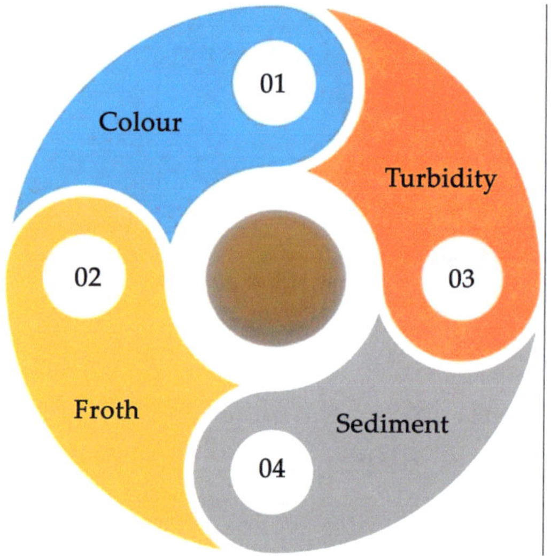

Figure 12.16. Factors affecting accuracy of results of urinalysis.

Source: https://www.frontiersin.org/files/Articles/812301/frans-01-812301-HTML-r1/image_m/frans-01-812301-g001.jpg.

12.6.2. Misinterpretation of Findings

Interpretation of urinalysis results plays a key role in the making of informed decisions in patient treatment. The interplay of test methods, like application of the trustworthy urine dipstick, occasionally clouding the issue if doctors lack the complete clinical backdrop. For instance, the dipstick—so widely used as a rapid screening test—can produce results that are not necessarily cut and dried, especially when protein is below normal. This may lead some doctors to miss important signs of protein in the urine or be overly cautious when choosing a treatment. Failure to thoroughly appreciate the idiosyncrasies of the dipstick and that it may produce false positives or false negatives can inadvertently compromise patient care, as previous studies (Björkman et al., 2020) have indicated in preeclampsia and other renal diseases. Errors can furthermore snowball because healthcare practitioners possess different degrees of experience. Junior practitioners, for example, may misread the subtle pointers in dipstick results, which will skew their choice. Research in general noted that the relationship between dipstick measurements and 24-hour protein levels was good (r = 0.634), while the relationship with protein-creatinine ratio was slightly lower (r = 0.401)—a reminder that the situation is everything. Under the pressure of high-pressure cases, such as pregnancy, even an insignificant misinterpretation can hide critical protein issues, so a painstaking but flexible approach is usually in order (Pallavee et al., 2017). Another hindrance occurs when physicians overdepend on dipstick results without ancillary testing. Much too frequently, normal habits or personal inclinations take over, overpowering hard realities and resulting in a kind of systemic mistake when diagnosing issues. Different tests can provide ambiguous results; a 1+ dipstick, for example, can indicate mild proteinuria but not detect underlying renal disease short of further questioning. Such are the oversimplifications that make it more difficult to assess patients, especially those who need extra monitoring—such as pregnant women at risk of complications. In short, small misreads in urinalysis can pose enormous risks, something that's why it's rather essential for medical professionals to keep on updating their knowledge and skills while utilizing these devices (Björkman et al., 2020) (Figure 12.17).

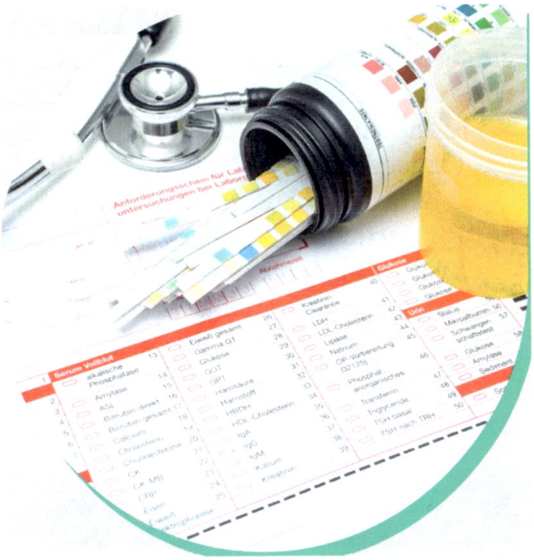

Figure 12.17. Interpreting urinalysis results.

Source: https://alborgdx.com/ksa/wp-content/uploads/2023/02/%D8%AA%D8%AD%D9%84%D9%8A%D9%84-%D8%A7%D9%84%D8%A8%D9%88%D9%84-%D9%85%D8%A7%D8%B0%D8%A7-%D9%8A%D9%83%D8%B4%D9%81%D8%9F-banner.webp

12.6.3. Ethical Considerations in Urinalysis

Urinalysis ethics is a messy pot—patient consent, confidentiality of information, personal impact from test results all mix together. Patients need to be told upfront what the test is, it's risk, and what might happen; this honesty, in most cases, preserves their right to choose and builds trust with the doctor. When individuals are not sufficiently informed, things do not go as planned, and sometimes serious issues if unintended side effects materialize suddenly. Basically, the way the diagnostic data are presented depends on ethical practices that enable individuals to make well-informed choices. And then there is the spin involved in processing and distributing the test results itself. The data from a urinalysis can spill pretty intimate secrets—like proof of drug consumption or hints of metabolic issues—and keeping that data safe from snoopers is essential. Data breaches, even tiny ones, can expose patients to stigma or discrimination; hospitals and clinics are therefore encouraged to take robust data protective steps and to stay close to health information standards. Shortcuts on these protections undermine not only patient confidentiality but possibly also trust in the conduct of diagnostics. Finally, interpretation of test results is complex in itself, especially as medical standards and social norms continuously evolve. Think, for example, about how glycosuria in pregnancy is evaluated; doctors must constantly redefine their threshold, weighing potential gains against risks like misdiagnosis or overdiagnosis. Usually, new research keeps the balance in a state of continuous change. Overall, healthcare professionals grapple with balancing scientific advancement and ethical responsibility—attempting to deliver equal, fair care while continually prioritizing patient health and safety (Maranga et al., 2019; Rose et al., 2024).

Test Your Knowledge

1. How can improper urine collection lead to inaccurate urinalysis results?
2. Why is urinalysis sometimes insufficient for definitive diagnosis of systemic diseases?

Summary

Urinalysis studies have been spreading into unsuspected areas, indicating its future utility in a wide range of clinical situations. It's now fairly obvious that this test is not only routine practice—it can identify conditions such as chronic kidney disease (CKD), but a real problem also particularly when resources are scarce. Consider, for example, parts of sub-Saharan Africa, where approximately 6.8% of some populations are challenged by CKD; combine that with the combination of local genetic peculiarities and outside adversity, and you truly realize why earlier detection and better health plans are needed in order to identify kidney issues before they spiral out of control (Atukunda et al., 2020). With urinary tract infections (UTIs), urinalysis again comes into its own. UTIs are still a common issue, but newer automated devices like the Sysmex UF-5000 have, in most circumstances, operated quite well compared to the earlier manual protocols. Research has a tendency to indicate that some urinary markers, such as renal tubular epithelial cells, are helpful in the ability to discern between upper and lower UTIs. Having this advanced technology integrated into everyday usage helps to streamline treatment options and, ultimately, enhances patient care (Boelens et al., 2020). As a whole, urinalysis is poised to be a central component of modern medicine. It's not just a case of finding CKD or diagnosing UTIs; early intervention with the assistance of this device seems to cut down on major issues down the line. As researchers dig deeper into urinary biomarkers, it appears increasingly a natural progression to incorporate these findings into clinical care. In many cases, the shift brings more accurate diagnoses and encourages the creation of targeted treatment regimens, cementing urinalysis as a vital part of preventive medicine and patient-tailored care (Atukunda et al., 2020; Boelens et al., 2020).

Urinalysis plays an important role in detecting urinary tract infections in young children. Quick tests can really initiate treatment decisions, and further studies continue to highlight the utility of that haste. For example, when a dipstick test is positive for leukocyte esterase and nitrite, the LR+ is approximately 28.2—essentially, that's a pretty good sign a UTI is present. But if both of them are negative, the overall LR-drops to approximately 0.20, something that practically ensures that there is no infection there. Such rapid decision-making not only enables physicians to act expeditiously but also cuts down on the risk of kidney complications for children (Doley et al., 2005). It doesn't stop there, however. Microscopical examination of urine for white cells and bacteria, i.e., pyuria and bacteriuria, yields equally impressive results. In most cases, a positive result on microscopical examination offers a pooled LR+ of about 37.0, significantly increasing the probability of an accurate diagnosis of UTI. Conversely, a negative microscopy decreases the LR- to approximately 0.11, a sure way of exclusion without unnecessarily overtesting once more. Through the use of these methods together, especially in the busy pediatric environment, true differences can be made (Doley et al., 2005). In total, approaching urinalysis not only enlightens present practice but also offers avenues for future investigation and development. The solid evidence in favor of dipstick as well as microscopic testing points out that rapid and efficient diagnostic tools are the priority when dealing with child UTIs. However, it should be noted that the majority of the methods widely used today have been around for over 30 years already. That obviously says a lot about the need for new research and new test methodologies to enhance diagnostic efficacy. Possessing a dynamic, ongoing review of such protocols may be what is needed to close the gap on urinalysis in everyday practice.

Critical Thinking Questions

1. **Which of the following is most commonly tested during a routine urinalysis?**
   a. Glucose
   b. Protein
   c. Bilirubin
   d. All of the above
2. **A positive result for glucose in urine (glucosuria) may indicate which of the following conditions?**
   a. Dehydration
   b. Diabetes mellitus
   c. Kidney disease
   d. Liver dysfunction
3. **The presence of protein in the urine (proteinuria) could be indicative of which of the following?**
   a. Normal kidney function
   b. Urinary tract infection (UTI)
   c. Kidney damage or disease
   d. Dehydration
4. **The urine specific gravity test is used to assess which of the following?**
   a. The pH level of urine
   b. The concentration of urine
   c. The presence of glucose in urine
   d. The amount of protein in urine
5. **Which of the following is a possible cause for a positive result for bilirubin in urine?**
   a. Diabetes
   b. Liver disease or jaundice
   c. Urinary tract infection
   d. Excessive water intake

Answers to Critical Thinking Questions

1. (d); 2. (b); 3. (c); 4. (b); 5. (b)

Short Answer Questions

1. What is the primary purpose of a urinalysis, and what does it assess?
2. What are the three main components of a standard urinalysis?
3. What can an abnormal urine color indicate in terms of health conditions?
4. What do casts in urine typically indicate, and what are some types of casts that may be seen in different conditions?
5. What is the clinical significance of protein in urine, and what conditions can lead to proteinuria?
6. How does the presence of red blood cells (RBCs) in urine relate to possible kidney or urinary tract issues?

References

1. Abrahamson, M., DiBartola, S. P., DiBartola, S. P., Finney, H., Kyhse-Andersen, J., Levey, A. S., Lulich, J. P., et al. (2016). Evaluation of cystatin C for the detection of chronic kidney disease in cats. https://core.ac.uk/download/84043650.pdf (accessed on 1st July 2025).
2. Adu-Oppong, B., Burnham, C. A. D., Dantas, G., Thänert, R., et al. (2022). Substantial overlap between symptomatic and asymptomatic genitourinary microbiota states. https://core.ac.uk/download/604217371.pdf (accessed on 1st July 2025).
3. Al Thani, A., Alhussain, H., Doiphode, S., Eltai, S., et al. (2019). Urine tests for diagnosis of infectious diseases and antibiotic-resistant pathogens. https://core.ac.uk/download/322444590.pdf (accessed on 1st July 2025).
4. Aldeal, M. J., Egido, P., Garcia-Lechuz, J. M., Lopez, J., et al. (2018). Comparing two automated techniques for the primary screening-out of urine culture. https://core.ac.uk/download/289996165.pdf (accessed on 1st July 2025).
5. Allen, K. (2023). Exploration of the implementation of an integrated electronic laboratory information management system on quality diagnostics service indicators at a county level public hospital in Western Kenya. https://core.ac.uk/download/591723462.pdf (accessed on 1st July 2025).
6. Anantharam, P., Burrough, E., Imerman, P. M., Rumbeiha, W., et al. (2016). Improved tissue-based analytical test methods for orellanine, a biomarker of *Cortinarius* mushroom intoxication. https://core.ac.uk/download/287623839.pdf (accessed on 1st July 2025).
7. Anger, J. T., Lee, U., Ackerman, A. L., Chou, R., Chughtai, B., Clemens, J. Q., Hickling, D., et al. (2019). Recurrent uncomplicated urinary tract infections in women: AUA/CUA/SUFU Guideline. *The Journal of Urology, 202*, 282–289. https://doi.org/10.1097/ju.0000000000000296 (accessed on 1st July 2025).
8. Assimos, D. G., Krambeck, A. E., Miller, N. L., Monga, M., Murad, M. H., Nelson, C. P., Pace, K. T., et al. (2016). Surgical management of stones: American Urological Association/Endourological Society Guideline, Part I. *The Journal of Urology, 196*, 1153–1160. https://doi.org/10.1016/j.juro.2016.05.090 (accessed on 1st July 2025).
9. Atukunda, M., Balzer, L. B., Black, D., Charlebois, E., et al. (2020). The epidemiology of chronic kidney disease (CKD) in rural East Africa: A population-based study. https://core.ac.uk/download/323062882.pdf (accessed on 1st July 2025).
10. Barbano, B., Cianci, R., Gasperini, M. L., Gigante, A., et al. (2018). Prognostic factors of renal involvement in systemic sclerosis. https://core.ac.uk/download/159268972.pdf (accessed on 1st July 2025).
11. Bartosiński, R., Dutkiewicz, J., Kaźmierczak, J., Kąpa, M., et al. (2025). Urolithiasis: Comprehensive review of etiology, diagnosis and treatment. https://core.ac.uk/download/646079976.pdf (accessed on 1st July 2025).
12. Bergstrom, M., Fox-Lewis, A., Gaskell, K., Noursadeghi, M., et al. (2017). Mismatch between suspected pyelonephritis and microbiological diagnosis: A cohort study from a UK teaching hospital. https://core.ac.uk/download/96628650.pdf (accessed on 1st July 2025).
13. Bidgoli, H. (2023). Integrating information technology to healthcare and healthcare

management: Improving quality, access, efficiency, equity, and healthy lives. https://core.ac.uk/download/611820415.pdf (accessed on 1st July 2025).

14. Biggi, A., Fretzayas, A., Gervaix, A., Haberlik, A., Hitzel, A., Hitzel, A., Hoberman, A., et al. (2005). How does study quality affect the results of a diagnostic meta-analysis? https://core.ac.uk/download/57953.pdf (accessed on 1st July 2025).
15. Björkman, S., Grahofer, A., & Peltoniemi, O. (2020). Diagnosis of endometritis and cystitis in sows: Use of biomarkers. https://core.ac.uk/download/479167809.pdf (accessed on 1st July 2025).
16. Black, C., Marks, A., & Sawhney, S. (2016). Discharge after acute kidney injury: Recognising and managing risk. https://core.ac.uk/download/42130561.pdf (accessed on 1st July 2025).
17. Boelens, J., Delanghe, J., Oyaert, M., Speeckaert, M., et al. (2020). Renal tubular epithelial cells add value in the diagnosis of upper urinary tract pathology. https://core.ac.uk/download/286086400.pdf (accessed on 1st July 2025).
18. Bonaconsa, C., Centner, C. M., Ferreyra, C., Hermans, S., et al. (2024). Point-of-care diagnostics for infection and antimicrobial resistance in Sub-Saharan Africa–A narrative review. https://core.ac.uk/download/610608466.pdf (accessed on 1st July 2025).
19. Braeckman, L., Haak, E., & Peremans, L. (2012). Routine dipstick urinalysis in daily practice of Belgian occupational physicians. https://core.ac.uk/download/55801809.pdf (accessed on 1st July 2025).
20. Brubaker, L., Carberry, C., Nardos, R., Carter-Brooks, C. M., & Lowder, J. L. (2018). American Urogynecology Society best-practice statement: Recurrent urinary tract infection in adult women. *Female Pelvic Medicine & Reconstructive Surgery, 24*, 321–335. https://doi.org/10.1097/spv.0000000000000550 (accessed on 1st July 2025).
21. Campbell, S. C., Uzzo, R. G., Allaf, M. E., Bass, E. B., Cadeddu, J. A., Chang, A., Clark, P. E., et al. (2017). Renal mass and localized renal cancer: AUA guideline. *The Journal of Urology, 198*, 520–529. https://doi.org/10.1016/j.juro.2017.04.100 (accessed on 1st July 2025).
22. Carson, A. L., Jackups, R., McMullen, K. M., Munigala, S., et al. (2017). Inpatient urine cultures are frequently performed without urinalysis or microscopy: Findings from a large academic medical center. https://core.ac.uk/download/83100994.pdf (accessed on 1st July 2025).
23. Chew, D. J., Daniels, J. B., Irom, S., Keil, D., et al. (2012). Evaluation of the efficacy and safety of high-dose short-duration enrofloxacin treatment regimen for uncomplicated urinary tract infections in dogs. https://core.ac.uk/download/323068657.pdf (accessed on 1st July 2025).
24. Contreras-Sanz, A., Farmer, C. K., Peppiatt-Wildman, C. M., Courtneidge, H. R., Malone-Lee, J., Durodie, J., Kelley, et al. (2014). Urinary ATP and visualization of intracellular bacteria: A superior diagnostic marker for recurrent UTI in renal transplant recipients? https://core.ac.uk/download/30706795.pdf (accessed on 1st July 2025).
25. Delanghe, J., & Speeckaert, M. (2014). Preanalytical requirements of urinalysis. https://core.ac.uk/download/19544928.pdf (accessed on 1st July 2025).
26. Doley, A., Hoberman, A., Hoberman, A., Hoberman, A., Weinberg, A. G., Rodriguez Caballero, A. M., Aronson, A. S., et al. (2005). Rapid tests and urine sampling techniques for the diagnosis of urinary tract infection (UTI) in children under five years: A systematic review. https://core.ac.uk/download/57944.pdf (accessed on 1st July 2025).

27. Dugusheva, V., Kotova, J., Groitsky, D., Volkova, A., Zarechny, P., & Kulakov, E. (2025). The diagnostic significance of discrepancies in the results of urinalysis obtained using the methods of "dry chemistry" and microscopic examination. *Medical Scientific Bulletin of Central Chernozemye (Naučno-medicinskij vestnik Central'nogo Černozem'â)*. https://www.semanticscholar.org/paper/e6afe85b497f4926a2591f407d662d203847a087 (accessed on 1st July 2025).

28. Esclarin De Ruz, A., Drummond, A. J., Pieretti, B., Cardenas, D. D., Chi, E. Y., Manoni, F., Neidhardt, F. C., et al. (2011). Clinical validation of integrated nucleic acid and protein detection on an electrochemical biosensor array for urinary tract infection diagnosis. https://core.ac.uk/download/pdf/8636310.pdf (accessed on 1st July 2025).

29. Garner, O. B., Ismagilov, R. F., Liaw, E. J., Savela, K., et al. (2020). Differential DNA accessibility to polymerase enables 30-minute phenotypic β-lactam antibiotic susceptibility testing of carbapenem-resistant *Enterobacteriaceae*. https://core.ac.uk/download/288435712.pdf (accessed on 1st July 2025).

30. Gyamfi, N. K. A., Osei, G. N., Brenyah, R. C., Agyemang, L. D., Ampomah, P., Darkwah, K. O., Toboh, E., et al. (2024). Assessing concordance of results: A comparative study of the manual and automated urinalysis methods. *BioMed Research International, 2024*. https://www.semanticscholar.org/paper/fe15f4ed146132fd6c8d6662f5d15bbff3264fbf (accessed on 1st July 2025).

31. He, X., Ren, F., Wang, Y., Zhang, Z., Zhou, J., Huang, J., Cao, S., et al. (2024). Acoustofluidic-based microscopic examination for automated and point-of-care urinalysis. *Lab on a Chip*. https://www.semanticscholar.org/paper/da9ebe61bcaca5d743b015007a72a2456a281930 (accessed on 1st July 2025).

32. Lamond, E. (2006). Toward new criteria for the laboratory, clinical, and presumptive diagnosis of UTI. https://core.ac.uk/download/159565075.pdf (accessed on 1st July 2025).

33. Mansoria, P., Singh, S. B., & Hada, S. S. (2023). Urine analysis in Ayurveda and modern medicine: Exploring convergence and divergence. https://core.ac.uk/download/617189589.pdf (accessed on 1st July 2025).

34. Maranga, J. (2019). The predictive value of urine dipstick glucose test in the screening for gestational diabetes mellitus in a tertiary private hospital in Kenya. https://core.ac.uk/download/597995970.pdf (accessed on 1st July 2025).

35. Marcantonio, E. R. (2017). Delirium in hospitalized older adults. *New England Journal of Medicine, 377*, 1456–1466. https://doi.org/10.1056/nejmcp1605501 (accessed on 1st July 2025).

36. Martinez, A. W., Noxon, I. C., Schultz, S. A., Sisley, C., et al. (2017). Paper-based diagnostic devices. https://core.ac.uk/download/231901328.pdf (accessed on 1st July 2025).

37. Mehrkens, L. R., Mohr, F. C., & Sykes, J. E. (2016). Clinicopathologic and histopathologic renal abnormalities in dogs with coccidioidomycosis. https://core.ac.uk/download/323070128.pdf (accessed on 1st July 2025).

38. Nasir, N. (2020). Electrical characterization and detection of blood cells and stones in urine. https://core.ac.uk/download/479074980.pdf (accessed on 1st July 2025).

39. Niijima, K. (2019). Prevalence of and risk factors for paroxysmal atrial fibrillation in patients

with cardiovascular disease but without diagnosed atrial fibrillation. https://core.ac.uk/download/237217629.pdf (accessed on 1st July 2025).

40. Omuro, A. (2013). Glioblastoma and other malignant gliomas. *JAMA, 310*, 1842–1842. https://doi.org/10.1001/jama.2013.280319 (accessed on 1st July 2025).

41. Pallavee, P., & Nischintha, S. (2017). A comparison of urine dipstick test with spot urine protein-creatinine ratio and 24-hour urine protein excretion in women with preeclampsia. https://core.ac.uk/download/543135513.pdf (accessed on 1st July 2025).

42. Peter, P. (2011). Urinc microscopy findings predict outcomes in hospitalized patients with acute kidney injury. https://core.ac.uk/download/232769570.pdf (accessed on 1st July 2025).

43. Qiao, X., Chu, T., Krell, E., Tissot, P., Holland, S., Ahmed, M., Smilovsky, D., et al. (2024). Interpretation and attribution of coastal land subsidence: An InSAR and machine learning perspective. *IEEE Journal of Selected Topics in Applied Earth Observations and Remote Sensing, 17*, 4768–4783. https://www.semanticscholar.org/paper/16c4d6316e44e44962c28ae2919ea86f38958064 (accessed on 1st July 2025).

44. Rose, D. (2024). FAA medical reform. https://core.ac.uk/download/616983264.pdf (accessed on 1st July 2025).

45. Summers, B. M. Y. (2017). Sexually transmitted infection or urinary tract infection? Misdiagnosis of *Chlamydia trachomatis* and *Neisseria gonorrhoeae* infections in primary care practice. https://core.ac.uk/download/217308149.pdf (accessed on 1st July 2025).

46. Taha, A. M., Abdulrazzaq, R. A., Hayyawi, A. H., Jameel, S. K., Khashea, M. R., et al. (2024). Seasonal variances in general urine examination findings among Al-Yarmouk Teaching Hospital patients. https://core.ac.uk/download/616974680.pdf (accessed on 1st July 2025).

47. Zimbardi, G. (2005). Workplace substance use, the risk of occupational injury, and testing. https://core.ac.uk/download/12208113.pdf (accessed on 1st July 2025).

EXAMINATION OF CEREBROSPINAL FLUID (CSF)

13

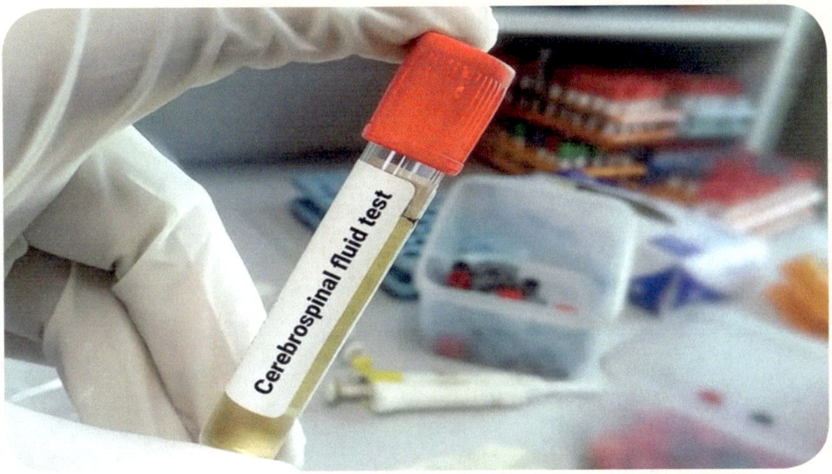

LEARNING OBJECTIVES

After studying this chapter, you will be able to:

1. Explain the composition of cerebrospinal fluid;
2. Discuss the production and circulation of CSF;
3. Describe the functions of cerebrospinal fluid;
4. Explore the Clinical significance of CSF analysis;
5. Focus on the pathologies associated with CSF;
6. Identify the advances in CSF research.

Introduction

Cerebrospinal fluid (CSF) comes in handy when we try to do problem-solving in the spinal cord and brain. It is not just a shock absorber—it is also a window to diagnosing and keeping pace with central nervous system problems. Infections, autoimmune diseases and other such conditions like to shake its makeup in ways that are hard to ignore. Research today highlights that certain of these markers, like the B cell chemoattractant CXCL13 (chemokine ligand 13), are able to actually shed light on what is happening inside. For instance, patients with neuroborreliosis have higher concentrations of CXCL13 in their CSF, a feature which is consistent with the activity of the disease and successful treatments (Brettschneider et al., 2009). For the most part, these changes in CSF seem to point toward a diagnostic utility that's somewhat intriguing to researchers. Brain functioning also relies on a whole lot of metabolic processes being in good working order—and when they're not, all kinds of problems can crop up. Take neuroglycopenia, for example, where the brain simply doesn't get enough glucose; it's a simple example of what happens when energy balance breaks down. Notably, even though we think of this in humans, horses too have demonstrated the same indicator signs when faced with extreme hypoglycemia, along with notably low CSF glucose levels (Aleman et al., 2018). These observations, in most cases, help reinforce the idea that changes in CSF are not mere indicators of disease—they even help quantify how deep or severe these metabolic hiccups are. Fundamentally, the exploration of CSF matters because it does a lot more than just protect our nervous system; it also enables biochemical transactions between our brain and the remainder of the body. The study of CSF gives scientists an insight into both the norm and the abnormalities that emerge, whether infection, inflammation, or even neurodegenerative diseases. By looking at biomarkers, fluid volumes, and cell components, researchers are able to learn about a plethora of disorders. And with each new diagnostic tool that emerges—sometimes seemingly out of nowhere—the dance between CSF results and current methods continues to remind us of how crucial it is to continue to explore its numerous functions in our health (Figure 13.1).

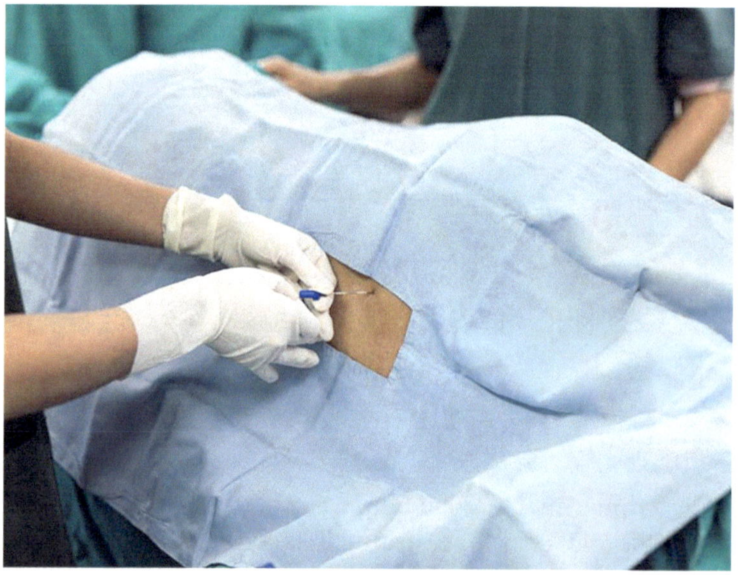

Figure 13.1. Examination of cerebrospinal fluid (CSF).

Source: https://external-content.duckduckgo.com/iu/?u=https%3A%2F%2Fwww.healthline.com%2Fhlcmsresource%2Fimages%2Ftopic_centers%2FCerebrospinal_Fluid_Smear-732x549-thumbnail.jpg&f=1&nofb=1&ipt=656c52c444a0627fe1b93fbfd2896b31ac0606cdb3723c58458ef6a5eada3bdb.

Definition of Cerebrospinal Fluid

CSF is a vital aspect of our brain's daily work, although it typically goes without appreciation. It's that clear, almost colorless liquid that drifts through the ventricles of the brain and adheres to the spinal cord, quietly working to give nerves a bit of cushioned protection. You might view it as merely a shock absorber, but actually it's busy working to help maintain balance through a process of trading nutrients and wastes between nerve tissue and blood vessels. The makeup of this fluid will usually mirror what is occurring within the brain, so doctors trust it in exams. In most cases, knowing more about CSF can provide clues to general brain health and even indicate troubles when there are problems. Studying CSF can be a turning point in diagnosing brain illnesses; it will usually reveal information regarding normal and unhealthy states. At some points, fluid markers specify infections, inflammation lumps, or even declining brain function. Take, for example, the protein neurogranin—its level in CSF has been associated with issues in the brain's wiring, such as those evident in Alzheimer's disease. Research, attempting to determine normal levels of neurogranin, even found elevated levels with lapses in cognitive patients (Agnello et al., 2021). This evidence really puts into perspective how important it is to check CSF in clinical practice, paving the way for timely treatment and even tailored treatment to a patient's individual needs. New and emerging diagnostic techniques are constantly rattling our understanding of CSF, adding new turns to how we perceive brain health. Improved imaging and laboratory work now allow us to chart how this fluid flows and what it's made of more accurately than ever previously. And invasive fungal disease pushing us to rethink our outmoded classifications, experts are updating definitions as new methods become available (Donnelly et al., 2019). These changes not only aid in the identification of conditions directly affecting CSF but also broaden our understanding of secondary complications from primary conditions. In general, the monitoring of CSF is crucial—it informs clinical research and can be a decision-maker of outcomes for individuals at risk for severe neurological issues.

Significance of CSF in the Central Nervous System

CSF is not just an inactive cushioning of liquid around our brain and spine—but it's rather crucial to keeping things even and avoiding nerve injury. This nearly invisible, watery liquid surrounds our central structures, mopping up shocks when we get hurt. While it also in the meantime performs its own type of janitorial work by clearing out waste and toxins that build up by the day through normal cell activity, which is essential for healthy neurons. Evidence generally indicates that when movement of this fluid becomes uncontrolled, sloppy inflammation or even chronic neurodegenerative issues might result. It also trades nutrients and chemical messages in a way that keeps the nervous system's complex internal operations on track. Beyond acting as a shock absorber, CSF is also humbly supporting our immune systems. It is an immune cell and other molecule corridor, enabling them to cruise by and check if there's any possible mischief. You can liken it to an early warning system—with vigilant immune cells in the mix ready to call out infections before they're a problem. To state it differently, in one such case that has been reported, a patient suffering from Guillain-Barré Syndrome was found to be HIV-positive upon a sensible inspection of her CSF, silently indicating the extent to which our immune status is enmeshed with neurological health. Such an observation points to the necessity of early intervention and diagnosis of central nervous system conditions. There also exists an intriguing twist wherein CSF seems to influence what we think and remember, possibly because it is connected with the gut-brain axis. There are new findings now that suggest there is an imbalance of bacteria in the gut—called dysbiosis—to change the CSF composition and may even influence cognitive functions, especially in HIV-positive individuals. Probiotic supplements, for instance, have shown some promise in restoring this balance by modifying the gut-brain dialogue, which further appears to affect CSF dynamics. Some evidence points to the fact that combining enhanced measures of lifestyle with antiretroviral therapy would improve cognitive functioning as well as immune function. In summary, these facts remind us that CSF is not just a passive fluid—it's an active participant in a broad, distributed system that bridges immune function and brain health (Figure 13.2).

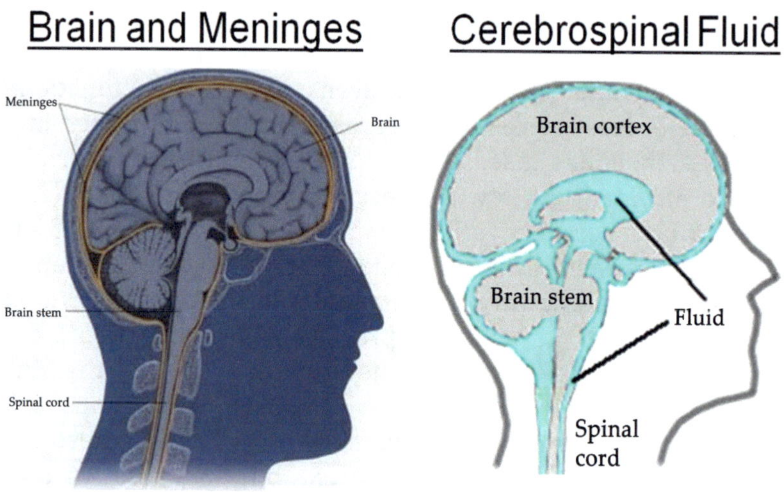

Figure 13.2. CSF in the central nervous system.

Source: https://external-content.duckduckgo.com/iu/?u=http%3A%2F%2Fbiology4isc.weebly.com%2Fuploads%2F9%2F0%2F8%2F0%2F9080078%2F743082317.jpg&f=1&nofb=1&ipt=6bb932062471169977f09ea34c9e30a7c294501151c2b88bf0fd8951a9489910.

13.1. Composition of Cerebrospinal Fluid

Learning Outcome

- Chemical components of CSF;
- Comparison with blood plasma;
- Role of electrolytes in CSF function.

CSF is a complicated little cocktail that keeps the central nervous system in harmony. It's mostly water, but you get a mix of electrolytes, proteins, and glucose joining in on the fun too. Sodium, potassium, calcium, and magnesium—each one has its role to play in keeping the neurons fired up and fluids in homeostasis. Which ions show up and how they show up is a good clue to the body's dicky control of its inner life. Proteins, far from floating aimlessly, help keep brain tissues safe and enable neurons to "talk" to each other. Most of the time, when things are not as they ought, the chemistry of the CSF is affected, giving us a glimpse of what is going on down in the CNS. More often than not, scrutinizing this mixture can indicate possible neurological issues. A look at the cells suspended in CSF gives us another window into its story. Lymphocytes, neutrophils, and so on can reveal infections, inflammation, or even malignancy in ways that may not necessarily be immediately apparent—every now and again, the very same cell types crop up in differing situations. Laboratories now generally depend upon automated machines to count up these cells, which appear to speed things along, yet there is still a wee catch. Studies had a tendency to show that while machines take care of efficiency, true accuracy—in that critical range of 5–30 cells/μL—still has a tendency to rely on someone manually checking. Realistically, this means that while automation is on the job, it remains wise to have confidence in good old microscopy for making good conclusions (Wick et al., 2021). When proteins in the CSF are considered, they too possess a complicated history—and especially that of neurological disorders such as Alzheimer's. Proteins such as beta-amyloid and tau are biomarkers that, in most cases, provide cues toward what disease could be progressing. Traditional means of identifying such biomarkers were intrusive, but this is no longer the case with newer imaging technologies on the scene. Others have even linked structural MRI with those quantitatively predicting the levels of amyloid and tau, presenting a quite tidy non-invasive option for ongoing follow-up (Wu et al., 2022). In conclusion, peeling away the layers of CSF composition not only helps diagnose finicky brain diseases but also informs us on how we plan to approach treatment and managing them in the future (Figure 13.3).

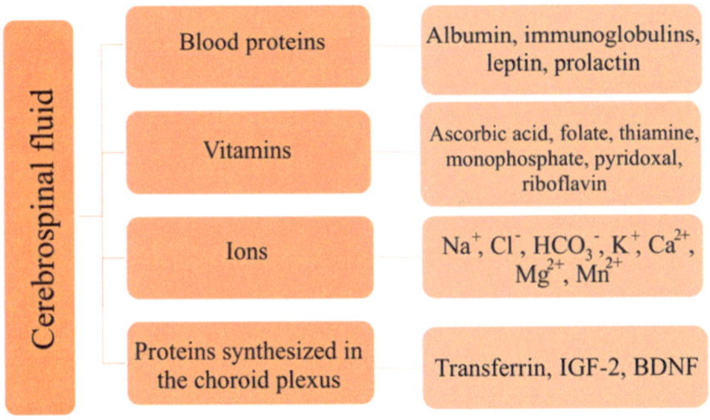

Figure 13.3. Composition of cerebrospinal fluid.

Source: https://pub.mdpi-res.com/biomedicines/biomedicines-11-01461/article_deploy/html/images/biomedicines-11-01461-g003.png?1684302191.

13.1.1. Chemical Components of Cerebrospinal Fluid

The chemical make-up of CSF truly makes a difference in the diagnosis and treatment of patients. Now, from all its components, certain metabolites—like neopterin and 5-hydroxytryptophan—have emerged as worthy signals. Neopterin, however, is traditionally seen as a marker for inflammation; elevated levels within the CSF generally suggest a shift from an early stage of illness to a later one in conditions such as human African trypanosomiasis, where an elevation tells us about the shift from stage 1 to stage 2. In the meantime, 5-hydroxytryptophan is involved in the creation of serotonin, which has already been linked to sleep disorders and other neurological issues, and so suggests broader effects on the body at large (Barrett et al., 2016). Proteins that float in CSF also provide big clues about neurologic disease and health. Think of clusterin—a protein that many researchers highlight for its ability to help cells manage stress and prevent the formation of protein aggregates. Some studies, in most instances, have shown that clusterin levels are increased in diseases like canine degenerative myelopathy versus idiopathic epilepsy. This recurring phenomenon suggests clusterin may be an effective marker to differentiate different brain disorders and ultimately improve the manner in which diagnoses are being made. Its occurrence rather underscores the messy, but fascinating, complexity of CSF and its role in unravelling central nervous system complications (Brodbelt et al., 2014).

Having a closer examination of the CSF's chemical shifts not only broadens our knowledge of neurological illnesses but also paves new ways for specific treatments. Raised levels of specific proteins and metabolites can improve diagnostic accuracy and even indicate individualized therapies for individual conditions. For example, the identification of specific biomarkers may reduce the number of invasive tests—such as lumbar punctures—rendering life slightly less complicated in the clinic. And, for the most part, how the composition of the CSF varies with the progression of a disease reminds us that continued research is necessary to decipher these biochemical messages. In general, delving further into the CSF components seems to give us vital information about challenging neurological diseases, ultimately contributing to better patient care through smarter diagnoses and more effective treatments (Barrett et al., 2016; Brodbelt et al., 2014) (Figure 13.4).

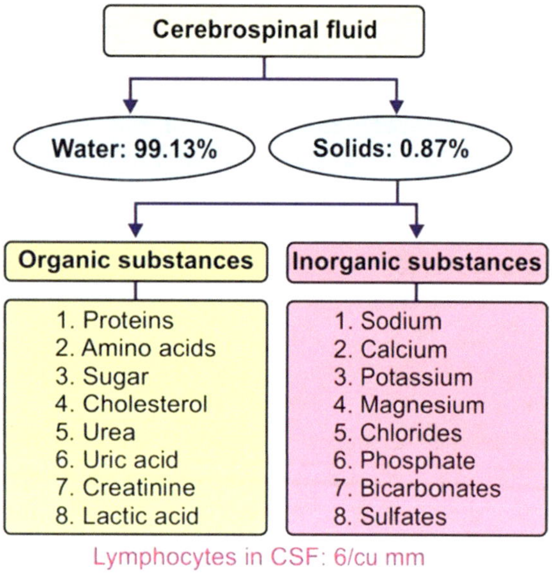

Figure 13.4. Chemical components of CSF.

Source: https://d45jl3w9libvn.cloudfront.net/jaypee/static/books/9789385999468/Chapters/images/680-1.jpg.

13.1.2. Comparison with Blood Plasma

CSF and blood plasma arise in the debates of science as unlikely partners—with CSF playing its own special part and blood plasma doing most of the heavy lifting in circulating nutrients, hormones, and waste products around to keep things in balance. Blood plasma carries the good stuff all over the body, and CSF offers protection for the central nervous system and even helps carry nutrients from the blood into nerve tissue. CSF isn't a passive fluid, either; it forms its own biochemical barrier and regulates ion levels so synapses and neurons are able to operate properly. Looking at these differences side by side, you can get a sense of how each system runs its affairs and what might mean for brain health and susceptibility to disease. If you examine the biochemistry closely, there are some eye-opening contrasts. Blood plasma is filled with proteins—albumin, immunoglobulins, etc.—while CSF, due to the finickiness of the blood-brain barrier, contains lots fewer proteins. Electrolyte ratios such as those of sodium, potassium, and chloride in CSF do not mirror those of blood plasma, a difference that's critical to keeping nerve cells functioning and synapses in tip-top working condition. Usually when these imbalances are present, they indicate a very specialized environment of the CNS, and even relatively small departures from normal have at times been found to imply underlying neurological abnormalities. Finally, comparing CSF and plasma gives us a glimpse of the brain's function, and it also puts lipid metabolism on the table. More recent studies have been found to demonstrate that certain facts are linked to proteins such as α-synuclein and could play a role in inciting neurological diseases. For example, phospholipids have been seen to aggravate conditions that follow α-synuclein aggregation, opening the way for novel therapeutic methods. All of this suggests that lipid composition within CSF may be as critical as in plasma blood, having great impact on CNS health in total. Examining lipid profiles in-depth thus remains to fuel controversy on neurodegenerative diseases and how necessary it is to maintain an even lipid profile (N/A, 2022) (Figure 13.5).

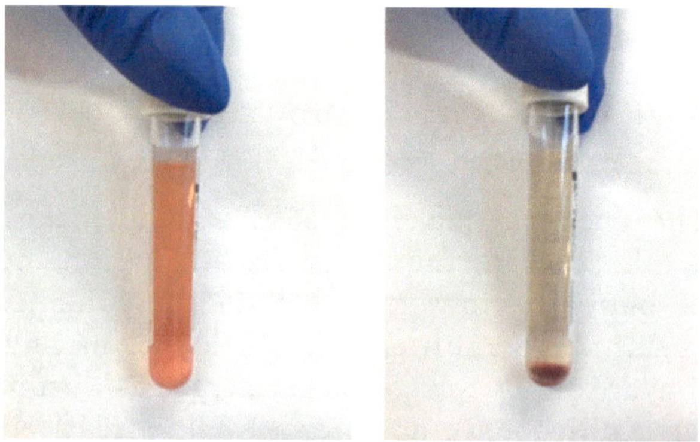

Figure 13.5. CSF comparison with blood plasma.

Source: https://ars.els-cdn.com/content/image/1-s2.0-S1752928X21001165-gr2.jpg.

13.1.3. Role of Electrolytes in Cerebrospinal Fluid Function

Electrolytes are CSF—take sodium, potassium, calcium, and chloride—are significant biggies when it comes to keeping neurons firing properly and the brain's overall balance in check. Oftentimes, these ions help deal with managing osmotic pressure, which is partially significant for protecting the strength of the brain's blood-brain barrier. The mixture of CSF, significantly altered by these minerals, serves two roles: it carries nutrients to nerve cells and dissolves metabolic waste, thus ensuring that communication in the neural system continues uninterrupted. Mild disturbances in amounts of electrolytes can lead to severe neurological issues, so obviously there must be precision in regulation. Aside from simply conveying nutrients and taking out waste, the role of these ions spills over into the realm of nerve message transmission. For example, the difference between sodium and potassium levels is what triggers the electrical impulses—action potentials—that enable nerve cells to "talk" to each other. If this delicate ionic balance is disrupted, you may have seizures, episodes of unconsciousness, or other neurological mishaps. If you have diseases like post-polio syndrome in which nerve function is already compromised, maintaining electrolyte levels tightly controlled is crucial. For the most part, therapies aimed at re-establishing this chemical balance (Bakhti et al., 2024) could be of immense benefit. In medicine, though, it is a whole lot more complex. Intrathecal pressure change in surgery can potentially confound the composition of the CSF, and transsphenoidal surgery for pituitary adenomas is susceptible to CSF leakage—a complication that can interfere with electrolyte homeostasis (Davi et al., 2024). Postoperative maintenance of such levels occasionally provides premonitory indications of complications so that interventions can be performed in a timely fashion. Overall, this comprehension of the various roles of such electrolytes in CSF not only enriches our knowledge of neurological function but also enhances our response to surgical challenges, suggesting that further investigation in this vital area is worthy of consideration (Figure 13.6).

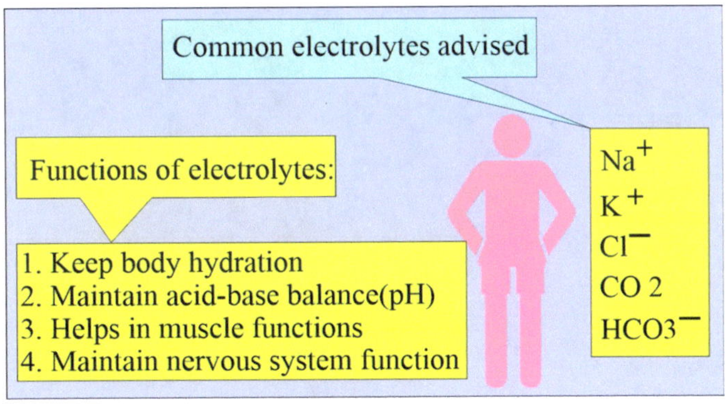

Figure 13.6. Role of electrolytes in CSF function.

Source: https://labpedia.net/wp-content/uploads/2020/01/electrolytes-advised-1.jpg.

Test Your Knowledge

1. What are the main chemical components of CSF, and how do they differ from blood plasma?
2. How does the electrolyte balance in CSF contribute to neuronal function?

13.2. Production and Circulation of Cerebrospinal Fluid

Learning Outcome

- Sites of CSF production;
- Pathways of CSF circulation;
- Mechanisms of CSF absorption.

CSF is essential to keeping our central nervous system functioning properly. It starts in the choroid plexus, that tiny tissue found within the lateral, third, and fourth ventricles, which produces a clear, electrolyte- and glucose-rich fluid. CSF is not just a passive padding covering the brain and spinal cord—it is also a carrier of nutrients and a waste remover. Our own bodies tend to make about 500 milliliters of it every day, which quite literally shows just how frantic and important the process is. The fluid passes through a maze-like network of ventricles: beginning at the laterals, then into the third and fourth, and then being absorbed by the blood through arachnoid granulations. Once it leaves those ventricles, CSF is spread into the subarachnoid space to bathe the brain and spinal cord, essentially an inbuilt shock absorber.

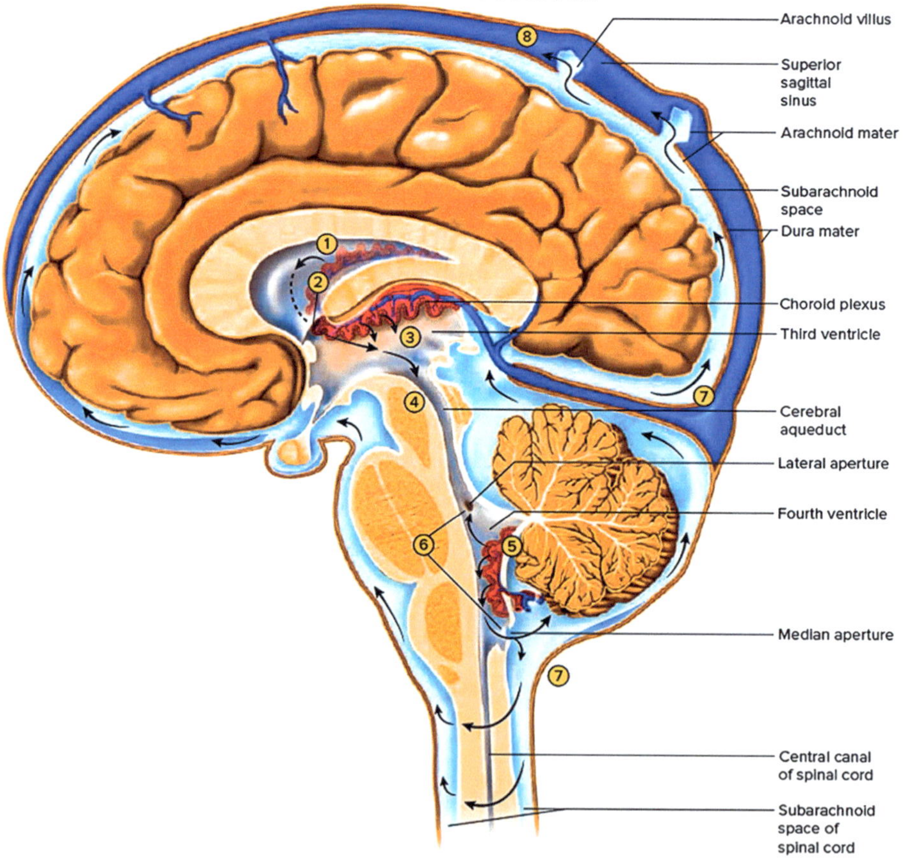

Figure 13.7. Cerebrospinal fluid formation, absorption and circulation.

Source: https://www.researchgate.net/profile/Licia-Romagnoli/publication/342149030/figure/fig1/AS:916010429329409@1595405313494/Cerebrospinal-fluid-formation-absorption-and-circulation-around-and-within-the-brain-1.png.

Its circulation serves to distribute neuroactive substances while keeping intracranial pressure in check—a balance that's extremely critical. Various factors can disrupt this circulation, such as changes in total perfusion or subtle variations in intracranial pressure. Take pediatric hydrocephalus as an example; in these conditions, even subtle hydrostatic changes may contribute to reduced blood flow and mild edema. Physicians would generally rely on devices such as transcranial Doppler sonography in order to monitor such dynamics, especially when they are treating high-risk groups such as neonates with hydrocephalus (Kolarovszki et al., 2019).

CSF regulation also plays a significant role in normal brain functioning. Where production and absorption are not quite in equilibrium, such conditions as hydrocephalus can arise—with too much fluid building up in the ventricles and increasing pressure in the head. That excess pressure may inhibit the circulation of blood, with possible symptoms of headaches or mild mental impairment. On a general basis, it's apparent that an exact balance in CSF dynamics matters since any error can contribute to the acceleration of neurological decline in patients with conditions like Alzheimer's. Research, funded by Alzheimer's Research UK, is probing these very processes, with a view to opening up better diagnostics and treatments for a range of brain diseases (Kelleher et al., 2013) (Figure 13.7).

13.2.1. Sites of Cerebrospinal Fluid Production

The central nervous system isn't just a neat diagram—it has sacs actually responsible for creating and circulating CSF. Take the choroid plexus concealed in the lateral, third, and fourth ventricles; this is really the CSF factory. The spaces are lined by ependymal cells that actively secrete the fluid, and the fluid itself controls ionic concentration and eliminates metabolic products of waste. The entire process relies on a delicate balance between production and absorption to maintain constant intracranial pressure and provide neurons with a constant environment. When that balance is disrupted even a little, problems may ensue; it just goes to show how crucial these places are for proper brain functioning.

It's also worthwhile to consider that CSF is not necessarily produced from the choroid plexus. More recent research indicates that perhaps there might be contributions extra-choroidal – perhaps areas like sections of spinal cord or meningeal components assisting, but less so. This multi-layered image makes the classic image look a bit too reductionist. In most cases, delving into these other sources might be able to disentangle CSF dynamics complexities and even shed light on inflammation-based neurological disorders, say. Take a neuroinvasive West Nile virus infection, for instance: alterations of biochemical CSF parameters indicate changes at various levels of the CNS (Balogh et al., 2015). A nearer look at the CSF itself gives us informative clues regarding neurodegenerative disease.

There is mounting evidence that genetics may also affect the content of CSF. For example, polymorphisms in CDC2 genes have been found to be involved with changes in biomarkers in CSF, including elevated levels of tau proteins and altered amyloid-beta levels—markers that may be indicative of the formation of neurofibrillary tangles. In general terms, this implies that both the locations of CSF production and the underlying genetic mechanisms must be taken into account. As scientists gradually begin to understand how these production points are connected with neurodegenerative activity, specifically directed therapeutic interventions may become more feasible, perhaps reorienting our treatment of these difficult disorders (Andreasen et al., 2005) (Figure 13.8).

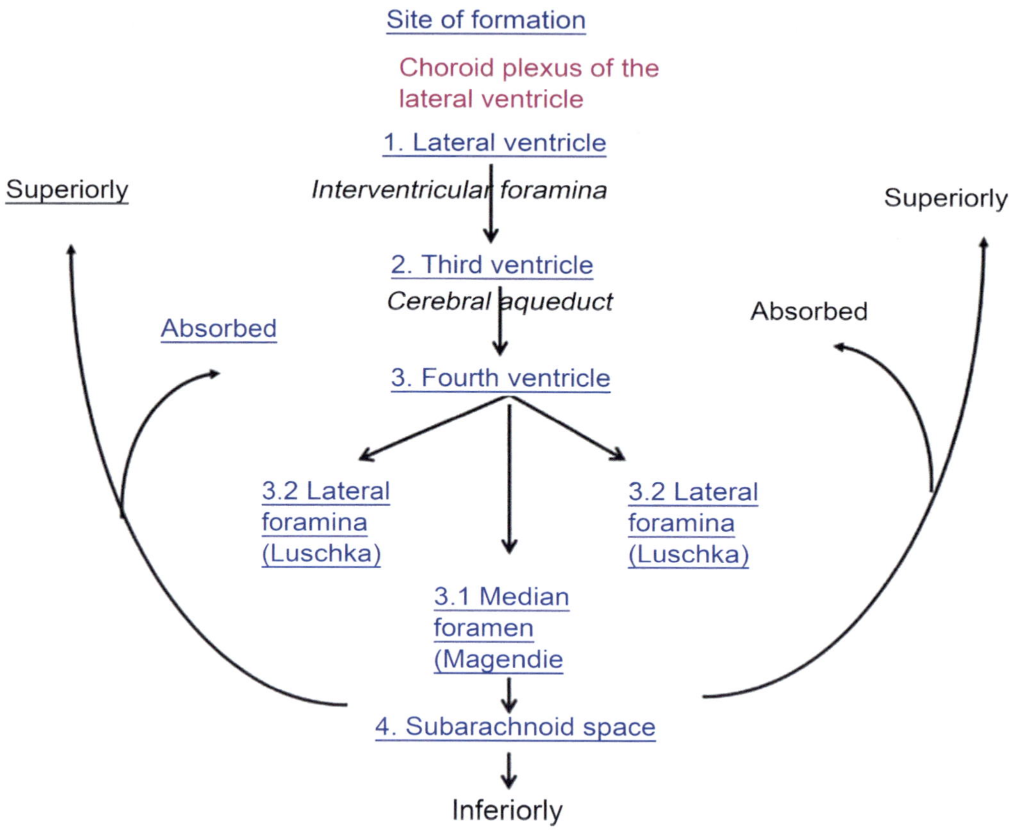

Figure 13.8. Sites of CSF production.

Source: https://external-content.duckduckgo.com/iu/?u=https%3A%2F%2Fimage.slidesharecdn.com%2Fcsfpptunni-120218102339-phpapp02%2F95%2Fphysiology-of-csf-production-and-circulation-alterations-in-various-pathology-22-728.jpg%3Fcb%3D1330220076&f=1&nofb=1&ipt=7f6d73ee63c9b398d6b8235978c515cdf9c6bdd7221c9ab1b7d939162f316b8e.

13.2.2. Pathways of Cerebrospinal Fluid Circulation

CSF circulation isn't a simple business—it's how our central nervous system is kept in line in unexpected manners. A majority of the liquid is supplied by the brain's ventricles, thanks to the choroid plexus; these specialized cells secrete salts and other needed pieces, roughly akin to tiny, controllable factories. Once it's formed, the CSF moves in an unpredictable manner: from the lateral ventricles, it drifts into the third ventricle, flows through the cerebral aqueduct into the fourth ventricle, then spills over into the subarachnoid space surrounding both the brain and spinal cord, kind of cushioning them while also providing a site for nutrient and waste exchange. In total, this continuous flow helps the neurons to function properly and alleviates pressure inside the skull, which is quite necessary for avoiding damage. Once the fluid has cycled around the subarachnoid space, it's mostly reabsorbed by the arachnoid villi back into the venous system. As a rule, maintaining a balance between CSF production and absorption is crucial because excess fluid can cause issues such as hydrocephalus. Sometimes, if something is blocking the way or the process of absorption is not ideal, the eventual outcome can be an intracranial pressure surge, potentially leading to severe neurological issues. In most cases, understanding these convoluted routes is key to furthering therapies - current studies are even investigating the causes of congenital hydrocephalus, showing how much it does matter to have a correct understanding of CSF dynamics. On another front, scientists are getting innovative by studying how CSF's normal circulation could be used as a drug-delivery route, particularly for recalcitrant brain tumors. There is increasing interest in using the fluid as a sort of conveyer belt that evades the notorious blood-brain barrier.

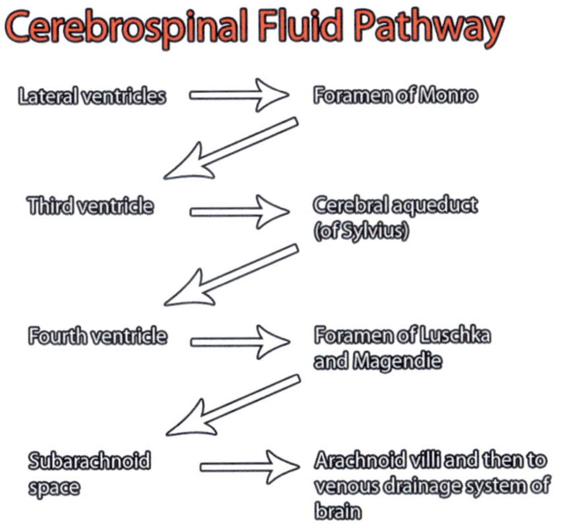

Figure 13.9. Pathways of CSF circulation.

Source: https://external-content.duckduckgo.com/iu/?u=http%3A%2F%2Fwww.virtualmedstudent.com%2Fimages%2Fcerebrospinal_fluid_pathway.jpg&f=1&nofb=1&ipt=864d60b3ccef4fa69041fbd6b05e1a7c0408f2aea9af53b57874ea8fbc202808.

Current research—even that which treated boronophenylalanine in boron neutron capture therapy (BNCT)—demonstrated that drugs administered through the CSF can reach tumors while restricting total exposure. These preliminary results suggest that harnessing the body's own CSF channels could radically transform how treatments are being created for various neurological conditions. As more and more research develops, it is certain that continuing to study these natural pathways could uncover safer and more effective treatments (Figure 13.9).

13.2.3. Mechanisms of Cerebrospinal Fluid Absorption

CSF absorption is serious business when it comes to keeping the central nervous system in proportion. Different processes work together in a pretty whimsical manner to maintain the CSF at the proper level and eliminate metabolic waste. One very obvious pathway is through those tiny ridges on the arachnoid membrane, the arachnoid granulations. They function very much like one-way gates—letting the fluid trickle into the venous sinuses but not back out. In the majority of cases, this open flow is what averts such issues as hydrocephalus, where CSF builds up and pressure goes through the roof. It's also significant to researchers trying to identify the root causes of many neurologic maladies and, in the end, to improve treatments. Venous pulsations also play a part in driving the CSF along, and one that is no less important. The regular, rhythmic muscle contractions of the brain veins create small changes in pressure which help to drive the CSF from the subarachnoid space into the venous system. Venous pulsations help to control the amount of fluid and ensure it does not build up in the ventricles, and so compromise neuronal activity. Existing studies, with the exception of a few, show that such factors as age and certain brain pathologies can interfere with pulsations. When this happens, the whole process of CSF absorption proceeds at a much-reduced rate, at times causing issues such as cerebral edema—which, naturally, underscores the all the more significant importance of further research into this subject. In addition to all of that, there is increasing interest in whether CSF absorption is linked to our lymph system. New studies suggest that the lymph vessels found within the meninges could be helping clear both CSF and interstitial fluid, thereby affecting CSF dynamics as well as immune responses. With these vessels lying there in the brain coverings, we have a fairly novel view on how fluid balance is maintained and immune functions are supported simultaneously. Discovery of this relationship makes new therapeutic options for various CNS disorders of both fluid and immune dysregulation available. All things being equal, untangling these intersecting pathways is crucial, not only to deal with current conditions but also to discover creative solutions that could someday result in improved patient outcomes (Figure 13.10).

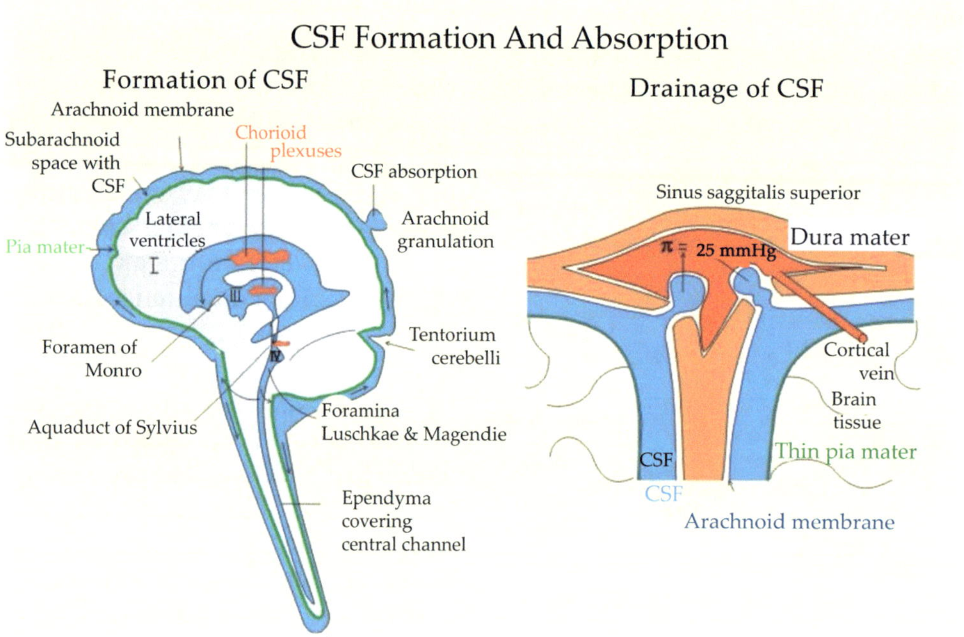

Figure 13.10. Mechanisms of CSF absorption.

Source: https://external-content.duckduckgo.com/iu/?u=https%3A%2F%2Fwww.zuniv.net%2Fphysiology%2Fbook%2Fimages%2Ffp3-7.jpg&f=1&nofb=1&ipt=bf3496d7b21b4d1c59bc585080f574ea8a9a4e580dc2c2da7287e80f7346a13c.

Test Your Knowledge

1. Which structures in the brain are primarily responsible for CSF production?
2. How does CSF circulate through the ventricles, subarachnoid space, and spinal cord?

13.3. Functions of Cerebrospinal Fluid

Learning Outcome

- Protection of the brain and spinal cord;
- Nutritional support for neural tissue;
- Removal of metabolic waste.

CSF's not just there to let the brain simply float around—no way. It does a whole lot more than that, actually. It works as a soft buffer for our central nervous system, diffusing the force of ordinary bumps and calming the damage, and delivering nutrients and taking out waste. Its chemistry can be quite unstable, supporting brain cells in a stable chemical environment, which is quite essential to the unimpeded passing of neurons. In most cases, a disturbance of this balance would indicate something wrong, and therefore doctors will do a more detailed scrutiny. CSF essentially provides physical support as well as ensures to maintain the typical biochemical composition required for optimal brain performance in daily activities, and also during disease. Besides physical support, CSF is responsible for carrying chemical messages within the central nervous system. It houses molecules such as hormones and neurotransmitters that help the brain talk to the rest of the body, controlling everything from mood to basic metabolic functions. It's fair to say it works in a way like some kind of "intermediary," especially in something like neuroinflammation, where it can mirror immune activity and sometimes even inform us that there are pathogens present. For instance, research at times discovers that changes in CSF composition can serve as early indicators of neurological pathology and report on both cognitive function and overall brain health. From the disease model, however, CSF has an even larger function when neurological illnesses and infections are at stake. Neuroscience studies, for example, have found that when such pathogens as *Trypanosoma brucei* gain entry into the CSF, they tend to cause severe aberrations, i.e., impairing sleep patterns or intellectual functions. The invasion of such agents not only destabilizes the physical composition of the brain but, along with the entry of contaminants, initiates a chain of physiological effects. Overall, therefore, these discoveries urge researchers to investigate the connections between disease pathology and CSF alterations further. Overall, in the context of neurocognitive well-being, analyzing CSF in more detail can actually help tailor treatments as well as improve patient outcomes.

13.3.1. Protection of the Brain and Spinal Cord

Our brain and spinal cord—our nervous system's core center—they need serious defense, and nature has an easy solution for it. CSF, that squishy pillow-like liquid, isn't hanging around doing nothing; it keeps the neurons in order by controlling ions and eliminating waste. It even acts as a built-in shock absorber, cushioning outside forces' blows. Nearly all the time, when the composition of CSF changes, it is a red flag that something is not quite right inside, so doctors do hurry to break it down for signs of infection or bleeding, supporting treatments that keep our neural circuits in functioning condition. In addition to serving as a physical cushion, CSF also plays an extremely significant role in biochemical defense. It contains a mix of signaling proteins and molecules that make certain that the neurons survive and trigger repairs when damage has occurred. Minimal variation in the concentrations of molecules such as glucose or lactate can reflect the status of the blood-brain barrier and overall brain metabolism. For instance, Bisdas et al. (2015) observed that patients who showed remarkable variations in CSF gas tensions after surgery were likely to have an impaired BBB. Pinpointing these chemical signals—when they are everywhere and nowhere at all—is the key for clinicians who are trying to predict complications and come up with treatments that protect our precious nerve cells. Inflammation comes into play, too, presenting yet another hurdle when it comes to protecting the brain and spinal cord. We know pro-inflammatory cytokines have been shown to speed along nerve damage, especially following ischemic events.

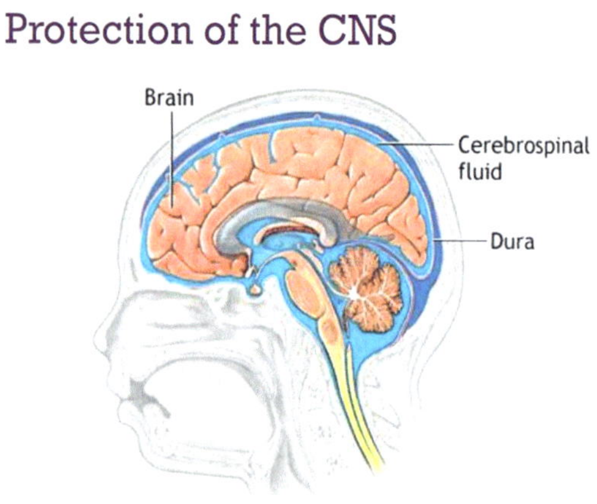

Figure 13.11. Protection of the brain and spinal cord.

Source: https://external-content.duckduckgo.com/iu/?u=https%3A%2F%2Fimage1.slideserve.com%2F2665023%2Fprotection-of-the-cns4-l.jpg&f=1&nofb=1&ipt=940a6562fba4f3f6b6985c8c62f0e972621f0e27eb5e02702aad2485f3504097.

An example of such research is the demonstration that treatment with an IL-1 receptor antagonist resulted in reduced loss of neurons following spinal cord ischemia (Akuzawa et al., 2008), suggesting that modulation of the inflammatory response may improve prognosis. Since inflammation speeds up damage, it should make sense to look for drugs that would reduce such harmful effects. There's even speculation regarding employing CSF to bring treatments right to the point of damage, which could quite possibly revolutionize how we repair the brain. In sum, these varied viewpoints remind us that it is not a one-dimensional narrative to defend our nervous system—there's the CSF both protecting and guiding the way to keep neurons safe (Figure 13.11).

13.3.2. Nutritional Support for Neural Tissue

Nutrition does matter when we're talking about our brain cells and the fluid that surrounds them, CSF. Tissue in the brain is not built around one food item—it's a blend of nutrients like fatty acids, proteins, and vitamins that makes everything work just right. Omega-3 fatty acids, in most cases, build neuron membranes and stimulate neurotransmitter production, which ultimately dictates how we see things and feel. Occasionally, if our nutrition gets derailed, even the CSF can shift in ways that can slow down the normal functioning of nerves. A diet rich in antioxidants and polyunsaturated fats can combat some of that cellular stress and aid in the recovery of neurons. In brief, understanding how our food supports neural function is crucial for allowing CSF to function and for keeping neurological problems at bay. There is also growing commotion about how not getting certain micronutrients is fueling brain deterioration. Vitamins B12, thiamine, and folate each play a vital role in nerve metabolism and in the maintenance of the insulating myelin sheath on our nerves—but deficiencies of them can be nerve-wracking for nerve function. The CSF, as a biochemical snapshot, will usually reflect these nutritional fluctuations. Thus, nutritional strategies to enhance such vitamins can indeed enhance CSF composition. Some studies, for example, have found that high levels of homocysteine, typically due to insufficiency of B vitamins, are correlated with faster cognitive decline. Generally, keeping your vitamin levels in check can go a long way to minimizing the risk of cognitive issues related to CSF alterations. New studies also indicate that normal dietary habits contribute a great deal to maintaining brain tissue robust, primarily through the impacts on CSF. Diets rich in fruits, vegetables, whole grains, and healthy fats appear to enhance brain function and even reduce the likelihood of neurodegeneration. These foods boost the body's own antioxidants and enable an anti-inflammatory environment to be established, perhaps to prod the CSF towards better balance. Worth noting, however, is that exposure to neurotoxic chemicals will disturb that delicate balance—studies using CSF biomarker measures have even attributed exposure to heavy metals as a cause of diseases like amyotrophic lateral sclerosis (ALS) (Bargellini et al., 2017). Overall, it is not just that the consumption of protective foods enriches neural tissue but also maintains the CSF under control, potentially staving off a range of neurological conditions (Creighton et al., 2016).

13.3.3. Removal of Metabolic Waste

Clearing out the rubbish in the brain is not white noise—it's crucial to running operations at full throttle. Neurons are firing activity, and that makes byproducts happen naturally, which, if they stay around, will build up to become toxic culprits that make us miss a step and feel our overall brain function suffering. Scientists now point out that CSF is not just drifting around; it collaborates with the blood-brain barrier, interstitial fluid, and perivascular spaces to help move waste either into the blood or directly into the CSF (Chopp et al., 2021).

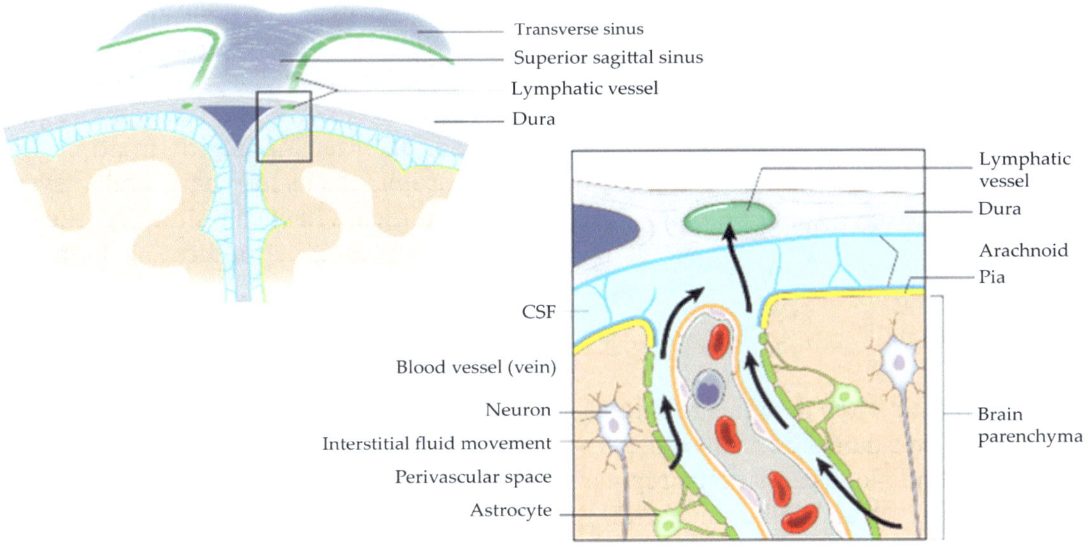

Figure 13.12. Removal of metabolic waste.

Source: https://spikesandbursts.wordpress.com/wp-content/uploads/2018/09/nature14432-sf10b.png.

This fluid motion not only keeps cells healthy but also maintains the tiny synapses so vital to optimal brain performance. Sleep is not just flipping a switch at night—most of the time, it acts more like the brain's own nightly cleaning crew. In slow-wave sleep (SWS), for example, the glymphatic system (a system of channels in which CSF moves) actually ramps up at high speeds, essentially sweeping up noxious metabolites like amyloid-beta, which has been associated with neurodegenerative conditions like Alzheimer's disease (Bovy et al., 2024). Yes, it sounds sort of redundant, but if the sleep is disrupted—say with cortisol surges—the brain's ability to clean out these toxins seems to break down, leaving those vital neurons exposed. There is also a contentious, and sometimes grimy, argument about exactly how the brain ships its trash. Other scientists refer to the operations of the glymphatic system and meningeal lymphatic vessels—these are the structures that not only drain interstitial fluid but also control CSF dynamics. In fact, waste removal isn't a one-stage process; it serves protection and repair functions at the same time. Subsequent research will even decide how to strengthen these CSF pathways to open up new lines of therapy, particularly for older individuals or those suffering from neurodegenerative diseases (Chopp et al., 2021). With more emphasis on all these mechanisms of clearance, the possible therapeutic potential for cognitive aging and disease prevention is fast becoming one of the most sizzling fields in neuroscience (Figure 13.12).

Test Your Knowledge

1. How does CSF provide mechanical protection to the brain and spinal cord?
2. What role does CSF play in maintaining chemical stability of the central nervous system?

13.4. Clinical Significance of Cerebrospinal Fluid Analysis

Learning Outcome

- Diagnostic procedures involving CSF;
- Common conditions detected through CSF analysis;
- Interpretation of CSF findings.

CSF is very important when it comes to finding evidence of neurological disorders like epilepsy. It can sometimes find biomarkers that a regular scan cannot identify, which can be the deciding factor. New studies even suggest that analyzing CSF is helpful when dealing with dog idiopathic epilepsy—a condition that has been hard to diagnose because it can show up in many different ways. With new developments in biomarkers and other diagnostic procedures, there's the sense that our whole strategy is going to shift a bit, with better means of predicting and treating the condition." In most cases, this will mean that CSF testing can actually significantly delineate the differences between types of epilepsy and guide more individualized treatment protocols in neurodiagnostics. CSF analysis isn't only useful for solving some specific issue, though. It also assists in the diagnosis of a neurological issue as a root cause or a secondary consequence of another disorder. Meningitis, multiple sclerosis, and encephalitis usually have similar symptoms, so it is difficult. In such a situation, the contents in CSF - sometimes indicating high levels of protein or abnormal cell numbers - can point towards an infection or inflammation. Throw in some of the more advanced functional neuroimaging with CSF tests, and you have a considerably better understanding of both acute and chronic disease. This sort of combined approach not only assists in diagnosing the problem but also in monitoring how well a treatment is working and how the disease might be progressing. Human and veterinary neurology are changing. So too is the need for standard CSF test protocols. Different approaches and interpretations can in fact muddy the waters and leave medical professionals stumped—especially with conditions like with canine idiopathic epilepsy. Some studies show that while established methodologies still give us useful information, lacking clear-cut criteria does hold up effective treatment. Combine more recent techniques like EEG and modern neuroimaging with CSF analysis and may just reveal superior approaches to defining diagnostic criteria and treatment protocols. For most cases, having firmer guidelines—backed by new evidence—may help clinicians better treat the complexity of neurological diseases and provide care that's better tailored to the unique needs of each patient (Brodbelt et al., 2016; Brodbelt et al., 2016) (Figure 13.13).

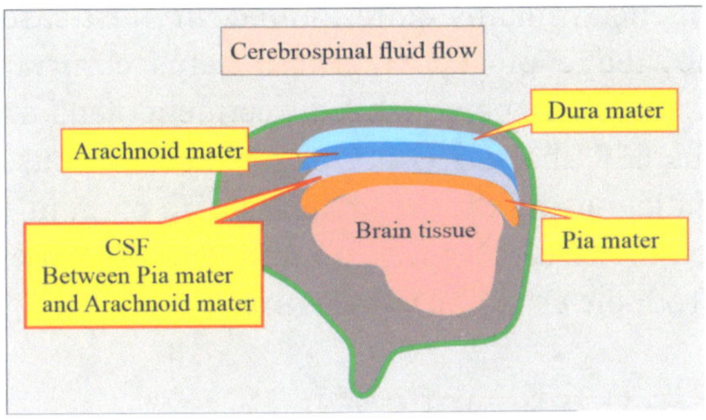

Figure 13.13. Cerebrospinal fluid analysis.

Source: https://labpedia.net/wp-content/uploads/2020/01/CSF-flow-in-arachnoidal-space-1.jpg.

13.4.1. Diagnostic Procedures Involving Cerebrospinal Fluid

CSF is a major issue when doctors suspect any type of neurological issue. Vets, for instance, will usually test a dog's CSF when idiopathic epilepsy is suspected. By drawing a sample, they can analyze its content of chemicals, cells, and immune messages that might be indicative of infections, inflammation, or even tumors. A quick look at the cells—occasionally through cytology—might identify unusual types that don't fit, and that little tidbit could be what tells you idiopathic epilepsy apart from diseases in some respects similar. For others, this simple test opens the door to more solid diagnostics and affects the treatment protocol. In recent times, the methods we utilize CSF in diagnosis have headed in a few interesting directions. Instead of merely relying on what one sees on scans or in clinical presentation, doctors are now complementing with CSF biomarkers so that they can better understand. Research today is, for the most part, moving everyone toward a better understanding of these markers and their role in conditions like epilepsy. More sophisticated neuroimaging now sometimes couples up with CSF testing, offering a kind-of multi-angle view that seems to further improve patient care overall. Effectively, these emerging developments are changing the practice of the norm, and that change will have its effects on future clinical decision-making. In idiopathic epilepsy, having a trustworthy CSF testing protocol matters more and more. Researchers are always digging around for potential biomarkers and winnowing out the criteria, often insisting that using simple signal checks in conjunction with full neurological examinations offers stronger indications. Old ways have their limitations, and these new CSF-based techniques are ready to offer superior alternatives. Existing studies, for example, recognize the need to dispel the current cloud of uncertainty over clear, useful guidelines for diagnosing canine idiopathic epilepsy (Brodbelt et al., 2016). Considering everything, many veterinary clinics seem open to trying newer more rational ways of recognizing different epileptic patterns, something that can have a direct effect on treatment plans and patient care (Brodbelt et al., 2016).

13.4.2. Common Conditions Diagnosed by Cerebrospinal Fluid Analysis

Analysis of the CSF has emerged as a key component in delivering precise neurological diagnosis. The majority of clinicians rely on it, especially in conditions like MS, when symptoms are totally unpredictable and render the detection of an issue difficult. An MS diagnosis generally entails combining clinical signs, neuroimaging, and laboratory examinations—and the CSF to reveal evidence of central nervous system inflammation. Perhaps the most fascinating discovery in most MS cases is the presence of oligoclonal bands (OCBs), technically the "gold standard" of laboratory testing, yet occasionally challenging to interpret due to analytical fails. In general, it underscores our ongoing need for better CSF biomarker studies and new diagnostic tests (Sasso et al., 2019).

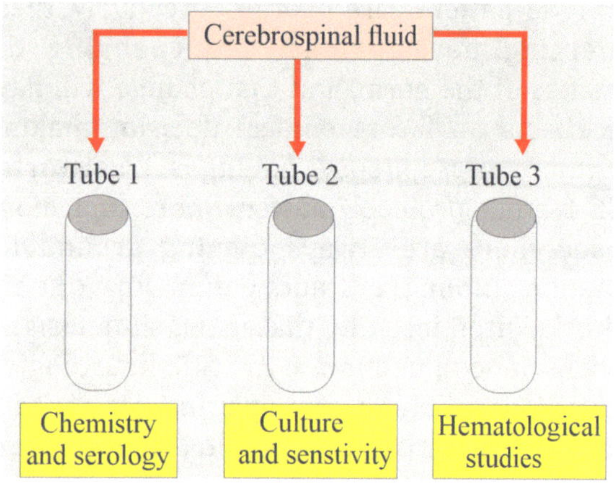

Figure 13.14. Common conditions detected through CSF analysis.

Source: https://labpedia.net/wp-content/uploads/2020/01/CSF-tubes-collection.jpg.

Aside from MS, testing of CSF also reveals clues for other neurological conditions like infections and tumors. Take conditions like meningitis, encephalitis or even certain brain cancers—sometimes they may be detected by the chemical makeup of the fluid. Abnormally high white blood cell counts, abnormal proteins and even traces of some pathogens all help point the diagnosis in the appropriate direction. In others, if doctors suspect a central nervous system cancer, CSF abnormals guide diagnosis and treatment. With these results, not only is there aid in the acute case but also long-term care of patients, demonstrating just how important CSF analysis is in practice. CSF analysis does not cease after diagnosis; it gives some insight into therapy too. In others, highly sensitive biomarkers in the CSF shed light on disease mechanisms, then on more personalized therapies. For example, quantifying free light chains (FLC) in the CSF has been gaining attention for its potential use to simplify diagnosis and monitoring of MS, a welcome alternative to previous techniques. At the same time, however, certain research studies have isolated some biomarkers which potentially are linked to epileptic diseases even as overall evidence remains quite limited. In most cases, knowledge of such markers helps clinicians develop more personalized treatment plans, and thus CSF analysis is no longer merely focused on diagnosing the problem but also on guiding treatment of complex neurological disorders (Brodbelt et al., 2016) (Figure 13.14).

13.4.3. Interpretation of Cerebrospinal Fluid Findings

Gaining a clear understanding of the complex realm of cerebrospinal fluid (CSF) testing is crucial when attempting to address a wide range of neurological issues. You discover that finding oligoclonal bands (OCBs) typically winds up implicating multiple sclerosis (MS) by implying an inflammatory kick in the central system. The process of diagnosing MS has changed over time—a mix of CSF markers, neurological exams, and imaging now directs the process, in general. Operating these bands is more a matter of confirming a diagnosis than anything else; they even sometimes help estimate how the disease might be progressing. However, it must be remembered that interpreting OCBs is not necessarily black-and-white since laboratory methods and operator skill can vary significantly. All that sophistication really supports the fact that we need more standardized protocols and fresh research on new biomarkers to sharpen diagnostic accuracy (Sasso et al., 2019). Beyond the historic tie to MS, deciphering CSF findings can reveal truly interesting signs about Alzheimer's as well as other neurodegenerative illnesses. Proteins in the middle like tau and amyloid-beta are increasingly used to follow disease progression and even early signs of cognitive decline. Other studies show a reasonable correlation between alterations in tau levels and what scans, including amyloid PET scans, show—this correlation demonstrates just how closely CSF data relates to what we can see on scans. With this, healthcare professionals have a more holistic and balanced picture of a patient's condition and disease progression. A latent time joint mixed-effects model, one that new research has examined, also makes us more capable of discerning long-term trajectories in cognition and pathology on the basis of a more firmly grounded interpretation of those CSF signals (Aisen et al., 2018). Aside from the usual method for the investigation of CSF, pursuing new biomarkers is key to advancing our diagnostic to the next level. For example, measurement of free light chains (FLC) in CSF has become a possible means to differentiate between different neuroinflammatory disorders. Unlike OCBs, which may take a bit longer and rely on whoever is doing the test, measurement of FLC level could speed up the process and give some added insight into the immune behavior in the central nervous system. In addition, as research keeps improving, clinicians' understanding of the specificity and sensitivity of these novel markers becomes increasingly relevant. This ongoing quest for ever more precise diagnostic tools is all about optimizing patient care through the provision of ensuring that CSF readouts are done both rapidly and accurately, which precisely highlights the relevance of interdisciplinary cooperation in neuroscience (Sasso et al., 2019).

Test Your Knowledge

1. What types of diseases can be diagnosed through lumbar puncture and CSF analysis?
2. How do changes in CSF cell count and glucose levels indicate infection?

13.5. Pathologies Associated with Cerebrospinal Fluid

Learning Outcome

- Hydrocephalus and its implications;
- Meningitis and its impact on CSF;
- Multiple sclerosis and CSF biomarkers.

CSF keeps coming up in brain research, mostly because it tells us something about what may be wrong in neurological disease. Take multiple sclerosis, for example – an immunologically related illness that progressively robs the insulating covering of nerve cells. CSF tests allow physicians to observe the way that the immune system is functioning within the brain, and detecting those protein clusters, or oligoclonal bands, has essentially become the gold standard for diagnosing MS. Sasso et al. (2019) goes on to note, however, that the methods for detecting these bands are currently highly dependent on operator expertise and training and can be extremely time-consuming. Meanwhile, test indicators such as free light chains in CSF are turning out to be novel interesting prospects for accelerating diagnosis. The function of CSF also involves testing the integrity of the blood-brain barrier. The ratio of CSF/serum albumin, or QAlb, ultimately measures how tight that barrier actually is. Recent studies seem to suggest that QAlb readings should consider age and sex differences – after all, evidence shows that males are more likely to experience issues with this barrier than females. That being the case, it suggests the potential for refining more accurate thresholds. In most cases, the optimization of these QAlb thresholds can result in more focused testing for neuroinflammatory disease, as Alessi et al. (2020) implies. It's not just MS or barrier problems that make doctors curious about CSF.

Meningitis, encephalitis, and inflammatory or infectious conditions can virtually turn the protein balance, sugar level, and immune cells within the fluid on its head. Such transformations typically offer important clues that guide clinicians on whether an infection is viral or bacterial – in the direction of the appropriate treatment pathway.

As our understanding of CSF biomarkers improves, it is possible that future research may unveil fresh signals that can track the progression of disease and quantify a patient's reaction to treatment, thus improving the management of various neurological disorders.

13.5.1. Hydrocephalus and Its Implications

Hydrocephalus is not just about mere neurological setbacks—it has an entire range of issues lying beneath. Most of the time, as normal pressure hydrocephalus (NPH) slowly takes its toll, people begin to realize some cognitive decline that can go entirely to spoil their everyday lives. Doctors use a mix of high-tech scans and doctor's checklists, with CSF tests forming a key consideration. Some of the CSF markers also seem to differentiate NPH from other conditions of brain wasting, something that is significant because NPH can be reversed if addressed in time.

A better understanding of these indicators may in the end result in more accurate ways of diagnosis and treatment of the disease. However, predicting the degree to which someone will get better following surgery remains an obstinate issue; present studies even link higher levels of P-tau in CSF with lesser chances of improvement after shunt surgery – illustrating that further excavation for beneficial biomarkers is needed (Saadaldeen et al., 2022). At another level, how exactly CSF flows and interacts with brain tissue has a huge role to play with hydrocephalus' vexatious nature. When that balance in absorbing and transmitting CSF is disturbed, the ventricles become filled, and that increased pressure can disorganize surrounding brain cells. New technologies in imaging—e.g., PET scans and DTI—have revealed some hints about how brain blood flow changes and even how its small structures survive the years. Often, a breakdown of blood supply in areas such as the basal ganglia and thalamus seems to match up with symptoms such as tripping on walks or general mental slowing. These signs not only provide us with a clearer picture of what's really going on in the brain, but also tell us how to make treatments more effective and improve patient care (Owler et al., 2004).

Essentially, treatment of hydrocephalus depends on a mix of smart clinical practice and ongoing examination of how CSF functions and what evidence it presents. Currently, we have research that focuses on the fact that we need to have more acute models in order to forecast outcomes resulting from treatment—more specifically, the success of shunt surgery. New studies into the CSF markers that are associated with symptoms can eventually offer more reliable diagnostic methods, so interventions can be conducted in a timely way. Additionally, attention to confounding brain-degenerative issues is essential in order to distinguish NPH from other disorders with similar symptoms. Remaining close to the CSF composition will certainly guide the way of future treatment, thereby improving the general management of individuals battling hydrocephalus (Saadaldeen et al., 2022) (Figure 13.15).

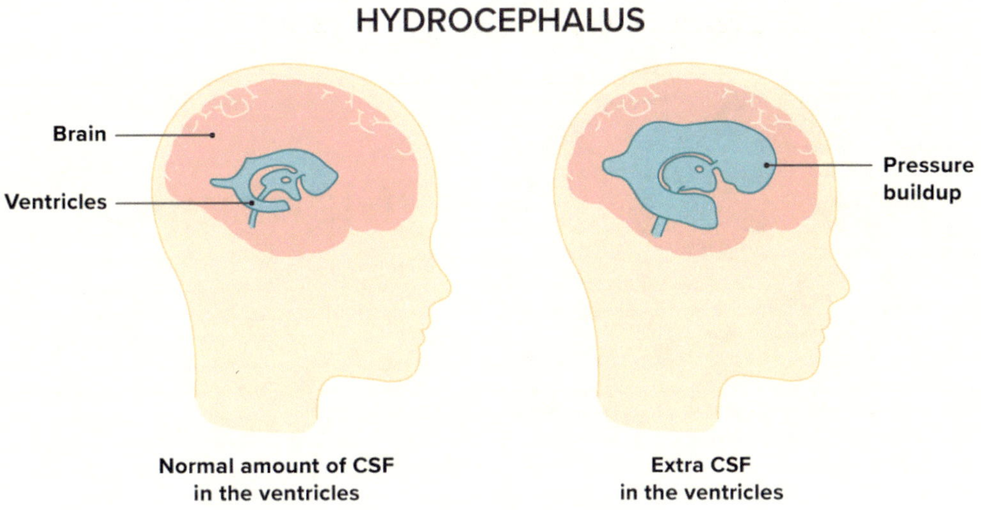

Figure 13.15. Hydrocephalus.

Source: https://external-content.duckduckgo.com/iu/?u=https%3A%2F%2Fpost.healthline.com%2Fwp-content%2Fuploads%2F2021%2F12%2F1830155-Hydrocephalus.png&f=1&nofb=1&ipt=a0fc2ff25b4283534efc08cc15d405181a334a6860f6eb62cd18a86af4f111b3.

13.5.2. Meningitis and Its Impact on Cerebrospinal Fluid

Meningitis diagnosis is not what it once was; it's completely different now due to newer methods of testing CSF. A particular stand-out test is PCR—particularly helpful when enteroviruses, thought by many to be the primary viral offenders, are at fault. In one recent look, RT-PCR found a sensitivity of 97% (in the majority of cases), a tremendous jump compared with the around 54.5% by standard culture methods for detecting enteroviruses in CSF samples (Gartzonika et al., 2005). A shift in method like this not only makes us better at being able to detect pathogens in the fluid, but it also makes care faster for patients, eliminating delays that might cause further complications. When you consider the clinical presentation of meningitis—more specifically the aseptic variety linked with enteroviruses—the constellation of symptoms and laboratory clues from CSF becomes very intriguing. A retrospective review proved that children present with fever, headache, and vomiting, and a number of cases even had a clear presence of polymorphonuclear cells in the CSF (Ahmed et al., 2007). The cell count was at the median of $201/mm^3$, which really emphasizes how much inflammation there is, varying with what triggered it. Aside from making an absolute diagnosis, identification of enterovirus RNA in CSF also appears to be associated with shorter hospital stay, suggesting that improved, quicker tests can result in better outcomes overall. More intriguing, however, is the fact that these findings do not merely enhance diagnosis—They seem to change the entire treatment approach to meningitis. With PCR on the agenda, doctors can rapidly isolate the bug causing the illness and adjust therapies accordingly. In fact, children suffering from enterovirus meningitis actually stayed shorter periods in the hospital, an indication that early treatment might decrease the overall healthcare load (Ahmed et al., 2007). Further, the decline in serious complications and fatalities suggests that contemporary testing is indeed pointing the way to treatment in the right direction. In summary, the employment of sophisticated CSF tests—most notably PCR—is a significant step in meningitis knowledge and treatment, providing a deeper insight into how brain fluid reacts during infection (Figure 13.16).

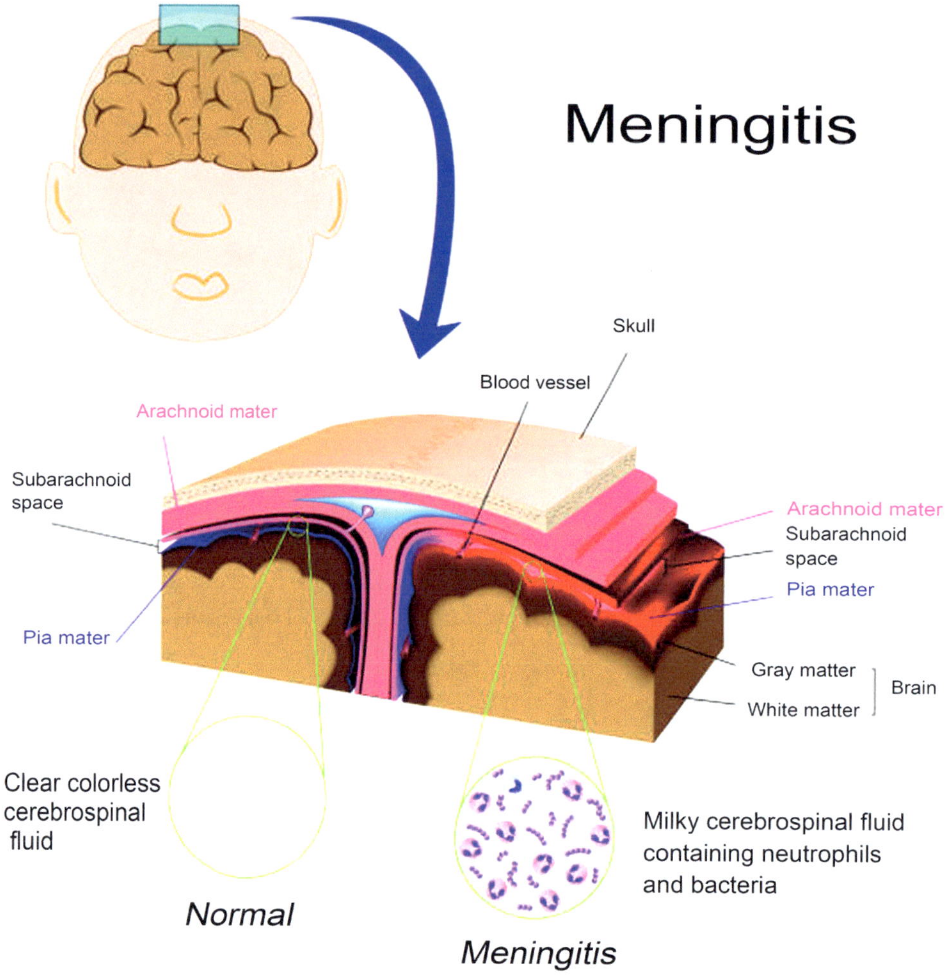

Figure 13.16. Meningitis and its impact on CSF.

Source: https://external-content.duckduckgo.com/iu/?u=https%3A%2F%2Fwww.headway.org.uk%2Fmedia%2F6538%2Fdiagram-showing-how-meningitis-affects-the-brain-including-the-meninges-around-the-brain-copyright-shutterstock_89870962.jpg&f=1&nofb=1&ipt=6731688f40e7b8164ebba6227c1948673e9e33c1ae1e691f9d4a6dc56b182b16.

13.5.3. Multiple Sclerosis (MS) and Cerebrospinal Fluid Biomarkers

Multiple sclerosis (MS) appears as a bundle of immune breakdowns, brain inflammation, and ongoing loss of nerve cells—a combination that undoubtedly calls for a wide-ranging effort to get it all out. More recent studies have turned to analyzing CSF in an attempt to find out what's really going on. Often, you'll find markers like oligoclonal bands in the CSF, which hint at local immune protein production that many doctors see as a classic sign of MS. People have also started keeping an eye on neurofilament light chain (NFL) levels; when these go up, it usually tracks with nerve damage and the activity of the disease. In the majority of cases, incorporating these markers into routine practice can potentially make diagnoses more precise and help tailor treatments to the specific needs of individual patients. Ongoing research still tries to improve these profiles in order to better predict the course of the disease and guide treatment decisions (Lorenzut et al., 2025). In diagnosing MS, it's not just a question of clinical examinations—high-level markers in the CSF actually play their part. Critical chemicals like matrix metalloproteinases (MMPs) and even cytokines like interleukin-17 (IL-17) give us a glimpse into the inflammatory environment of the disease. MMPs, for example, cause the opening up of the blood-brain barrier, an action whose significance is appreciated in terms of when and where lesions in the central nervous system begin to develop. In the same way, higher levels of IL-17 tend to signal that the immune system is functioning optimally, which leads to demyelination. Such information not only facilitates the distinction between MS and other of its kind—it also opens doors for earlier detection. In addition, linking CSF markers with neuroimaging (e.g., MRI) introduces a new, layered aspect to MS's messy pathology (Coulthard et al., 2023). As MS treatment continues to evolve, CSF biomarkers are becoming more clearly defined. Determining those patients potentially racing toward speeding up disease progression enables therapies to commence earlier and in a more aggressive manner. Sometimes a cut-and-dried pattern among these markers is seen as indicating a higher possibility of relapses—or even conversion into the more difficult secondary progressive course—encouraging doctors to move toward more tailored treatment plans. Concurrently, several clinical trials are assessing newer drugs that target specifically the inflammatory processes emphasized by such CSF markers, all in an effort to protect against the long-term consequences of the disease. This unification of biomarker information and treatment techniques really shows the potency of personalized medicine in the treatment of MS. Finally, digging deeper into CSF data not only makes our diagnosis more accurate but also allows for greater patient outcomes through more targeted and tailored treatments (Lorenzut et al., 2025).

Test Your Knowledge

1. How does bacterial meningitis alter the composition of CSF?
2. What CSF abnormalities are commonly observed in subarachnoid hemorrhage?

13.6. Advances in Cerebrospinal Fluid Research

Learning Outcome

- Innovations in CSF collection techniques;
- Emerging biomarkers in neurological disorders;
- Future directions in CSF studies.

Surgical techniques really did shift with our growing knowledge of CSF. More modern technologies, like those more minimally invasive procedures, just keep coming as studies and observations from CSF further increase our knowledge. Now, doctors increasingly employ rigid scopes—devices that enable them to look at parts of the body previously out of reach—to enhance surgery success and offer new options in neurological care. These advancements not only help tackle really tough conditions but also remind us just how essential CSF is in recognizing and understanding brain conditions. All too frequently, the way we sharpen surgery and investigate CSF data blur together naturally, indicating us to more smart ways of diagnosing and treating conditions that affect the central nervous system, ultimately at the benefit of the patient in better care. Today's research is incorporating genetic studies into the care of CSF-related conditions. A series of recent papers in general state that even such unusual genetic problems—problems that even stump practitioners—can be resolved a bit better by seeing what CSF might have to say. These intricate disorders take a form with a combination of neurological symptoms that become more complex with the passage of time, making it difficult for scientists to delve into what exactly is occurring at the cell level. By examining CSF's chemistry very closely, scientists have begun to identify specific gene mutations and how mutations affect cell behavior, which in most cases makes treatment more feasible to customize more specifically. For example, the progress in lipid metabolism has shed some light on the mechanisms that cause conditions like Niemann-Pick disease (Naffadi et al., 2024), opening the door for newer methods of diagnosis and potentially managing them. It's a dynamic arena where genetic clues and CSF secrets seem to be having a discussion step by step, both adding to the complex picture of neurological therapy. And then there's the whole world of high-tech imaging and biomarker studies that are creating another level of CSF consciousness. Techniques like mass spectrometry and MRI, for instance, have given researchers the tools to pick out barely detectable markers in CSF that indicate diseases such as multiple sclerosis or Alzheimer's. This not only aids in the early diagnosis of these conditions, but also brings us closer to specific treatments for each case. Ongoing research still reminds us that CSF is no passive fluid; it is an active player in balancing activities of the brain and can signal the onset of diseases. Overall, the constant flow of CSF studies continues to redefine our concepts of diagnosing and managing neurological disease, steadily laying the groundwork for improved patient outcomes-even if the specifics sometimes appear a tad randomized (Figure 13.17).

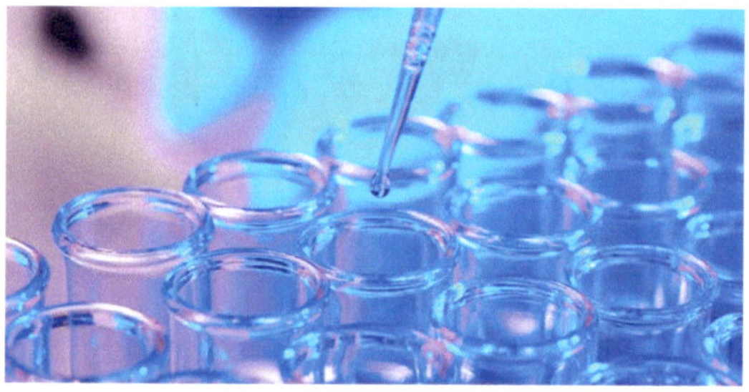

Figure 13.17. The precision and care involved in clinical and biomedical research workflows.

Source: https://external-content.duckduckgo.com/iu/?u=https%3A%2F%2Fwww.targetals.org%2Fwp-content%2Fuploads%2F2022%2F09%2FTALS-Blog-Image_CSF-2-1024x512.jpg&f=1&nofb=1&ipt=e2092ba8fc6816f141f7b61823be0d5a9133d784d0d8aafc43e2adb1ad8a5b8f.

13.6.1. Innovations in Cerebrospinal Fluid Collection Techniques

Methods for CSF collection have changed—present changes are an indication of a true shift from the invasive techniques of the past. In the majority of cases, previous techniques were harsh on patients, often involving perilous, invasive interventions that could lead to complications and protracted recoveries. Presently, thanks to advances, doctors opt for far less brutal techniques but no less effective in diagnosing and curing diseases. Look at endoscopic methods, say for instance; they've improved the management of CSF leaks, with fewer post-op complications and fewer days spent in the hospital, and that does matter significantly. Specialists now have precision-designed tools and work together across departments, and with this collective strength, they not only discover a cure for today's problem but lay the groundwork for future achievement in CSF harvesting and treatment—a landmark shift in neuroscience procedures (Galli et al., 2021).

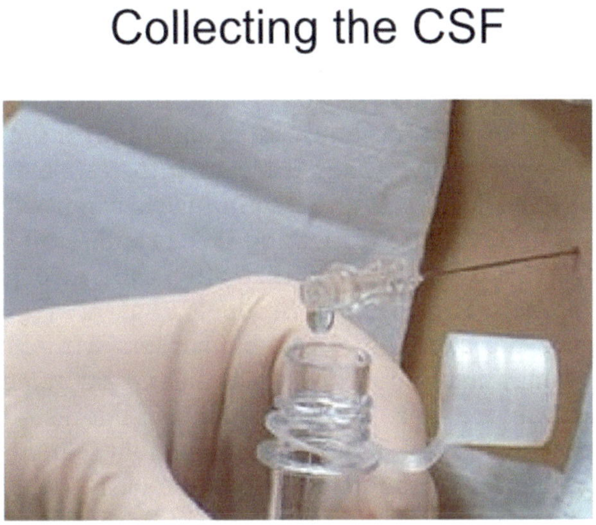

Figure 13.18. CSF collection techniques.

Source: https://external-content.duckduckgo.com/iu/?u=https%3A%2F%2Fimage.slidesharecdn.com%2Fcerebrospinalfluid-111019052744-phpapp01%2F95%2Fcerebrospinal-fluid-51-728.jpg%3Fcb%3D1319002129&f=1&nofb=1&ipt=2b1da6e222aab8c13f4b6a0a1fc625df2b8afc720329abc92fd59e3325308737.

Technological advances in CSF testing have also made great strides, particularly in the fight against blood cancers. Advances in equipment—flow cytometry and automated hematology analyzers—now are essential for identifying leukemia blasts in specimens, supplanting the outdated manual cell count that too frequently struggled with inconsistencies and subpar turnaround times. Recent research, overall, identifies the way flow cytometry is able to separate blast cells from the rest distinctly, giving a more accurate diagnosis in acute leukemias. By integrating these machines in routine clinical practice, doctors can assess risk in real-time and plan treatment options more effectively than before, something that can ultimately translate into an enormous advantage in patient care. Researchers are constantly refining such methods, and overall, CSF analytics as an art is set to be even more refined. In the meantime, there is more buzz about biomaterial advancements for applications in CSF. Nowadays, specifically designed, biocompatible materials are being used for procedures that strive to reduce invasiveness—accelerating the collection procedure and ensuring sample quality. When you combine sophisticated materials and clever instrumentation, the outcomes for both treatment and diagnosis become much better. In addition, neurosurgeons, neuroradiologists, and other specialists are pooling their collective expertise to tailor these approaches so they're better suited to each patient's unique requirements. As they continue to gain traction and evolve, they have the potential to reshape what best practice in dealing with CSF issues looks like, paving the way for an even more personalized system of neurological treatment (Galli et al., 2021) (Figure 13.18).

13.6.2. Emerging Biomarkers in Neurological Disorders

Diagnosis of neurological disease is changing fast these days, causing much excitement about new biomarkers—especially those obtained from CSF. Setting absolute diagnostic criteria has always been a bit of a headache, as researchers and clinicians don't usually "see eye to eye." New methods of diagnosis are now causing ripples in ways no one could have envisioned. CSF biomarkers may be able to sift through different neurological issues more conclusively, and this would be able to make treatments hit the nail more directly on the head. It is especially important because the way symptoms emerge can be so fluid and changeable, and this makes epilepsy especially hard to pinpoint with our sloppily applied limited treatments. New biomarkers, incidentally, are offering a glimpse of hope when it comes to detecting such conditions as idiopathic epilepsy. Some recent studies even promise that investigating CSF profiles can give us a clue about the underlying biological idiosyncrasies—knowledge that often falls through the cracks amidst the morass of cross-cutting symptoms. For example, Brodbelt et al. (2016) points out that although diagnosis remains challenging, the coupling of CSF biomarkers with cutting-edge neuroimaging and electroencephalography may indeed sharpen our diagnostic game significantly. This dual approach not only paves the way for more rapid intervention but also encourages us to develop treatment plans that are individually fine-tuned to each patient's own story. For the most part, investigating CSF biomarkers appears to be a necessity if we wish to truly understand something about neurological disease and enhance patient care. Beyond providing us with better diagnostic capabilities, these new biomarkers may completely change the manner in which we administer treatments. Brodbelt et al. (2016) reminds us that while the classic anti-epileptic medicines have their virtues, there is a variation response that leaves some boxes unopened, specifically where certain phenotypes are involved. Biomarkers that are currently emerging can potentially account for why variations do occur and shed important light on pharmacogenomics—thus allowing us to tailor treatments wiser. In total, this change illustrates the importance of ongoing research in biomarker fields, particularly those of CSF origin. Shedding light on the biochemical processes implicated in neurological disease via these biomarkers may well set us on the course toward the next generation of treatments—ones that are not only more effective but also oddly tailored.

13.6.3. Future Directions in Cerebrospinal Fluid Studies

CSF is in the spotlight these days as an important element in the diagnosis of brain diseases. The latest studies keep unfolding that the mysterious biomarkers in CSF could just uncover what's happening in the brain, especially in conditions such as Alzheimer's. Some studies indicate that protein levels—take Aβ1-42 and tau—could be associated with the speed of decline in thinking abilities, and even foretell neurodegeneration. To illustrate, you continually find that where there are heightened concentrations of Aβ1-42, there is also a sort of psychological resilience, partially because of what has been termed cognitive reserve (Allegri et al., 2015). While scientists hone their methods and techniques, there's a growing likelihood that CSF biomarker signatures will ultimately be helpful in informing the establishment of therapies more accurately tailored to specific patients—a relatively gigantic leap for diagnosis and prognosis in neurology. More sophisticated statistical models, including latent time joint mixed-effects models, seem to be leading the way in upcoming CSF research. Researchers are already using these models so that they can combine measurements of memory, daily life functioning, and biomarkers simultaneously, which allows them to better establish how neurodegeneration is advancing (Aisen et al., 2018). Not only does this process dictate the order of pathological changes, but it also allows for speculation about when symptoms will develop. By putting together CSF analysis with imaging and cognitive testing, scientists are piecing together a kind of layered story about the course of disease. It's innovative, one that actually highlights the value of interdisciplinarity—because sometimes taking a step back to get some perspective is what brings research forward. CSF research in the future may indeed depend on breakthroughs in new technology, particularly when it comes to finding and analyzing biomarkers. High-throughput metabolomics and proteomics, for example, are pushing it to the next level by providing an almost comprehensive inventory of what is present in the CSF. Because the usual biomarkers might not reveal the full picture of the complicated details of neurologic conditions, adding new molecules to the mix might unleash hidden links to cognitive decline or other impairments. More often than not, this research casts lighter on the role of CSF and advances personalized medicine by bringing treatment regimens closer to whatever particular patient is required. Generally, all these trends show real promise to turn neurological science and practice on its head and in the not-too-distant future, offer more precise diagnostics and treatments.

Test Your Knowledge

1. How are biomarkers in CSF being studied for early detection of neurodegenerative diseases like Alzheimer's?
2. What role does proteomics and metabolomics play in advancing CSF research?

Summary

CSF has been revolutionary in the manner in which we not only make a diagnosis but decide on the best treatment for a wide range of neurological disorders. Take spontaneous intracranial hypotension (SIH), for instance—when a patient presents with headaches that intensify upon standing, these symptoms often point directly to issues rooted in the cerebrospinal fluid (CSF). Sometimes, an MRI with a little added contrast to the equation doesn't stand alone. Rather, it supports the information the fluid study provides helping doctors put all the pieces together. This blend of imaging and lab work makes it probable that it will build a sound diagnosis stressing the central role of CSF in modern neurology (Alexis et al., 2018). Looking closer, it turns out that CSF isn't only about confirming what's wrong – it also nudges treatment choices in a big way. In a lot of SIH cases, sticking to basics like bed rest coupled with oral steroids has often helped ease the symptoms, suggesting that the pressure measured in CSF works double duty: it flags the issue and points toward a fix. It's as though the liquid is wedded to the diagnosis of the disorder and being a target for treatment. And if you dig far enough into the mechanisms by which CSF functions, you might even extract tips for other disorders; for instance, in epilepsy the personal biochemical make-up of the CSF could decide how successful anti-epileptic medication proves (Brodbelt et al., 2016). In most cases, that's why ongoing research is so timely—there's still much more to sort through regarding the intricacies of CSF's involvement with neurological disease. Pairing precise imaging with detailed CSF analysis isn't just clarifying the fluid's current importance; it's also paving the way for what comes next. Future studies will likely reveal increasingly nuanced hints at CSF's role in a wide range of diseases, laying the groundwork for more tailored treatments. As we come to realize better just how complexly involved neurological disorders can be, it would only stand to reason that digging deeply into CSF data can refine diagnostic accuracy and make management strategies more effective. The achievements already realized—and the promise held out by new imaging technology—point to an extremely rosy future for diagnosing and treating brain and nerve disease. In many ways, a careful inspection of CSF is going to remain a cornerstone on which to build better therapies and achieve better patient outcomes.

Advanced imaging is today at the forefront of diagnosing and treating brain disorders. Numbers taken from such scans are replacing conventional, qualitative assessments. The Cortical Asymmetry Index (CAI) has been touted in most recent studies as a valid tool in distinguishing between illness states like Alzheimer's disease and Frontotemporal dementia. Researchers, using the instruments of information theory, have created a system that not only translates subjective visual impressions into objective ones but also permits patients to be categorized into distinct clinical clusters. This shift, in most cases, creates the opportunity for earlier diagnosis and more highly individualized interventions. Importantly, correlating the CAI to fluid biomarkers—such as neurofilament-light (NfL) and glial fibrillary acidic protein (GFAP)—gives a more accurate representation of disease development and validates the utility of the convergence of imaging and laboratory testing in clinical settings (Agnès et al., 2025). Testing CSF, another factor being examined is the stability of its contents once the sample has been collected. Glucose levels in CSF, for example, are pivotal when it comes to diagnosing illnesses such as meningitis, but they decrease significantly even within a matter of hours after being drawn. One study recently showed that they drop relatively sharply over a short period of time, making it even more necessary to have quick analysis. Small changes in these figures can make a big difference in terms of diagnostic outcomes, so it's absolutely imperative that clinicians get to testing in a timely manner. This reality highlights the challenge of sampling CSF and underscores the need for standardized protocols to ensure the validity of data to aid in informed clinical practice decisions (Haryando et al., 2024). Essentially, neurological practice is evolving into a more interfused field where imaging and biochemical testing work in tandem. The application of technologies like the CAI not only demystifies how we differentiate among the neurodegenerative diseases but may also be a tool for tracking their progression over time. Meanwhile, however, the clear demands for direct, routine testing for elements of CSF—especially in emergency conditions like meningitis—have a tendency to bring out the multi-angled nature of these tests. All these innovations, in aggregate, are pushing us toward a more unifying diagnostic approach that integrates imaging, biomarkers, and timely testing, ultimately yielding better patient outcomes and clinical practices.

KEY TERMS FROM THIS CHAPTER

- Appearance
- Blood-CSF barrier
- Cerebrospinal fluid (CSF)
- Clarity (clear, cloudy, or bloody)
- CSF culture
- CSF pressure
- Cytology
- Differential count
- Glucose concentration
- Gram stain
- IgG index
- Lactate
- Lumbar puncture (spinal tap)
- Oligoclonal bands
- Opening pressure
- PCR (polymerase chain reaction)
- Protein concentration
- Red blood cell count (RBC)
- White blood cell count (WBC)
- Xanthochromia

Critical Thinking Questions

1. **Which of the following is a common cause for the presence of white blood cells in cerebrospinal fluid (CSF)?**
   a. Brain tumor
   b. Meningitis
   c. Stroke
   d. Multiple sclerosis
2. **A clear and colorless CSF sample is considered normal. What would a cloudy or turbid appearance of CSF most likely indicate?**
   a. Presence of blood
   b. Infection or inflammation
   c. Increased protein concentration
   d. Normal CSF variation
3. **In the examination of cerebrospinal fluid, what is the significance of an increased protein level?**
   a. Indicates bacterial infection or inflammation
   b. Indicates normal CSF composition
   c. Signifies a decrease in white blood cells
   d. Suggests brain hemorrhage
4. **Which of the following tests is most commonly used to detect bacterial infection in CSF?**
   a. Gram stain
   b. Glucose test
   c. Protein electrophoresis
   d. Culture and sensitivity
5. **Which of the following conditions would be most likely associated with low glucose levels in cerebrospinal fluid?**
   a. Viral meningitis
   b. Bacterial meningitis
   c. Multiple sclerosis
   d. Brain injury

Answers to Critical Thinking Questions

1. (b); 2. (b); 3. (a); 4. (a); 5. (b)

Short Answer Questions

1. What is the primary purpose of cerebrospinal fluid (CSF) examination, and what does it help diagnose?
2. What are the normal physical characteristics (appearance, color, clarity) of CSF?
3. What does xanthochromia in CSF indicate, and how is it identified?
4. What is the significance of an elevated white blood cell count (pleocytosis) in CSF, and what conditions can cause it?
5. How is glucose measured in CSF, and what does a low glucose level suggest?
6. What can the presence of red blood cells (RBCs) in CSF indicate, and how is it differentiated from traumatic lumbar puncture?

References

1. Agnello, L., Lo Sasso, B., Vidali, M., Scazzone, C., Piccoli, T., Gambino, C. M., Bivona, G., et al. (2021). Neurogranin as a reliable biomarker for synaptic dysfunction in Alzheimer's disease. *Diagnostics, 11*, 2339–2339. https://doi.org/10.3390/diagnostics11122339 (accessed on 1st July 2025).
2. Ahmed, A., Michos, A. G., Lee, B. E., Ramers, C., Robinson, C. C., Hadjichristodoulou, C., Mylonakis, E., et al. (2007). Aseptic meningitis in children: Analysis of 506 cases. https://core.ac.uk/download/pdf/7658741.pdf (accessed on 1st July 2025).
3. Aisen, P. S., Donohue, M. C., Iddi, S., Li, Y., et al. (2018). Bayesian latent time joint mixed-effects model of progression in the Alzheimer's Disease Neuroimaging Initiative. https://core.ac.uk/download/323064943.pdf (accessed on 1st July 2025).
4. Akuzawa, S., Bashar, A. H. M., Kazui, T., Shi, Y., et al. (2008). Interleukin-1 receptor antagonist attenuates the severity of spinal cord ischemic injury in rabbits. https://core.ac.uk/download/pdf/82241369.pdf (accessed on 1st July 2025).
5. Aleman, M., Costa, L. R. R., Crowe, C., Kass, P. H., et al. (2018). Presumed neuroglycopenia caused by severe hypoglycemia in horses. https://core.ac.uk/download/323069529.pdf (accessed on 1st July 2025).
6. Alessi, F., Baldi, E., Bellini, T., Caniatti, M., et al. (2020). Increased age and male sex are independently associated with higher frequency of blood–cerebrospinal fluid barrier dysfunction using the albumin quotient. https://core.ac.uk/download/287848476.pdf (accessed on 1st July 2025).
7. Allegri, R. F., Campos, J., Chrem Mendez, P. A., Clarens, C. M., et al. (2015). Cognitive reserve and Aβl-42 in mild cognitive impairment (Argentina–Alzheimer's Disease Neuroimaging Initiative). https://core.ac.uk/download/159284131.pdf (accessed on 1st July 2025).
8. Andreasen, N., Johansson, A., Blennow, K., Braak, E., Bybee, A., Donovan, N., Dranovsky, A., et al. (2005). Genetic association of CDC2 with cerebrospinal fluid tau in Alzheimer's disease. https://core.ac.uk/download/16432819.pdf (accessed on 1st July 2025).
9. Anukam, C., Barletta-Rodolfi, C., Belleville, S., Bianchi, F., Bressi, S., Carabotti, M., Cryan, J., et al. (2017). A pilot study on the effects of probiotic supplementation on neuropsychological performance and microRNA-29a-c levels in antiretroviral-treated HIV-1-infected patients. https://core.ac.uk/download/141694702.pdf (accessed on 1st July 2025).
10. Back, W., Bastiaansen, J. W. M., Boegheim, I. J. M., Dibbits, B., et al. (2015). A nonsense mutation in *B3GALNT2* is concordant with hydrocephalus in Friesian horses. https://core.ac.uk/download/55765719.pdf (accessed on 1st July 2025).
11. Bailey, R., Bradshaw, J., Foley, K., Gruendl, S., Gunn-Moore, D., Kipar, A., Laubner, H., et al. (2017). Clinicopathologic features and magnetic resonance imaging findings in 24 cats with histopathological confirmed neurologic feline infectious peritonitis. https://core.ac.uk/download/96600371.pdf (accessed on 1st July 2025).
12. Bakhti, K., Duflos, C., Gelis, A., Hirtz, D., et al. (2024). Post-polio syndrome is not a dysimmune condition. https://core.ac.uk/download/604467731.pdf (accessed on 1st July 2025).
13. Balogh, N., Bódai, E., Joó, K., Kutasi, F., et al. (2015). Cerebrospinal fluid parameters of horses

with West Nile virus neuroinvasive disease. https://core.ac.uk/download/42938104.pdf (accessed on 1st July 2025).

14. Bargellini, A., Filippini, T., Fini, N., Grill, P., et al. (2017). Lead, cadmium and mercury in cerebrospinal fluid and risk of amyotrophic lateral sclerosis: A case-control study. https://core.ac.uk/download/84493536.pdf (accessed on 1st July 2025).
15. Barrett, M. P., Bisser, S., Biéler, S., Cattanach, K., et al. (2016). Metabolomics identifies multiple candidate biomarkers to diagnose and stage human African trypanosomiasis. https://core.ac.uk/download/74231142.pdf (accessed on 1st July 2025).
16. Bentivoglio, M., Bradley, B., Etet, P. F. S., Grassi-Zucconi, G., et al. (2016). *Trypanosoma brucei brucei* invasion and T-cell infiltration of the brain parenchyma in experimental sleeping sickness: Timing and correlation with functional changes. https://core.ac.uk/download/74231018.pdf (accessed on 1st July 2025).
17. Bianchi, L., Cavallari, E. N., Ceccarelli, G., Corano Scheri, S., et al. (2017). Improvement of neuropsychological performances and reduction of immune-activation markers after probiotic supplementation and change of lifestyle in an HIV-positive male: Targeting the microbiota to act on the gut-brain axis. https://core.ac.uk/download/141694703.pdf (accessed on 1st July 2025).
18. Bisdas, T., Boeck, A. L., Fleissner, F., Haverich, A., et al. (2015). Intraoperative changes in cerebrospinal fluid gas tensions reflect paraplegia during thoracoabdominal aortic surgery. https://core.ac.uk/download/211705679.pdf (accessed on 1st July 2025).
19. Black, H., Gunson, R. N., Shepherd, S. J., Thomson, E., et al. (2017). HIV-positive patient with GBS-like syndrome. https://core.ac.uk/download/84915802.pdf (accessed on 1st July 2025).
20. Bovy, L., Claassen, J. A. H. R., de Wolff, T., Dresler, M., et al. (2024). Divergent associations of slow-wave sleep versus rapid eye movement sleep with plasma amyloid-beta. https://core.ac.uk/download/624077847.pdf (accessed on 1st July 2025).
21. Brettschneider, J., Ludolph, A. C., Pfister, H. W., Rupprecht, T., et al. (2009). The chemokine CXCL13 in acute neuroborreliosis. https://core.ac.uk/download/19450594.pdf (accessed on 1st July 2025).
22. Brodbelt, A., Felbecker, A., Lidstrom, A. M., Nilselid, A. M., Szoor, B., Sihlbom, C., et al. (2014). The chaperone protein clustering may serve as a cerebrospinal fluid biomarker for chronic spinal cord disorders in the dog. https://core.ac.uk/download/16462793.pdf (accessed on 1st July 2025).
23. Brodbelt, D. C., Charalambous, M., & Volk, H. A. (2016). The evidence behind the treatment of canine idiopathic epilepsy. https://core.ac.uk/download/36779227.pdf (accessed on 1st July 2025).
24. Brodbelt, D. C., Charalambous, M., & Volk, H. A. (2016). The evidence behind the diagnostic investigation of canine idiopathic epilepsy. https://core.ac.uk/download/36779228.pdf (accessed on 1st July 2025).
25. Chopp, M., Davoodi-Bojd, E., Ding, G., Fahmy, L., et al. (2021). Waste clearance in the brain. https://core.ac.uk/download/478539342.pdf (accessed on 1st July 2025).
26. Coulthard, E., & Hosseini, A. A. (2023). Blood biomarkers: Ready for clinical practice? *Journal of Neurology, Neurosurgery, and Psychiatry, 94*, 409–410. https://www.semanticscholar.org/

paper/690f31c61712304d835869d31b80588c8204d2f6 (accessed on 1st July 2025).

27. Creighton, E. K., Keating, M. K., Lyons, L. A., Sisó, S., et al. (2016). Characterization of an inherited neurologic syndrome in Toyger cats with forebrain commissural malformations, ventriculomegaly and interhemispheric cysts. https://core.ac.uk/download/323069548.pdf (accessed on 1st July 2025).

28. Davi, D., Ibrahim, S., & Savitri, A. A. (2024). Transsphenoidal approach for seller region tumor: A case series. https://core.ac.uk/download/617167825.pdf (accessed on 1st July 2025).

29. Donnelly, J. P., Chen, S., Kauffman, C. A., Steinbach, W. J., Baddley, J. W., Verweij, P. E., Clancy, C. J., et al. (2019). Revision and update of the consensus definitions of invasive fungal disease from the European Organization for Research and Treatment of Cancer and the Mycoses Study Group Education and Research Consortium. *Clinical Infectious Diseases, 71*, 1367–1376. https://doi.org/10.1093/cid/ciz1008 (accessed on 1st July 2025).

30. Galli, J., Morelli, F., Paludetti, G., Rigante, D., et al. (2021). Management of cerebrospinal fluid leak: The importance of multidisciplinary approach. https://core.ac.uk/download/479163469.pdf (accessed on 1st July 2025).

31. Gartzonika, C., Levidiotou, S., & Vrioni, G. (2005). Evaluation of a commercially available reverse transcription-PCR enzyme immunoassay (Enterovirus Consensus kit) for the diagnosis of enterovirus central nervous system infections. https://core.ac.uk/download/pdf/82001809.pdf (accessed on 1st July 2025).

32. Haryando, H. S., Yusri, E., & Desywar. (2024). Differences in cerebrospinal fluid glucose levels in meningitis patients based on examination time: A single center observational study at Dr. M. Djamil General Hospital, Padang, Indonesia. *Bio Scientia Medicina: Journal of Biomedicine and Translational Research.* https://www.semanticscholar.org/paper/f6e1ad0e7c685a8941e47aa420d658498d72a81b (accessed on 1st July 2025).

33. Jolly, K. (2024). Endoscopic anterior skull base surgery and reconstruction. https://core.ac.uk/download/620188742.pdf (accessed on 1st July 2025).

34. Kelleher, R. J., & Soiza, R. L. (2013). Evidence of endothelial dysfunction in the development of Alzheimer's disease: Is Alzheimer's a vascular disorder? https://core.ac.uk/download/153513708.pdf (accessed on 1st July 2025).

35. Kolarovszki, B. (2019). The role of transcranial Doppler sonography in the management of pediatric hydrocephalus. https://core.ac.uk/download/322444490.pdf (accessed on 1st July 2025).

36. Kusaka, S., Voulgaris, N., Onishi, K., Ueda, J., Saito, S., Tamaki, S., Murata, I., et al. (2024). Therapeutic effect of boron neutron capture therapy on boronophenylalanine administration via cerebrospinal fluid circulation in glioma rat models. *Cells, 13.* https://www.semanticscholar.org/paper/e23d466e93f77989c4063c778b94be73a3bb197e (accessed on 1st July 2025).

37. Lo Sasso, B., Bellia, C., Bivona, G., Agnello, L., & Ciaccio, M. (2019). Cerebrospinal fluid analysis in multiple sclerosis diagnosis: An update. https://core.ac.uk/download/224993428.pdf (accessed on 1st July 2025).

38. Lorenzut, S., Del Negro, I., Pauletto, G., Verriello, L., Spadea, L., Salati, C., Musa, M., et al. (2025). Exploring the pathophysiology, diagnosis, and treatment options of multiple sclerosis. *Journal of Integrative Neuroscience, 24*(1), 25081. https://www.semanticscholar.org/paper/2381862f6d0210a66b03150611c574e89a15269e (accessed on 1st July 2025).

39. N/A (2015). Poster session. *Rinsho Shinkeigaku, 55*, S242–S467. https://doi.org/10.5692/clinicalneurol.55_supplement_s242 (accessed on 1st July 2025).

40. N/A. (2025). *International Journal of Laboratory Hematology*. https://core.ac.uk/download/556253840.pdf (accessed on 1st July 2025).

41. Naffadi, H. M. (2024). Neimann-Pick diseases: Beyond lipid accumulation–Genetic, diagnostics, and therapeutic strategies. https://core.ac.uk/download/622109115.pdf (accessed on 1st July 2025).

42. Owler, B. K. (2004). Pathophysiology of normal pressure hydrocephalus. https://core.ac.uk/download/41229769.pdf (accessed on 1st July 2025).

43. Pérez-Millan, A., Lal-Trehan Estrada, U. M., Falgàs, N., Guillén, N., Borrego-Écija, S., Juncà-Parella, J., Bosch, B., et al. (2025). The cortical asymmetry index for subtyping dementia patients. *European Radiology*. https://www.semanticscholar.org/paper/8a97f0e1d20fc05819d2de027b1a389e2aa47365 (accessed on 1st July 2025).

44. Saadaldeen, M. (2022). Idiopathic normal pressure hydrocephalus: Associations between CSF biomarkers, clinical symptoms and outcome after shunt surgery. https://core.ac.uk/download/491190213.pdf (accessed on 1st July 2025).

45. Wick, M., Gross, C., Tumani, H., Wildemann, B., Stangel, M., & German Society of CSF Diagnostics. (2021). Automated analysis of cerebrospinal fluid cells using commercially available blood cell analysis devices—A critical appraisal. *Cells, 10*. https://www.semanticscholar.org/paper/1f03fd3030210a735b938a62f094986a4c6a0d24 (accessed on 1st July 2025).

46. Wu, J., Su, Y., Zhu, W., Mallak, N., Lepore, N., Reiman, E., Caselli, R., et al. (2022). Improved prediction of beta-amyloid and tau burden using hippocampal surface multivariate morphometry statistics and sparse coding. *ArXiv, abs/2211.05235*. https://www.semanticscholar.org/paper/958dc28c6fa66ae28ec876f733a6a87c2cbf59e3 (accessed on 1st July 2025).

47. Zandolino, A., Manto, A., Serino, A., Camilla, C., et al. (2018). Spontaneous intracranial hypotension: Two steroid-responsive cases. https://core.ac.uk/download/160736714.pdf (accessed on 1st July 2025).

48. Zhang, M., Hu, X., & Wang, L. (2024). A review of cerebrospinal fluid circulation and the pathogenesis of congenital hydrocephalus. *Neurochemical Research, 49*, 1123–1136. https://www.semanticscholar.org/paper/be1a60bfb64338c56b89291f8b04e919cb49c37b (accessed on 1st July 2025).

SEMEN, SYNOVIAL, AND SEROUS FLUIDS

14

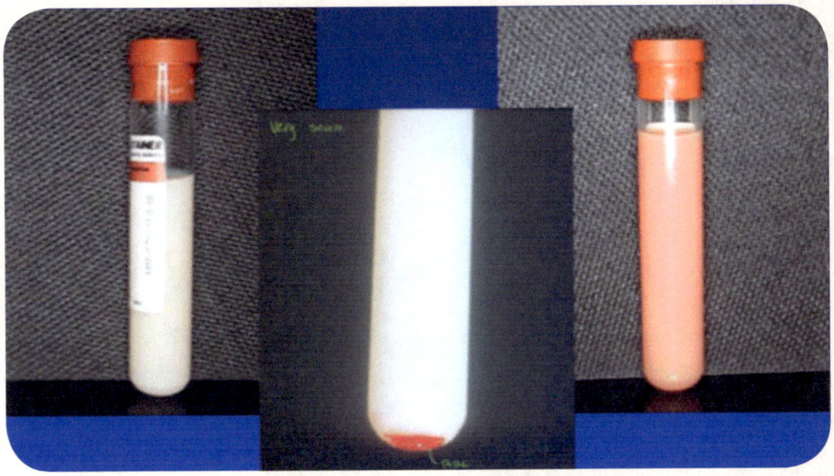

LEARNING OBJECTIVES

After studying this chapter, you will be able to:

1. Discuss about semen;
2. Define synovial fluid;
3. Explain about Serous fluid;
4. List the Comparison of semen, synovial, and serous fluids;
5. Explore the diagnostic importance of semen, synovial, and serous fluids;
6. Focus on the treatment and management of semen, synovial, and serous fluids.

Introduction

Body fluid knowledge is important to understanding how our bodies function, both in health and when they are not. Semen, synovial fluid, and serous fluid each possess their own quirks and purposes, and all work to keep us in motion in various ways. They have us do things like lubricate our joints so they can slide easily, help move things around our body, and even clean out waste; and in addition to, that, give us clues about what's happening in our body when disease strikes. It's more about recording facts to gain insight into these fluids—more like exploring how our system reflects and affects our general health. Consider semen, for example. It's not just a case of transporting the sperm; it also supplies nutrients and a degree of immune protection, so it's a significant figure in reproduction. Synovial fluid, which we use to lubricate our joints and prevent friction whenever we move, in most cases has a surprisingly crucial role to play in joint health. And then there's serous fluid, which can be found in places like the pleural and peritoneal cavities, enabling our organs to move smoothly past each other. Studying chemical behavior and composition of these fluids can, in general, yield a treasure of useful information about health that is pertinent to both the diagnosis and management of disease. Health care practitioners—nurses, physical therapists, etc.—can indeed benefit from knowledge of these facts. Changes in fluid dynamics, like changes in synovial fluid, might signal a propensity for joint issues, and abnormal values of serous fluid might indicate infection or inflammation. This insight, while sometimes elusive or inconsistent, helps caregivers deal with the multifaceted changes of aging and disease. In most cases, a more detailed examination of these fluids not only enhances our scientific understanding but also provides health practitioners with practical wisdom for better patient care (Allen et al., 1994; Ellerton et al., 2023) (Figure 14.1).

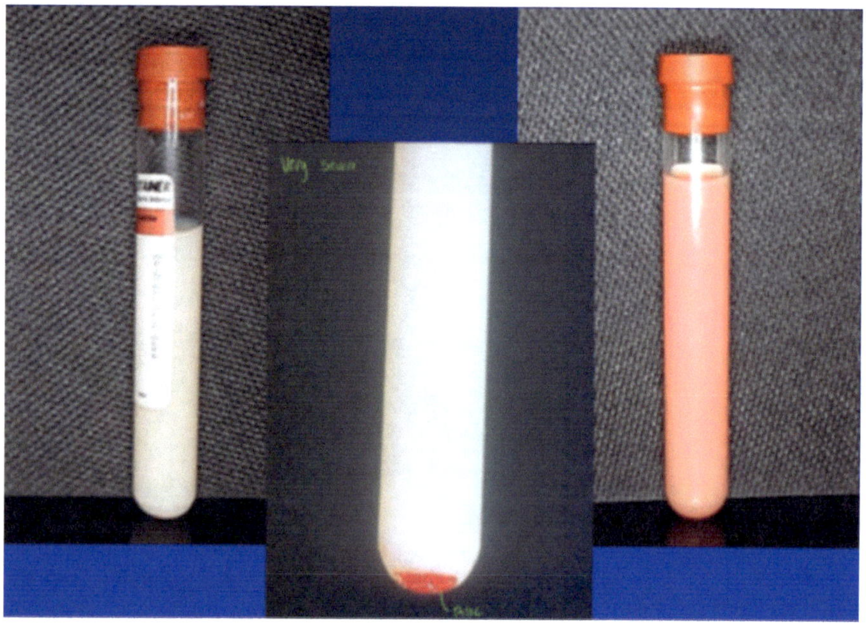

Figure 14.1. Body fluids: Serous, seminal, synovial.

Source: https://external-content.duckduckgo.com/iu/?u=https%3A%2F%2Fo.quizlet.com%2F30CtwhXP0Y1YP2yP5WXlVA.png&f=1&nofb=1&ipt=b8ae5e7b2875d28a97e01c921c90050fb9fa3ad11eef59afc1e0a3348cbb4dfe.

Definition of Bodily Fluids

Body fluids have a pretty impressive way of keeping things in balance in our systems, all assisting each other so everything works as it should. They don't get the job done by way of one fluid alone—each has a purpose, from delivering nutrients and removing waste to cushioning joints and covering organs. Instead of being merely lumped together, these fluids can be sorted into what they're made of and what they do. For example, you have blood, interstitial fluid, and lymph mixed with more specialized ones like semen, synovial, and serous fluids. Understanding these functions, in general, provides us with an insight into how they contribute towards good health and disease resistance. As we age, these fluids may change slightly, so that we must reassess their function and their impact on our overall health (Allen et al., 1994). If you take a closer look, you can sort these fluids into three big groups: those in the spaces between cells, those inside cells, and a special group known as transcellular fluids. Extracellular fluids (think of blood plasma and fluid between cells) are very important to get material from place to place. Then there's intracellular fluid, hidden away in each cell, driving metabolism and conveying messages between. And don't leave out transcellular fluids like cerebrospinal fluid and certain serous fluids, which are key in the protection and lubrication of tissues. In most cases, even mild shifts in these fluids' constitution will be reflective of states of disease, and therefore, it's crucial to have a clear grasp of their functions when it comes to clinical evaluation (Ellerton et al., 2023). Take semen, synovial, and serous fluids, for instance. Semen is not all about reproduction; it transports sperm, feeds them, and even protects them along the way. Synovial fluid, nestled within our joint cavities, reduces friction and absorbs shock with movement. And while serous fluids inhabit the areas surrounding organs, they create a slippery surface that makes everything slide around easily, avoiding unnecessary wear and tear. Every fluid's set of unique biochemical properties and functions illustrates how clever the architecture of the body is—despite the fact that, every so often, the particulars can occasionally look slightly sloppy (Allen et al., 1994).

Importance of Learning Various Types of Fluids

Body fluids give us a unique insight into how our bodies work. Take semen, synovial, and serous fluids—each one performs a distinct duty, and when their natural balance is affected, it could indicate underlying health issues. Like examining synovial fluid in joint disorders typically gives clues to inflammation or even degenerative wear. Oftener than not, examining such fluids more closely not only helps trace and detect diseases but also recommends improved treatment. It is as if these fluids all hold a tale to tell, which is why studying their finer points still remains so important to scientists. Methods used to study these fluids, however, must be very specific. With serous fluids, for instance, guidelines set by the Working group for extravascular body fluid samples (WG EBFS) help coordinate different testing procedures—while doing its best to reduce errors in the process. Overall, pre-, during, and post-testing phases are all equally significant pieces. If careless handling at some stage can skew results, then a bit of extra care here will make an enormous difference in the manner clinical data are collected and interpreted by clinicians and consequently end up affecting patient care. Fresh developments in biofluid flow sensors have also presented exciting research avenues. Recent reviews indicate such advanced instruments can measure the state of fluids with greater accuracy, providing another dimension of understanding of how diseases alter the nature of such vital substances. It appears that once disease alters the properties of semen, synovial, or serous fluids, there is a need for timely analysis to allow early intervention. Overall, this intersection of technologies and biological information is the basis of medical breakthroughs—allowing researchers to engineer treatments that closely match the complex challenges of human disease (Gim et al., 2022; Jokic et al., 2020).

14.1. Semen

Learning Outcome

- Composition of semen;
- Functions of semen in reproduction;
- Factors affecting semen quality.

Body fluids have intrigued us throughout, and semen is no exception to that complexity. It comes straight out of the male system, mixing not only sperm cells but also fluids from organs like the seminal vesicles and the prostate—a very strange mix. Most of the time, this fluid is not just about the transportation of sperm but also has proteins, enzymes, and nutrients which ensure sperm remain alive and swim well. These factors, in a kind of careless synergy, create an environment within the female tract that's ideal for fertilization—so much so that they deflect even the acidic bite of the vaginal canal and thereby enhance the chances of conception. Aside from its well-documented reproductive purpose, researchers have started to examine semen's physical and biochemical characteristics. Rather than following a precise order, scientists combine their techniques, testing the chemical makeup of every type of fluid, including semen. For example, when techniques like inductively coupled plasma source mass spectrometry come onto the scene, trace minerals such as boron and calcium will become apparent; interestingly, these minerals crop up in other body fluids like synovial fluid and blood (Havercroft et al., 2018). For the most part, trace components can have an insidious function in influencing sperm quality and male general fertility—suggesting that semen, as fluids, play a function to keep the body in balance. Coming to terms with semen's many functions requires an examination of how it behaves in both healthy and pathological states. Changes in its elemental content at times mirror underlying disease or even nutritional disorders, making it an intriguing tool in clinical diagnosis. One could note that findings from seminal fluid analysis at times are hand-in-hand with findings from synovial fluid, with changes in elemental content being linked to diseases such as rheumatoid arthritis (Bingham et al., 1938). By exploring these intersections, scientists are gradually uncovering potential biomarkers for fertility issues and other diseases, slowly piecing together how men's reproductive health contributes to the broader picture of overall well-being (Figure 14.2).

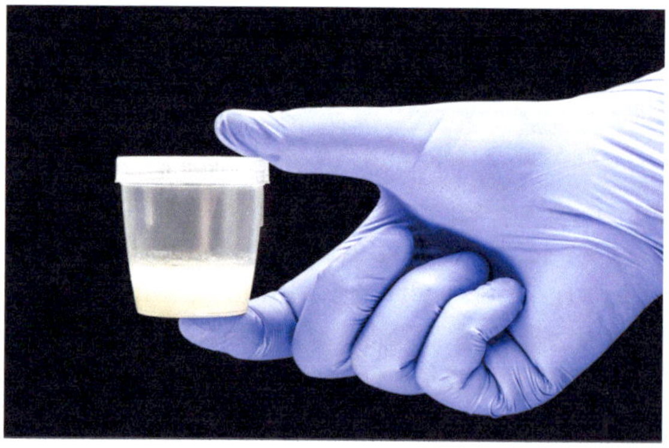

Figure 14.2. Semen.

Source: https://external-content.duckduckgo.com/iu/?u=https%3A%2F%2Fmedia.wired.com%2Fphotos%2F63042924f06d7dee6f53bbc4%2Fmaster%2Fw_2560%252Cc_limit%2Fspermdonor_science_GettyImages-1365858707-(1).jpeg&f=1&nofb=1&ipt=5bb89b637c4f763e3c223c32e6b359b65a68170f32e4b38ec75d1b21368c67eb.

14.1.1. Composition of Semen

In reproductive biology, the semen composition is significant—it doesn't just carry sperm; it really gets the stage ready for fertilization. Semen usually comes in two forms—a batch of sperm and a huge fluid known as seminal plasma, making up about 90% of the composition. The fluid is not a simple liquid; it is a blend of secretions from some glands, including the seminal vesicles, the prostate gland, and the bulbourethral glands. These liquids, in many cases, add the nutrients, pH balance, and just the right conditions for sperm to swim and survive. They are also filled with enzymes, prostaglandins, and hormones that influence not only how reproduction is achieved but also participate in the quality of the female reproductive system. In most cases, the precise combination can play a huge role in fertility outcomes, making the importance of knowing the composition of semen both clinically and biologically relevant. The seminal vesicles add the majority of the fluid, adding along the way such compounds as fructose and prostaglandins to help energize sperm motility and even cause uterine contractions that facilitate their transport. The prostate, meanwhile, adds more fluid packed with citric acid, enzymes, and zinc—substances critical to keeping sperm healthy. Then there are, of course, the bulbourethral glands, which release a clear, mucous fluid that serves as a lubricant to aid the sperm's journey. In a way, these various fluids nourish and effectively move sperm towards the egg and demonstrate how seemingly simple a substance can be beneficial to reproduction. It's a complex interaction of factors that really emphasizes evolutionary adaptations designed to maximize reproductive success, and semen is more than a carrier of sperm. With extravascular body fluids like semen, biochemical examination plays a critical role in assessing male reproductive status. In broad terms, careful handling and analysis are necessary because any errors in preanalytical, analytical, and postanalytical steps can lead to biased results. Semen analysis techniques, like those embraced by studies in serous fluid (Jokic et al., 2020), must be accurately tested to determine if they're being properly interpreted and are still of clinical significance. Complicated as it is, semen definitely requires additional studies, especially because changes in its components can occur at the same time as other conditions like infertility. Everything considered, semen quality and sperm health are absolutely essential—not just for getting pregnant but also for giving hints regarding a man's overall health (Allen et al., 1994) (Figure 14.3).

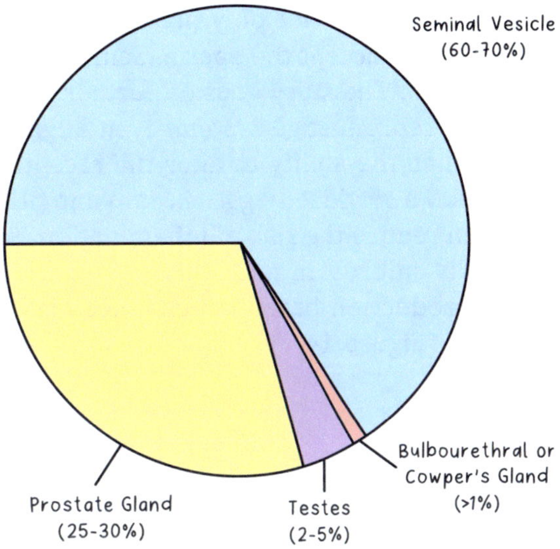

Figure 14.3. Composition of semen.

Source: https://images.squarespace-cdn.com/content/v1/6412bf3715e2d4255a53c869/5f1f5ddd-c361-4879-851a-b59f00584ceb/Composition+of+Semen.jpg.

14.1.2. Functions of Semen in Reproduction

Human reproduction is more complex than it seems. Much of what makes it a success is the liquid called semen. Manufactured by the male reproductive system, it is not just a sperm carrier; it carries necessary nutrition and protection factors that benefit the sperm in their quest. Seminal plasma, for example, harbors necessary enzymes and nutrients that support sperm during their passage down the female tract. The weakly adhesive nature of semen prefers to hold on to the sperm that remain sitting on the cervical mucus (Allen et al., 1994). In most cases, such a protective film also breaks the force of the female immune assault, so the sperm can survive with more facility. It is not restricted to transportation only, either. Semen provides hormones and signaling molecules that enhance fertility in subtle but important ways. By and large, these chemicals facilitate conditions favoring conception and even provide sperm with a little nudge in the right direction. Prostaglandins, for example, assist in initiating uterine contractions that channel sperm upward towards the ova (Ellerton et al., 2023). It can be said that this hormonal duet not only predigests the ground for fertilization but also gently prepares the female body to accept the sperm. Semen wonderfully acts as both a messenger and an accelerator to conception. The story goes on further. Bioactive agents in semen may exert subtle actions upon the female reproductive system, even augmenting and sometimes inhibiting the process. Seminal fluid also has the ability to alter the receptivity of the endometrium, which can affect the quality of how well a fertilized egg will implant (Allen et al., 1994). In addition, its immune-modulatory effects can reduce the risk of inflammation in the reproductive tract, creating a better environment for an early embryo. In total, this combination of biochemical messages means that semen not only starts reproduction but also helps keep going the subsequent processes involved in a successful pregnancy (Figure 14.4).

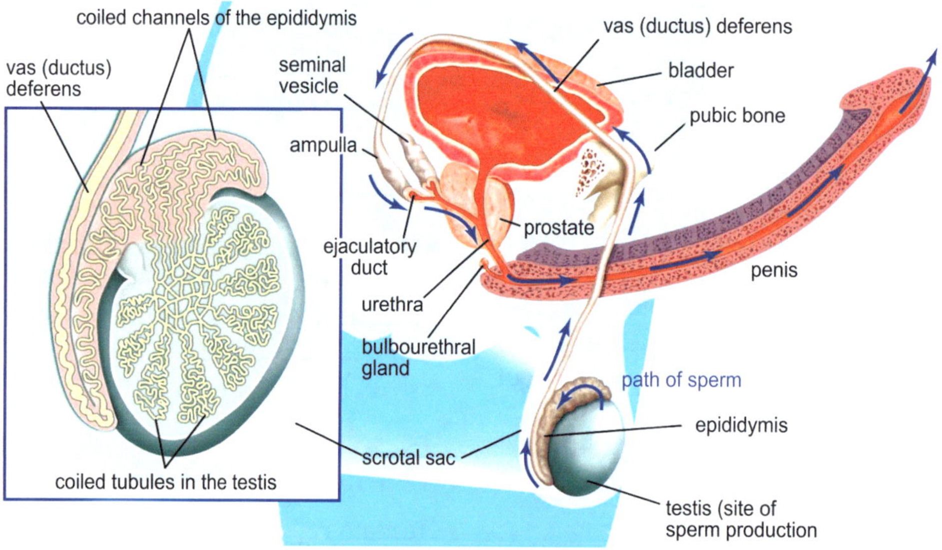

Figure 14.4. Functions of semen in reproduction.

Source: https://cdn.britannica.com/99/26999-050-B384ACC6/Structures-production-transport-semen.jpg.

14.1.3. Factors Affecting Semen Quality

Semen quality is not simply one thing—sperm quality is a mix of biology, environment, and everyday choices. Testosterone is needed to produce sperm; when balance to this hormone is lost, sperm levels fall and their mobility is impaired, and that is bad news for fertility. Age will also likely be a factor—in the majority of cases, studies show a decrease in sperm count and viability as men get older, illustrating the manner in which natural physiological shifts can affect the larger picture. Hormones and aging join forces and teach us that internal mechanisms are not always steady. What is happening in our environment becomes part of the equation. Pollutants, chemicals, and even heat—any and all of them have the potential to wreak havoc on sperm, sometimes in ways that are surprising. You might discover that farm pesticides and heavy metals alter the shape and mobility of sperm cells; frequent exposure to heat from saunas or even tight clothing could interfere with normal sperm production. It's a filthy interaction between our world and our bodies, so keeping an eye on our world is critical to reproductive health. And let's not overlook the way we live our lives on a day-to-day level. What we eat, how we move, and habits like smoking and too much booze all seem to make a big difference. A diet rich in antioxidants and essential nutrients can enhance sperm function, whereas obesity may disturb your hormonal balance, causing semen quality to decline. Smoking and excessive alcohol consumption, however, have been found to cause fewer, less mobile sperm. For the most part, healthier day-to-day choices may actually serve to improve overall reproductive results—though it could take some time to reap the benefits (Figure 14.5).

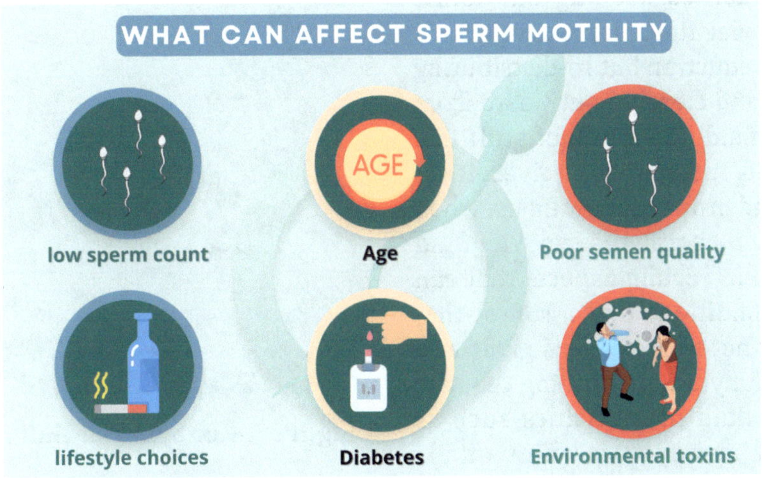

Figure 14.5. Factors affecting semen quality.

Source: https://androwash.in/wp-content/uploads/2023/01/sperm-motility.png.

Test Your Knowledge

1. What are the main components of semen and their physiological roles?
2. How do sperm count and motility affect male fertility?

14.2. Synovial Fluid

Learning Outcome

- Role Of Synovial fluid in joint health;
- Composition and properties of synovial fluid;
- Common disorders associated with synovial fluid.

Biofluids accomplish so much more than merely lubricate the joints; they're really the behind-the-scenes heroes keeping our joints running. Take synovial fluid, for example: it's not merely friction reduction but re-distributing essential nutrients and clearing out waste from the cartilage. This fluid has a mix of stuff like hyaluronic acid and lubricin that gives it its special stickiness and properties. At times, when there is compromised health, the synovial fluid formula is modified in certain aspects that can imply underlying conditions that a run-of-the-mill checkup might not pick up. This gives rise to the necessity of fully understanding the role played by synovial fluid in specialties such as rheumatology and orthopedics (Gim et al., 2022). When joints start getting under way, synovial fluid changes may arise as disease symptoms from osteoarthritis up through rheumatoid arthritis. You can see it in the thickness or volume of fluid, or even when the inflammatory cells first start appearing—all of which can mean a disease sneaking in or out. Physicians can obtain a sample by arthrocentesis in most instances, a procedure not only helpful in untangling diagnosis but also helpful in decreasing swelling and enhancing mobility. Technology is continually bringing new data on the character of synovial fluid and new ways to treat joint issues (Ellerton et al., 2023). Taking a closer examination, synovial fluid is not merely a daily lubricant—its examination bridges from basic science to routine practice in the medical world. An understanding of its physical and biochemical quirks helps in tailoring more efficient treatment regimens, especially for those who are coping with joint wear and tear. With medicine more and more shifting toward personalized therapy, the unique behavior of this fluid in each individual becomes significant. Advanced therapy and diagnostic technology more and more depend upon our deep understanding of synovial fluid, and it is a cornerstone of clinical application and research efforts to enhance joint health and overall well-being (Gim et al., 2022) (Figure 14.6).

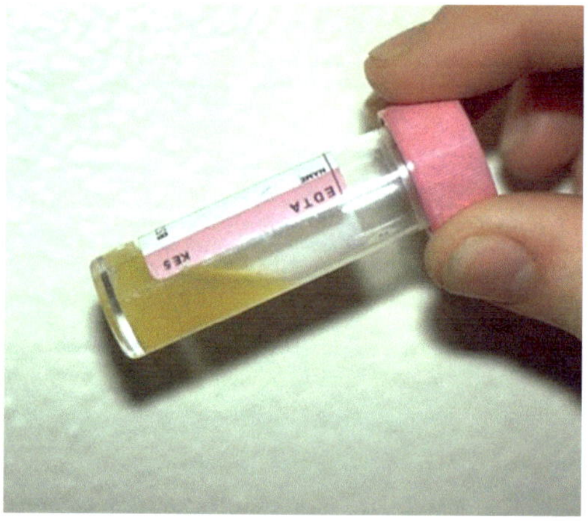

Figure 14.6. Synovial fluid.

Source: https://www.vetlexicon.com/wp-content/uploads/2023/05/7_5478.jpg.

14.2.1. Role of Synovial Fluid in Joint Health

It's an important job of what occurs in our synovial fluid. That thick, syrupy fluid actually does double duty—it's a natural lubricant that diminishes friction as our joint surfaces slide by each other, and it also cushions against impact so the joint structures aren't damaged. When lubricin and hyaluronic acid blend in there, they give the fluid a kind of elastic, springy quality that really improves joint function. Even a small change in its composition or amount has the power to speed stress and inflammation, which usually leads to pain—so it's kind of a no-brainer that a healthy joint depends on healthy fluid. Looking more closely, you can actually learn a great deal about what is happening in tissues throughout by analyzing the content of synovial fluid. Studies using advanced methodologies (Havercroft et al., 2018) have shown that elements such as boron, calcium, and iron can fluctuate, especially when conditions such as rheumatoid arthritis are present. Their levels also appear to oscillate back and forth in sync with inflammation markers, such as white blood cell counts, and even some of the crystalline deposits, suggesting that the fluid is not only lubricating the joints but also is painting a diagnostic picture of something being wrong. In summary, synovial fluid and its relationship to joint function is one that is complex yet critical, pertinent to everyday health as well as disease states. Ensuring this fluid is in its best state is paramount to the uninhibited functioning of joints and helps to avoid conditions like osteoarthritis or rheumatoid arthritis. As Ellerton et al. (2023) has noted, a more detailed look at synovial fluid science actually provides both clinicians and patients with an extra edge in managing joint issues. Ultimately, deciphering the code of this substance not only teaches us more about joint health but also holds the promise of unlocking new treatment paths that may yield true fruit in patient outcomes (Figure 14.7).

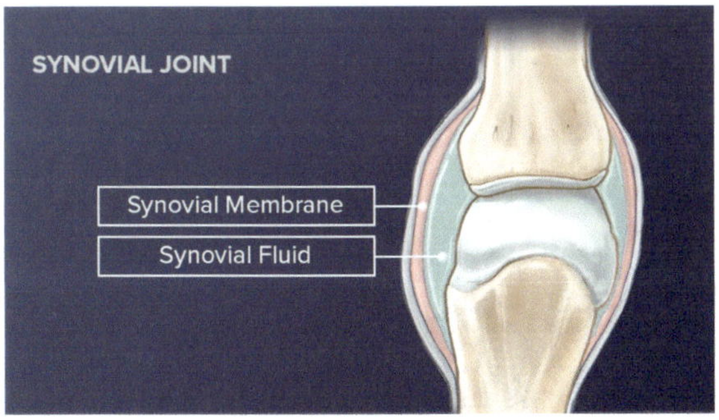

Figure 14.7. Role of synovial fluid in joint health.

Source: https://res.cloudinary.com/da1molee1/image/upload/w_1200,h_675/synovial-joint.webp.

14.2.2. Composition and Properties of Synovial Fluid

Synovial fluid is not a gooey lubricant—it's a diligent sidekick for our joints. It brings cartilage essential nutrients and flushes out waste, all the while smoothing surfaces. You get a blend of hyaluronic acid, lubricin, with a cocktail of electrolytes and proteins all working together to give the fluid it's odd, thick consistency. Hyaluronic acid, for instance, not only thickens joints but forms a protective barrier over the joints, lowering friction when we're moving. It even acts as a shock absorber by spreading stresses - sweet touch for keeping our joints in one piece when things heat up. Look closer and there's indeed more quirks. Trace minerals such as boron, calcium and a few others are found in this fluid, and their concentration indeed varies among healthy people and patients with joint diseases such as rheumatoid arthritis or osteoarthritis. In most situations, higher iron concentration is observed in the synovial fluid of osteoarthritis patients compared to that of rheumatoid arthritis, and that hints at some metabolic variations underlying. These variations underscore how valuable a simple fluid analysis can be to diagnosis, and reveal new avenues for exploring the biochemical processes of joint illness problems. But there are ingredients more than just ingredients to remember—how it behaves is affected also. Its behavior can vary with age, sex, and even disease. For example, inflammation might raise the number of white blood cells, which in turn would shift the balance of the fluid and might even cause further difficulties. Minor elevations of substances like magnesium and zinc are very frequently observed with inflammation; this means that examination of synovial fluid can be particularly valuable in tracking joint problems over time. Generally speaking, this fluid is more than just a natural grease, but also a thrilling diagnostic window onto joint disease and its treatment (Havercroft et al., 2018; Jokic et al., 2020).

14.2.3. Common Disorders Associated with Synovial Fluid

Synovial fluid makes our joints function by lubricating joint surfaces and nourishing the cartilage—a point easily taken for granted until something starts going wrong. If the fluid's composition alters, presto, the joints don't work as well, and a wide range of symptoms occur.

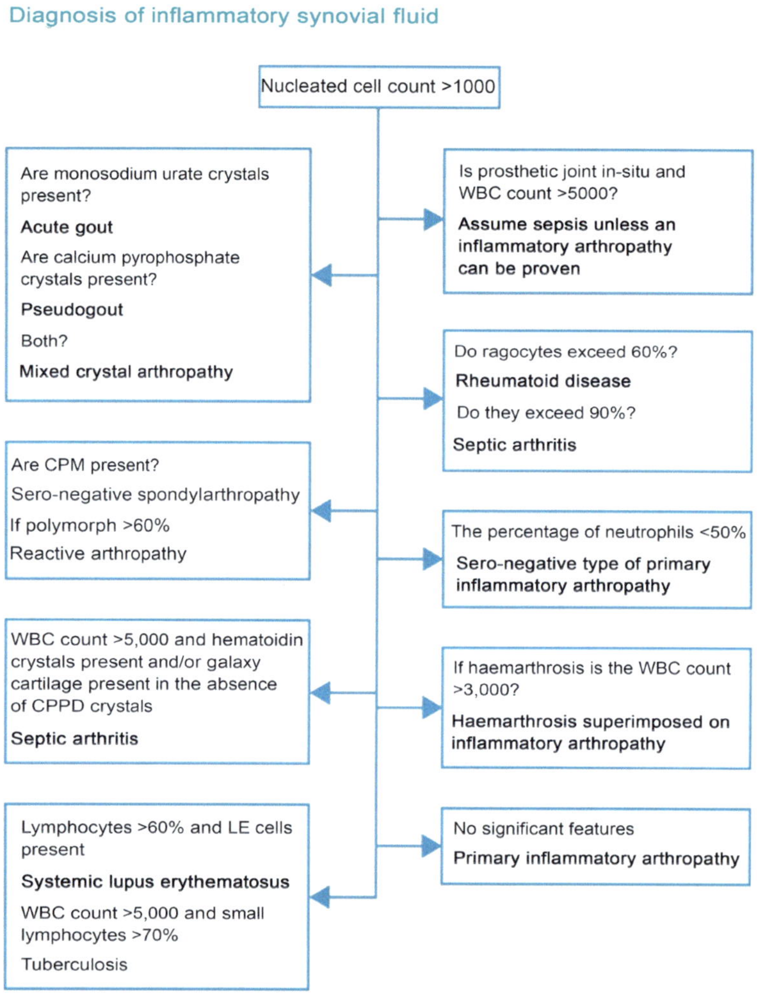

Figure 14.8. Common disorders associated with synovial fluid.

Source: https://ars.els-cdn.com/content/image/1-s2.0-S1756231717300531-gr15.jpg.

Take osteoarthritis, for example. When this condition arises, not just the cartilage but even the bone underneath it begins to deteriorate, and the fluid itself begins to thicken and undergo alterations in its chemical profile. The alterations cause an increase in inflammatory mediators, which stimulate pain and stiffness. Over time, the excess inflammation only quickens cartilage breakdown and wear, creating a type of self-sustaining cycle that gradually degrades overall joint health. Rheumatoid arthritis (RA) is a different kind of issue when it interferes with synovial fluid. Rather than the wear-and-tear involved in osteoarthritis, RA is an autoimmune condition that inflames the joint lining and changes the fluid properties in an essential way. Overall, studies suggest that people with RA tend to have significantly higher levels of white blood cells and pro-inflammatory cytokines lurking in their fluid—a double confirmation that the joint is flaring (Havercroft et al., 2018). Both of these findings, along with microscopic variations in trace elements such as iron, provide clues to the activity of the disease and can be utilized to steer treatment (Havercroft et al., 2018). It's a subtle photograph, with the hyperactivity of the immune system in the limelight. On some occasions, the presence of minute crystals within the synovial fluid does the talking. Gout is one such traditional example, arising when there is excess uric acid that leads to the formation of monosodium urate crystals that cause excruciating acute attacks of swelling and pain. In such episodes, the fluid usually shows a notable increase of white blood cells—with neutrophils, in particular, center stage—indicative of an acute inflammatory response. Quick but careful diagnosis is crucial here, as crystal-induced inflammation can rapidly result in joint damage. Moreover, scientists have reported that changes in such parameters as calcium and magnesium usually accompany these inflammatory peaks, and this suggests the necessity of careful biochemical examination in understanding common joint conditions (Jokic et al., 2020) (Figure 14.8).

Test Your Knowledge

1. What is the composition of synovial fluid, and how does it support joint function?
2. How does synovial fluid act as both a lubricant and a nutrient medium for articular cartilage?

14.3. Serous Fluid

Learning Outcome

- Definition and types of serous fluid;
- Functions of serous fluid in the body;
- Clinical significance of serous fluid analysis.

Body fluids are a mystery—really significant when we're trying to grasp both normal and pathologic body functions. Take serous fluid, for example; it's not just a sticky lubricant that permits tissues and organs to glide over one another, but it has a lot more of an advantage to it than most would probably suppose. Poured by serous membranes, it makes its home in places like the pleural, pericardial, and peritoneal cavities, where it not only aids movement but silently keeps the body's balance by providing means for nutrient exchange and waste removal. Its make-up—mainly water, electrolytes, and a dash of proteins—is generally optimal to keep things running, though sickness in most cases can clog these functions. Doctors routinely use this fluid's examination as an insight into what is wrong inside, and it is therefore a diagnostic asset (Gim et al., 2022). Besides reducing friction, serous fluid plays a real function in our immunological protection. It carries things like antibodies and enzymes that help the body catch and disable invaders—a kind of first line of defense against illness. When the body is injured or falls ill, you can observe the composition of the fluid change; e.g., rising inflammatory markers may indicate problems such as peritonitis or pleuritis. It is as if the fluid is complaining about the ailment and giving away deeper issues in minor changes. Even the methodologies of flow sensing and biochemistry assays are used by scientists to determine not only the amount of fluid present, but even its quality, which can enhance our understanding of the numerous conditions that occur with serous membranes (Ellerton et al., 2023). The current technological advancements in biomedicine have bettered our ability to analyze serous fluid much beyond that, leaving doctors with a better opportunity to diagnose severe illnesses. New sensing technologies enable continuous and sensitive monitoring, discerning even minor changes that can indicate such conditions as heart failure or liver disease in which fluid buildup can have considerable impact. With emerging technologies, more frequently in new ways, not only do they increase our understanding of disease mechanisms, but also how patients are treated on a daily basis. Overall, the use of modern sensor tools in conjunction with standard diagnostics would seem to refine accuracy and, ultimately, patient outcomes, emphasizing the critical significance of serous fluid in our global approach within the area of study of body fluids and clinical medicine (Gim et al., 2022) (Figure 14.9).

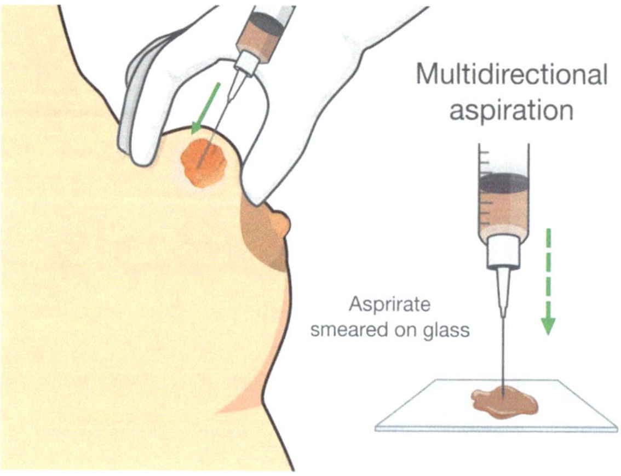

Figure 14.9. Serous fluid.

Source: https://external-content.duckduckgo.com/iu/?u=https%3A%2F%2Fcdn-prod.medicalnewstoday.com%2Fcontent%2Fimages%2Farticles%2F312%2F312875%2Ffine-needle-aspiration.jpg&f=1&nofb=1&ipt=31f38c72dca868a98b1343426160676f7b351f93c96cfd521a408b50b25bec72.

14.3.1. Definition and types of serous fluid

Serous fluids play a crucial role in maintaining our bodily balance and ensuring that a wide range of bodily processes run smoothly. These fluids, a type of transudate, usually show up with a clear, pale-yellow look and only a small amount of protein. You'll find them hanging out in areas like the pleural, peritoneal, and pericardial spaces where they naturally ease friction between organs that are on the move. When things go off track—say, if there's an abnormal buildup or signs of infection—it often points to bigger issues. Generally speaking, doctors rely on these analyses to steer diagnoses and treatments, making this kind of study a key part of clinical pathology (Jokic et al., 2020). Pleural, peritoneal, and pericardial fluids are the main types you'll encounter. Lying between the layers of pleura covering the lungs, pleural fluid is very necessary for smooth breathing motions. Peritoneal fluid allows digestive organs to slide against each other in the abdominal cavity, working somewhat as a cushion. Pericardial fluid, situated in the sac covering the heart, reduces friction every time the heart pumps. All fluids contain their own signs about our overall well-being, and therefore physicians examine them closely to detect issues that could otherwise go unnoticed (Allen et al., 1994). In diagnosing issues with regards to these fluids, the process occurs in several steps. First, there's the preanalytical stage where accurate collection works towards protecting the sample quality. Next, analytical testing like microscopic examination of cells or biochemical tests investigates what is really present in the fluid. Finally, postanalytical stage involves interpreting these findings as part of informed treatment and patient care. Professional guidelines generally stress good, sound methods of fluid analysis to leave patients better off in the long run. In most cases, information regarding the nature and importance of these fluids plays a vital role in enabling early detection and proper management of potential health complications (Jokic et al., 2020).

14.3.2. Functions of Serous Fluid in the Body

Human anatomy is full of fluids that labor diligently to sustain us. Take serous fluid, for instance—it plays a critical role in making sure our organs get to slide easily and get cushioned inside the body. You can find it tucked away inside membranes like the pleura, peritoneum, and pericardium; basically, it reduces friction between organs so motion will not be a scraping nightmare. Take breathing, for instance: in the pleural cavity, the fluid makes the lungs expand and contract with virtually no resistance, which serves to underline the value of lubrication in facilitating smooth respiration. It also, in the majority of instances, serves to keep everything in its place by maintaining the pressure just so and keeping organs well-positioned.

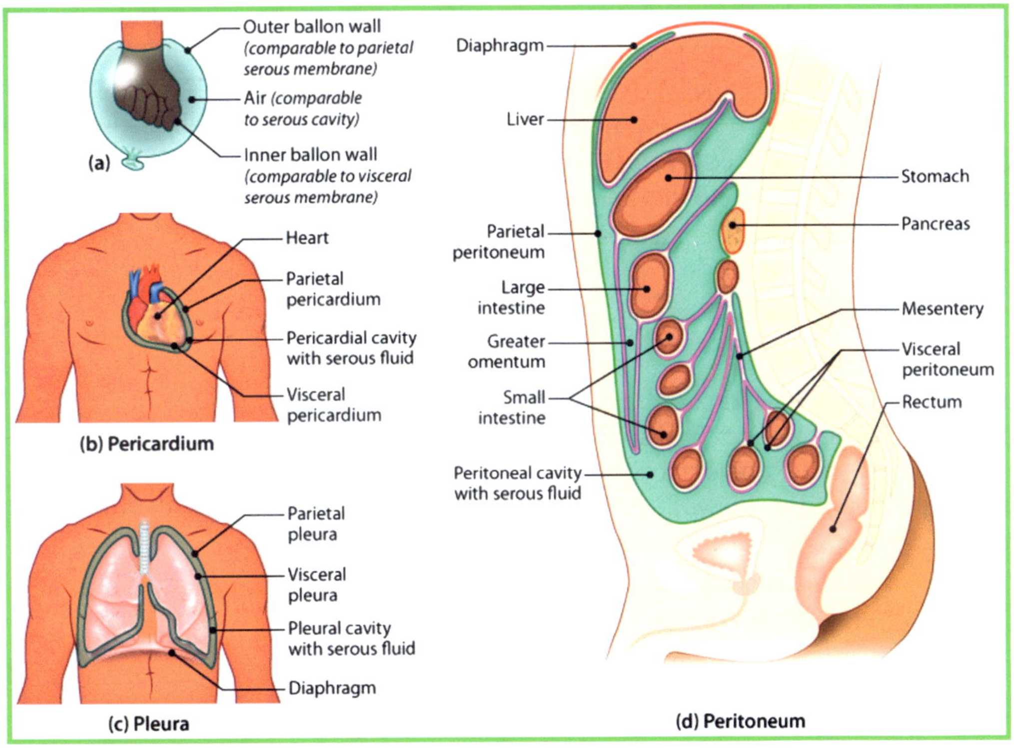

Figure 14.10. Functions of serous fluid in the body.

Source: https://qph.cf2.quoracdn.net/main-qimg-64e8449a0daf3dc739b22aeacace2bd2-pjlq.

But there's more to it than that. Serous fluid is also involved in nutrient exchange and waste removal. In the tiny crevices of its membranes, it actually shuttles nutrients from blood vessels to adjacent tissues—a very important function because many organs are relying upon this local environment for metabolic needs. Its makeup—a mix of electrolytes, enzymes, and proteins—is just so, and this blend even has some antimicrobial qualities that protect against infection in those tight spaces, ultimately boosting our natural immunity. Aside from that, serous fluid gets activated once inflammation is already taking place, and it works to seal and hold damage or infection. When tissues inside these cavities get damaged, the amount of fluid will increase to maybe eliminate debris and unwanted aggressors. This shows how it works both to act as a slippery lubricant and as a healing agent. Secondly, it is used to maintain pressure equilibrium in body cavities, a feature that is critical for the efficient function of the surrounding organs. Finally, in conclusion, identification of such varied functions serves to indicate just how serous fluid maximizes mechanical function as well as strengthens immune defenses and tissue integrity (Ellerton et al., 2023; Krause et al., 2005) (Figure 14.10).

14.3.3. Clinical Significance of Serous Fluid Analysis

Serous fluids in our body—i.e., those occupying the pleural, peritoneal, and pericardial spaces—play an important role in helping doctors decide on treatment. The knowing of what is going on with them can actually wake clinicians to hidden health issues, whether it is an infection, a malignancy, or an inflammatory aberration. Very often, a plan that speaks to all the way from how the sample is treated before being tested to what occurs after is what serves to minimize misdiagnoses. Using standard procedure of daily routine, results seem to be more trustworthy, which in most cases keeps treatments aligned with clinical guidelines (Jokic et al., 2020). It's not just an issue of deciding what's wrong. And then there's the practical benefit of enabling doctors to guide procedures like therapeutic thoracentesis or paracentesis by depending on the chemical and cellular clues in the fluid. When one takes into account both the amount of fluid as well as its composition, physicians can guide treatment plans that really hit the mark. Also, being extra careful to maintain electrolyte balance and fluid resuscitation—especially in very ill patients—certainly makes a significant difference because an error can often mean extra complications (Bingham et al., 1938). Getting everyone into sync on standard protocols for serous fluid testing is very important as well. Clear, easy guidelines reduce the risks of fluid accumulation and analysis. And truthfully, making sure that clinical staff and lab professionals are privy to these nitty-gritty facts fosters a safety-first culture of patient care. In the long run, reinforcing our hands-on knowledge of heavy-duty fluid analysis not only speeds up solid diagnoses but also enhances overall patient treatment effectiveness (Jokic et al., 2020).

Test Your Knowledge

1. Where in the body is serous fluid normally found, and what is its role?
2. How does serous fluid accumulation (effusion) indicate underlying pathology?

14.4. Comparison of Semen, Synovial, and Serous Fluids

Learning Outcome

- Similarities in composition;
- Differences in function;
- Variations in clinical significance.

Biofluids hold a lot more surprises than one might think. Different fluids in our body do unique jobs – they're not arranged in neat categories, they simply work together in a lively, somewhat unpredictable way. Take semen, for example. It's a thick, nutrient-rich liquid loaded with sperm cells and a plasma that fuels them along their journey, a detail that plays a key role in conception. Then there's synovial fluid, which hangs out in our joints. It reduces friction between cartilage surfaces—thanks largely to things like hyaluronic acid and lubricin—keeping our movements smooth even when we're in a hurry. And don't forget serous fluids. Found in areas like the pleura and peritoneum, these liquids act more like a protective cushion between organs, lightly preventing them from rubbing against each other. All of these varied roles, in most cases, give doctors a significant insight into our overall health, diagnosing and treating most disorders. Taking a closer look at such liquids really does give one an indication of human health. Semen analysis, in most respects, is a standard test under infertility testing; it checks such as sperm quality and motility, both critical to fertilization. Conversely, synovial fluid analysis is sometimes capable of uncovering signs of arthritis or joint infection, as its composition will become altered by inflammation or trauma. Serous fluid, too, has a story to tell—its examination can help detect infections, inflammatory conditions, or even malignancies, giving clues as to what is transpiring within. All of these fluids are not just taking up space quietly; they are replicating important signals from the body about how the body responds to damage and stress. The more our study continues, the more varied and precise ways of investigating these substances have become, and the more advanced the diagnostic and therapeutic options as a whole. Advances in biofluid analysis technology also are altering healthcare as we treat it. Techniques like flow sensing, which are continually optimized, enable scientists to record the fluid dynamics in real time; in the majority of cases, this yields information on how these fluids change when in diseased state. Gim et al. (2022) even underscores the necessity for ongoing efforts in advancing these flow sensing strategies to completely evaluate biofluids under different clinical conditions. Meanwhile, careful observation of the microscopic, or histological, nature of these fluids—examining their very composition (a process in some ways as complicated as it is basic)—helps to further inform us of their purposes. Krause et al. (2005) reminds that proper, quality training in histology remains paramount to comprehending these matters. By integrating new analytical methods with safer educational bases, researchers and clinicians together move forward toward more successful solutions to health that better engage the body's ever-changing, complex realities.

14.4.1. Similarities in Composition

Biological fluids in our body—even as different as semen, synovial, and serous—share more in common with one another than you would normally expect. You can examine all of them and see that they all do more than just take up space; they keep everything running properly by mixing together all kinds of ingredients like proteins, electrolytes, and small micronutrients that together really add up. In all but one case, they also have trace elements—like calcium and magnesium are found in synovial fluid in patterns that mirror what we find in the other two (Havercroft et al., 2018). This kind of communal recipe really predicts the body to sustain a fine balance, and it makes you wonder how these ingredients loosely interact in order to have an influence on overall health or even to induce, in some cases, disease. If you pay a second glance at the chemistry involved, you do start to see that the mixing of the elements present in these liquids is not an arbitrary happenstance. Generally, electrolytes like potassium and sodium play opposite roles: osmotic balance in serous fluid and alteration of fairly critical sperm functions within semen. And synovial fluid—its purpose in lubrication of the joints as well as cartilage cushioning depends on a complex blend comprising hyaluronic acid, to help mention only one, who is also present in the composition of seminal and serous fluid. This duplication seems to be the result of evolutionary fine-tuning, responding to similar physical needs across the body. Researchers began comparing these elemental profiles to try to determine how any imbalances would correlate with inflammatory or degenerative disease. Beyond the chemistry itself, how these fluids function in practice exhibits a dynamic relationship inherent to maintaining us healthy. All three classes of fluids carry out such functions as lubrication, nutrient transport, and allowing cells to communicate with each other without impeding each other. Take semen, for instance—the glycoproteins within allow it to adopt a gel or viscoelastic state, a property which shows up in synovial fluid too where it helps keep the joint stable. Serous fluid, on the other hand, is renowned for constructing a slippery film over organ surfaces, which allows it to move almost effortlessly. All these shared physical and chemical characteristics seem to justify an evolutionary approach to effective survival and gliding body processes—despite, in most cases, the specifics being somewhat unseemly and complex (Reinsalu et al., 2022) (Figure 14.11).

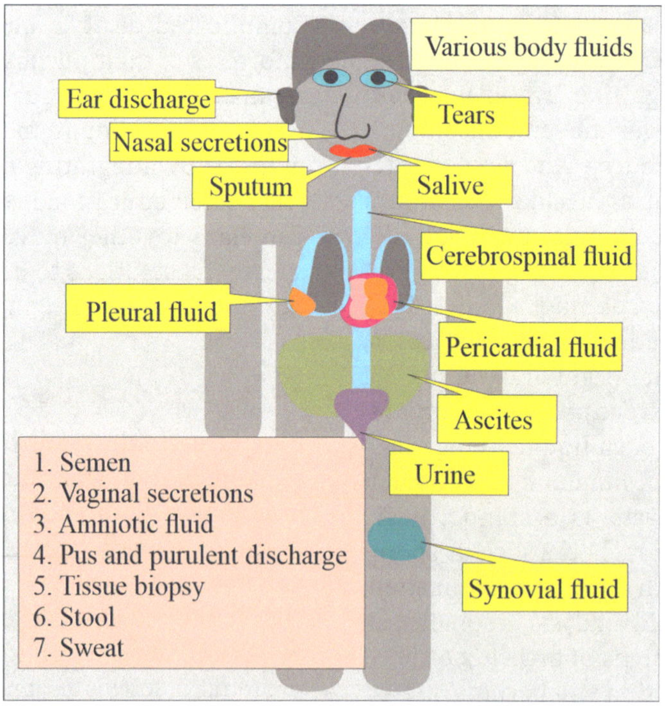

Figure 14.11. Similarities in semen, synovial, and serous fluids.

Source: https://labpedia.net/wp-content/uploads/2020/04/Body-fluids-various-2.jpg.

14.4.2. Differences in Function

The human body operates with a surprising mixture of biofluids that keep everything in equilibrium; each has its own specific function to help us keep our internal balance. Think of semen, synovial, and serous fluids—all three of which have a function that's essential but also quite unique. Semen is geared towards reproduction, carrying sperm down while nourishing them and protecting them through its makeup of seminal plasma proteins and nutrients. Synovial fluid, by contrast, resides in our joints, where it primarily functions as a natural lubricant, reducing friction during movement and even absorbing shocks during everyday activities.

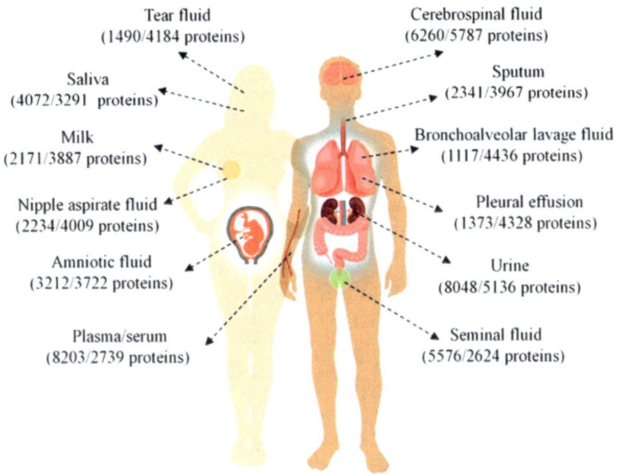

Figure 14.12. Differences in function of biofluids.

Source: https://www.creative-proteomics.com/upload/image/biological-fluids-functions-analysis-significance-1.jpg.

It's interesting how these fluids, each suited to specific tasks, show just how intricately our physiology is put together. From a clinical standpoint, knowing what each fluid does can really help in figuring out a range of health issues. Very often, when synovial fluid is abnormal in its content, it can be warning us of inflammatory or degenerative joint diseases that lead to pain in the joints. Similarly, more detailed inspection of serous fluid at times can predict infection, even malignancy, building up in body cavities. Study of these extravascular body fluids (EBF) is imperative—after all, they usually represent our overall health or signal more localized disease. Defining their roles on a daily basis does not only highlight their inherent value but also open up to more effective evaluations and treatment plans to enhance outcomes in patients, as noted by Jokic et al. (2020). New breakthroughs in the methods utilized to analyze these fluids are representative of the importance of their roles in a clinical setting. For instance, newer flow-sensing techniques have, in most cases, helped us quantify biofluids with greater accuracy under various medical conditions. Studies confirm that such developments directly strengthen the manner in which we conduct diagnostics and planning of therapy. With medical tech advancing, combined methods will likely further our understanding of how semen, synovial, and serous fluids operate in our bodies—resulting in more personalized medicine, as exemplified by Gim et al. (2022) (Figure 14.12).

14.4.3. Variations in Clinical Significance

Body fluids—semen, synovial, or serous types—bear on our conception of health in frequently unexpected ways. Differences in their elemental composition can inform us about underlying pathologic processes. The technique of inductively coupled plasma source mass spectrometry (ICP-MS) was used, for instance, to analyze how trace elements like boron and calcium differ in various tissues. Not surprisingly, the researchers compared synovial fluid and found that less boron was in RA bones (Havercroft et al., 2018). In most cases, this pairing of some of these elemental shifts with clinical findings leads you to conclude that you really do need to examine the situation of each fluid in order to know what's going on. The chemical makeup of synovial fluid is self-explanatory when it comes to inflammation. Studies have linked high white blood cell counts with trace element alterations, i.e., magnesium, phosphorus, and zinc—each of which may rise at times in tandem with markers of inflammation in conditions like osteoarthritis and RA (Havercroft et al., 2018). With few exceptions, these correlations explain how inflammation impacts joint function. It's as though these elemental changes act as fingerprints to guide diagnosis and treatment in the clinic. Electrolyte balance is equally crucial, especially in fluid management in the surgical setting. Proper hydration and electrolyte balancing is a must, as miscalculation, even the smallest, can exacerbate complications during or after surgery. For instance, sodium chloride administration protocols must be tightly controlled according to respective patients' own fluid loss in a timely manner in order to maintain homeostasis. This tailored, case-specific approach—based on extensive clinical observation—comes to be crucial for speeding recovery and reducing the rate of future complications. Briefly put, these small changes in the composition of body fluids not only assist in diagnosis but also inform treatment regimens, testifying to the inseparable interdependence of fluid balance and general well-being.

Test Your Knowledge

1. How do the compositions of semen, synovial fluid, and serous fluids differ in terms of cells and proteins?
2. What are the major diagnostic uses of semen analysis versus synovial and serous fluid analysis?

14.5. Diagnostic Importance

Learning Outcome

- Testing methods for semen analysis;
- Synovial fluid analysis in rheumatology;
- Serous fluid analysis in diagnosing diseases.

Body fluids are useful in giving doctors informative information about the overall condition of a person. Different fluids like semen, synovial, and serous liquids all give different types of information. Semen, for example, is useful not only in screening the male fertility but also in showing hormone issues, infection, or even genetic disease. The presence of cells and drugs together in the fluid in a joint (synovial) fluid typically means conditions like arthritis or infection. These exams were not merely routine lab tests - they inform treatment and management approaches as well as directly affect outcomes. By searching for specific biomarkers, doctors can find targeted interventions that accelerate and improve care. Examine carefully, and these biofluids too frequently whisper of underlying disease. Variations in the thickness or cell number of synovial fluid, for instance, typically indicate inflammatory or degenerative processes. In the same way, serous fluids, which sometimes accumulate as a result of illness, offer a kind of window into illness conditions that can even include cancer. Newer technologies grounded in advanced imaging and molecular examination continually enhance these examinations (Amaral et al., 2021). Generally, improved testing uncovers new biomarkers that can result in earlier diagnosis and a better prognosis for patients. With precision medicine the new paradigm in the modern age, fluid analysis leads diagnostics. Systematic, routine testing in clinical settings creates a broader, if sometimes incomplete, picture of complex disease. Newly published research—such as studies on new approaches to detection of infection in animal models—also sheds light on the prospect of cross-species surveillance and increased biosecurity measures (Annand et al., 2023). This not only increases diagnostic accuracy but also improves public health surveillance efforts. As more is learned about how these fluids are associated with overall health, research and updated clinical approaches are bound to bring significant advances in both diagnostic techniques and treatment strategies.

14.5.1. Methods of Semen Analysis Testing

Exploring body fluids has always been of interest to medicine, especially when tracking reproductive health. Sperm analysis is a big part of that—it measures the amount of sperm, how many, how they move, and even their shape. Sometimes small points suggest inherent issues, and doctors can detect the optimal therapy. Modern techniques are more precise and emphasize specific conditions, and they are based on tried and tested methodologies so that results are consistent within the field. Technology is today reshaping our understanding of sperm testing. Computer-aided sperm analysis (CASA) combines exact imaging with sophisticated algorithms to analyze movement and shape, reducing typical human errors while providing comprehensive data. And, you know, there are emerging sensors that have the ability to track fluid flow in real-time (Gim et al., 2022). Overall, this trend towards automation is slowly paving the way for personalized male fertility treatment. When you pair old-school testing with these advancements, you have a more comprehensive view of male reproductive health. Add in molecular tools, such as DNA fragmentation analysis—which gives extra insight into a sperm's genetic state (McLaughlin et al., 1988)—and you're looking at a method that seems to be gaining traction for tackling infertility. As research advances, further refining these tests will likely enhance diagnostic precision and, ultimately, lead to improved outcomes for individuals facing fertility challenges (Figure 14.13).

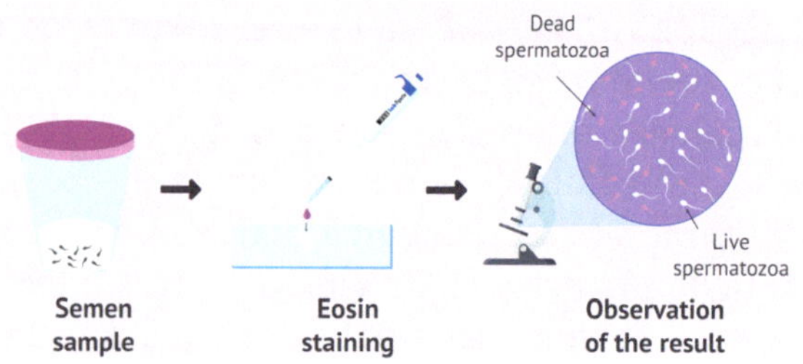

Figure 14.13. Testing methods for semen analysis.

Source: https://www.invitra.com/en/wp-content/uploads/2014/04/spermatozoa-vitality-analysis-staining.png.

14.5.2. Synovial fluid analysis in rheumatology

Rheumatology typically starts by examining very closely synovial fluid, since knowing its chemical makeup is rather significant in working with joint issues. This fluid is not just a slippery lubricant; it's more akin to a covert messenger, providing bits of information about joint inflammation and overall health. Physicians examine it to seek out signs of inflammatory markers, serum components, and other molecules that are typical of diseases such as rheumatoid arthritis or osteoarthritis. Studies – as some studies have generally shown – reveal that alterations in some trace elements would be more likely to concur with the severity of disease; e.g., differences mentioned between rheumatoid arthritis and osteoarthritis patients absolutely emphasize the value of the fluid as a diagnostic medium (Havercroft et al., 2018). Switching slightly from the previous direction, analysis of synovial fluid also gives some insight into the role that adipokines play in joint health. These bioactive messengers that combine daily metabolic signals with more technical clues of inflammation appear to play a significant role. Their levels can change and, in many scenarios, indicate the pathophysiology that is taking place within the joints, and at times point clinicians more specifically in the direction of treatment. Therefore, the combination of testing elemental content with characterizing adipokine profiles results in physicians that have a more robust, two-dimensional appreciation for the health of joints. This dual approach likely positions the stage for continued discovery of new pharmacological targets and ultimately, better patient outcomes (Büchler et al., 2020). Beyond that, the broader relevance of examining synovial fluid also includes the construction of new treatments.

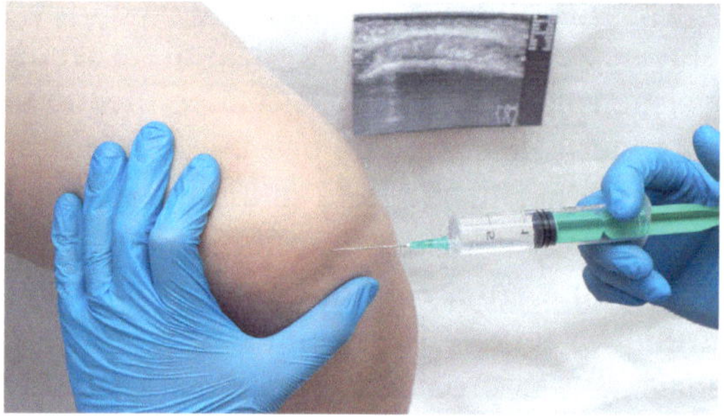

Figure 14.14. A healthcare professional administers an intra-articular injection into a patient's knee, commonly used to deliver corticosteroids or other therapeutic agents for joint inflammation and pain.

Source: https://www.verywellhealth.com/thmb/mhybIFjXz22ghCml68AN6YS8MsA=/2000x1333/filters:no_upscale():max_bytes(150000):strip_icc()/GettyImages-1174570027-d5ba663ef8bc4b5d823ede957a579100-82f2723256f1404284bb472a325bf177.jpg.

It is not just a question of identifying rheumatological disease that is already present; observation of changes in the fluid can also inform clinicians whether treatment is effective or if change is necessary. For instance, change in some of the inflammatory indices or trace elements can suggest that therapy is going along successfully—or possibly suggest that change is necessary. The fluid's dynamic properties render it a valuable puzzle piece in current research seeking to unravel the complex puzzle of joint disease, and incorporating its analysis with other clinic data will undoubtedly contribute significantly to our knowledge base regarding such diseases (Havercroft et al., 2018) (Figure 14.14).

14.5.3. Serous Fluid Analysis in Diagnosing Diseases

Serous fluid build-up—such as that which appears in pleura, peritoneum, or even pericardium—is a frequent indication in all types of health conditions. Indeed, infections, cancers, and even inflammatory disease are likely to put them on the case, so doctors have to get a second look. You'll often find that labs use these samples to decide if the fluid is more like a simple leak (what's called transudative) or if it's from an active problem (exudative), a split that really points to the underlying cause. It's typically essential to have rigorous testing protocols—to be adhered to from before the sample is taken, during the test, and even subsequently—just as the Working group for extravascular body fluid samples (WG EBFS) (Jokic et al., 2020) advises.

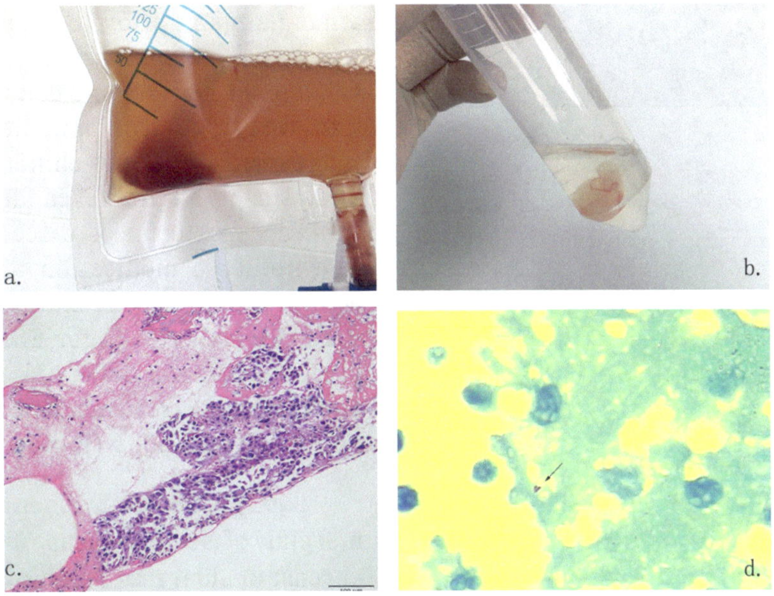

Figure 14.15. Increased diagnostic yield of tuberculous serositis.

Source: https://media.springernature.com/full/springer-static/image/art%3A10.1038%2Fs41598-018-35942-y/MediaObjects/41598_2018_35942_Fig1_HTML.png.

An understanding of the special nature of serous fluid, thus, helps medical professionals minimize risks and enhance patient safety overall. Spinning serous fluid isn't an one-piece procedure—it combines procedures like cell tests and chemical tests that suit the situation at hand. There might be a quick look at the microscope at other times and get malignant cells, or protein measurement and lactate dehydrogenase tests that can indicate why the fluid is too abundant. Laboratories test to find any bacteria or fungi that may be part of the process as well. This differential method of capturing infections and cancers, as well as monitoring disease change over time, gives physicians useful leads for management of treatment (Department A). It's a key part of everyday practice that makes a difference in enhancing healthcare outcomes. In sum, serous fluid analysis is more than just filling out diagnostic checklists—it's a pillar of personalized medicine. It gives doctors an inside look at healthy and unhealthy body functions, then directs more personalized treatment plans. With new testing equipment and a greater understanding of how fluids flow in the body, the benefits of these tests keep growing. For the most part, staying up to date and following guidelines—such as those set by the WG EBFS (Jokic et al., 2020)—ensures patients have the very best care. Last but not least, serous fluid analysis is a critical resource that enhances patient safety and overall healthcare efficiency (Figure 14.15).

Test Your Knowledge

1. How is semen analysis important in the evaluation of male infertility?
2. How can synovial fluid analysis differentiate between infectious, inflammatory, and degenerative arthritis?

14.6. Treatment and Management

Learning Outcome

- Interventions for semen-related issues;
- Management of joint disorders involving synovial fluid;
- Therapeutic approaches for serous fluid accumulation.

Human biofluids are a multifaceted subject, and to deal with them—semen issues, synovial or serous fluids—takes more than one solution at times. Arriving at the proper diagnosis is where it starts, and that usually involves taking a comprehensive analysis of these fluids to inform treatment measures. New sensor technology has really upped our game in tracking where these fluids go and what they're made of, giving us a clearer picture of what's really going on beneath the surface. For example, when biofluid tests are standard practice in healthcare, doctors can identify disease in a way that leads to treatments tailored directly to the patient (Gim et al., 2022). When the topic is synovial and serous fluids, sometimes specialists take a look at examination of extravascular body fluids (EBF) in order to assist them in deciding on the next step. Well-executed solid diagnosis plans encompass what happens prior to, during, and following the tests—this makes the data much more reliable. Proper sample collecting and handling minimizes risks for patients, which, naturally, is top-priority in any clinic. Take serious fluid analysis: it might be capable of sorting out different patterns of disease and then refer to whether a medication adjustment or even a joint aspiration is indicated. By embracing the standard criteria for EBF practice, medical professionals can make diagnosis more precise and formulate treatments according to different patients' conditions (Jokic et al., 2020).

Lastly, successful therapy hinges on the merging of several areas of study and staying abreast of emerging studies in biofluid analysis. Doctors should stay informed of new sensor technologies and updated EBF checking methods if patient care is to be preserved at an optimum level. Additionally, partnership—labs and medical folks hand in hand—is crucial in the simplification of the whole biofluid examination process and enhancing the overall quality of care. Being dedicated to finding the special features of semen, synovial and serous fluids may give rise to new thoughts in medicine, provide further paths of treatment, and in general aid patients to become better. As steadily developing research keeps going forward in this field, synergistically integrating practical clinical knowledge and technical knowledge will increasingly become essential in designing the treatment plans of the future.

14.6.1. Interventions for Semen-Related Issues

Semen issues can be tackled in numerous forms, and the initial consideration is where. Temperature, light, and nutrition in breeding conditions all have a significant effect on how sperm behaves. Even small modifications—like extreme temperature changes or an inadequate diet—can create unnecessary stress on creating sperm, potentially losing fertility in the process. There are plenty of tests to find these semen idiosyncrasies, which consequently sends clinicians (and vets) down the avenue of discovering treatments.

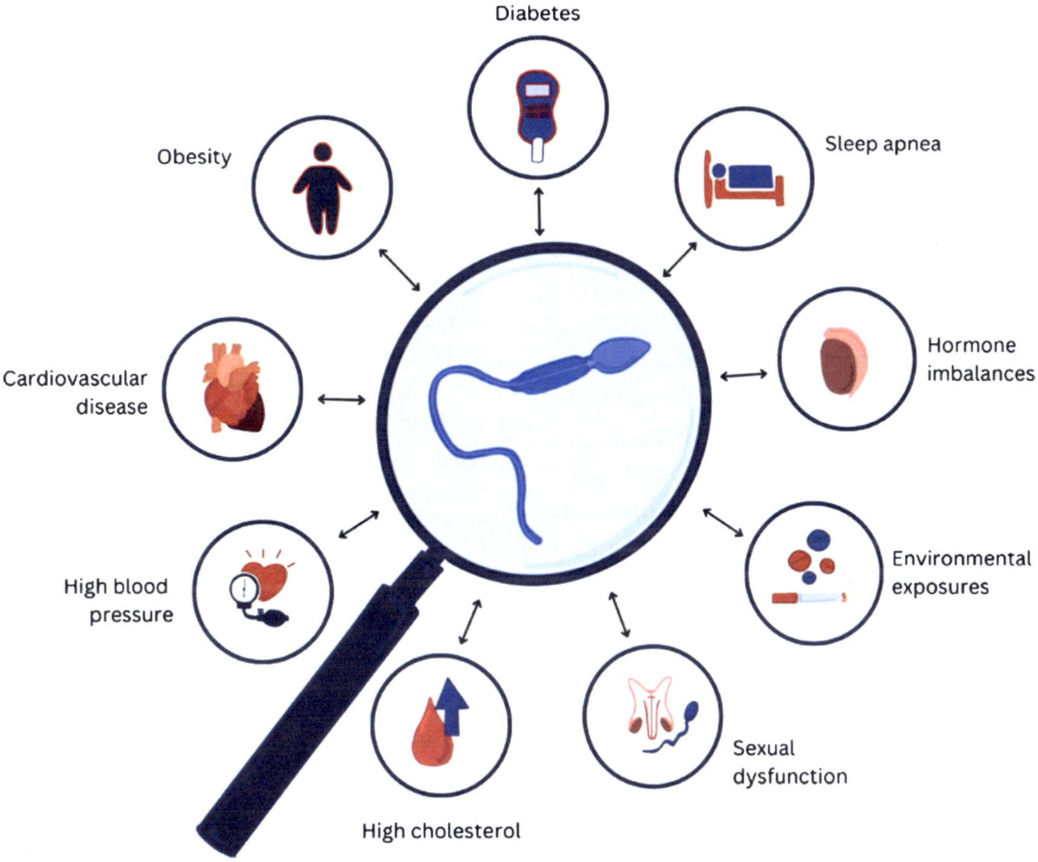

Figure 14.16. Interventions for semen-related issues.

Source: https://media.springernature.com/m685/springer-static/image/art%3A10.1038%2Fs41443-024-00949-9/MediaObjects/41443_2024_949_Fig1_HTML.png.

It would seem quite reasonable, then, that the relationship between your surroundings and how sperm move is more than one might think (Jokic et al., 2020). Medications also come into play, and quite often they can really help even when all other aspects feel out-of-kilter. Hormone therapy, for instance, is given when low testosterone or the similar causes and triggers practitioners also employ gonadotropin therapy to stimulate sperm production. Antioxidants also gain much attention since oxidative stress gets in the way sidelining sperm health. When you compound these hormone therapies with antioxidant supplements, the result seems to be some kind of synergy that enhances the quality of the semen while counteracting the negative effects of the environment. Taking a close look at how these therapies are implemented gives medical practitioners the freedom to tailor regimens to achieve optimal fertility outcomes (Annand et al., 2023). Reproductive medicine has also been progressing on its own uneven pace. Techniques like intrauterine insemination (IUI) and in vitro fertilization (IVF) allow doctors to bypass some of the natural barriers that go with lower-quality semen. In some cases, only the most powerful, most virile sperm are used, and in others, even this gives rise to a chance of genetic selection, making it more likely to conceive. And there's sperm washing—therapeutic technique to isolate active sperm from the remaining seminal fluid, which can increase pregnancy potential further. As more and more research continues to uncover more facts about sperm biochemistry, such techniques are gradually unmasking more information on tailoring treatment in human as well as animal medicine (Jokic et al., 2020) (Figure 14.16).

14.6.2. Management of joint disorders involving synovial fluid

Addressing issues of joint illness that involve the synovial fluid is more than a question of textbook terminology—it's really a matter of understanding how that fluid behaves when everything is in good shape and staying vigilant for any unusual changes that can happen within the joint. Synovial fluid doesn't merely allow for movement; it carries nutrients and eliminates waste as well. In conditions like rheumatoid arthritis or osteoarthritis, you will observe that the fluid becomes thicker or contains more inflammatory cells. These alterations generally lead to swelling, pain, and stiffness of the joints. With improved fluid analysis methods (which, more often than not, yield surprising specificity), doctors can identify exactly what type of joint problem they are dealing with—for instance, they can usually tell whether the swelling is due to an inflammatory process or not (Jokic et al., 2020). New technology is now integrating into how we screen synovial fluid kinematics, which is transforming the management of joint disorder. New developments in sensing biofluid flow have given health care practitioners convenient instruments that measure everything about the fluid's properties and its passage, sometimes even in real time. The tracking of these aspects of flow can significantly enhance our understanding of how joint diseases become established and how they respond to changes in treatment. Even as biofluids research continues to improve (and yes, there's always more to learn), researchers are encouraged to explore these methodologies further. All of these advances help clinicians develop better, upgraded treatment—more accurate checks lead, ultimately, to better decisions about the handling of many joint issues (Gim et al., 2022). To summarize, treatment of joint disorders with synovial fluid involves a far-reaching, multi-faceted strategy involving comprehensive fluid analysis, new technology breakthroughs, and sound clinical moves. Reliance on evidence-based guidelines for synovial fluid checkup not only educates treatment choices but also optimizes the validity of these diagnoses. It's fairly clear that teamwork amongst healthcare professionals—whether rheumatologists, physical therapists, or laboratory personnel—is a cornerstone on which advances toward joint disorder care can be established. With research in the area still plugging along, it is important to be flexible, including newer ways of researching synovial fluid, all in an effort to actually improve patient care (Gim et al., 2022; Jokic et al., 2020) (Figure 14.17).

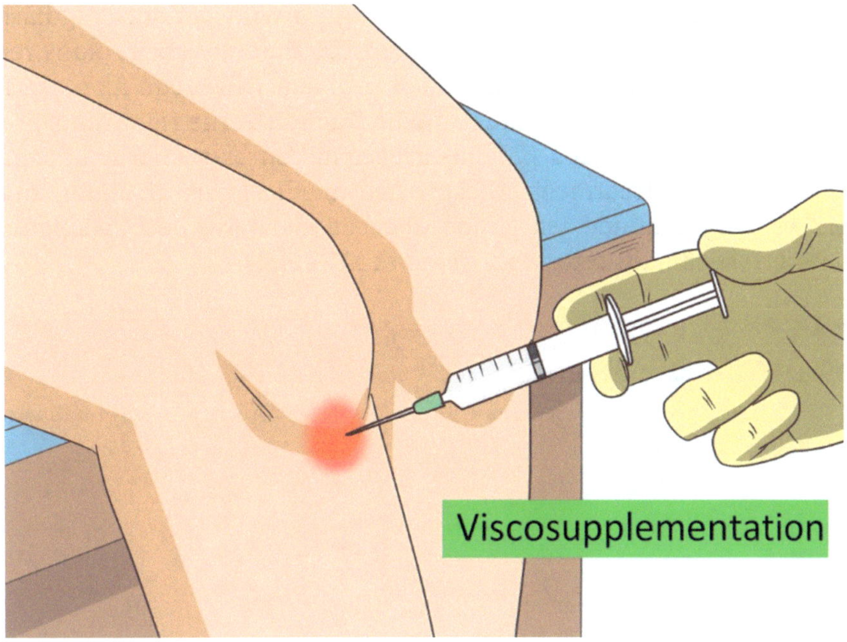

Figure 14.17. Management of joint disorders involving synovial fluid via Visco supplementation.

Source: https://www.wikihow.com/images/thumb/e/e2/Increase-Synovial-Fluid-Step-19-Version-2.jpg/aid9509300-v4-1200px-Increase-Synovial-Fluid-Step-19-Version-2.jpg.

14.6.3. Therapeutic approaches for serous fluid accumulation

When you're treating accumulation of serous fluid, figuring out what's causing it all is pretty important. You typically have to start by analyzing the fluid itself—its composition can actually guide you to the best treatment. You'll sometimes have pleural effusions or ascites, and these can occur due to infections, cancer, or even cardiac issues. Combining imaging tests and fluid work usually opens the proceedings in figuring out what intervention is best. Interventions may be as simple as low-level medications to some procedures, which means that one size does not fit all; the highly specific nature of the cause truly makes a difference. An inspection of the extravascular body fluids, oddly enough, gives further pointers that help augment these tactics, guiding choice in the right direction (Jokic et al., 2020). Management of this form of fluid build-up is almost always a cooperative endeavor. Pulmonologists, cardiologists, surgeons and their brethren tend to be drafted in most times so that efforts coordinate nicely with each other—even though sometimes it seems rather disorganized. Think, for example, of procedures like paracentesis or thoracentesis: they're not just about relieving the added load, but also about capturing samples to get a closer look. Procedures come with the advantage of relief of symptoms, as well as laying the groundwork for more accurate diagnosis and ongoing shifts in treatment. For the most part, being meticulous about working through preanalytical, analytical, and postanalytical processes is paramount to making sure the fluid is tested as precisely as it can be, with as few risks as possible along the way (Ellerton et al., 2023). The integration of acute management and longer-term approaches, like changes to lifestyle and repeated follow-up, really is the basis of the whole strategy. Ultimately, working patients actively does have a big difference. The better they understand why the fluid buildup occurs, and what their options are for treatment, the better they can take care of themselves—maybe even if the conversation isn't ever entirely smooth. Catching up with patients regularly and ensuring that patients engage well with their care teams can ensure that treatment plans remain on course, something that definitely reduces the likelihood the problem will recur. Also, possessing an acute sense of early warning signs at times can cause medical action at the right time, preventing further complications. Highlighting personalized, patient-focused measures-even when the path is not always linear-hence optimizes overall treatment efficacy. With medical care changing and developing on a day-to-day basis, keeping in mind such patient-focused measures becomes paramount to better results when treating serous fluid retention (Jokic et al., 2020).

Test Your Knowledge

1. What medical or surgical treatments are available for male infertility related to semen abnormalities?
2. How are synovial fluid–related disorders such as gout or septic arthritis managed?

Summary

Combining the various roles of semen, synovial, and serous fluids perfectly explains how complex human physiology is. Semen alone is not only tasked with reproduction but also with nourishing sperm with vital components; synovial fluid acts as a natural lubricant for joints, allowing gliding of joints, while serous fluid minimizes friction in body cavities. If you lay these functions side by side, it rapidly becomes apparent that our body is all about righting things in unexpected ways, a reminder that, more frequently than not, fluid dynamics contains some of the secrets of health and disease we're still chasing. We can't overstate how critical these fluids are especially in terms of healthcare. For instance, if the synovial fluid production becomes out of sync, it may trigger some quite uncomfortable joint issues, and excessive serous fluid is a sign something is amiss—like infections or even cancers. Clinical practices that work to restore balance to this are significant, and sometimes even tiny tuning tweaks reduce risks in surgeries. A closer look at the metabolism of these fluids—not to mention good electrolyte handling (Bingham et al., 1938)—far too often gives new clues, by and large, for improved therapy. Revisiting semen, synovial, and serous fluids offers an insight into human biology, revealing how these fluids regulate our body functions. They don't do a single task; each one mirrors wider principles that underlie health and disease. Research still seeks out their complex roles, and what we may learn could perhaps revolutionize the practice of medicine and our knowledge of the science of it. Overall, what we can learn about these fluids and their peculiarities reminds us of the robust connections which make life operate and the quite considerable need for balancing fluids to recover and live well (Ellerton et al., 2023).

Within our body, fluids surprisingly perform a wide range of functions. Consider semen, synovial fluid, and serous fluids – all have their own spin on getting things going. Semen, essentially sperm and its associated plasma, assists in carrying and feeding sperm to aid in reproduction. And then stored away in our joints, synovial fluid reduces friction and allows for smoother movement. Concurrently, within the body cavities, serous fluids—like the ones found within cavities such as the pleural and peritoneal spaces—constitute slippery padding whereby organs can slide over each other with ease. These functions point to the close relationship between each fluid's composition and its specific function. The contents of the fluids differ significantly from each other in line with the special functions each one performs. Such as seminal plasma contains proteins, enzymes, and even a burst of fructose to increase motility and viability of sperm, and synovial fluid that loads up hyaluronic acid and lubricin, which is very crucial in minimizing wear on joints. And also, serous fluids that consist mostly of water, electrolytes and proteins, serving as a cushion for protection around organs. Generally speaking, this particular mix isn't just about working with a given job – it also helps maintain the balance of our body's health. Examining the composition of each may at times yield important information about various sicknesses and cures. Studying these bodily liquids becomes vital because they're related to both treatment and diagnosis. Minor alterations in semen composition may affect fertility, and deviations in synovial fluid may signal joint diseases like arthritis. Examination of serous fluids sometimes yields information about infection, cancer or other diseases. With knowledge of the most significant constituents and purposes of semen, synovial, and serous fluids, health care professionals can generally diagnose and manage related disorders more competently. In most cases, but a few excepted, texts such as Essentials of Human Histology and the OER course Human Anatomy and Physiology equip students with a good footing to venture into the depths of human biology (Ellerton et al., 2023; Krause et al., 2005).

KEY TERMS FROM THIS CHAPTER

Crystal analysis
Glucose
Peritoneal fluid
Pleural fluid
Seminal fluid volume
Sperm count
Sperm motility
Synovial fluid analysis
Viscosity
Fructose concentration
Pericardial fluid
pH of semen
Semen
Serous fluid
Sperm morphology
Synovial fluid
Synovial fluid aspiration

Critical Thinking Questions

1. **Which of the following is the primary component of synovial fluid?**
   a. Red blood cells
   b. White blood cells
   c. Hyaluronic acid
   d. Glucose
2. **The presence of sperm in semen analysis is an indication of:**
   a. Low sperm count
   b. Presence of infection
   c. Normal fertility in males
   d. High testosterone levels
3. **What is the primary function of synovial fluid in joints?**
   a. To nourish cartilage and reduce friction
   b. To promote immune response
   c. To transport oxygen to tissues
   d. To produce red blood cells
4. **A decrease in the volume of serous fluid in body cavities can be an indicator of:**
   a. Infection or inflammation
   b. Dehydration
   c. Increased white blood cell count
   d. Normal fluid balance
5. **What is the most common finding in the semen of a man diagnosed with azoospermia?**
   a. Presence of spermatozoa
   b. Absence of spermatozoa
   c. High sperm count
   d. High semen viscosity

Answers to Critical Thinking Questions

1. (c); 2. (c); 3. (a); 4. (a); 5. (b)

Short Answer Questions

1. What are the main components assessed in a semen analysis, and why are each important for fertility evaluation?
2. What is the significance of sperm count, and what range is considered normal for fertility purposes?
3. How does sperm motility affect the chances of fertilization, and what levels are considered normal?
4. What does the morphology of sperm indicate about male reproductive health?
5. What factors might influence semen volume, and how does a low volume impact fertility?
6. What is the purpose of synovial fluid analysis, and what conditions can it help diagnose?
7. What are the normal physical characteristics of synovial fluid, and how does the appearance change in joint diseases?

References

1. AHBS Department. (2025). *MSO 102: Medical Terminology*. https://core.ac.uk/download/638988839.pdf (accessed on 1st July 2025).
2. Allen, M. C. (1994). *The Normal Physiological Aspects of Aging as They Relate to Nurse Aid Care*. https://core.ac.uk/download/560696978.pdf (accessed on 1st July 2025).
3. Amaral, T., Audisio, R., Dopazo Taboada, C., Sandrucci, S., et al. (2021). The ESSO core curriculum committee update on surgical oncology. https://core.ac.uk/download/534957948.pdf (accessed on 1st July 2025).
4. Annand, E. J. (2023). *Horses as Sentinels of Emerging Infectious Disease*. https://core.ac.uk/download/576836830.pdf (accessed on 1st July 2025).
5. Bingham, D. L. C. (1938). *The Surgical Aspects of Water and Salt Metabolism*. https://core.ac.uk/download/429705752.pdf (accessed on 1st July 2025).
6. Büchler, C. (2020). *Adipokines 2.0*. https://core.ac.uk/download/478098132.pdf (accessed on 1st July 2025).
7. Ellerton, S. S., & Roblodowski, C. (2023). *Introduction to Human Biology*. https://core.ac.uk/download/571402331.pdf (accessed on 1st July 2025).
8. Havercroft, J. M. (2018). *Boron and Other Trace Elements in Human Tissues and Fluids*. https://core.ac.uk/download/528159584.pdf (accessed on 1st July 2025).
9. Jokic, A., Kocijan, I., Culej, J., Kopcinovic, L. M., & Bozovic, M. (2020). Laboratory testing of extravascular body fluids: National recommendations on behalf of the Croatian Society of Medical Biochemistry and Laboratory Medicine. Part I–Serous fluids. https://core.ac.uk/download/481972806.pdf (accessed on 1st July 2025).
10. Krause, W. J., II. (2005). *Krause's Essential Human Histology for Medical Students*. https://core.ac.uk/download/62770592.pdf (accessed on 1st July 2025).
11. Mas Giménez, G. de, Royo Royo, S., & Yáñez Alvarado, C. R. (2022). Overview of biofluids and flow sensing techniques applied in clinical practice. https://core.ac.uk/download/541513760.pdf (accessed on 1st July 2025).
12. McLaughlin, C. A. (1988). Legal issues in the healthcare settings AIDS: Current state of the law–An overview. https://core.ac.uk/download/216931467.pdf (accessed on 1st July 2025).
13. Reinsalu, O. (2022). Vähi-testis antigeen MAGE-A4 inkorporeeritakse ekstratsellulaarsetesse vesiikulitesse ja on eksponeeritud selle pinnal. https://core.ac.uk/download/532377244.pdf (accessed on 1st July 2025).

SEROLOGICAL AND IMMUNOLOGICAL TESTS

15

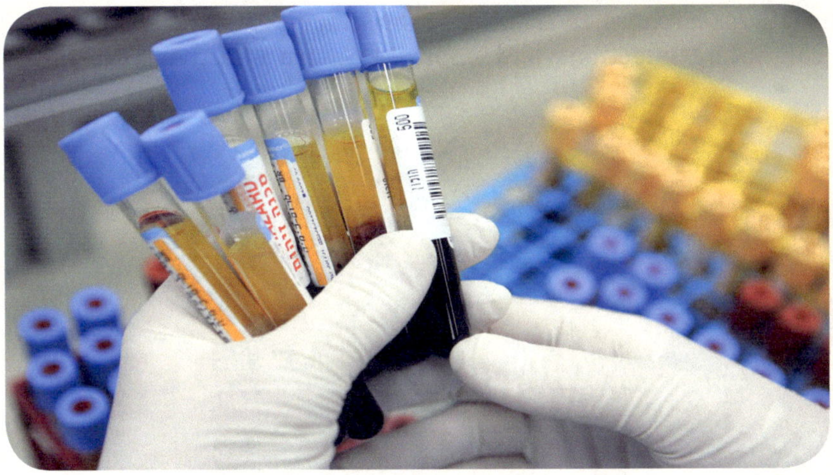

LEARNING OBJECTIVES

After studying this chapter, you will be able to:

1. Give historical background serological and immunological tests;
2. List the types of serological tests;
3. Explain the types of immunological tests;
4. Explore the applications in disease diagnosis for serological and immunological tests;
5. Identify the advantages of serological and immunological tests;
6. Focus on the limitations and challenges serological and immunological tests.

Introduction

Disease detection and surveillance has, in essence, changed over the years—gratified, no less, by recent breakthroughs in biology. You now have diagnostics that scan blood components—serological and immunological ones—employed by researchers and doctors to understand how we bodies are overpowering germs. They detect things like certain antibodies and antigens, which give insights into infections, autoimmune disease, and even vaccine effectiveness. Sometimes these tests appear in other random locations too; veterinary service, for example, where they track bugs like *Salmonella gallinarum* in chickens. It is most common that this means that these tests play an important role a lot, not just for human beings but also for keeping farms and the economy on track. As more attention is given to these blood tests, having established rules is normally becoming a requirement. The complexity of these tests normally demands strict guidelines so that they can be replicable and reliable. For instance, the European Medicines Agency usually demands strict standards for tests used in new vaccine formulations, especially flu vaccines. Techniques like Hemagglutination Inhibition and Virus Neutralization tests, for example, need to reach set targets before any approval of a flu vaccine is given. This kind of regulatory approach has a monolithic effect, not just on proving the effectiveness of a vaccine, but on building public trust, even if there is still buzz among researchers about exploring other possible avenues. Merging serological and immunological testing into our wider health monitoring systems could really flip things on their head. Using a blend of old methods and new tests, public health officials get a better sense of how diseases spread. A serological survey might detect, say, how widespread an infection is among a specific population, whereas an immune assay tells them how well a vaccine works—like in some flu studies. Further research, combined with new technological advances, should strengthen these testing methods even further. Efforts to fine-tune the procedures will ultimately benefit many people—from lab researchers to healthcare providers—ensuring these tests continue to play a key role in combating infections and informing more effective health policies (Figure 15.1).

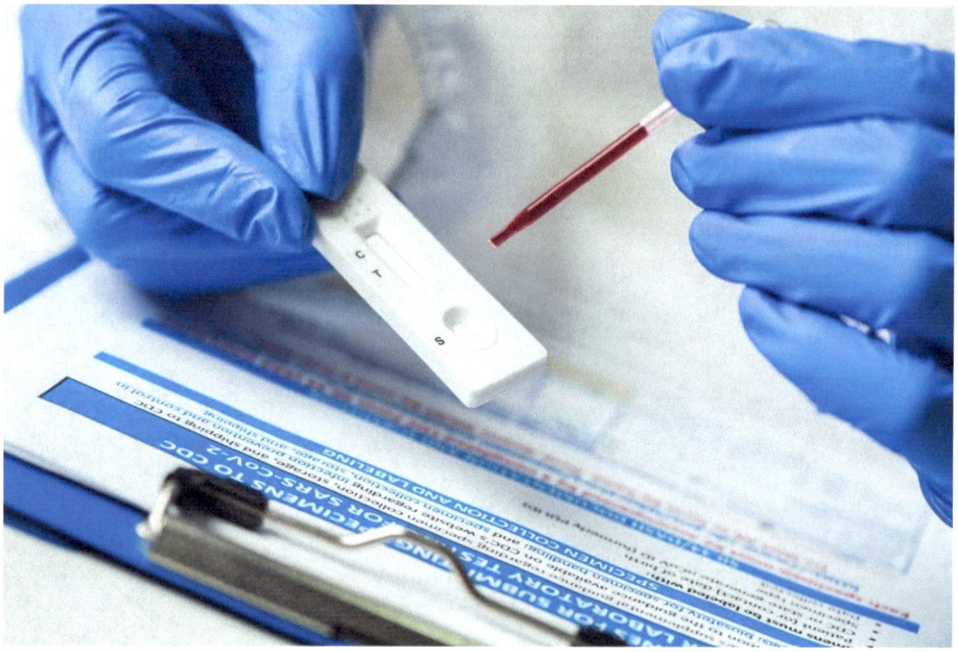

Figure 15.1. Serological test.

Source: https://d2jx2rerrg6sh3.cloudfront.net/images/news/ImageForNews_705943_16462272081747550.jpg.

Definition of Serological Tests

Serological testing gives us a window into the manner in which our immune systems respond to invaders. Tests for antibodies or antigens in a patient's serum—typically revealing to us what happens subsequent to infection or immunization. Practically in all cases, they inform decisions in the management of infections, autoimmune diseases, and allergies. For example, autoantibody detection in autoimmune disorders can reveal hidden processes in the body and even aid in tailoring treatments. Current technological developments have largely translated into more accurate assays with greater sensitivity and specificity and therefore better patient outcomes. All of this speaks to how such tests have evolved to be indispensable tools for routine clinical practice and research. In routine clinical practice, their use goes beyond the identification of diagnosis. Such tests can also serve as important markers in the epidemiology of disease prevalence as well as in the assistance of epidemiological studies. In public health, seroprevalence surveys also rely on such measurements to be able to estimate community immunity, with implications for immunization policy and public health policy. Take tuberculosis, for instance—rapid antibody detection here can prove a major aid in controlling outbreaks. But problems like cross-reactivity and differential immune response according to groups of people still perplex interpretation. In most cases, ongoing research must not only optimize current methods but also look for new immunological markers, as has been noted in recent reviews of the diagnosis of tuberculosis. Linking serological testing with broader immune investigation enhances our general understanding of complex immune interactions. The way test reaction relates to clinical course suggests the need for further investigation. By examining specificity and sensitivity against one another in various contexts, researchers have found room for what current diagnostic tools are unable to do. Development of point-of-care tests—despite a few potholes in the process—holds the promise to disrupt disease detection, especially in resource-limited settings where intervention on a timely basis can decrease morbidity and even mortality. Generalov et al. (2014), the promise of an augmented diagnostic approach that provides more detailed insight into disease development and immunity is strong, as highlighted in efforts surrounding challenging cases such as tuberculosis (Harari et al., 2012).

Definition of Immunological Tests

Immunologic tests are integral to what we're familiar with as to how the body is reacting. They're not necessarily lab tests, but rather aid in finding and measuring antibodies and antigens for certain bugs. Overall, these tools utilize our own immune system to check whether infections are active or whether vaccines have activated our defenses into responding. Scientists use such methods as enzyme-linked immunosorbent assays (ELISA) and western blotting—terms that sound unnecessarily cutting-edge but are actually descriptive of simple ideas—to identify reactions that tell us about one's overall state of health. You see such tests appearing in all manner of contexts, ranging from the diagnosis of infections to the identification of autoimmune issues, thus attesting to their very importance in modern medicine. Serological tests, a category falling under this broader immune toolkit, are designed with accuracy to quantify the amount of antibodies produced as a result of exposures like infection, vaccines, or even allergens. In the majority of research activity, techniques such as Hemagglutination Inhibition (HI) and Single Radial Hemolysis (SRH) have been used, especially when measuring reaction to influenza vaccines – a testament to the reason why agencies like the European Medicines Agency (EMA) demand strict protocol. More often than not, such assays not only assist clinicians to determine what could be impacting a patient but also aid public health initiatives by monitoring immune markers within groups. In the majority of instances, the gradual development of such techniques requires revisiting outdated standards, something that's typically necessary for vaccine research refinement and successful disease management (Callow et al., 2014). However, immunology is not exclusively characterized by the conventional serology tests. The field today includes a mix of experimental approaches that dig deeper into the complexity of our immune system – sometimes in a gaudy, somewhat haphazard way. In cell-mediated responses, measurement approaches and more recently pseudo type-based neutralization assays bring new information, particularly when determining whether or not vaccines are effective. As our understanding of immune processes deepens, it is increasingly obvious that incorporating these sophisticated tests into routine practice is more critical than ever. They don't simply broaden our perspective on immune responses; they also open the door to more individualized care and precision medicine. Taking all this into account, the expansion of accepted immunological tests is a crucial step toward advancing the development of clinical practice and research in the field (Generalov et al., 2014) (Figure 15.2).

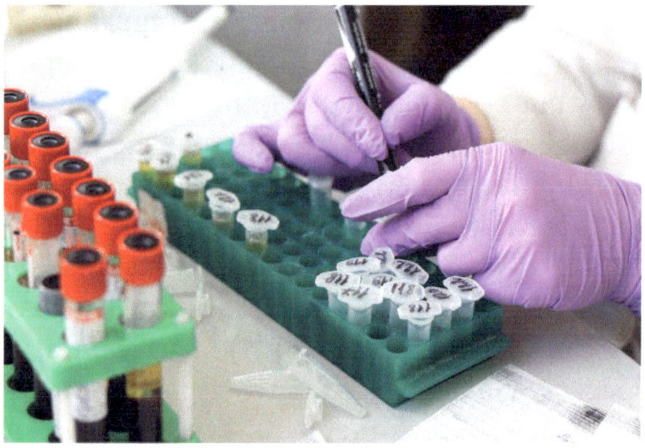

Figure 15.2. Immunological tests.

Source: https://medical.thearcgroup.co.uk/wp-content/uploads/2024/12/Immunology-Blood-Testing.jpg.

Importance of These Tests in Modern Medicine

Serology and immune system screenings essentially changed the way doctors today diagnose illnesses. These tests detect disease symptoms by looking for antibodies or antigens in the blood—a process that became an unexpected game-changer. For example, methods like enzyme-linked immunosorbent assays (ELISA) and Western blotting enable doctors to trace the origins of mysterious symptoms back to the culprit, giving them a more direct route to treatment. As far as possible, the fast pace of development in these testing technologies seems to reflect a trend towards personalized treatment, in which the treatments are tailored to a person's unique immune profile, and frankly, it sounds like a logical step in modern medicine. At other times, the impact of these tests goes beyond simply detecting an infection early on. In fact, detection of some markers can guide treatment for long-term or autoimmune disease patients. You might even discover such practices in vet communities—where once an elimination diet was strictly the rule for allergies, today serum antibody tests (Dunn et al., 2020) have joined the fray to speed up identifying actual culprits. This adoption of new techniques into regular health check-ups shows, in a quite evident way, that these tests are becoming an integral component in instant diagnosis and ongoing care. In retrospect, it's difficult not to admire the history behind these diagnostic tests. The early pioneers such as Schaudinn and Wassermann paved the way for understanding difficult conditions such as syphilis and left behind hints that continue to shape the industry today (Duff et al., 1935). Their contributions have a lasting reverberation that reminds us how far medical testing has evolved—even if the evolution often feels somewhat uneven. As researchers discover more about how our immune systems truly work, these tests continue to reveal the intricate relationships between diseases of all kinds, and generally speaking, they shed new light on public health concerns. Generally speaking, the relentless march of serological and immunological testing continues to show us how vital they are both in everyday healthcare and in managing major epidemics.

15.1. Historical Background

Learning Outcome

- Development of serological testing;
- Key milestones in immunological testing;
- Evolution of diagnostic techniques.

Serological and immunological testing evolved over time in ways that illustrate the tendency of scientific progress to provide in advance for actual public health needs. Initially, people had naive notions of immunity and infection but not yet the technology that now enables modern diagnostics. The leaders of the science of microbiology and immunology got the process underway when they began identifying antibodies and antigens with relatively crude methods. And that early groundwork eventually gave rise to further sophisticated techniques—techniques that would allow doctors to pinpoint specific pathogens and quantify immune responses across different populations of people. Those advances were especially crucial during periods of health emergencies like pandemics; rapid analysis and prudent tracking, as exemplified in certain studies on COVID-19 serological testing (Porru et al., 2021), really counted. In hindsight, the history of immunological testing is not just about awesome technology—it's also about learning about disease spread by looking at who has antibodies. For example, research on healthcare workers was especially enlightening about how humans respond to SARS-CoV-2, not only informing care for individuals but also public health policy. Test protocols became increasingly sophisticated through time, taking into account such aspects as sensitivity and specificity, allowing scientists a clearer insight into bacterial and viral threats. These results most commonly led to better methods of avoiding infections from gaining a foothold, protecting medical staff along with the broader community from arising diseases (Rüggeberg et al., 2003).

The history of the tests also shows an ongoing conversation between what is happening at a patient's bedside and broader trends being seen in populations. New challenges—new germs and antibiotic resistance—continued to challenge new thinking for diagnostics. Meanwhile, inequalities in who can access testing, often founded on socio-economic status, have had real-world implications for the impact of public health measures. Scientists, in some cases even found a correlation between socio-economic status and disease incidence such as anaphylaxis, indicating more equitable healthcare might have a bearing. Generally, this varied exploration of serological and immunological testing illustrates that these tools are valuable not merely in patient diagnosis, but also in co-coordinating more extensive public health measures (Rüggeberg et al., 2003).

15.1.1. Development of Serological Testing

Serological investigations have come a long way since it was prompted by the need for truly accurate reagents for diagnosis in clinical immunology. When tests were just simple blood tests, they've gradually become sophisticated techniques that are capable of detecting particular antibodies against a whole range of infectious agents. This development has been required to untangle disease mechanisms and understand how patients react. Researchers have always pointed out the pivotal role of such serological indicators—especially in chronic disease and autoimmune disease. For example, studies on marine turtle fibro papillomatosis unexpectedly led to the construction of tests for herpesvirus, postulating that tailored assays in wildlife may eventually be a factor in human health initiatives (Bjorndal et al., 2000). The application of recombinant technology really put the cat among the pigeons in the case of such tests—it made it possible to identify a wide combination of antigens. Techniques such as immunoblotting now drive sensitivity and specificity upwards, something that is especially noticeable in conditions such as Lyme borreliosis. Various research has noticed that varying antibody patterns closely follow clinical manifestations; this further emphasizes the crucial role of serological analysis in disease management. In particular, assays which target distinctive proteins—such as VlsE and OspC in *Borrelia burgdorferi*—may determine treatment and even predict prognosis (Aguero-Rosenfeld et al., 2008). Their applicability to a variety of pathogens makes them virtually indispensable in medical practice. In the future, serological testing will be capable of incorporating next-generation technologies, such as nanotechnology and microfluidics, which can produce results sooner and with higher throughput. The updating is essential, in general, in outbreak settings where speed is paramount to patient care and public health intervention. Increasingly, immunologists and biotechnologists are working together to create assays that not only detect immune responses but also characterize them at a molecular level. As implicated by the marine turtle research, these new techniques will broaden the use of serological tests and make them essential tools to employ when monitoring viral persistence and evaluating how environmental factors impact immune health (Bjorndal et al., 2000) (Figure 15.3).

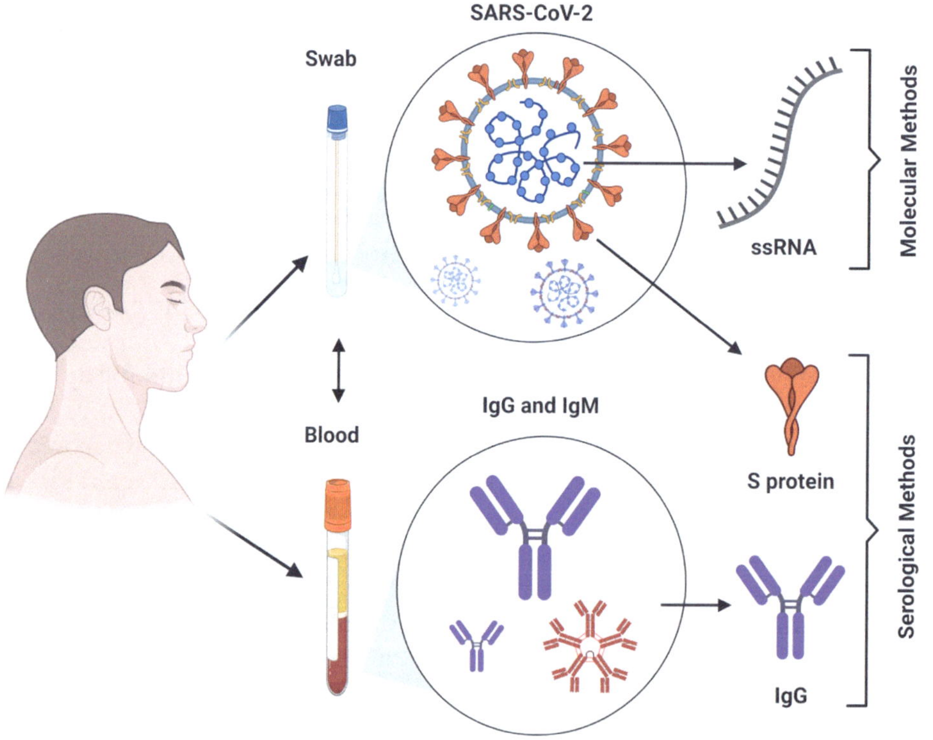

Figure 15.3. Development of serological testing.

Source: https://dfzljdn9uc3pi.cloudfront.net/2020/10180/1/fig-1-full.png.

15.1.2. Key Milestones in Immunological Testing

Immunological testing has come a long way, really shaking up how diagnoses get made. One big turning point was tweaking the serological tests for celiac disease—a change spurred on by a growing buzz among patients and healthcare folks alike. Over the last three decades, we've seen a pretty steep rise in diagnosed cases, mostly because clinical insights have sharpened and our tests got super sensitive. But still, it is worrisome that nearly 95% of all individuals with celiac disease go undiagnosed, which, in general terms, translates to needing more education and better screening practices. Additionally, the insidious nature of histopathological examinations at times produces false negatives, and thus our serological examinations have to keep up with the varied clinical indicators across various patients (Ali et al., 2022). One other highlight moment was when health crises—like COVID-19—pushed us into developing diagnostic tests at breakneck speed. Mostly, the emergency need for fast, precise tests gave a big boost to advanced techniques like polymerase chain reaction (PCR) and lateral flow assays. These measures not only increased the sensitivity of diagnostics but also ushered in a faster testing age, which enabled health systems to view emerging infections early. All this notwithstanding, moving from innovative ideas into practice on a daily basis is not always unproblematic, as with ultra-cutting-edge technologies like nano-biosensors, which, as great as they promise in terms of quicker and cheaper outcomes, have not yet caught up broadly based on regulatory and market issues (Canudo et al., 2021). Serological testing is now standard in clinical practice, another leap forward for immunology. Being able to detect autoimmune diseases and infections early on has basically turned patient care on its head, enabling doctors to get in ahead of severe complications. With the tests concentrating on specific antibodies, there is a closer look at immune responses, paving the way for targeted treatments. Look, for example, to the rheumatoid arthritis and other autoimmune conditions screening; improved diagnostics therein have equated to improved patient outcomes. As the science advances, so the bringing together of new technological advancements and experiential medicine remains fundamental in order to ensure that new diagnostic methods do not only emerge but are implemented fairly, with a perceptible impact upon immunological testing as a whole (Ali et al., 2022) (Figure 15.4).

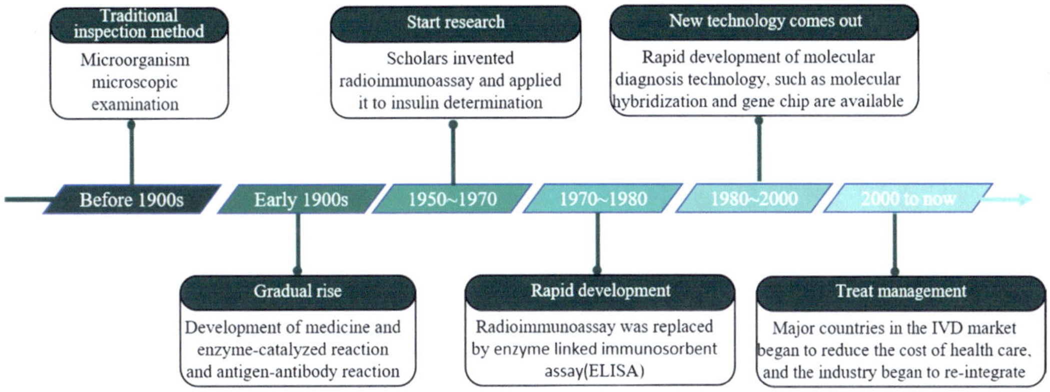

Figure 15.4. Key milestones in immunological testing.

Source: https://pub.mdpi-res.com/processes/processes-11-00403/article_deploy/html/images/processes-11-00403-g001.png?1674972845.

15.1.3. Evolution of diagnostic techniques

Medical diagnostic methods have come a long way, and you can literally see that in the way we test for disease these days. Such antiquated methods as looking under a microscope or culturing simply couldn't catch all the wily germs. Now, tests that search for antibodies or antigens in a patient sample have boosted our accuracy way, way up. High-throughput screening and the discovery of new biomarkers enable us to quickly identify pathogenic pathogens. This shift, which you might say hastens the whole diagnostic process, also enables us to diagnose such illnesses as Chagas disease earlier in the game. New diagnostic tools are seeking to outdo previous limitations by providing consistent, reproducible results for every kind of patient and clinical setting (Balouz et al., 2016). Immunological tests also made it into the spotlight as technology improved. ELISAs and PCR—those very same ones—are now deemed essential for diagnostic purposes, reconciling sensitivity with specificity in a manner that no traditional methods could. They work magic even on complicated issues like trypanosomiasis, a disease which keeps us in our toes due to ever-mutating strains of the pathogen and mercurial host responses. As a general principle, how such tests identify antibody production and immune suppression, like in Trypanosoma infections, reminds us that adapting testing practices to accommodate the unique differences of the patient is most important (Desquesnes et al., 2008). Refining such techniques over time not only makes us more accurate with tests, but in some way, they also help improve patient care and treatment planning. And then there is the sweeping vision of under-funded areas where healthcare systems fall behind. The majority of the neglected diseases—Chagas, say—are too often denied the proper diagnostic tools, and that does permanent damage to the populations. The latest developments in point-of-care diagnostics, which are simple to employ and robust, are working to turn that around. New biomarkers that can even detect early congenital transmission or measure the effectiveness of treatments are a testament to how much we need new approaches to diagnostics. Generally, through the integration of such innovative approaches into regular healthcare, public health challenges can be managed more effectively, paving the way for improved results and improved quality of life for patients battling chronic disease like Chagas (Balouz et al., 2016).

Test Your Knowledge

1. How did the discovery of antibodies contribute to the development of serological testing?
2. What role did the Wassermann test play in the early history of serological diagnostics?

15.2. Types of Serological Tests

Learning Outcome

- Enzyme-linked immunosorbent assay (ELISA);
- Western blotting;
- Radioimmunoassay (RIA).

Serological diagnosis has actually revolutionized infectious disease diagnosis. ELISA is a fine example—it's a workhorse nowadays for diagnosing diseases like schistosomiasis. Researchers normally follow a standard procedure and commonly notice that ELISA is more sensitive and specific than older methods like complement fixation tests or even skin tests. In some studies, small adjustments—such as performing ultracentrifugation on antigens and refining quality control—have increased its dependability in various epidemiological contexts. This all demonstrates, in most instances, why it's worthwhile to continue refining serological methods to enhance research and patient care (McLaren et al., 2025).

Blood work isn't reserved solely for infections, however. It does make a difference in the case of autoimmune conditions such as childhood-onset idiopathic inflammatory myopathies (IIMs). A national registry and biobank have been formed in the majority of cases to collect biological samples from children who are struggling with these extremely rare conditions, which enables researchers to study and track them more strictly. Collaborative effort is likely to illuminate disease mechanisms, quantify the effectiveness of therapy, and monitor long-term outcomes. By following standardized procedures for testing and sample collection, researchers essentially provide a better picture of juvenile myositis and its various presentations. Serial sampling with clinical databases only means to complement the overall resource so that fresh ideas about therapy and subsequently better patient management are obtained (Bohan et al., 2011). There's another dimension in the equation with rapid diagnostic tests beyond ELISA or autoimmune markers. Rapid tests yield results virtually immediately in a clinical environment, which is extremely valuable for deployment where resources are scarce, allowing practitioners to initiate treatment without delay. Lateral flow assays, for example, make it easier by allowing timely intervention while offloading the burden from healthcare systems. All the same, such rapid tests are often less specific and less sensitive than their more complex relatives and need to be fully tested when selecting an appropriate diagnostic technique. In general, the wide range of serological tests available serves to underscore just how essential these tools are to improving diagnostic accuracy and guiding patient management in infectious as well as non-infectious illness (Figure 15.5).

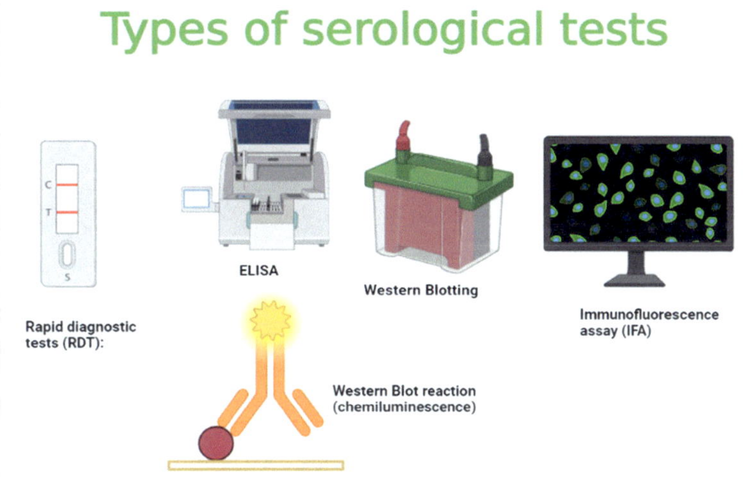

Figure 15.5. Types of serological tests.

Source: https://external-content.duckduckgo.com/iu/?u=https%3A%2F%2Fsciencevivid.com%2Fwp-content%2Fuploads%2F2022%2F12%2FTypes-of-Serological-Tests.png&f=1&nofb=1&ipt=abb6612db44f4a21f10275031b65805a0948bf34cfb511f095e604d3d58b95a6.

15.2.1. Enzyme-Linked Immunosorbent Assay (ELISA)

Serological tests can be very generalizable – think about how ELISA works. Enzyme-based and antibody-based, this method uses these devices in a fairly straightforward way to target pathogens. Instead of relying on complicated definitions, think of the ELISA as being a test in which target antibodies bind to specific antigens, and it enables us to measure immune responses in many different animals. I recall a study on *Trypanosoma evansi* which demonstrated, very interestingly indeed, how ELISA could distinguish infected camels from ones that were not due to a collection of custom antisera. Identifying that difference is actually very important to livestock disease control because it can detect infection early, which then dictates the decision to treat. And then, too, there's the issue that ELISA can detect both circulating antibodies and antigens – a double-barreled stunt that highlights its status as a fundamental reagent in the field of serodiagnosis; this is a truth that is patent in veterinary and clinical laboratories alike (Aitken et al., 1989). But it doesn't stop there. Eventually, the use of ELISA in the diagnosis of viral infections has come quite a distance, overall terms, bragging of its versatility. In some recent work, researchers even identified a few herpesviruses from marine turtles – which would seem surprising initially. For instance, data on the LETV herpesvirus not only puts focus on ELISA's capacity to detect infectious agents but also forms the first basis for conservation. It is highly fascinating how the antigenic proteins of reptilian herpesviruses turned out to be immunogenic, significantly expanding the potential for wildlife health and veterinary virology. Slowly but surely, all these findings, directly born out of ELISA's applications, confirm its crucial role concerning the understanding of host-pathogen interactions within a range of ecosystems (Jacobson et al., 2001).

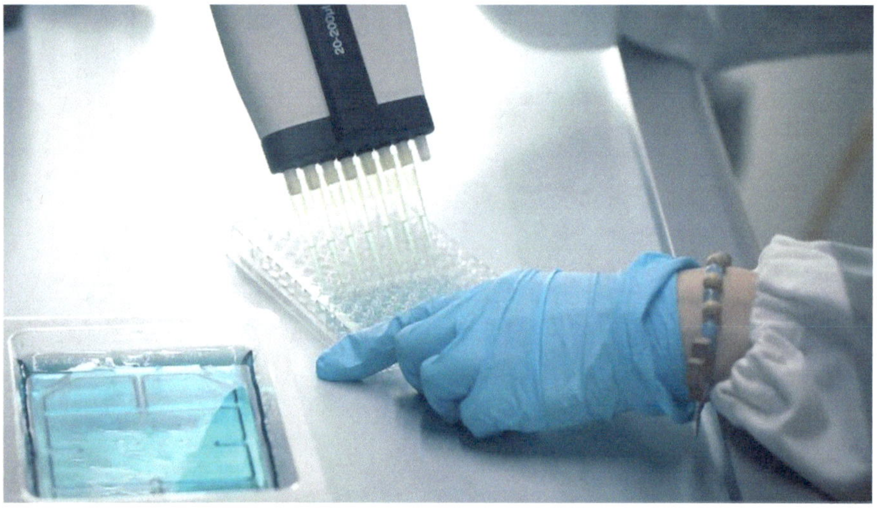

Figure 15.6. Enzyme-linked immunosorbent assay (ELISA) test.

Source: https://external-content.duckduckgo.com/iu/?u=https%3A%2F%2Fassets.technologynetworks.com%2Fproduction%2Fdynamic%2Fimages%2Fcontent%2F350024%2Fan-introduction-to-the-enzyme-linked-immunosorbent-assay-elisa-test-350024-960x540.jpg%3Fcb%3D11908166&f=1&nofb=1&ipt=1fa78ff989022ac13ef1a7220d396baeda9e26f27dfae94db0dea1cb1e8bb939.

Beyond diagnostics, ELISA is still an arena that can enable more immunological research. It enables scientists to measure antibodies after an infection—a pivotal detail that also creates the potential for tracking the effectiveness of vaccines and the humoral immune response in general. This data proves especially useful when designing strategies against infectious diseases, as it captures a snapshot of how organisms respond to various pathogens over time. Practically, the enzyme-linked immunosorbent assay (ELISA) enhances not only our serodiagnostic capabilities but also public health by generating data that may eventually influence vaccination campaigns and therapeutic decisions. Since so much is continually being done to expand the limits, for the majority of uses, ELISA's long-standing value in serological and immunological studies continues to be the basis for progressing the prevention and treatment of disease in many fields (Figure 15.6).

15.2.2. Western Blotting

Western blotting shows up in immunological diagnostics as a handy method of exploring proteins—especially when antibodies and antigens interact. Scientists initially separate proteins by size with electrophoresis and then transfer them onto a membrane to create a platform for antibodies to bind. This makes it possible for researchers to isolate and even measure target proteins from a soiled mixture, giving them leads about cell function and disease contributors. Sometimes you see a very distinct band at the 64–70 kDa range, and that in the majority of cases means that the method can actually highlight certain immune responses that are involved in pathogen recognition (Maria et al., 2024). Western blotting is not just limited to human research laboratories either; its applicability spills over to veterinary and wildlife science. Recent research has started to test the method with wild animals in an effort to ensnare pathogens and create serological tests sensitive to species-specific immune subtleties. Working with varied animals, such as various marsupials, requires that researchers find out about how different reagents adhere to their immunoglobulins. Overall, even though taxonomic differences are created, a large majority of reagents seem to work broadly throughout species, enabling the technique to aid in tracking disease patterns and even help conservation by showing infections that could reverberate into zoonotic epidemics (Liyanage et al., 2023). In immunological and serological work, Western blotting is a strong diagnostic standard—consistent and mostly reliable. It nicely complements traditional ELISAs, particularly if a double confirmation of antigen-antibody interactions is necessary. Doctors will typically use the apparent, visible protein bands to not only diagnose infection but also monitor treatment response and vaccine efficacy. Seeing these definitive bands gives an added degree of interpretive capability that directs the decision on treatment in relation to how the patient's immune system is reacting. By incorporating Western blotting into routine testing, scientists and doctors are further able to clarify immune dynamics and overall physiological status, although ignorance of some sort still exists (Maria et al., 2024) (Figure 15.7).

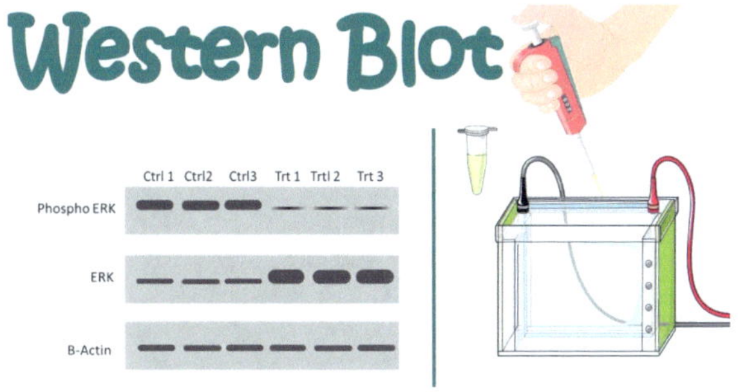

Figure 15.7. Western blotting.

Source: https://external-content.duckduckgo.com/iu/?u=https%3A%2F%2Fi.ytimg.com%2Fvi%2FYh69yHJMWPc%2Fmaxresdefault.jpg&f=1&nofb=1&ipt=a934c7052793c308c2b642619b2d1067f7d9bcde9e7cea11ce606e365d23841b.

15.2.3. Radioimmunoassay (RIA)

Antigen and hormone measurement has actually prompted immunologists to come up with some ingenious means. RIA has the tendency to receive much credit for being even more sensitive and specific in detecting minute amounts of biological material. It accomplishes this by competing radiolabeled antigens with their non-radiolabeled counterparts for antibody binding, and in most cases gives us fairly good estimates of such things as hormones, drugs, and even individual proteins. This neat method isn't limited to one type of study—it's been used far and wide in clinical research labs and investigation, where it's been used over and over to study serum samples with RIA to uncover how hormones are controlled and our immune system reacts, even sometimes finding a new way of treating disease. RIA's capability also manifests when checking antibody response, an important part of checking infectious disease. For instance, research on *Mycobacterium leprae*—the organism responsible for leprosy—have involved the measurement of IgM antibodies via RIA, and the tests usually show that individuals more vulnerable to the disease have a strong, continuing antibody signal, while naturally resistant persons possess little or none at all. In most cases, these differences enable researchers to distinguish between various immune profiles, providing clues on how infections start and then disseminate over time. This kind of specificity in following immune responses has helped establish the credibility of RIA as a significant tool in serological research. RIA has evolved alongside other immunoassay methods over time. Traditional RIA techniques depend extensively on radioactive substances, but growing concerns about the risks of radiation and environmental contamination have stimulated interest in alternatives like enzyme-linked immunosorbent assays (ELISA). However, RIA's unmatched sensitivity still holds its position in situations where infinitesimally small concentration is of paramount significance. Modern refinements in the original process aim to maintain its strengths while minimizing some of its limitations. The ongoing developments in both immunological and serological assays—like the continued use of RIA—demonstrate the way scientific investigation and clinical realities are constantly jostling together, extending our understanding of immune mechanisms and disease processes in numerous fields (Basit et al., 2018; Truman et al., 1985) (Figure 15.8).

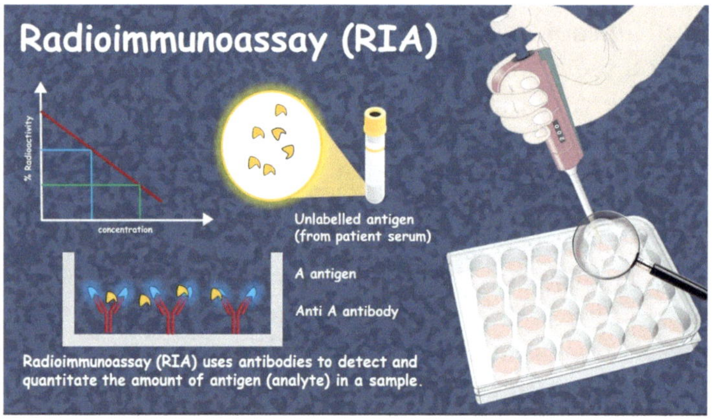

Figure 15.8. Radioimmunoassay(RIA).

Source: https://external-content.duckduckgo.com/iu/?u=https%3A%2F%2Fi.ytimg.com%2Fvi%2FJtbcqkiFf7w%2Fmaxresdefault.jpg&f=1&nofb=1&ipt=ce265f94d22d11ee0e9619c9ecf4f6dc2095c61f9aa383d64eaad10a1dccc4a0.

Test Your Knowledge

1. What are the main differences between agglutination, precipitation, and complement fixation tests?
2. How do enzyme-linked immunosorbent assays (ELISA) function as a serological method?

15.3. Types of Immunological Tests

Learning Outcome

- Complement fixation test;
- Agglutination tests;
- Flow cytometry.

Immunological tests have a taste for all seasons, all of which are designed to find disease and further research. ELISA is one that really stands out because it measures minute levels of antigens or antibodies in different samples with amazing sensitivity. Such an assay is especially useful in remote circumstances, such as space exploration, where it is crucial to identify microbial agents in order to be secure. Some studies even show that, to meet the extremely stringent standards of human spaceflight, scientists developed custom solid-phase, membrane-supported ELISA systems (Hejtmancik et al., 2025). Overall, with advancing science, we can see ELISA being created for even more challenging environments, and this is a testament to how innovative immunological testing can be. When conducting research on viral infections, serological tests add another dimension to our knowledge of our body's defenses. Methods such as Hemagglutination Inhibition (HI), Single Radial Hemolysis (SRH) and Virus Neutralization (VN) tests help to reveal how our immune system responds to viruses. Generally speaking, HI and SRH are the default methods of quantifying influenza-specific antibodies—a vital step in tracking vaccine effectiveness. Regulatory bodies like the European Medicines Agency (EMA) closely track these tests to ensure that new vaccines meet high standards of safety and efficacy. As a matter of course, while these assays are chiefly for use among healthy adults and elderly, still there is a missing link in the testing for children, with the need for improved testing standards (Callow et al., 2014). Recent developments in immunological assays are not only about developing vaccines—occasionally, but they also merely decode the subtle processes of our immune system. The new techniques, including pseudo type-based neutralization assays and neuraminidase tests, represent a direction towards more detailed, high-resolution methods. These approaches probe deeper into antibody-dependent and cell-mediated immunity, presenting a richer picture of the protective elements induced by vaccines. Most importantly, authorities like the EMA have started recognizing these newer methods to make sure that vaccine candidates are analyzed using today's correct measures. In general, as immunotesting continues to advance, it will likely influence public health policies and shape the direction of future research, offering significant potential for global health benefits (Figure 15.9).

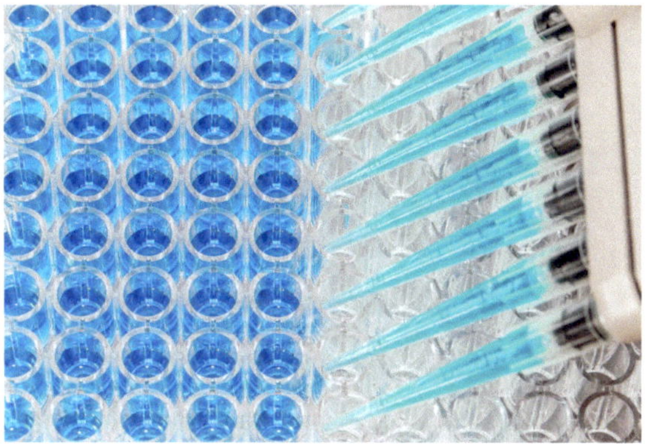

Figure 15.9. A multichannel pipette dispenses liquid into a 96-well microplate, commonly used in high-throughput assays for biochemical and clinical laboratory testing.

Source: https://external-content.duckduckgo.com/iu/?u=https%3A%2F%2Fcdn.britannica.com%2F53%2F193053-050-8DEBAA0B%2Fassay-laboratory.jpg&f=1&nofb=1&ipt=fa8c326651a413d4560c7ccf1afa8415160cb41488d4ca66584e7f721d7283ef.

15.3.1. Complement Fixation Test

The complement fixation test (CFT) is a time-honored diagnostic test—it essentially finds antibodies in patient serum by exploiting how the complement system works. The system is just a set of proteins that help antibodies eliminate foreign invaders. For the most part, if you mix a patient's serum with an antigen, whatever antibodies are present activate the complement proteins; if the proteins are consumed, they are rendered ineffective at causing indicator red blood cells to hemolyze, which is an indication of a positive test. Doctors utilize this process for detecting infections and autoimmune disease and screening for certain cancers. Aside from its diagnostic applications, the test also provides information regarding our immune responses. By examining how much of the complement is consumed, researchers can make a rough approximation of antibody levels—something that not only shows active infection but sometimes even implies previous immune activity. In general terms, an improved understanding of complement interactions makes us more well-rounded in our general comprehension of immunological diseases and could even lead to more specific treatments; it's a matter of fitting into a puzzle how our bodies combat diseases (N/A, 2004). That being said, the CFT is not without its idiosyncrasies. Problems such as unavailability of some antigens, immune response heterogeneity from different subjects, and risk of cross-reactivity can all make things harder and undermine precision. Moreover, the test is quite technically demanding—something that might be hard to keep up with in poor-resource settings. While newer molecular techniques like enzyme-linked immunosorbent assays (ELISA) and polymerase chain reaction (PCR) are starting to make limelight, the CFT remains rock-solid as a cornerstone technique. Its combination of advantages and disadvantages is still fascinating, even as the frontier of diagnostics unfolds (Figure 15.10).

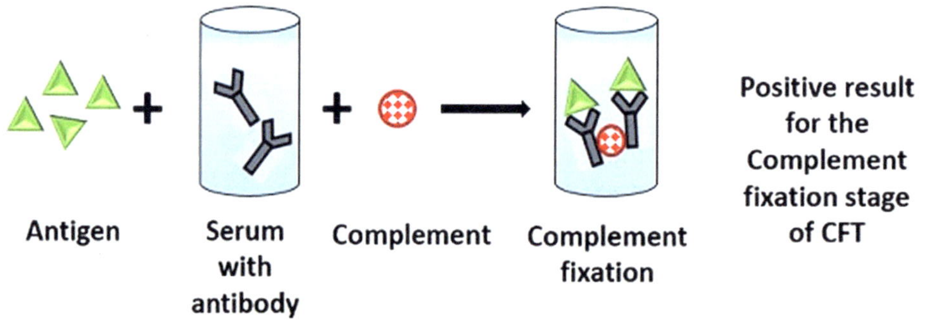

Figure 15.10. Complement fixation test.

Source: https://external-content.duckduckgo.com/iu/?u=https%3A%2F%2Fbiologyreader.com%2Fwp-content%2Fuploads%2F2019%2F07%2Fpositive-result-for-the-complement-fixation-stage.jpg&f=1&nofb=1&ipt=49e748078674568cca7b532de6dfee6f994010b87f3ebb0bc30fa34a323c6d89.

15.3.2. Agglutination Tests

Agglutination tests are an old standby of serological and immunological analysis – their potential to do everything really comes into its own when you need results fast and accurately. They work by bringing particles, be they bacterial cells or even latex beads, together in the presence of the right antibodies. Essentially, antigens on these particles meet up with their matching antibodies, and that interaction creates clumps that you can view by the naked eye. This is a simple-to-use technique and, in most uses, gives rapid results, and is thus a mainstay in medical clinics (e.g., streptococcal infection screening). Scientists also can manipulate some of the test parameters to maximize sensitivity and specificity, adding an extra layer of control that can enhance the accuracy of diagnoses. Advances in immunoassay techniques have given the tests a new lease on life. Traditional assays have, nonetheless, been supplemented with modern advances over the years – in the majority of instances, techniques like enzyme immunoassays (EIAs) now arrive on the scene to enhance sensitivity and specificity. For example, some EIA approaches that hunt down pathogens like *Salmonella* show visible improvements from the previous setups. A well-planned combination of modified protocols and purified antibody conjugates usually has the effect of reducing cross-reactivity but pushing detection levels upwards, as is the situation in food safety analysis (Minnich et al., 1981). Such flexibility not only optimizes laboratory procedures but also offers possibilities for novel applications in a wide variety of fields from clinical diagnosis to environmental monitoring. Beyond medicine, agglutination assays are also expected to find practical uses in plant pathology and agriculture. Crop integrity is most often threatened by viral pathogens, and they have been developed to detect such threats at a fast pace and enhance food safety. They can quickly sort and identify different pathogens, providing the critical information necessary to implement effective control measures (Alemu et al., 2015). Coupled with new molecular methods, they are another boost in terms of specificity—a luxury compared to conventional diagnostics. Together, these combinations of traditional and new techniques place these tests not only as independent diagnostic tools, but also as key players in a broader, multifaceted effort to monitor and maintain plant health, and thus obtain enhanced outcomes in agriculture (Figure 15.11).

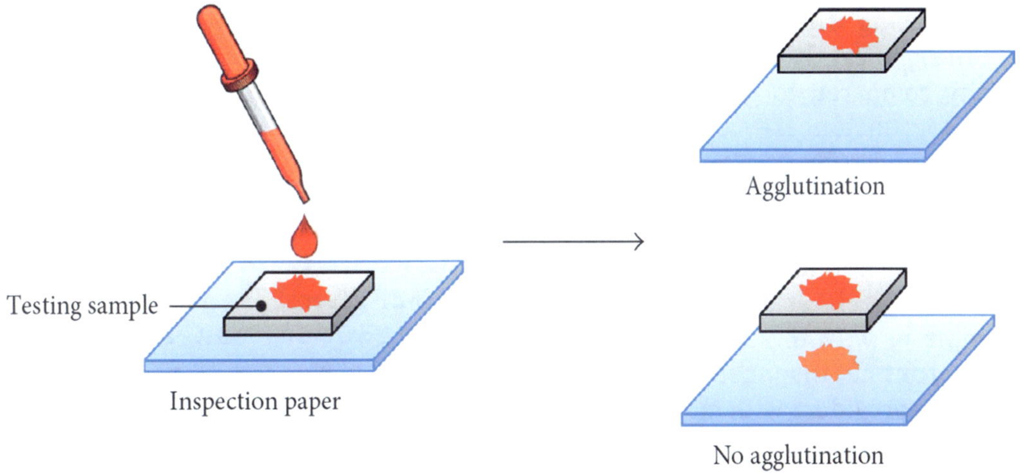

Figure 15.11. Agglutination tests.

Source: https://external-content.duckduckgo.com/iu/?u=https%3A%2F%2Fwww.researchgate.net%2Fpublication%2F326152115%2Ffigure%2Ffig2%2FAS%3A1086429253906436%401636036327481%2FA-schematic-diagram-of-the-blood-agglutination-test.jpg&f=1&nofb=1&ipt=12018bc5ffa11041bda521d05512d07ab4282a80b81bbd912344c074237478ff.

15.3.3. Flow Cytometry

New laboratory techniques have highly accelerated the speed and accuracy of serological and immunological tests. Flow cytometry, for example, seems like a highly valuable technique—it enables researchers to analyze several characteristics of cells at once. You can measure things like cell size, how speckly they are, and even how brightly they fluoresce in a given light. In the clinical setting, this is about being able to guide the proper treatment choices in a glance. It's now required for immune response screening, recognizing specific cell populations, and characterizing tumor properties—giving clues to intricate diseases that older serological methods do not identify (Gorshunov et al., 2019). The field of immunodiagnosis keeps evolving, and flow cytometry seems to be squarely in the middle of streamlining how we diagnose so many ailments. Overall, its capacity to detect specific biomarkers and low-level cell signals comes a great distance towards diagnosing autoimmune diseases, infections, and cancers. For example, using fluorescently labeled antibodies can significantly enhance sensitivity and specificity compared to traditional blood testing. In a few instances—consider celiac disease, for example—flow cytometry is able to identify gluten-specific T-cells, which could potentially provide the answer to why certain patients don't neatly fit into standard diagnostic categories (Costa-García et al., 2010). This is a good example of why the addition of flow cytometry in routine diagnostics generally grants healthcare providers with more accurate instruments. Data analysis has also changed with flow cytometry's technological advancements. High-parameter cytometers and sophisticated software now enter the picture, broadening what we can uncover. We're not just discussing identifying a large panel of cell markers; these developments also permit us to track down small populations of cells that may be lost in standard tests. With continued refinement in serological and immunologic testing approaches, flow cytometry remains an integral part of insight into disease mechanisms and tailoring therapy to individual patients (Gorshunov et al., 2019). Even when the details do become somewhat complex, this synergy of advanced hardware and enhanced analysis still propels diagnostic potential forward (Figure 15.12).

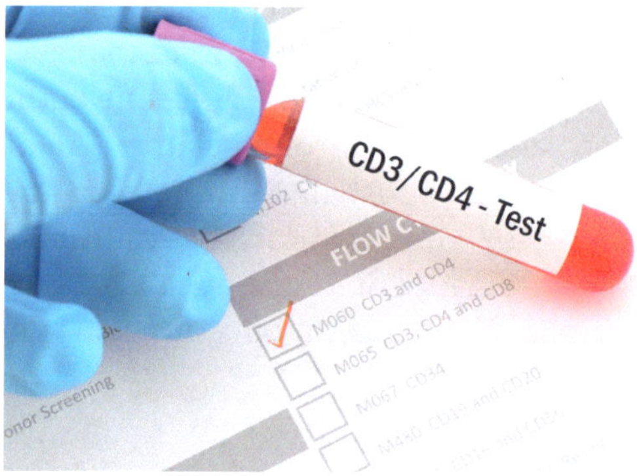

Figure 15.12. Flow cytometry.

Source: https://external-content.duckduckgo.com/iu/?u=https%3A%2F%2Fwww.verywellhealth.com%2Fthmb%2FN63TWHNAG3ykjnJvHwjTvLuTTtA%3D%2F2656x1771%2Ffilters%3Ano_upscale()%3Amax_bytes(150000)%3Astrip_icc()%2Fcd3-cd4-test-856641352-bf6832835209469eb3a77ab99d90eb8c.jpg&f=1&nofb=1&ipt=11be72f86c8c78621202e896e4be2f3592f529961b34688672adcaef494318d7.

Test Your Knowledge

1. How do direct and indirect immunofluorescence assays differ in principle and application?
2. What is the role of flow cytometry in immunological testing?

15.4. Applications in Disease Diagnosis

Learning Outcome

- Infectious diseases;
- Autoimmune disorders;
- Allergies and hypersensitivity reactions.

Serology and immunological assays have truly changed how diagnoses occur, particularly for diseases that simply don't receive the attention they should—consider Chagas disease. There is an increasing demand for diagnostics that really perform well with all types of communities, as the ones in use now tend to fall short. In the majority of cases, researchers are now investigating novel biological markers in hopes that these clues will warn us of an illness sooner, indicate the effectiveness of treatments, and even suggest where the disease will progress. It is increasingly important in parts of the world where access to quality health care is limited, so utilizing more specific diagnostic tools may actually level the playing field for Chagas victims (Balouz et al., 2016). And then again, these tests aren't just sticking to everyday environments—these are being re-engineered for off-the-wall ones such as space. Yes, scientists are experimenting with advanced serological techniques on missions where resources are scarce and the stakes are astronomical. Take ELISA, for example: it's currently being adapted to identify bacterial or fungal threats even in microgravity. This change not only highlights how adaptable these processes are but also points to the need to include coverage even for the most extreme of cases, such that astronauts and others who work in other extreme environments get proper health check-ups (Hejtmancik et al., 2025). Immunological testing also extends beyond immediate disease detection. Early detection by such tests is usually an important part of the wider view of public health. Smiting an outbreak at an early time enables administrators to scramble and deploy targeted vaccinations or treatment protocols—an action priceless, particularly in under-funded regions. In a vast majority of cases, new serological approaches enable decision-makers to have more data to make quick decisions, ultimately leading to enhanced all-around health results by keeping disease from spreading too far, as with Chagas (Balouz et al., 2016).

15.4.1. Infectious Diseases

Global health wages the war against infectious diseases, and it's a hard, ever-evolving battle. Laboratory tests that dip straight into our immune system—serological and immunological tests, say—are now becoming true workhorses at catching mischievous pathogens. They basically test for antigens or antibodies that show up when our body weds with an infection, helping doctors decide if an illness is starting or already making inroads. Occasionally, scientists are left with surprising clues; look at the case when proteins of reptilian herpesviruses gave indications of how Florida's sea turtles, those wonderful creatures, deal with a variety of viruses. Such a finding not only brings down precious clues regarding how often infections might be occurring but also suggests that human and wildlife health are mysteriously interrelated (Jacobson et al., 2001). It's a reminder that enhanced surveillance and rapid diagnosis are, in most cases, purely vital. These tests aren't just for garden-variety bugs—they're a broad-screening test involving very minute protozoa. Take the case of Trypanosoma evansi: a 38-year-old Vietnamese patient presented symptoms similar to trypanosomiasis, which prompted a rather divergent set of diagnostic tests. With the use of techniques like polymerase chain reaction (PCR) amplification and serological testing, clinicians were ultimately able to pinpoint the perpetrators. This case, in which cattle were suspected to be the likely source, is not only a testament to what modern tests can do but also to the enigmatic ways in which diseases sometimes spread from animals to humans (Baker et al., 2016). It is a good example of how an expanded diagnostic approach can be helpful in addressing new dangers. Today, with infectious disease epidemiology unpredictably shifting, the role of serological and immunological tests simply cannot be ignored. They play a central role in following the spread of disease, in streamlining treatment protocols, and in informing public health response. Through our constant attempts to revolutionize testing methods, early infection detection is improving incrementally, which can serve to prevent outbreaks from spiraling out of control. Constant study—whether it's in wild animals like those incredible sea-dwelling turtles or even in humans like that Trypanosoma epidemic—is proof that infectious disease research continues to expand. The understanding that we gain through these various studies enriches scientific knowledge, as well as enhances public health interventions and ultimately improves global health outcomes (Baker et al., 2016; Jacobson et al., 2001) (Figure 15.13).

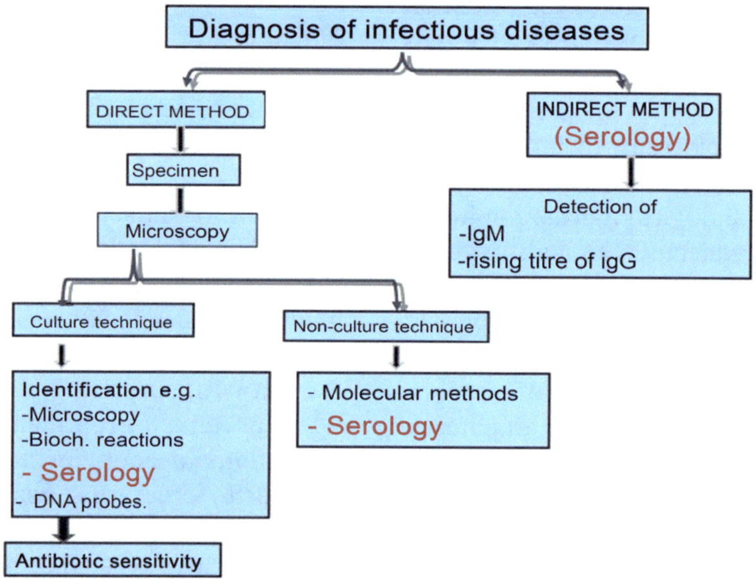

Figure 15.13. Diagnose infectious diseases.

Source: https://external-content.duckduckgo.com/iu/?u=http%3A%2F%2Fimage.slidesharecdn.com%2Fserologypractical-131125100403-phpapp02%2F95%2Fserology-prac-microbiology-1-638.jpg%3Fcb%3D1385395473&f=1&nofb=1&ipt=fc6807ce909d65a8a4a1dffe7178dc547e1c136d917071c780f32442bebfc160.

15.4.2. Autoimmune Disorders

Autoimmune illnesses are inherently multifaceted; they cannot be diagnosed on an across-the-board basis. Serological and immunologic tests come into play here, these being the usual suspects in detecting autoantibodies seen with various autoimmune disorders. Let's take thyroid problems, for example. Hashimoto's thyroiditis and Graves' disease would generally demonstrate the presence of anti-TPO and anti-TSH-receptor markers. When such markers appear, doctors feel safer identifying a diagnosis and going for treatment procedures. With some teething troubles in recent times, advances in technology have made these tests more sensitive and specific – that in most cases enables detection at an earlier point and permits treatments to be tailored. In conditions like dermatitis herpetiformis, blood tests become even more essential as it is linked to gluten-sensitive enteropathy.

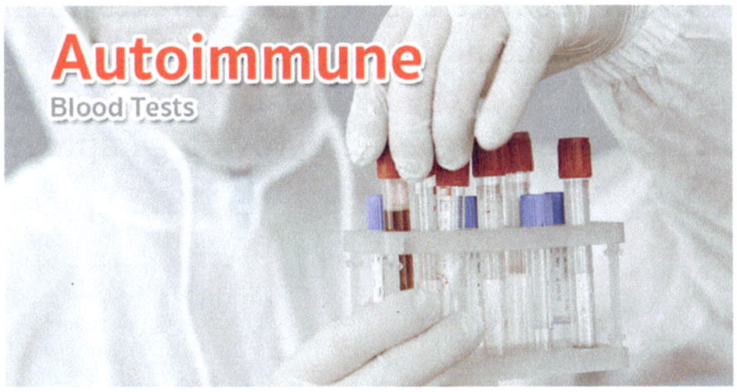

Figure 15.14. Autoimmune blood tests.

Source: https://external-content.duckduckgo.com/iu/?u=https%3A%2F%2Fdrorawan.com%2Fwp-content%2Fuploads%2F2020%2F08%2F1200x628_Autoimmune-Blood-Tests.jpg&f=1&nofb=1&ipt=f206397911eb70d04b19bc7ee911343954419321862 5ff6893b3d16f57349880.

In this place, the tests will be predisposed to elevate the presence of particular autoantibodies (such as anti-TG2 and anti-TG3) as meaningful indications. Direct immunofluorescence—while somewhat involved—helps by recognizing those granular IgA deposits in dermal papillae; this method does not just establish the condition but also differentiates the condition from other skin disorders, giving a broader diagnostic picture (Kapciak et al., 2024). Combining the results of blood tests with an examination of tissue samples provides physicians a richer, sometimes more complex, but more comprehensive diagnosis. Autoimmune illnesses do not typically fly solo, however; they are paired with other autoimmune issues, which complicate matters further. Patients with dermatitis herpetiformis, for example, usually have other illnesses to deal with as well, including type 1 diabetes or autoimmune thyroid disease. Finding these overlaps really does bring home the need for a serological test above and beyond that of an individual disorder. These broad screenings can also uncover underlying comorbidities and identify potential risks—like non-Hodgkin lymphoma in certain groups. As a whole, it is recognizing the depth of these serological profiles that could be necessary in order to develop balanced treatment and diagnostic regimens that consider all facets of a patient's health (Górny et al., 2024) (Figure 15.14).

15.4.3. Allergies and Hypersensitivity Reactions

Hypersensitivity reactions are stealthy and need a more detailed look at how our immune system handles allergens. Allergic reactions typically occur in four forms, but those that are IgE antibody-mediated are most common. When an allergen is introduced into the picture, B cells come into play and start manufacturing IgE antibodies that have a specific affinity for that given allergen. Later on, when the person is exposed to the allergen again, those antibodies attach themselves to the allergen, causing mast cells and basophils to release histamines and other chemicals that trigger the classic symptoms of an allergy. It's helpful to understand this process for successful allergy diagnosis and treatment. Blood IgE level tests are an excellent help with this, prompting doctors to tailor treatments that minimize symptoms and maximize quality of life. Working environments can also have latent hazards from time to time—molds in damp buildings, for example, can badly affect employees' health. A recent case study established a clear link between workers' complaints and mold exposure, employing specific serum tests to look for hypersensitive reactions. The majority of exposed workers were atopic, and increased IgG antibody levels were a sign of an immune reaction to fungi like *Cladosporium* and *Alternaria alternata*. All this does serve to show how using these serological tests can be quite useful in detecting would-be allergen contact. It also serves to highlight a need for standard reference values so that laboratory tests would be simpler, considering both the blood tests and the environmental markers (Matuka et al., 2023). Food allergies add another factor to the equation, leading to severe health hazards for children and adults. About 6% of children and 3.7% of adults are affected, thus a major problem. The diagnostic procedure would usually begin with a patient history, followed by skin tests or laboratory tests to identify food-specific IgE antibodies if presenting symptoms are suspicious. Controlled food challenges are performed in others to get an absolute answer. It's also interesting to understand how IgE antibodies are going to cross-react with homologous proteins and how to chart out what specific portions of the food cause the reaction. With the newer diagnostics in the pipeline, they have the potential for a more lucid insight into food allergies and providing improved results for patients (Eckman et al., 2009) (Figure 15.15).

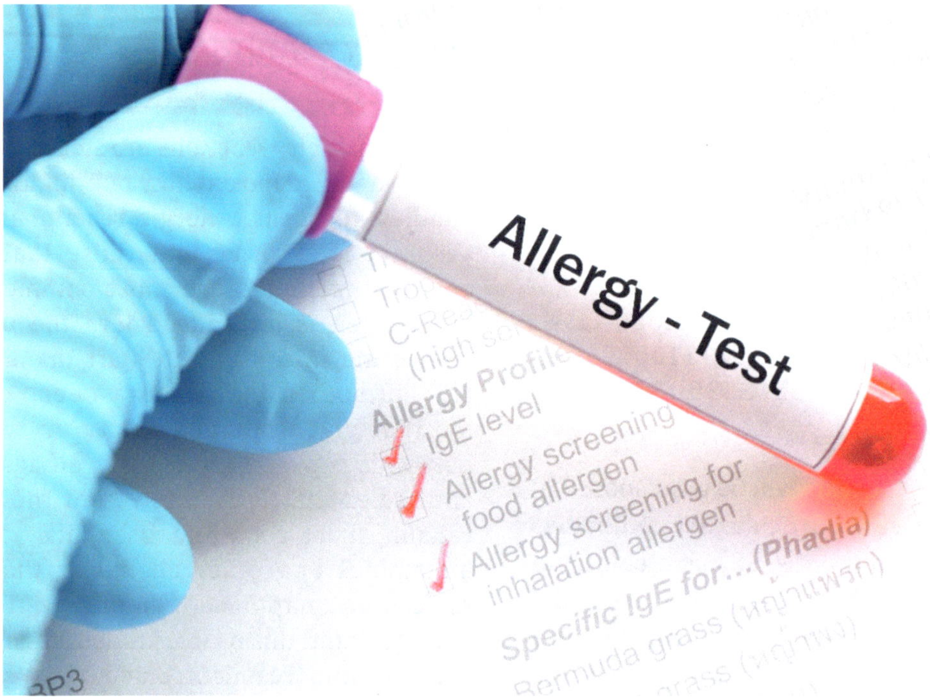

Figure 15.15. A blood sample labeled for allergy testing is shown alongside a checklist for IgE level and allergen screenings, used to identify sensitivities to food and environmental allergens.

Source: https://external-content.duckduckgo.com/iu/?u=https%3A%2F%2Fhealthclinicgroup.com%2Fwp-content%2Fuploads%2F2020%2F07%2FAllergy-test-866279392.jpg&f=1&nofb=1&ipt=fa441d7a82ab8b70a0fbe8090f116ecdcbc1cf8efd6a5669b7c6bdcd01697ce4.

Test Your Knowledge

1. How are serological tests used in the diagnosis of infectious diseases such as HIV and hepatitis?
2. What role do immunological tests play in detecting autoimmune disorders?

15.5. Advantages of Serological and Immunological Tests

Learning Outcome

- High sensitivity and specificity;
- Rapid results and turnaround time;
- Non-invasive sample collection.

Serological and immunological examinations have truly transformed modern diagnosis. They tap into our own immune reactions to warn us of pathogens or antibodies, which can flag disease in its early stages—ELISA tests, for example, are a common method of registering infection-causing antigens with great accuracy. These tests not only give us an immediate answer but also allow us to track the way a disease takes hold or fades with time. New technologies, such as mimetic peptides—yes, a bit of an oddity—push the envelope further by improving diagnostic precision, especially where working with diseases like leprosy and mycobacterial infection. Not infrequently, the steady refinement of these assays puts us in mind of just how vital biotechnology is to robust public health initiatives (Lima et al., 2019). Another neat feature is the way that these tests work out in the field. Rapid, deployable technologies such as point-of-care tests and lateral flow assays enable medical workers to receive immediate results even in remote or limited-resource settings. This is particularly useful when standard culture and molecular testing, which can take time and may involve advanced laboratory facilities, simply cannot be arranged for the control of mycobacterial infections. By streamlining the testing process, these assays allow practitioners to take critical decisions quickly – a true lifesaver in the context of outbreak conditions and an excellent addition to community-level health gains. The real-time factor, with its concomitant flexibilities, says it all about their transformative role in modern diagnostics (Eda et al., 2012). The second breakthrough is achieved through the development of multi-antigen serodiagnostic tests. Recent studies, in most cases, reveal that combining species-specific protein antigens can significantly increase diagnostic sensitivity for diseases like tuberculosis and Johnes disease. There is also growing interest in the detection of new nonprotein molecules from mycobacteria, which provides more knowledge about immune responses and could lead to even more accurate tests. This combined approach of this kind facilitates early detection but also provides avenues for more efficient treatment strategies. With researchers further advancing these serological methods, the addition of intricate antigenic components seems poised to introduce next-generation diagnostic tools—tools that will remain crucial in our struggle against infectious disease (Lima et al., 2019).

15.5.1. High Sensitivity and Specificity

Serological and immunological assays rely significantly on whether or not they are able to detect the faintest of whispers—that is, they must be highly sensitive and absolutely specific. Even with only a whisper of the target, such as trace levels of antibodies or antigens, showing up, a sensitive assay is able to detect it, minimizing false negatives. This is especially important in real clinical settings where detection of infections early on actually makes the difference in treatment. For example, research comparing Jembrana disease virus (JDV) found that with real-time PCR combined with ELISA, an impressive 98.6% concordance between the two techniques was obtained. But the issues of seroconversion lag and cross-reactive epitopes have a tendency to render it problematic—a reminder, in general, that finding the perfect balance between sensitivity and specificity is no simple feat (Desport et al., 2009). Specificity alone concerns trying to identify the people who really don't have the disease and eliminating them, thereby minimizing false positives. It prevents people from being misdiagnosed simply due to similar reactions, which sometimes lead to unnecessary treatment. In a peculiar but fascinating example, when space missions sought dependable serological tests, scientists developed an ELISA to detect *Legionella pneumophila*. Scientists employed solid-phase, membrane-supported systems—methods that served to limit cross-reactivity while identifying the presence of the pathogen. This approach illustrates that by adjusting specificity to exactly the right level, not only do tests get more specific but they get more generally applicable in challenging or unconventional contexts (Hejtmancik et al., 2025). In essence, optimizing for both sensitivity and specificity is a delicate dance that really influences how we go about diagnosing illnesses. The balance versus imbalance between detecting all true positives and reducing false alarms can inform everything from public health policy to patient care on an individual basis. Particularly in the case of emerging infectious disease, when minutes are the difference between detection and failure, making tests that walk this tightrope is essential. The experiences of JDV research and novel methods utilized in Legionella testing are excellent examples that there should be continuous fine-tuning and field testing—whether here on Terra or out there in the vast expanse of space's wilderness (Desport et al., 2009; Hejtmancik et al., 2025) (Figure 15.16).

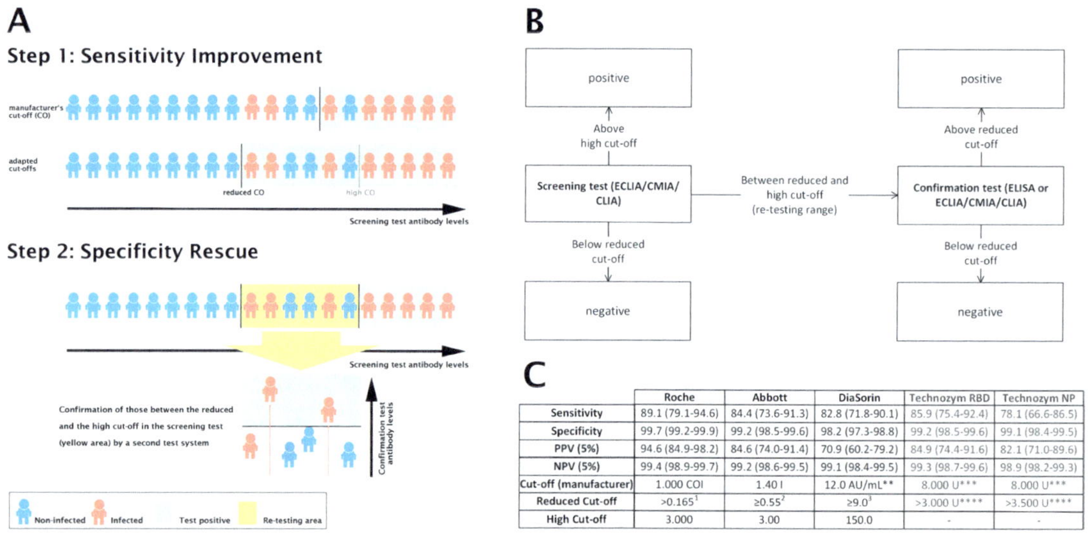

	Roche	Abbott	DiaSorin	Technozym RBD	Technozym NP
Sensitivity	89.1 (79.1-94.6)	84.4 (73.6-91.3)	82.8 (71.8-90.1)	85.9 (75.4-92.4)	78.1 (66.6-86.5)
Specificity	99.7 (99.2-99.9)	99.2 (98.5-99.6)	98.2 (97.3-98.8)	99.2 (98.5-99.6)	99.1 (98.4-99.5)
PPV (5%)	94.6 (84.9-98.2)	84.6 (74.0-91.4)	70.9 (60.2-79.2)	84.9 (74.4-91.6)	82.1 (71.0-89.6)
NPV (5%)	99.4 (98.9-99.7)	99.2 (98.6-99.5)	99.1 (98.4-99.5)	99.3 (98.7-99.6)	98.9 (98.2-99.3)
Cut-off (manufacturer)	1.000 COI	1.40 I	12.0 AU/mL**	8.000 U***	8.000 U***
Reduced Cut-off	>0.165[1]	≥0.55[2]	≥9.0[3]	>3.000 U****	>3.500 U****
High Cut-off	3.000	3.00	150.0	-	-

Figure 15.16. High sensitivity and specificity.

Source: https://jcp.bmj.com/content/jclinpath/76/11/770/F1.large.jpg.

15.5.2. Rapid Results and Turnaround Time

Rapid, efficient testing is absolutely crucial when infections come on hard and fast. Take, for instance, routine blood tests for Chagas disease—cold storage and trained laboratory staff are needed, something easily to make results run weeks behind. Such lengthy delay, typically several weeks, risks denying many patients follow-up care. Rapid tests, on the other hand, can yield results in an hour or so. This shift not only hastens on-time treatment decisions in clinics but also helps in managing patients in heavily affected areas of the disease. In most cases, those immediate results deliver the holes in healthcare systems with what they require, ultimately offering patients a greater chance for on-time treatment (Alonso-Padilla et al., 2023). Rapid tests offer something more than speed. They free themselves from the awkward logistics of traditional serological methods, which tend to necessitate much—wound-up specimen handling and troublesome outcome interpretation as well. Most often, these kinds of procedures simply are not possible in settings that lack resources. These rapid tests, by contrast, demand very little; a tiny drop of blood after a brief finger prick is all that is needed. This simplicity enables them to be used in remote and under-resourced locations, taking much-needed care nearer to more individuals. Campaigns that incorporate swift tests into standard practice for diseases such as Chagas are providing initial outcomes in identifying the issue in time—a downright crucial process for efficient disease control. As doctors slowly adopt these advances, offering prompt, precise diagnosis becomes progressively within reach (Padilla et al., 2023). Rapid diagnostic testing has broader significance than assisting individual patients; it can also reshape public health. Rapid infection detection is, overall, crucial to preventing outbreaks from spiraling out of control. Where disease burden is great and healthcare infrastructure is often stretched thin, rapid tests are quite handy. When test results come in immediately, it encourages a more proactive approach to care and strengthens overall healthcare response—even if the progress sometimes feels a bit uneven. A steady commitment to checking these tests across different places and clinics is essential if we're to tap into their full benefits. By incorporating quick testing into regular practice, there is genuine hope for improved health outcomes and decreased instances of diseases such as Chagas (Alonso-Padilla et al., 2023).

15.5.3. Non-Invasive Sample Collection

Diagnostic technologies in immunology and serology have come to a level where they are now inclined towards avoiding the conventional invasive techniques. Contemporary laboratories are now searching for means of sample taking without discomfort to patients, such as needles—in general, fewer complications and less hassle. For example, some studies have investigated the use of milk instead of blood to test for antibodies for Capri poxvirus. In one test, ELISA assays were performed on milk and serum, and the milk had an average sensitivity of 88 to 91%—a neat proof that it could perhaps be a good surrogate in immunologic research. Indeed, these new methods not only enhance the accuracy of diagnosis, but they also widen the scope of samples we can tap into for tracking livestock disease (Dietze et al., 2020). The advantages of non-invasive sampling do not end at the animal's health; they've even spilled over into human diagnostics, especially where budgets are tight. Take visceral leishmaniasis (VL) as an example: diagnosing VL previously entailed enduring invasive tissue aspirations, which, to be frank, aren't exactly patient-friendly. In most instances, shifting to urine-based assays—which have the double bonus of being less painful and less invasive—has turned the world around. Studies, such as those conducted with the use of ELISA and dipstick tests, have shown that the urine tests have been successful in identifying anti-Leishmania antibodies. This is a reliable alternative for VL and even its consequences, like post kala-azar dermal leishmaniasis (PKDL). All these help in improved patient compliance and can lead to early diagnosis and treatment in challenging cases (Das et al., 2016). Sample acquisition by non-invasive methods not only makes it easier for patients—it also opens up new avenues for public health research and epidemiologic study. When researchers can obtain samples from diverse populations without the impediments of invasive procedures, the resultant data sets are richer and more representative. Consider how the use of milk to screen capripoxvirus in cattle has benefited disease surveillance on a more general level: the idea of expanding diagnostic tools naturally supports additional research. It's a message that, by continuing to push for better non-invasive technologies, we incite additional research and eventually direct public health interventions towards more effective interventions (Das et al., 2016; Dietze et al., 2020) (Figure 15.17).

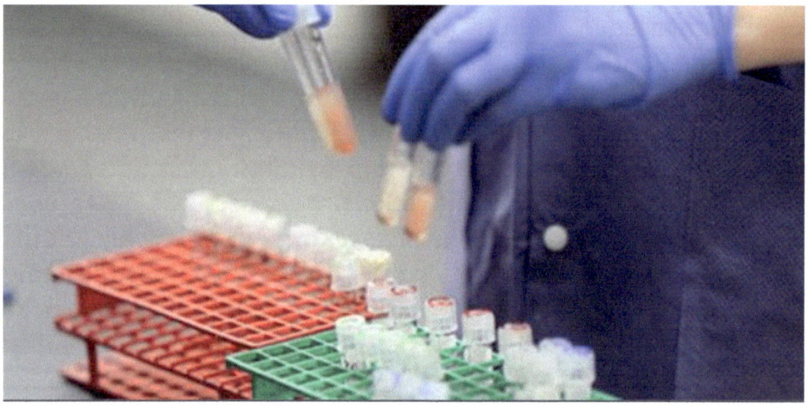

Figure 15.17. A laboratory technician handles blood samples in test tubes, preparing them for analysis using organized tube racks. This step is essential for maintaining sample integrity and accurate diagnostics.

Source: https://external-content.duckduckgo.com/iu/?u=https%3A%2F%2Ftse3.mm.bing.net%2Fth%2Fid%2FOIP.9dzf9HBtj2pd2FwZ8HFmhwHaDf% 3Fpid%3DApi&f=1&ipt=4780897c9725d56ecfd4c5665f7cea2538df40198e13bf7787fb42af1f9fcad4.

Test Your Knowledge

1. What are the main advantages of serological tests compared to traditional culture-based methods?
2. How do immunological tests provide rapid and specific diagnosis?

15.6. Limitations and Challenges

Learning Outcome

- False positives and negatives;
- Cross-reactivity issues;
- Interpretation of results.

Serological and immunological tests fall into trouble not only because they are so inherently complicated but also because of the antiquated methods still in use. Different populations tend to behave in a manner which you cannot predict—genetic quirks, the phase of a disease, and overall health all intersect and twist data from tests. In diseases like Chagas, you especially value having stable, consistent biomarkers which stand up under fluctuating conditions. The problem, in most cases, is then compounded by a lack of sufficient investment in R&D, creating a substantial shortfall between what is needed in order to make an accurate diagnosis and what current technology can deliver (Balouz et al., 2016). The problems persist when we turn our attention to viral infections, as was the case with the COVID-19 pandemic. A variety of antibody tests were introduced, but they did not all concur as they ought to have done and provided us with confusing data on whether a subject was immune to an infection or vaccine. For example, one comparison of different SARS-CoV-2 immunoassay systems concluded that they agreed just moderately and that there was sufficient variability to raise real clinical concern. And to top it all, if the samples are taken at different points in the disease process, timing can be a spanner in the works—sometimes creating false positives or false negatives. Without grasping these constraints to an absolute extent, rolling out such tests on a mass scale could lead to incorrect conclusions about individual health and community immunity (Napoli et al., 2023). In practice, rolling out such tests isn't exactly that easy. Much of today's testing is highly technical and involves special equipment and trained personnel—factors not always easily available in poor or remote areas, where the neglected diseases will most likely break out. In many cases, the issue isn't so much performing the test as it is interpreting what the test actually tells us for patient care. There is a growing need for easy yet accurate point-of-care tests, but developing them is risky in balancing ease of handling and ensuring sound results for numerous patients and physicians in real life (Balouz et al., 2016).

15.6.1. False Positives and False Negatives

Infections are dirty to diagnose. Often, the dirty character of serological and immunological tests means that results can be a jumble of this and that—sometimes detecting a disease when it's not actually present, and sometimes failing to detect it at all. A false-positive outcome may be a mistake, leading to unwarranted treatment and unwarranted worry; a negative test is just as dangerous in that it permits a true disease to silently progress.

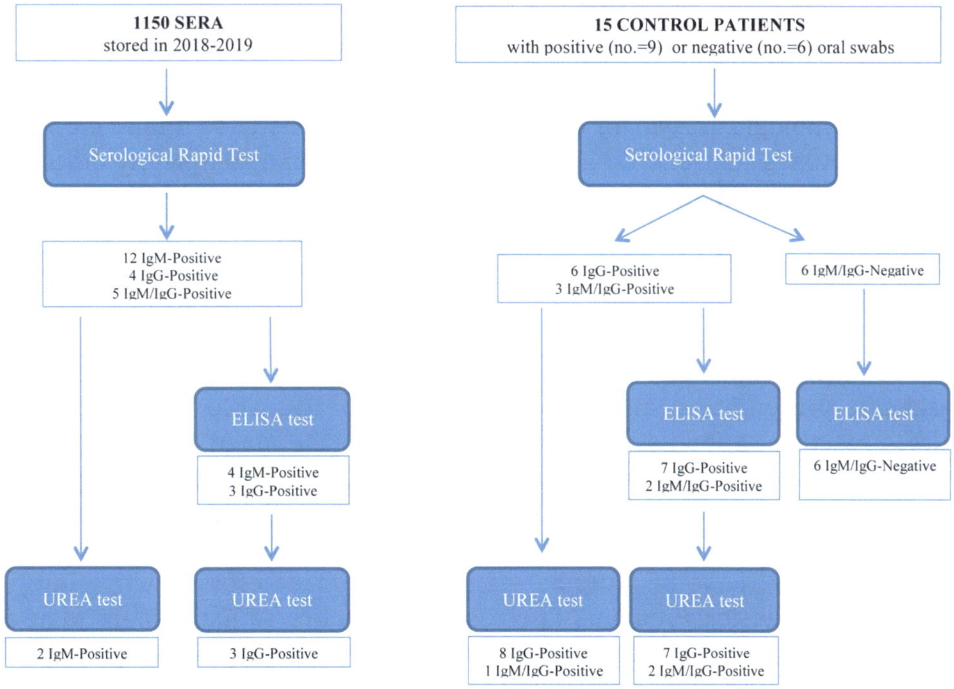

Figure 15.18. False positives and negatives.

Source: https://www.ijidonline.com/cms/10.1016/j.ijid.2020.12.067/asset/36180a09-c23a-461c-b893-65c4b2c724f5/main.assets/gr1_lrg.jpg.

Take gambiense human *African trypanosomiasis* (HAT) as an illustration—the algorithm for its diagnosis is particularly complicated, in considerable part because sensitivity and specificity of tests may be extremely variable. All of that actually does need a firmer confirmation step in screening to really diminish both types of errors (Cox et al., 2011). Errors in tests are not merely screwing up care for one person—there are ripple effects to other public health on a larger scale. Misleading test outcomes can throw off our understanding of disease transmission by modifying epidemiological information and undermining control measures. For example, a number of studies have established that a high number of commercially bought serological tests for diseases such as tuberculosis do not perform well, adding to the issue. False negatives cause delays in initiating effective treatment, while false positives may increase resource consumption and result in unnecessary interventions. In general, having good tests is important when monitoring disease and guiding policy choices; thus, it's of paramount importance that these diagnostic tests are thoroughly tested to improve both specificity and sensitivity (Dendukuri et al., 2011). Emerging technology is gradually meeting these challenges by targeting increased precision in diagnostic tests. In everyday practice, blending various methods of testing—like combining serological tests with follow-up diagnoses—would avoid those pesky errors. Health workers would be able to utilize the more holistic approach, which not only accounts for individual cases but also helps to closely monitor for outbreaks. Provided that testing procedures get continuously updated and bettered, reliability will improve with time. Lastly, removal of false positives and false negatives at source makes better not just care for persons but also makes public health intervention more focused and precise, enhancing its impact in the control of disease (Figure 15.18).

15.6.2. Cross-Reactivity Issues

Serological and immunologic assays are also difficult—antibodies have a tendency not to bind to just one target. Sometimes they end up binding to antigens from a completely different source, so assays can produce false positives or confusing results. Take, for example, Chagas disease caused by *Trypanosoma cruzi*. Tests designed to detect specific antibodies often get thrown off by similar antigens coming from other parasitic infections or even non-infectious conditions (Dumonteil et al., 2019). In areas where multiple infections are common, these overlaps significantly challenge our ability to obtain a clear diagnosis, highlighting the urgent need for more targeted testing methods. Chagas disease really highlights this problem. The disease is subtle and can be readily overlooked due to non-specific presentation, and the vast majority of available tests aim at anti–*T. cruzi* antibodies. Cross-reactive antibodies obscure the picture in the majority of cases, so one cannot be sure whether the test is truly positive because of *T. cruzi* or not. It was only in recent times that researchers took a broad overview of *T. cruzi* proteins, finding some markers that enhance the sensitivity of the detection of antibodies (Ho et al., 2008). Such a more targeted strategy—by weeding out from a wide range of proteins—is likely to reduce cross-reactive interference and make test interpretation easier. Problems of cross-reactivity are so many more than one disease. When lab testing goes wrong, the effects filter down to affect public health programs, treatment guidelines, and even drive-up costs as misdiagnoses pile up. It's only natural that there would be extra training for lab personnel in interpreting these flawed tests, and for rigorous protocols—including follow-up testing—to be in place. With the majority of instances, embracing these innovations is capable of reducing errors and ensure that customized care as well as global health efforts are on firm ground (Ho et al., 2008) (Figure 15.19).

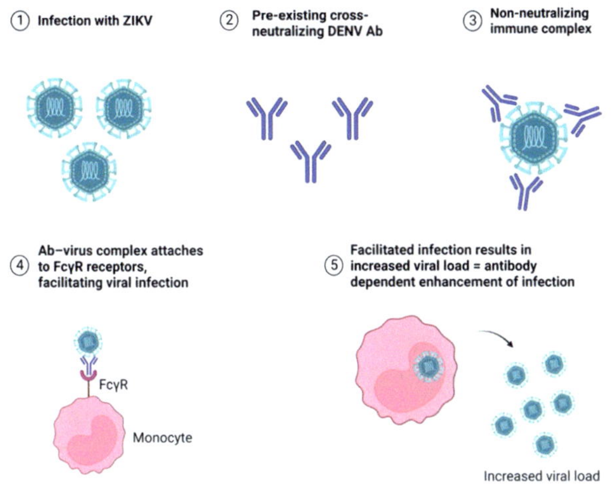

Figure 15.19. Cross-reactivity issues.

Source: https://www.mdpi.com/antibodies/antibodies-12-00018/article_deploy/html/images/antibodies-12-00018-g005.png.

15.6.3. Interpretation of Results

Serological and immunologic testing often play a significant role in deciding what to do next. Enzyme immunoassays, for example, might give some solid clues as to whether or not an infectious agent might exist or how advanced a disease process might have reached. You can have a test that detects trypanosomal antibodies due to the use of a particular anti-camel IgG conjugate – a tidy little trick that, in most instances, enables us to observe the various stages of an infection without complications. At times, seeing how frequently particular results appear informs us whether an ongoing infection is present or whether it's residual antibodies from a long, long time ago. And in fact, when an ELISA cannot be clever enough to pick out an infected from a similarly hanging-around animal, only that is why choosing the right test matters so much (Aitken et al., 1989). When you move on to vaccines, it is equally crucial to test immune responses. Take the case of a gp120/V3-consensus peptide that has been designed to elicit some neutralizing immune responses against HIV-1. How the serological findings were – nearly 90% of patient sera showed recognition of the peptide – truly is a hallmark of a strong immunogenic wallop. Findings like this not only reinforce the notion that certain immunogens work, but also imply that these breadcrumbs are the ticket to the future for diagnostics and vaccine development. It is like saying, broadly speaking, that correlating immunologic data with vaccine approaches makes it possible for us to wrap our brains around the varied way that people react (Böltz et al., 1992). Stepping back, it's not any given test result; it's about the overall picture. Variation in serological findings, for instance, can signify trends across groups, shed light on variations in pathogens, or even imply clever immune avoidance mechanisms. Take T-cell epitopes: discovering them and seeing how certain cytotoxic T-lymphocytes jump at the chance to pick them out can shape vaccine and therapeutic strategies. Discovering the delicate interplay between serological and immunological data enables clinicians and researchers to build better public health programs and even tailor so-called personalized medicine approaches. Finally, putting it all together truly promotes our clinical practices as well as vaccine research (Aitken et al., 1989; Böltz et al., 1992).

Test Your Knowledge

1. How can cross-reactivity lead to false-positive results in serological testing?
2. What challenges exist in ensuring sensitivity and specificity of immunological tests?

Summary

Different studies illustrate how serological and immunological tests are significant in deciphering ambiguous disease data—take diseases like SLE or even chronic hepatitis B, for instance. How they find disease, such as recognizing anti-C1q antibodies with kidney markers in lupus nephritis, is significant when doctors are trying to figure out the best course of action. For example, higher levels of anti-C1qAb are more likely to be associated with kidney flares, indicating that such tests in routine basis can actually enhance patient care (Calatroni et al., 2025). Using baseline tests and seeing what occurs with the passage of time, it can typically help physicians make adjustments to treatment better. Serological markers aren't merely employed to identify what is not quite right; they also help track the manner in which diseases evolve, and the efficacy of treatment in patients. With chronic hepatitis B, low HBsAg levels at times create particular problems—potentially suggesting more severe fibrotic alterations within the liver. In most cases, determining how different indicators relate to the disease is crucial. Take the cue of preS2 deletion mutations for avoiding the immune system and modifying viral behavior; this development somehow necessitates re-evaluation of treatment protocols for some individuals. These nuances in testing can redefine treatment protocols, suggesting the tests carry more weight than a preliminary diagnosis (Chen et al., 2024). Generally, inclusion of serological and immunological testing within the everyday practice not only makes diagnosis more acute but also lays the ground for more individualized treatment. Further development of these tests may ultimately enhance diagnostic accuracy as well as how accurately we can predict outcome. As our understanding of disease progression improves, the value of these immune markers increases—although, admittedly, at some point it does seem a little wild-card like in terms of predicting flares or complications. This gradual progression highlights why there needs to be further research to get a better idea of just how useful these tests are for different patient populations. Bottom line, optimizing the value of these tests can drive up the quality of care so patients receive well-timed, well-informed treatments based on good, evidence-based facts (Calatroni et al., 2025; Chen et al., 2024).

Serological and immunological tests are not so cut and dry. To diagnose a condition such as gambiense human *African trypanosomiasis* (HAT), it means performing more than one activity simultaneously—screening, confirming, then staging—just because the tests that exist are not sensitive and specific enough. In areas such as the Republic of Congo, South Sudan, and Uganda, Médecins Sans Frontières has evaluated these multi-step methods and concluded that their effectiveness can be inconsistent (Cox et al., 2011). Evaluations such as those, in this case, help with improving protocols and acceleration of treatment, which really emphasizes the importance of good serological techniques in public health. Nature occasionally throws in another monkey wrench to throw into the pot. Take bats, for example—they host a rich diversity of viruses, and their periodic life events alter patterns of infection in unforeseen ways, amplifying zoonotic spillover risks when you least expect. By tracking henipavirus antibodies in a captive *E. helvum* colony over a prolonged period, researchers have uncovered variables such as lingering maternal antibodies. This observation illustrates, in most cases, that biological and environmental factors play a fundamental role in viral transmission, and such observations are essential in developing effective serological tests (Baker et al., 2014). It is a reminder that having a vague idea of nature's quirks can sometimes lead to gaps in public health policy. Blending old methods with new, newer fresh serological tests can enhance diagnostic accuracy and, in the end, improved patient outcomes. An understanding of these complex infections also reveals gaps in what we do know and suggests that a more standardized approach might be needed in different areas. When you consider how knowing the ecological and biological properties of reservoir hosts enables us to tailor tests better, it makes sense that every scrap of information counts. As our knowledge of these nuances builds—step by step but surely—so too does our ability to counteract threats emerging, in vindicating the central role that serological and immunological investigations play in modern medicine and the prevention of disease.

KEY TERMS FROM THIS CHAPTER

- Agglutination
- Antibody
- Antigen
- Antigen-antibody reaction
- Complement fixation test
- Cytokine assay
- Enzyme-linked immunosorbent assay
- Flow cytometry
- Hematologic crossmatch
- Immunofluorescence
- Immunoglobulin (Ig)
- Immunohistochemistry
- Lateral flow assay
- PCR (polymerase chain reaction)
- Radioimmunoassay (RIA)
- Seroconversion
- Serology
- Vaccination titer

Critical Thinking Questions

1. **Which of the following is the primary purpose of serological tests?**
   a. To identify genetic mutations
   b. To detect specific antibodies or antigens in the blood
   c. To analyze blood cell counts
   d. To measure hormone levels
2. **In an enzyme-linked immunosorbent assay (ELISA), what is the key element that helps detect the presence of an antigen or antibody?**
   a. Enzyme-substrate reaction
   b. DNA hybridization
   c. PCR amplification
   d. Fluorescence markers
3. **The Rhesus factor (Rh factor) in blood is typically tested to determine:**
   a. Blood glucose levels
   b. Antigen-antibody reaction in transfusions
   c. Risk for cancer
   d. Blood type compatibility for organ transplants
4. **Which of the following tests is used to confirm HIV infection?**
   a. Western blot test
   b. Complete blood count (CBC)
   c. Urine test
   d. MRI scan
5. **Which immunological test is used to determine the presence of tuberculosis (TB)?**
   a. Skin test (Mantoux test)
   b. ELISA
   c. Western blot test
   d. Urinalysis

Answers to Critical Thinking Questions

1. (b); 2. (a); 3. (b); 4. (a); 5. (a)

Short Answer Questions

1. What is the primary purpose of serological testing, and how is it different from other diagnostic tests?
2. What are antibodies, and how are they involved in the immune response that is assessed in serological tests?
3. Explain the difference between active immunization and passive immunization in the context of serology.
4. What is the purpose of the Enzyme-Linked Immunosorbent Assay (ELISA), and how does it differ from other serological tests?
5. How is polymerase chain reaction (PCR) related to serology, and when is it used in conjunction with antibody testing?
6. What does a titer measure in serological testing, and how can it be used to assess immunity or infection?

References

1. Adetunji, J. A., Hashimu, G. A., Junaid, S. A., Okeke, O., et al. (2007). Serological survey of *Salmonella gallinarum* antibody in chickens around Jos, Plateau State, Nigeria. https://core.ac.uk/download/pdf/86948.pdf (accessed on 1st July 2025).
2. Aguero-Rosenfeld, M. E., Bacon, R. M., Wilske, B., Bono, J. L., Bruckbauer, H. R., et al. (2008). Immunoblot analysis of the seroreactivity to recombinant *Borrelia burgdorferi* sensu lato antigens, including VlsE, in the long-term course of treated patients with erythema migrans. https://core.ac.uk/download/16432785.pdf (accessed on 1st July 2025).
3. Aitken, C. G., Higgins, A., Jones, T. W., Luckins, A. G., et al. (1989). Evaluation of enzyme immunoassays in the diagnosis of camel (*Camelus dromedarius*) trypanosomiasis: A preliminary investigation. https://core.ac.uk/download/28971946.pdf (accessed on 1st July 2025).
4. Alemu, K. (2015). *Detection of Diseases, Identification and Diversity of Viruses: A Review*. https://core.ac.uk/download/234660577.pdf (accessed on 1st July 2025).
5. Ali, M. K. M. (2022). Article review: The approach to celiac disease in children. https://core.ac.uk/download/597862205.pdf (accessed on 1st July 2025).
6. Alonso Padilla, J., Gascón i Brustenga, J., Gállego Culleré, M. M., Schijman, A., et al. (2023). Molecular diagnostics for Chagas disease: Up to date and novel methodologies. https://core.ac.uk/download/595479408.pdf (accessed on 1st July 2025).
7. Alonso-Padilla, J., Gascon, J., & Pinazo, M. J. (2023). How effective are rapid diagnostic tests for Chagas disease? https://diposit.ub.edu/dspace/bitstream/2445/202886/1/8.%20How_effective_are_RDTs_for_Chagas_disease_v2_cleared.pdf (accessed on 1st July 2025).
8. Aquino de Sá, M. C., Raynal, J., Alcântara, M. E., Lima, G. A. R., Santos, R. M., Ribeiro, M., Trindade, S., et al. (2024). Interferon gamma kinetics associated with immunodiagnostic techniques in experimental goats infected with biofilm producer and non-biofilm producer strains of *Corynebacterium pseudotuberculosis*. *Brazilian Journal of Veterinary Research and Animal Science*. https://www.semanticscholar.org/paper/2cca4e648bdbc581abe2cfd087cdf4118b513e48 (accessed on 1st July 2025).
9. Baker, K. S., Barr, J., Boots, M., Broder, S., et al. (2014). Viral antibody dynamics in a chiropteran host. https://core.ac.uk/download/9357743.pdf (accessed on 1st July 2025).
10. Baker, S., Berto, A., Campbell, J. I., Carrique-Mas, J., et al. (2016). A clinical and epidemiological investigation of the first reported human infection with the zoonotic parasite *Trypanosoma evansi* in Southeast Asia. https://core.ac.uk/download/77019010.pdf (accessed on 1st July 2025).
11. Balouz, V., Buscaglia, C. A., & Fernandez Aguero, M. J. (2016). Chagas disease diagnostic applications: Present knowledge and future steps. https://core.ac.uk/download/159295515.pdf (accessed on 1st July 2025).
12. Basit, M. H., Malik, K., Sadia, S., & Haleema, H. (2018). Protein-based detection methods for genetically modified crops. https://core.ac.uk/download/322436239.pdf (accessed on 1st July 2025).
13. Batdorj, D. (2018). *Studies on the Development of Dourine Specific Diagnostic Methods*. https://core.ac.uk/download/636356791.pdf (accessed on 1st July 2025).

14. Bergua Canudo, J. F., Calucho, E., De Carvalho Castro Silva, C., Delamarche, C., et al. (2021). Nano diagnostics to face SARS-CoV-2 and future pandemics: From an idea to the market and beyond. https://core.ac.uk/download/491372323.pdf (accessed on 1st July 2025).
15. Bjorndal, K. A., Bolten, A., Brown, D. R., Coberley, C., et al. (2000). Pathogenic, molecular, and immunological properties of a virus associated with sea turtle fibro papillomatosis. Phase II: Viral pathogenesis and development of diagnostic assays. https://core.ac.uk/download/11017010.pdf (accessed on 1st July 2025).
16. Bohan, B., Brown, G., Chinoy, H., Christen-Zaech, S., Pilkington, C. A., et al. (2011). A national registry for juvenile dermatomyositis and other pediatric idiopathic inflammatory myopathies: 10 years' experience; the Juvenile Dermatomyositis National (UK and Ireland) Cohort Biomarker Study and Repository. https://core.ac.uk/download/10413.pdf (accessed on 1st July 2025).
17. Böltz, T., Fliessbach, H., Modrow, S., Niedrig, M., et al. (1992). Immunological reactivity of a human immunodeficiency virus types I derived peptide representing a consensus sequence of the GP120 major neutralizing region V3. https://core.ac.uk/download/11549714.pdf (accessed on 1st July 2025).
18. Calatroni, M., Conte, E., Stella, M., De Liso, F., Reggiani, F., & Moroni, G. (2025). Clinical and immunological biomarkers can identify proliferative changes and predict renal flares in lupus nephritis. *Arthritis Research & Therapy*, *27*. https://www.semanticscholar.org/paper/379c5898090b6b98095bfc9a1812129dae546519 (accessed on 1st July 2025).
19. Callow, K. A., Calza, L., Chan, K. H., De Jong, M. D., Farrohi, M., Ferrara, F., et al. (2014). Overview of serological techniques for influenza vaccine evaluation: Past, present and future. https://core.ac.uk/download/30704521.pdf (accessed on 1st July 2025).
20. Chen, Y., Wang, G., Li, M., Wang, J., Gu, J., Huang, R., Wu, C., et al. (2024). Virological and immunological characteristics of HBeAg-positive chronic hepatitis B patients with low HBsAg levels. *Alimentary Pharmacology & Therapeutics*. https://www.semanticscholar.org/paper/556d947759acd14b2d0a34d8a08a48f8623441c6 (accessed on 1st July 2025).
21. Costa-García, A., Delerue-Matos, C., González-García, M. B., Neves, M. G. P. M. S., et al. (2010). Celiac disease diagnosis and gluten-free food analytical control. https://core.ac.uk/download/47138081.pdf (accessed on 1st July 2025).
22. Cox, A., Garcia, A., Courtioux, B., de Clare Bronsvoort, B. M., Burri, C., Enoe, C., Paquet, C., et al. (2011). Accuracy of five algorithms to diagnose gambiense human African trypanosomiasis. https://core.ac.uk/download/pdf/9418044.pdf (accessed on 1st July 2025).
23. Das, A., Vallur, A. C., Ahmad Mumtaz, A., Abeijon, C., Mukhopadhyay, D., et al. (2016). Noninvasive diagnosis of visceral leishmaniasis: Development and evaluation of two urine-based immunoassays for detection of *Leishmania donovani* infection in India. https://core.ac.uk/download/148352507.pdf (accessed on 1st July 2025).
24. Dendukuri, N., Flores, L. L., Hopewell, P. C., Laal, S., et al. (2011). Commercial serological tests for the diagnosis of active pulmonary and extrapulmonary tuberculosis: An updated systematic review and meta-analysis. https://core.ac.uk/download/pdf/8605266.pdf (accessed on 1st July 2025).
25. Desport, M., Hartaningsih, N., Lewis, J. R., McNab, T., et al. (2009). Comparison of immunoassay and real-time PCR methods for the detection of Jembrana disease virus infection in Bali cattle. https://core.ac.uk/download/11235481.pdf (accessed on 1st July 2025).

26. Desquesnes, M., Gonçalves da Costa, S. C., Madruga, C. R., Osorio, A. L., et al. (2008). *Trypanosoma (Duttonella) vivax*: Its biology, epidemiology, pathogenesis, and introduction in the New World–A review. http://agritrop.cirad.fr/546874/1/document_546874.pdf (accessed on 1st July 2025).

27. Dietze, K., Hoffmann, B., Milićević, V., Milovanović, A., et al. (2020). Suitability of individual and bulk milk samples to investigate the humoral immune response to lumpy skin disease vaccination by ELISA. https://core.ac.uk/download/326438744.pdf (accessed on 1st July 2025).

28. Duff, E. H. (1935). *Modern Conceptions in Syphilology with Special Reference to Serological Diagnosis and Treatment by The Aryl Arsonates and Bismuth*. https://core.ac.uk/download/429724246.pdf (accessed on 1st July 2025).

29. Dumonteil, E., López-Monteon, A., & Ramos-Ligonio, A. (2019). More than a hundred years in the search for an accurate diagnosis for Chagas disease: Current panorama and expectations. https://core.ac.uk/download/322442976.pdf (accessed on 1st July 2025).

30. Dunn, S. (2020). *Development and Management of Canine Adverse Food Reactions and Its Connections to The Grain-Free Dog Food Movement*. https://core.ac.uk/download/304169066.pdf (accessed on 1st July 2025).

31. Eckman, J., Hamilton, R. G., & Saini, S. S. (2009). Diagnostic evaluation of food-related allergic diseases. https://core.ac.uk/download/pdf/8347937.pdf (accessed on 1st July 2025).

32. Eda, S., Hickling, G. J., & Wadhwa, A. (2012). Opportunities for improved serodiagnosis of human tuberculosis, bovine tuberculosis, and paratuberculosis. https://core.ac.uk/download/pdf/8740257.pdf (accessed on 1st July 2025).

33. Generalov, I. I., Sencovich, S. A., & Zheleznyak, N. V. (2014). *Instructions for Laboratory Training in General Microbiology & Immunology*. https://core.ac.uk/download/80150439.pdf (accessed on 1st July 2025).

34. Górny, J., Hawajski, A., Jankowska, N., Kamieniecka, K., et al. (2024). Is a gluten-free diet sufficient in the treatment of Duhring's disease? –A review. https://core.ac.uk/download/636385543.pdf (accessed on 1st July 2025).

35. Gorshunov, Y. V., Komar, A. G., & Motronenko, V. V. (2019). Serological methods in modern biotechnologies and their bioanalytical standardization. https://core.ac.uk/download/323528090.pdf (accessed on 1st July 2025).

36. Harari, A., Zumla, A., Armand, A., Axelsson-Robertson, R., Banada, P., Marais, B., Betsou, F., et al. (2012). Tuberculosis diagnostics and biomarkers: Needs, challenges, recent advances, and opportunities. https://core.ac.uk/download/9839032.pdf (accessed on 1st July 2025).

37. Hejtmancik, K. E. (2025). A solid phase enzyme-linked immunosorbent assay for the antigenic detection of *Legionella pneumophila* (serogroup 1): A complement for the space station diagnostic capability. https://core.ac.uk/download/pdf/42833966.pdf (accessed on 1st July 2025).

38. Ho, A., Solari, A., Castro, A. M., Duarte, A. M., Bundy, B., Young, C., Chang, C. D., et al. (2008). High throughput selection of effective serodiagnostics for *Trypanosoma cruzi* infection. https://core.ac.uk/download/pdf/8195686.pdf (accessed on 1st July 2025).

39. Jacobson, E., & Klein, P. A. (2001). Sero epidemiological studies of herpesvirus-associated

diseases of marine turtles: Fibro papillomatosis and lung-eye-trachea disease. https://core.ac.uk/download/11017006.pdf (accessed on 1st July 2025).

40. Lima, M. I. S., Moraes, E. C. S., Pinho, J. D., Santos, J. B., et al. (2019). Molecular and biotechnological approaches in the diagnosis of leprosy. https://core.ac.uk/download/322436707.pdf (accessed on 1st July 2025).

41. Liyanage, K. D., Vaz, P. K., Jabbar, A., & Hufschmid, J. (2023). Towards a pan marsupial sero-immunological tool in the demanding field of wildlife serology: Marsupial immunoglobulin-binding capability with protein A/G, protein L and anti-kangaroo antibody. *PLOS ONE, 18*. https://www.semanticscholar.org/paper/f1a94353c146090eb2992829bec346e5bb8abe80 (accessed on 1st July 2025).

42. Matuka, D. O., Muleba, L., Muvhali, M., Ratshikhopha, T., et al. (2023). Navigating the complexities of mould exposure in damp buildings: A case report on challenges and potential solutions. https://core.ac.uk/download/613869285.pdf (accessed on 1st July 2025).

43. McLaren, M. L. (2025). *The Development of The Enzyme Linked Immunosorbent Assay (Elisa) For Schistosomiasis and Its Epidemiological Applications.* https://core.ac.uk/download/287606756.pdf (accessed on 1st July 2025).

44. Minnich, S. A. (1981). *The Use of An Enzyme Immunoassay for The Detection of Salmonellae in Foods.* https://core.ac.uk/download/38898795.pdf (accessed on 1st July 2025).

45. N/A. (2004). Immunomodulatory activities of *Cordyceps sinensis* used as a single herb and in concoction. https://core.ac.uk/download/48536871.pdf (accessed on 1st July 2025).

46. Napoli, A., Farina, A., Angeloni, A., Gaeta, A., Pucci, B., Berardelli, E., Anastasi, E., et al. (2023). Anti-N SARS-CoV-2 assays for evaluation of natural viral infection. https://core.ac.uk/download/577149899.pdf (accessed on 1st July 2025).

47. Porru, S., Monaco, M., Carta, A., Spiteri, G., Parpaiola, M., Battaggia, A., Galligioni, G., et al. (2021). SARS-CoV-2 infection in health workers: Analysis from Verona SIEROEPID study during the pre-vaccination era. *International Journal of Environmental Research and Public Health, 18*. https://www.semanticscholar.org/paper/0a9b0d16cede8cbdc7175650f9d386a696890fb1 (accessed on 1st July 2025).

48. Rüggeberg, J., Collins, C., Balfour, G., Tighe, H., Archer, M., Diggle, L., Borrow, R., et al. (2003). Allergy, immunity, and infection. *Archives of Disease in Childhood, 88*, A54–A57. https://www.semanticscholar.org/paper/eeb54378b1bce0ff8ed1cbb19c94900eff547cf5 (accessed on 1st July 2025).

49. Truman, R. W. (1985). Host responses to the phenolic-glycolipid-1 antigen of *Mycobacterium leprae* (ELISA, leprosy, epidemiology, armadillo, human). https://core.ac.uk/download/217387118.pdf (accessed on 1st July 2025).

INDEX

C

D

E

F

G

H

I

K

L

M

T

U

V

W